T0182000

Scalable Computing and Communications

Series editor

Albert Y. Zomaya, University of Sydney, Darlington, New South Wales, Australia

Editorial Board

Jiannong Cao, The Hong Kong Polytechnic University, HongKong
Samee U. Khan, North Dakota State University, USA
Rajiv Ranjan, CSIRO, Australia
Sartaj Sahni, University of Florida, USA
Lizhe Wang, Chinese Academy of Science, China
Paul Watson, University of Newcastle, UK

Scalable computing lies at the core of all complex applications. Topics on scalability include environments, such as autonomic, cloud, cluster, distributed, energy-aware, parallel, peer-to-peer, greed, grid and utility computing. These paradigms are necessary to promote collaboration between entities and resources, which are necessary and beneficial to complex scientific, industrial, and business applications. Such applications include weather forecasting, computational biology, telemedicine, drug synthesis, vehicular technology, design and fabrication, finance, and simulations.

The Scalable Computing and Communications Book Series combines countless scalability topics in areas such as circuit and component design, software, operating systems, networking and mobile computing, cloud computing, computational grids, peer-to-peer systems, and high-performance computing.

Topics of proposals as they apply to scalability include, but are not limited to:

Autonomic computing
Big Data computing
Data center computing
Grid computing
Cloud computing
Green computing and energy-aware computing
Volunteer computing and Peer-to-Peer computing
Multi-core and many-core computing
Parallel, distributed and high-performance simulation
Workflow computing
Unconventional computing paradigms
Pervasive computing, mobile computing and sensor networking
Service computing, Internet computing, Web based computing
Data centric computing and data intensive computing
Cluster computing
Unconventional computation
Scalable wireless communications
Scalability in networking infrastructures
Scalable databases
Scalable cyber infrastructures and e-Science
Smart City computing

More information about this series at http://www.springer.com/series/15044

Samee U. Khan · Albert Y. Zomaya
Assad Abbas
Editors

Handbook of Large-Scale Distributed Computing in Smart Healthcare

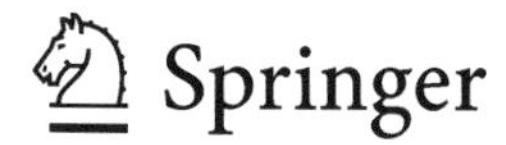

Editors
Samee U. Khan
Department of Electrical and Computer Engineering
North Dakota State University
Fargo, ND
USA

Assad Abbas
Department of Computer Science
COMSATS Institute of Information Technology
Islamabad
Pakistan

Albert Y. Zomaya
School of Information Technologies
University of Sydney
Sydney, NSW
Australia

ISSN 2520-8632 ISSN 2364-9496 (electronic)
Scalable Computing and Communications
ISBN 978-3-319-86364-1 ISBN 978-3-319-58280-1 (eBook)
DOI 10.1007/978-3-319-58280-1

© Springer International Publishing AG 2017
Softcover reprint of the hardcover 1st edition 2017
This work is subject to copyright. All rights are reserved by the Publisher, whether the whole or part of the material is concerned, specifically the rights of translation, reprinting, reuse of illustrations, recitation, broadcasting, reproduction on microfilms or in any other physical way, and transmission or information storage and retrieval, electronic adaptation, computer software, or by similar or dissimilar methodology now known or hereafter developed.
The use of general descriptive names, registered names, trademarks, service marks, etc. in this publication does not imply, even in the absence of a specific statement, that such names are exempt from the relevant protective laws and regulations and therefore free for general use.
The publisher, the authors and the editors are safe to assume that the advice and information in this book are believed to be true and accurate at the date of publication. Neither the publisher nor the authors or the editors give a warranty, express or implied, with respect to the material contained herein or for any errors or omissions that may have been made. The publisher remains neutral with regard to jurisdictional claims in published maps and institutional affiliations.

Printed on acid-free paper

This Springer imprint is published by Springer Nature
The registered company is Springer International Publishing AG
The registered company address is: Gewerbestrasse 11, 6330 Cham, Switzerland

Preface

The demand for deployment of large-scale distributed computing technologies in healthcare domain has increased due to the enormous growth in healthcare data. Millions of devices are unceasingly generating healthcare data every day, which depicts the evolving nature of smart healthcare services. Moreover, numerous research works emphasizing on patient monitoring, fall detection, activity recognition, and Body Area Networks (BAN) have been carried out in the recent past. However, it has become evident that integration of traditional healthcare practices with large-scale distributed computing technologies ensures the efficient provision of smart health services and is also instrumental to their widespread acceptance.

Currently there are several books that cover the topics related to pervasive health care and mobile health. However, to the best of our knowledge there is no specific book that comprehensively reports the efforts made to integrate pervasive healthcare with the large-scale and distributed computing approaches. This book provides advanced perspectives and visions for the cutting-edge research in ubiquitous health care with emphasis on large-scale computing techniques. The topics covered in the book mainly emphasize on large-scale architectures and high-performance solutions for smart healthcare, healthcare monitoring using large-scale computing techniques, Internet-of-Things (IoT) and big data analytics for healthcare, Fog Computing, mobile health, large-scale medical data mining, advanced machine learning methods for mining multidimensional sensor data, smart homes, and resource allocation methods for the BANs.

This book covers the topics ranging from the theory, concept, and systems, to the applications of large-scale healthcare systems for ubiquitous healthcare services. The book contains high quality chapters contributed by internationally renowned researchers working in domains, such as e-Health, pervasive and context-aware computing, cloud, grid, cluster, and big data computing. We are optimistic that the topics included in this book will provide a multidisciplinary research platform to the researchers, practitioners, and students from biomedical engineering, health informatics, computer science, and computer engineering.

Fargo, USA
Sydney, Australia
Islamabad, Pakistan

Samee U. Khan
Albert Y. Zomaya
Assad Abbas

About the Book

1. This book includes the latest research efforts in the field of smart healthcare. To maximize the readers' insight into the domain, integration of smart healthcare services with large-scale distributed computing systems has been emphasized.
2. Particular consideration has been devoted to the theoretical and practical aspects of wide array of emerging large-scale healthcare applications and architectures, including the remote health monitoring, wearable devices, activity recognition for rehabilitation, mobile health, and cloud computing.
3. The book explains the concept of healthcare big data in great details and includes several chapters focusing on data quality in large-scale healthcare datasets.
4. The book includes several case studies which will provide readers a real perspective of the smart healthcare domain.
5. The book will be an exceptional resource for diverse types of readers including academics and researchers from several disciplines, such as health informatics, computer science, and computer engineering.

Keywords: Pervasive health, Cloud computing, Distributed systems, Fall detection, Activity recognition, Home health monitoring, Body area networks, Wearable sensors, Dimension reduction, Scalability, Sensor data management, Internet-of-Things, Mobile health (m-health), Data quality.

Contents

Introduction to Large-Scale Distributed Computing in Smart Healthcare

Assad Abbas, Samee U. Khan and Albert Y. Zomaya

1 Background Information

Conventional healthcare services have seamlessly been integrated with the pervasive computing paradigm and consequently cost-effective and dependable smart healthcare services and systems have emerged [1]. Currently, the smart healthcare systems employ Body Area Networks (BANs) and wearable devices for pervasive health monitoring and Ambient-Assisted Living (AAL). The BANs utilize smart phones and numerous handheld devices to ensure pervasive access to the healthcare information and services [2]. However, due to the intrinsic limitations in terms of the CPU speed, storage, and memory, the mobile and several smart computing devices appear scanty to handle huge volumes of unceasingly generated sensor data [3]. The collected data is used for multiple purposes, such as tele monitoring, activity recognition tasks, and therapies. In addition, the aforementioned data is highly complex and multi-dimensional and consequently is difficult to handle using the conventional computing procedures. Therefore, integrating the BANs with large-scale and distributed computing paradigms, such as the cloud, cluster, and grid computing is inevitable to handle the processing and storage needs arising due to continuously originating data from the BANs [1, 4].

Moreover, the contemporary research efforts mostly focus on health information delivery methods to ensure the information exchange across various devices at a

A. Abbas (✉)
COMSATS Institute of Information Technology, Islamabad, Pakistan
e-mail: assadabbas@comsats.edu.pk

S.U. Khan
North Dakota State University, Fargo, USA
e-mail: samee.khan@ndsu.edu

A.Y. Zomaya
The University of Sydney, Sydney, Australia
e-mail: albert.zomya@sydney.edu.au

© Springer International Publishing AG 2017

S.U. Khan et al. (eds.), *Handbook of Large-Scale Distributed Computing in Smart Healthcare*, Scalable Computing and Communications,
DOI 10.1007/978-3-319-58280-1_1

small scale. Consequently, the efforts have been very limited in connecting several BANs remotely through the servers. Therefore, the need to develop large scale solutions, such as Internet of Things (IoT), Cloud Computing, and Fog Computing to connect heterogeneous devices to transmit and process large amounts of data without requiring rigorous explicit human-to-human and human-to-machine interactions increases manifold [5]. Moreover, integrating the High Performance Computing (HPC) paradigms with the BANs and smart healthcare services brings several key benefits including scalability, storage, and processing to handle online and offline streams of data [6].

2 New Research Methods to Integrate the Smart Healthcare and Large-Scale and Distributed Computing Paradigm

In the recent past, plentiful research has been carried out pertaining to human activity recognition for rehabilitation, fall detection, mobile health, pervasive computing, and home health monitoring. However, very few researchers have only considered utilizing large-scale distributed computing methodologies in conjunction with smart healthcare systems. Considering the high growth of healthcare data flowing into the systems, this is the appropriate time to devise methodologies that are capable enough to proficiently deal with the data from its origination to processing and from processing to storage. Currently, there is no specific book that comprehensively reports the efforts made to integrate pervasive healthcare and BANs with the large-scale distributed computing approaches. Therefore, this book provides advanced perspectives and visions for the cutting edge research in smart healthcare with emphasis on large-scale and distributed computing systems in smart healthcare, QoS and resource allocation issues of BANs, healthcare IoT, Fog Computing, data quality and big data analytics for healthcare, machine learning methods, and models for multidimensional data.

This book explores the intersection of e-health services and distributed computing paradigm to improve the overall delivery of healthcare services. The book explains several recently emerged topics, such as IoT, Fog Computing, and big data in context of their large-scale implementation in healthcare domain.

The topics in the book have been mainly divided into five parts. Part I includes chapters on High Performance Computing and Large-Scale Healthcare Architectures. Part II of the book contains chapters on Data Quality and Large-Scale Machine Learning Models for Smart Healthcare whereas chapter on the IoT, Fog Computing, and mobile and connected health are included in Part III of the book. Part IV contains chapters that establish the connection between wearable devices and distributed computing for activity recognition and patient monitoring. Part V contains chapters on resource allocation, Quality of Service (QoS), and context-awareness in smart healthcare. A brief description of each of the chapters is given below.

Part I: **High Performance Computing and Large-Scale Healthcare Architectures**

Part I of the book comprises of four chapters mainly focusing on high performance computing and big data architectures for smart healthcare. Chapter 2 discusses the challenges in designing algorithms and systems for healthcare systems followed by a survey on various relevant solutions. The chapter also discusses next-generation healthcare applications, services, and systems related to big healthcare data analytics. Chapter 3 proposes a task-level adaptive MapReduce Framework to process streaming data in healthcare. This framework extends the generic MapReduce architecture by designing each Map and Reduce task as a scalable daemon process. The proposed architecture is claimed to be capable of scaling up and scaling down the resources as per real-time demands.

Chapter 4 presents a brief introduction of optical brain imaging techniques and highlights challenges specific to such techniques. Moreover, this chapter also introduces a massively parallel GPU based Monte Carlo simulation framework. Furthermore, the chapter explores a number of optimization techniques to improve computational efficiency and discusses the current and potential applications of this technique in biomedical imaging. Chapter 5 gives a concise review of Building Automation and Control Systems (BACS) addressing healthcare issues in the home environments. The strong aspect of the chapter is that it emphasizes on the effects of the BACS on well-being and health. The BACS can be considered as a large-scale network of distributed, interacting, and autonomous components where the size (scale) of the network is depending on the number of components, such as heating, ventilating, air-conditioning and refrigeration (HVAC&R), lighting, and window blinds/shades control. As a result, a BACS can contribute to the optimization of the physical environment toward individual users' needs, health, and well-being.

Part II: **Data Quality and Large-Scale Machine Learning Models for Smart Healthcare**

Part II comprises of four chapters on the importance of data quality and large-scale machine learning models for smart healthcare. Chapter 6 presents a detailed discussion on the data quality issues in Electronic Health Records (EHRs) and highlights the challenges pertinent to data that are crucial for the interoperability and standards across healthcare organizations. In particular, the discussion focuses on the large-scale Database Management Systems (DBMSs) and the importance of data quality for intelligent interfaces, structured data entry, and mobile computing. Chapter 7 covers all aspects of large-scale knowledge mining for medical and diseases investigation. A genome-wide association study is used in the chapter to determine the interactions and relationships for Alzheimer disease (AD). The chapter is a useful resource for details on mining the large-scale medical datasets for accurate diagnosis using big data methods.

Chapter 8 gives an overview of machine learning methods for analysis of heterogeneous and high dimensional healthcare data and also describes the effects of dimension reduction on the computational efficiency. The chapter reviews two case studies to evaluate the patients' health related concerns through data-driven models. Chapter 9 discusses the major issues related to large-scale and distributed architectures involving mobile sensing data for healthcare research, data curation, data provenance, and the data quality.

Part III: Internet-of-Things, Fog Computing, and m-Health

Part III of the book contains chapters on Internet-of-Things (IoT), Fog Computing, and mobile and connected health. Chapter 10 analyzes the ideas and impacts of the based healthcare systems on the design of new e-health solutions and also highlights various challenges, for example privacy and confidentiality to estimate the successful adoption of the IoT based e-health system. To ensure the widespread acceptance of the e-health systems, the chapter establishes six objectives and suggests that the development of future healthcare systems should primarily be based on the IoT, big data, and cloud computing. Chapter 11 defines and explores Fog Computing (FC) in the context of medical IoT. The chapter presents discussion on the FC as a service-oriented intermediate layer in IoT, providing an interface between the sensors and cloud servers for orchestrating connectivity, data transfer, and providing a queryable local database. The experimental results demonstrate that the FC can minimize the obstacles of existing cloud-driven medical IoT solutions and can significantly enhance the overall performance of the system in terms of computing intelligence, transmission, storage, configurability, and security.

Chapter 12 presents an innovative medical image cloud solution that enables accessible mobile healthcare and supports the hierarchical medical care services in China. A real scenario of regional medical imaging centers is also presented to compare its operational feasibility in comparison with traditional Picture Archiving and Communication Systems (PACS) services. Chapter 13 describes issues of the innovative large-scale technological developments for the community healthcare and well-being in context of developing nations with particular emphasis on receivers' perspective. The chapter presents discussion on utilizing large-scale technologies and their effective provision in community support and also highlights the benefits of Software-as-a-Service (SaaS) and mobile health infrastructure.

Part IV: Wearable Computing for Smart Healthcare

Part IV of the book comprises of six chapters that present variety of information on wearable devices and distributed computing for activity recognition and patient monitoring. Chapter 14 proposes a wearable system for recognition of American Sign Language (ASL). The proposed system design is an example of fusing different sensor modalities and addressing computation cost challenge of wearable computer based Sign Language Recognition (SLR) due to the high-dimensional data. The study is claimed to be the first American Sign Language recognition system fusing Inertial Measurement Unit (IMU) sensor and surface Electromyography (sEMG) signals which are complementary to each other. Chapter 15 introduces a novel ECG anomaly detection technique to be implemented in the cloud. The proposed technique which works by comparing the beat segments against a normal beat, succeeds in fulfilling all the necessary prerequisites for large-scale monitoring. The complexities of such systems are also highlighted and real-time signal processing methods and heuristics are applied in the chapter to estimate the boundary limits of individual beats from the streaming ECG data.

Chapter 16 presents a motion recognition method to the upper-limb prosthetic and robotic devices with emphasis on myoelectric pattern recognition techniques. The potential of distributed computing in healthcare with particular focus on the design and development of robust upper-limb rehabilitation devices has been discussed in the chapter. Chapter 17 proposes a novel data segmentation technique that harnesses the power of change point detection algorithm to detect and quantify any abrupt changes in sensor data streams of smart earrings. The presented framework is evaluated on two wearable sensor-based daily activity benchmark datasets to attest the scalability and adaptation of the presented techniques for other activity and large-scale participatory sensing health applications.

Chapter 18 outlines several challenges that developers, patients, and providers face in recent times. Several commercial platforms for health monitoring are reviewed and their impacts are discussed. The chapter also includes recently developed Berkeley Telemonitoring Framework and Android-based open source solution for development of health-monitoring applications. Chapter 19 describes the exploitation of physiological sensors and related signal processing methods to enhance monitoring care in patients with mental disorders. The authors in this chapter describe a pervasive and wearable system comprising of a comfortable t-shirt with integrated electrodes to monitor bipolar patients to support the diagnosis in clinical settings.

Part V: Resource Allocation, Quality of Service (QoS), and Context-awareness in Smart Healthcare

Part V of the book contains chapters on resource allocation in large-scale smart healthcare systems, QoS, and context-awareness. Chapter 20 reviews recent progress on multiple energy sources for BANs and the corresponding energy harvesting techniques. In particular, discussion on multi-node communications with energy harvesting for large-scale BANs where complicated network structures are employed is presented. Apart from conventional energy sources, for example photovoltaic, thermoelectric, and electromagnetic energy harvesting that can be applied in BAN, the chapter also describes the energy sources, such as kinetic and biochemical energy harvesting that are exclusively adopted on human body for BAN. Chapter 21 proposes an Analytic Hierarchy Process (AHP) based algorithm to manage m-QoS based on Telemedicine service selection, evaluation, and assessment on the priority and urgency basis by randomly selecting three decision parameters namely throughput, delay and jitter, to provide cost-effective and quality life to emergency patients at remote location in the hospital.

Chapter 22 presents an ontology based system to collect the contextual data, before, during, and after a digestive surgery. The proposed system is used in a clinical setting as a part of the E-care medical monitoring platform and is applied to the rehabilitation process after a digestive surgery to collect the data. The collected data are subsequently statistically analyzed to make decisions regarding the patients' health status. Chapter 23 presents a methodology to design a multi-agent telemonitoring platform. The preliminary results show that this platform is able to assist health professionals in providing an automated processing of data sent from the sensors and automatically generating alerts in order to detect and report risk situations.

3 Perspective on Future Research Directions

Despite the effectiveness of large-scale computing techniques in healthcare delivery methods and services, there are certain areas that need further investigation. The first possible direction for future research is to investigate the potentials of deploying the IoT based solutions for epidemic control and predict possible disease breakouts. The aforementioned solutions can definitely be beneficial for community healthcare in general and for developing economies in particular because despite all of the economic and financial issues still large number of people possess smartphones. Devising techniques that emphasize on epidemic data collection through smartphones can help government agencies in efficiently identifying the affected areas. Off course at individual and consumer level, implementation of such methods is challenging due to high involved costs but is certainly possible at government level.

The second potential area to be emphasize on is the curation of healthcare datasets. Veracity of healthcare data not only ensures the accuracy of the monitoring procedures but can also lead to energy efficiency if effective dimension reduction techniques are applied on the healthcare data. In fact, the inception of BANs and the IoT in healthcare have resulted in excessive data volumes and thereby increased number of features. Therefore, to truly benefit from the parallelism offered by big data tools and techniques, the machine learning methods capable of optimizing the datasets while preserving the accuracy are needed.

Another direction worth exploring in context of smart healthcare services is the privacy and security of healthcare data. Although the health data privacy and security in general attained significant attention of the researchers in past, measures are needed to ensure the privacy of the healthcare applications and methodologies typically designed for smartphones and several other handheld devices.

References

1. M. U. S. Khan, A. Abbas, M. Ali, M. Jawad, S. U. Khan, K. Li, and A. Zomaya, "On the Correlation of Sensor Location and Human Activity Recognition in Body Area Networks (BANs)," *IEEE Systems Journal*, doi:10.1109/JSYST.2016.2610188.
2. J. Wan, C. Zou, S. Ullah, C.-F. Lai, M. Zhou, and X. Wang, "Cloud-enabled wireless body area networks for pervasive healthcare," *IEEE Network*, 27, no. 5, 2013, pp. 56–61.
3. Wang, Xiaoliang, Qiong Gui, Bingwei Liu, Zhanpeng Jin, and Yu Chen. "Enabling smart personalized healthcare: a hybrid mobile-cloud approach for ECG telemonitoring." IEEE journal of biomedical and health informatics 18, no. 3 (2014): 739–745.

4. Bellifemine, G. Fortino, R. Giannantonio, R. Gravina, A. Guerrieri, M. Sgroi, "SPINE: A domain-specific framework for rapid prototyping of WBSN applications" *Software Practice and Experience*, Wiley, 41(3), 2011, pp. 237–265.
5. "Internet of Things," http://internetofthingsagenda.techtarget.com/definition/Internet-of-Things-IoT.
6. Fortino, Giancarlo, Mukaddim Pathan, and Giuseppe Di Fatta, "BodyCloud: Integration of Cloud Computing and body sensor networks," in *4th IEEE International Conference on Cloud Computing Technology and Science (CloudCom)*, pp. 851–856, 2012.

Part I
High Performance Computing and Large-Scale Healthcare Architectures

Big Healthcare Data Analytics: Challenges and Applications

Chonho Lee, Zhaojing Luo, Kee Yuan Ngiam, Meihui Zhang, Kaiping Zheng, Gang Chen, Beng Chin Ooi and Wei Luen James Yip

Abstract Increasing demand and costs for healthcare, exacerbated by ageing populations and a great shortage of doctors, are serious concerns worldwide. Consequently, this has generated a great amount of motivation in providing better healthcare through smarter healthcare systems. Management and processing of healthcare data are challenging due to various factors that are inherent in the data itself such as high-dimensionality, irregularity and sparsity. A long stream of research has been proposed to address these problems and provide more efficient and scalable healthcare systems and solutions. In this chapter, we shall examine the challenges in

Chonho Lee's work was done while he was at National University of Singapore.

C. Lee
Osaka University, Suita, Japan
e-mail: leech@cmc.osaka-u.ac.jp

Z. Luo · K.Y. Ngiam · K. Zheng · B.C. Ooi · W.L.J. Yip
National University of Singapore, Singapore, Singapore
e-mail: zhaojing@comp.nus.edu.sg

K.Y. Ngiam
e-mail: kee_yuan_ngiam@nuhs.edu.sg

K. Zheng
e-mail: kaiping@comp.nus.edu.sg

B.C. Ooi
e-mail: ooibc@comp.nus.edu.sg

W.L.J. Yip
e-mail: james_yip@nuhs.edu.sg

K.Y. Ngiam · W.L.J. Yip
National University Hospital, Singapore, Singapore

M. Zhang (✉)
Singapore University of Technology and Design, Singapore, Singapore
e-mail: meihui_zhang@sutd.edu.sg

G. Chen
Zhejiang University, Hangzhou, China
e-mail: cg@zju.edu.cn

© Springer International Publishing AG 2017

S.U. Khan et al. (eds.), *Handbook of Large-Scale Distributed Computing in Smart Healthcare*, Scalable Computing and Communications,
DOI 10.1007/978-3-319-58280-1_2

designing algorithms and systems for healthcare analytics and applications, followed by a survey on various relevant solutions. We shall also discuss next-generation healthcare applications, services and systems, that are related to big healthcare data analytics.

Keywords Healthcare · Data analytics · Big data · Machine learning

1 Introduction

Large amounts of heterogeneous medical data have become available in various healthcare organizations and sensors (e.g. wearable devices). Such data, which is called Electronic Health Records (EHR), is the fundamental resource to support medical practice or help derive healthcare insights. Previously, most of the medical practices were completed by medical professionals backed by their experiences, and clinical researches were conducted by researchers via painstakingly designed and costly experiments. However, nowadays the rapidly increasing availability of EHR is becoming the driving force for the adoption of data-driven approaches, bringing the opportunities to automate healthcare related tasks. The benefits may include earlier disease detection, more accurate prognosis, faster clinical research advance and better fit for patient management.

While the promise of Big Healthcare Analytics is materializing, there is still a non-negligible gap between its potential and usability in practice. Heterogeneity, timeliness, complexity, noise and incompleteness with big data impede the progress of creating value from data. Big Healthcare Analytics is no different in general. To make the best from EHR, all the information in EHR must be collected, integrated, cleaned, stored, analyzed and interpreted in a suitable manner. The whole process is a data analysis pipeline where different algorithms or systems focus on different specific targets and are coupled together to deliver an end-to-end solution. It can also be viewed as a software stack where in each phase there are multiple solutions and the actual choice depends on the data type (e.g. sensor data or text data) or application requirements (e.g. predictive models or cohort analysis).

There are mainly two types of EHR data, namely electronic medical records (EMR) and sensor data. There are two major directions of the advancement of Big Healthcare Analytics related to EMR data and sensor data respectively. One is to provide better understanding and interpretation about the basic EMR from hospitals. The key challenges are to detect the specific characteristics of EMR data and build customized solutions for every phase of the data analysis pipeline. The other is to benefit from the development of new technologies of sensors (e.g. capturing devices, wearable sensors, and mobile devices) by getting more medical related data sources. The key challenges are to support real time data processing and real time predictive models.

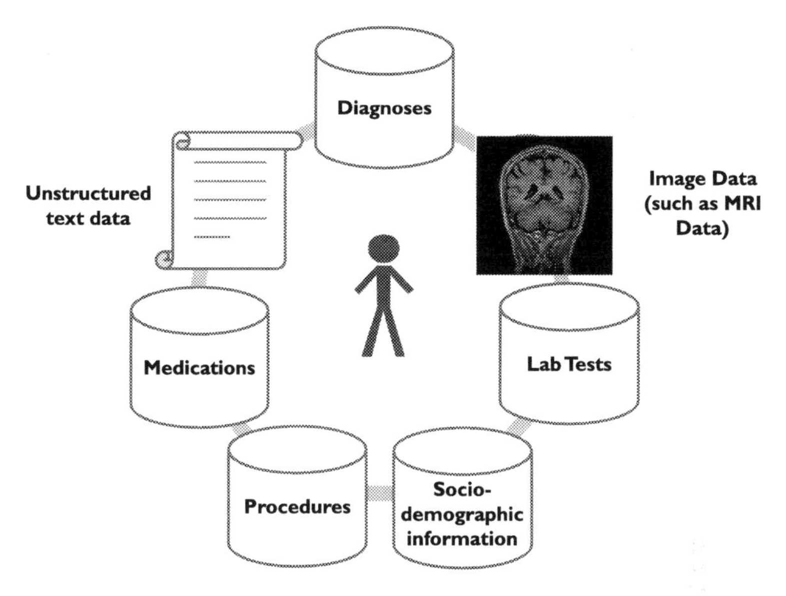

Fig. 1 EMR data consisting of structured data, unstructured text data and image data etc. *Source* http://adni.loni.usc.edu/data-samples/

EMR Data: With the development of electronic healthcare information systems, more and more EMR data is collected from hospitals and ready to be analyzed. EMR data is time series data that records patients' visits to hospitals. As shown in Fig. 1, EMR data typically includes socio-demographic information, patients' medical history and heterogeneous medical features such as diagnoses, lab tests, medications, procedures, unstructured text data (e.g., doctors' notes), image data (e.g., magnetic resonance imaging (MRI) data) and so on. The effective use of EMR can be extremely helpful in data analytics tasks such as disease progression modelling, phenotyping, similar patient and code clustering [54] and so on. However, mining from EMR data is challenging due to the following reasons. First, EMR data is high-dimensional as a large number of medical features have to be captured. Second, EMR data is often dirty or incomplete due to the collection being done over a long period of time; consequently, this data has to be treated before it can be used. Third, EMR data is typically collected irregularly by hospitals as patients tend to visit the hospital only when necessary. Consequently, we have to address challenges such as high-dimensionality, sparsity, noise, missing data, irregularity and bias when we design analytics solutions.

Sensor Data: With the wide use of sensors in collecting data for monitoring and better responding to the situational needs, sensor signals or data streams are also common in healthcare data. From a big data perspective, such sensor signals exhibit some unique characteristics. The signals originate from millions of users and sensor/mobile devices, form an extremely large volume of heterogeneous data streams in real time. Figure 2 shows example networks with various sensors/mobile devices, where the data streams are generated.

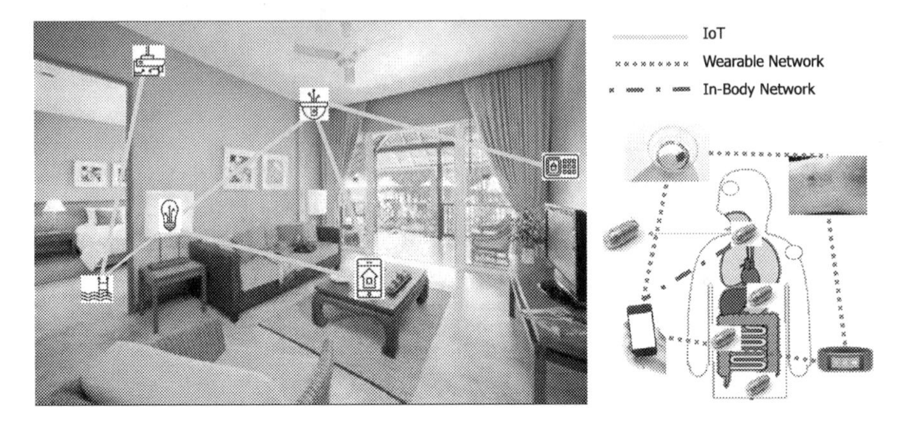

Fig. 2 Network of interconnected sensors (e.g., mobile phones, cameras, microphones, ambient sensors, smart watches, smart lenses, skin-embedded sensors [114], intestinal gas capsules [48]) that produce healthcare data streams

With the advancement in sensor technology and miniaturization of sensor devices, various types of tiny, energy-efficient and low-cost sensors are expected to be widely used for improving healthcare [2, 15, 29]. These sensors form wireless networks such as Internet of Things [21], wearable networks [5] and in-body nano-scale networks [67, 69], and generate massive and various types of data streams. Monitoring and analyzing such multi-modal data streams are useful for understanding the physical, psychological and physiological health conditions of patients. For examples, surveillance cameras, microphones, pressure sensors installed in a house can track the daily activities of elderly people remotely and can help detect falls[1]; EEG and ECG sensors can capture changes in patients' emotions and help control the severity of stress and depression [89, 91, 116]; Carbon nano-tube sensors measuring oxygen saturation and pH of the body, which are bio-markers to react against cancer tissues, help doctors to manage patients [55, 103]. For many healthcare applications, such data must be acquired, stored and processed in a real-time manner. However, there are limitations in implementing the real-time processing of enormous data streams with a conventional centralized solution that does not scale well to process trillions of tuples on-the-fly [21]. Instead, distributed architectures [1, 35, 47, 60, 75, 115] are more amenable to scalability and elasticity to cater to different workloads.

Implementing the next-generation smart healthcare systems, especially those for supporting Big Healthcare Analytics, requires us to carefully examine every phase in the data analysis pipeline, and adjust the methods by modelling the specific medical context. An overview of existing solutions would be of value to those who want to implement a new solution or application. With this in mind, we hereby provide an overview of healthcare data analytics and systems in this chapter. Based on the different types of EHR data and their characteristics introduced earlier, we next

[1]http://www.toptenreviews.com/health/senior-care.

outline several challenges in big healthcare data analytics and review various proposals with respect to these challenges in Sect. 2. Section 3 describes several key steps for processing healthcare data before doing data analytics. Section 4 presents various healthcare applications and services that can be supported by data analytics, and various healthcare systems. We summarize and discuss potential directions in Sect. 5.

2 Challenges

Mining EMR data is challenging because of the following reasons: high-dimensionality, irregularity, missing data as well as sparsity, noise and bias. Figure 3 shows a real-life patient matrix to help readers better understand different challenges in EMR data. Each challenge will be described in detail.

2.1 *High-Dimensionality*

EMR data typically consists of hundreds to thousands of medical features. This gives rise to the high-dimensionality problem. To illustrate, in a sample data set from a real-world longitudinal medical database of National University Hospital, for 10000 patients over a one year period, there are 4143 distinct diagnosis codes. However, nearly 80% of the patients have fewer than 10 diagnosis codes and about 70% of them have fewer than four visits to the hospital, which makes each patient's feature vector high-dimensional and sparse. Similar characteristics are observed from public

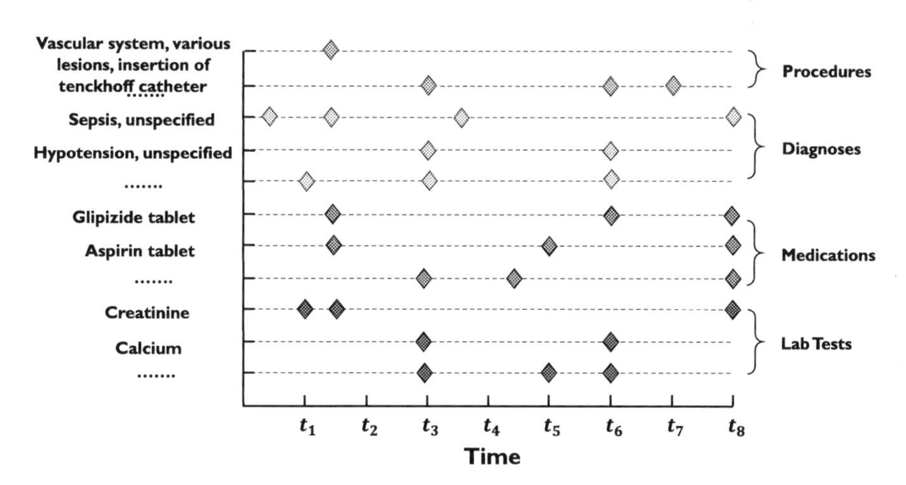

Fig. 3 EMR data of patients

data sets. In a diabetes readmission data set from UCI Machine learning Repository,[2] there are about 900 distinct diagnosis codes, but most patients are associated with fewer than three diagnosis codes. In a subsample of 10000 patients, extracted from a data set provided by Centers for Medicare and Medicaid Services (CMS) 2008–2010, we find nearly 88% of the patients have fewer than four diagnosis codes, although there are 153 distinct diagnosis codes in total.

Dealing with very high-dimensional data is challenging, as it introduces more parameters into the model, making the model much more complex. Also, high-dimensional data is highly likely to be associated with noise and sparsity problems. To address the high-dimensionality problem, there are two main categories of dimensionality reduction methods, namely feature selection and feature extraction.[3]

2.1.1 Feature Selection

Feature selection is the process of selecting a subset of relevant predictive features for model construction [34]. Common feature selection methods include filter methods, wrapper methods and embedded methods [34]. Filter methods select significant features independent of models. These methods will rank the features according to their relations to the predicted features and are usually univariate. Filter methods are computationally efficient and robust to over-fitting but the relations between features are neglected. Different from filter methods, wrapper methods take the relationships between features into consideration. A predictive model will be built to evaluate the combinations of features and a score will be assigned to each set of feature combinations based on the model accuracy. Wrapper methods take a much longer time since they need to search a large number of combinations of features. Also, if the data is not enough, this method will have over-fitting problem. Embedded feature selection methods shift the process of feature selection into the building process of the model. Embedded methods have the advantages of the previous two methods, fast and robust to over-fitting as well as considering relationships between features. Unfortunately, these methods are not generic as they are designed for specific tasks with certain underlying assumptions. For healthcare analytics, univariate analysis and stepwise regression are widely adopted. These two methods belong to filter methods and wrapper methods respectively.

In [68], a univariate analysis as well as a multivariate logistic regression with stepwise forward variable selection are implemented to perform feature selection. Among the initial 20 or so manually selected features, five of them are finally found to be significantly associated with readmission within 30 days for a population of general medicine patients in Singapore and are included in the final model. These features include age, Charlson comorbidity index, white cell count, serum albumin and number of emergency department (ED) visits in previous six months. In [53], a modified stepwise logistic regression is performed to do feature selection in order

[2]https://archive.ics.uci.edu/ml/datasets/Diabetes+130-US+hospitals+for+years+1999-2008.

[3]http://www.kdd.org/kdd2016/topics/view/dimensionality-reduction.

to predict heart failure readmissions. In this work, with the help of domain experts, 95 condition categories (CC), two demographic variables (age and gender) and two procedure codes are included as candidate features. After feature selection, 37 features are considered in the final model. In [106], a backward stepping feature selection method is used to select significant features for the final model. 48 patient-level and admission-level features are collected from 4812 patients that are discharged in Ontario. Among these variables, only four of them, namely, length of stay in days, acute (emergent) admission, comorbidity (Charlson comorbidity index score) as well as number of ED visits during previous six months, are finally found out to be significant to the readmission prediction task.

2.1.2 Feature Extraction

Apart from feature selection methods, we may perform feature extraction to learn low-dimensional latent representations of original features to reduce dimensionality. The main idea of feature extraction is to embed original features in a lower-dimensional space where each dimension corresponds to a combination of original features. Compared with the features derived by feature selection methods, the features learned by feature extraction are much more difficult to interpret. There are mainly two categories of feature extraction methods, depending on whether the transforming methods are linear or non-linear. Linear transforming methods may struggle in discovering complex non-linear relationships between the original features while non-linear transforming methods are much more difficult to optimize and are more likely to be trapped in local optima.

In [57], Gaussian process regression is used to infer longitudinal probability densities for uric acid sequences. Following this transforming step, an auto-encoder is then used to infer meaningful features from the transformed probability densities. When configuring the hidden layer of the deep learning model, the dimension of the hidden layer could be set smaller than the visible layer so as to avoid learning the identity transformation.

In [105], a modified Restricted Boltzmann Machine (RBM) is trained to embed medical objects in a low-dimensional vector space which works as a new representation for the raw high-dimensional medical feature vector. This new low-dimensional representation is then used for assessing suicide risk.

In addition to learning non-linear low-dimensional hidden representations using deep learning models, dimensionality reduction can also be achieved through principal component analysis (PCA). A stochastic convex sparse PCA method is developed in [7] to effectively perform sparse PCA on EMR data so that the derived representation is both low-dimensional and interpretable.

2.2 Irregularity

Irregularity is one of the bothersome characteristics of EMR data and provides challenges for EMR data analytics. Irregularity is caused by the fact that patients will only have EMR data recorded when they visit hospital. As a consequence, patients' EMR data is organized into a "longitudinal patient matrix" where one dimension represents various medical features and the other is time [108, 118], and the consecutive patients' EMR records will be scattered within uneven-spaced time spans. Moreover, for different patients, the granularity of medical records varies significantly and the time periods between visits also vary a lot.

Generally, there are three categories of methods to alleviate this irregularity issue. The details are demonstrated as follows.

2.2.1 Use of Baseline Features

The first kind of methods is to utilize patients' "baseline" features (i.e., the data recorded when patients visit hospital to perform examinations for the first time) for EMR data analytics tasks.

For instance, baseline MRI scans [100] are used to predict patients' clinical scores including Mini-Mental State Examination (MMSE), Dementia Rating Scale (DRS), Auditory Verbal Learning Test (AVLT) and Alzheimer's disease Assessment Scale-Cognitive Subtest (ADAS-Cog). In this work, a relevance vector regression, a novel sparse kernel method in a Bayesian network, is employed. Similarly, patients' baseline MRI features (together with baseline MMSE features, and some demographic features) [27] are used to predict the one-year changes in the MMSE feature. The whole process entails data collection and extraction from MRI data, feature dimensionality reduction via PCA, prediction of future MMSE changes via robust linear regression modelling. In [107], the association between patients' baseline features and changes in severity-related indicators is examined via linear mixed-effects models and the baseline features are used to predict the conversion time from amnestic mild cognitive impairment (aMCI) to Alzheimer's disease via Cox proportional hazards models. In [95], a risk score based on patients' baseline features and demographic features is proposed to predict the probability of developing Type 2 diabetes. Specifically, a multivariate Cox regression model is used to assign weights to different variables. In [26], Alzheimer's disease patients' baseline features are used to predict their probability for different class memberships representing different severity levels based on a multivariate ordinal regression model using Gaussian process that is implemented in a Bayesian network.

Another line of research focuses on multi-task learning [14]. Several works [80, 117, 119] choose Alzheimer's disease patients as the cohort and predict their future severity in terms of MMSE values and ADAS-Cog values in multiple timepoints. The prediction in each timepoint is modelled as a regression task. These works utilize patients' baseline features and employ multi-task learning to capture the relationships between tasks (i.e. the prediction tasks in multiple future timepoints), where all these tasks are trained together with constraints on the changes within consecutive timepoints. However, there are several minor differences between these two methods. Besides predicting patients' future severity, [119] manages to select a common set of features that are significant to all prediction tasks via a $l_{2,1}$-norm penalty term. [117] extends [119] in that it not only selects a common set of features for all tasks, but also selects task-specific bio-markers via a l_1-norm penalty term. [80] proposes a further improvement of regression performance to consider the consistency for prediction utilizing multi-modal data (i.e., multiple sources/forms of medical features), and handles the missing data in both modality data and label data via an adaptive matrix factorization approach.

The prediction performance of this category may be limited by only making use of baseline features. This is due to under-utilization of time-related features. Since patients' health conditions tend to change along with time, it is of vital importance to utilize as many time-related features available as possible other than just baseline features. Another limitation specific to multi-task learning methods is that they can only deal with linear relationships among features. However, in the medical area, relationships between medical features, relationships between medical features and labels can be quite complicated and may not be described using simple linear relationships.

2.2.2 Data Transformation

In regularly sampled series, lots of successful algorithms have been developed. However, there remain many challenging problems in handling irregular data. In the medical area, we are faced with longitudinal, irregularly collected EMR data. To alleviate this problem, some existing works organize patients' EMR data along with time and have divided such longitudinal data into "windows". For instance, in [110], a probabilistic disease progression model based on Markov jump process is proposed to model the transition of disease states for Chronic Obstructive Pulmonary Disease (COPD) patients. The EMR data is processed by segmenting the time dimension into non-overlapping windows (i.e., encounters) with a length of 90 days, and the regularly reorganized data is then used for further modelling and analysis.

Similarly, in [18], two kinds of features are used: daily recorded features and static features. These two kinds of features are exploited to distill knowledge from deep learning models (including Stacked Denoising Auto-encoder and Long Short-Term Memory (LSTM)) by making use of Gradient Boosting Trees.

In [62], training data is processed by resampling to an hourly rate, where the mean measurement is applied in each hourly window. The application task is to classify 128 medical diagnoses employing an LSTM model [40] to capture the dynamic patterns in input features. In [16], the dynamic changing trends are captured using an alternative approach. After preprocessing data into overlapping "windows", the occurrence of a certain disease is predicted based on Multi-Layer Perceptron (MLP) with prior domain knowledge.

While transforming irregular data into regular time series allows us to employ some efficient methods (such as linear algebra) directly, we need to be aware of the side effects associated with such method. For instance, the resampling method may possibly lead to the sparsity and missing data problems because for some features, there could be no observations during certain time windows. Moreover, by dividing longitudinal data into windows, the model may be less sensitive to capturing short-time feature patterns.

2.2.3 Direct Use of Irregular Data

Contrary to the methods mentioned above, there are approaches that make use of medical features with irregular, accurate time information directly. In [86], the computation of LSTM model is adapted by incorporating the time spans between consecutive medical features to handle the irregularity. The proposed model is applied to model disease progression, recommend interventions and predict patients' future risks. Similarly, models based on Gated Recurrent Units (GRU) [19] have been proposed which simultaneously consider the masking and time durations between consecutive medical features in a decay term [17]. Through this decay term, the proposed method is designed to handle irregular data directly.

This category of methods demonstrates the possibility of fully utilizing available data. However, when parameterizing time between consecutive medical features, these methods model the decay term using a heuristic method, such as a monotonically non-increasing function based on logarithm or a parametric method to learn a time weight matrix [86]. Such heuristic methods may cause either under-parameterization or over-parameterization.

2.3 Missing Data and Data Sparsity

Typically, missing EMR data can be caused by either insufficient data collection or lack of documentation. In data collection problem, patients are not checked specifically for a certain medical feature. In documentation problem, patients are checked for a certain feature, but either their outcomes are negative, which means that they are not needed to be documented, or the outcomes are positive but are not recorded due to human errors [112]. The missing data problem is further exacerbated by data sparsity due to the fact that most patients only pay a few visits to the hospital, and in most visits, only a couple of medical features are recorded. Fortunately, missing data and sparsity problems share many common techniques for solving them.

In [93], various imputation methods for handling missing data are described and broadly categorized into two categories. The first category is under the *missing at random* assumption, including methods from simple ones such as case deletion, mean imputation, to the advanced ones such as maximum likelihood and multiple imputation. The second category is under the assumption of *missing not at random*, which mainly includes selection models and pattern-mixture models.

In [18], a simple imputation strategy is adopted in solving missing temporal features: for features with binary values, the majority value is used for filling; for features with numerical values, the mean values are used for imputation. In [62], the forward-filling and back-filling methods are proposed to fill the missing data during a resampling process. For a feature that is totally missing, the clinically normal value suggested by medical experts is used instead.

Apart from solving the missing data problem through imputation in preprocessing phase, a recent work [17] addresses missing data by incorporating two missing patterns: masking and time duration inside the objective function of the deep learning model structure. The proposed method is designed to capture the informative missing EMR data.

For sparsity, the above-mentioned missing data imputation methods, such as mean imputation, forward-filling and back-filling, are also widely used to get a dense patient matrix in order to solve the sparsity problem. Matrix densification/completion is another method to solve the sparsity problem [118]. The basic idea of matrix completion is to recover unknown data from a few observed entries. The algorithm assumes that the completed data for each patient has the factorization form of two matrices. Thus the data can be completed by multiplying these two derived matrices to densify the raw patient matrix.

2.4 *Noise*

EMR data is usually noisy due to various reasons, such as coding inaccuracies, inconsistent naming conventions, etc. Many machine learning researchers tend to learn latent representations to derive more robust representations in order to solve this problem. These methods include Gaussian regression models, topic models or factorization-based methods. A Gaussian process regression is proposed in [57] to transform the raw noisy data (uric acid sequences) into a continuous longitudinal probability density function. This transforming step assumes that each uric acid sequence is a set of possibly noisy samples taken from the source function. Afterwards, instead of operating on the noisy raw data, an auto-encoder takes the mean vector of the learned Gaussian distribution to derive hidden representations. In [39], the noise problem is resolved by learning meaningful medical concepts (or phenotypes) in the form of tensors. Its insight is to map raw EMR data into medical concepts, learn latent bases of the raw data and perform predictive tasks in the latent space. Similar to [39], [111] factorizes the raw patient tensor into several interaction tensors, each representing a phenotype. Experimental results suggest that this method is robust to noise because it not only depends on the observed tensor but also on various other constraints to derive the phenotype tensors. Another latent variable model to solve the noise problem is proposed in [88], which leverages a topic modelling technique to handle noise in the raw EMR data by modelling the relationships between observations that are implicit in the raw data.

2.5 Bias

Bias is also an outstanding characteristic of EMR data, which is regarded as a non-negligible issue in healthcare data analytics [37, 41, 42, 87]. Bias is often considered as biased sampling, which means that the sampling rate is dependent on patients' states, and also dependent on doctors' judgment on patients. Consequently, patients are sampled more frequently when ill, but are sampled less frequently when comparatively healthier [42]. Other sources of bias include (i) the same patient may visit different healthcare organizations for medical help and different organizations do not share information between each other; (ii) patients fail to follow up in the whole medical examination process; (iii) the recorded data in one specific healthcare organization is incomplete [37].

In [87], bias in the lab tests of EMR data is modelled by examining the relationships between concrete lab test values and time intervals between consecutive tests, and exploiting the lab test time patterns to provide additional information. Furthermore, different lab test time patterns are identified so that they can be separately modelled when EMR data analytics and experiments are performed. The limitation of this method is that it can only model the bias based on coarse-grained patterns, and the intra-pattern biases remain to be unsolved.

The influence of time parametrization in EMR data analytics is studied in [42], in which three methods of parameterizing time are compared: sequence time (i.e., the sequence of measurements' occurrences after a specified start time), clock time (i.e., the absolute time of measurements) and an intermediate warped time which is a trade-off between the previous two. The study finds that the sequence time could perform the best among three methods, perhaps due to clinicians' tendency to change sampling rate according to patients' severity. However, the proposed time parameterization methods are heuristic in nature and may cause under-parameterization or over-parameterization.

2.6 Knowledge Base

Over the years, a large number of knowledge sources in the healthcare domain have been built and maintained to provide people with easy access to comprehensive medical information. Common knowledge sources include International Classification of Diseases (ICD-9 or ICD-10) for diagnoses, Healthcare Common Procedure Coding System (HCPCS) for procedures, Logical Observation Identifiers Names and Codes (LOINC) for laboratory tests. Besides, Unified Medical Language System (UMLS) maintains useful relationship knowledge, and Lab Tests Online [4] explains the relationships between lab tests. Incorporating structured medical knowledge provides a good basis to construct intelligent predictive models, which can then be used to improve healthcare data analytics in terms of interpretability and predictive ability.

---

[4]https://labtestsonline.org/.

In [111], existing medical knowledge is incorporated into the tensor factorization algorithm in order to derive more fine-grained phenotypes. In particular, the algorithm can derive different sub-phenotypes which fall into a broader phenotype. This can help to stratify patients into more specific subgroups.

Since knowledge has been successfully incorporated into deep learning models in natural language processing field [9], many deep learning researchers are heading towards incorporating existing medical knowledge into deep learning models in order to improve interpretability as well as performance of the model. In [16], medical ontology knowledge is incorporated into the MLP as a regularization term so as to improve the performance of the model. A similar approach is developed in [105], in which structural smoothness is incorporated into the RBM model via a regularization term. Its basic underlying assumption is that two diseases which share the same parent in the taxonomy are likely to possess similar characteristics.

3 Key Steps for Processing

Before EHR data (including EMR data and sensor data) is input into various models for analysis, data needs to go through several steps of processing. Figure 4 illustrates the pipeline for big data analysis [22, 45]. Firstly, EHR data needs to be recorded, accessed and acquired. Secondly, obtained raw EHR data is probably heterogeneous, composed of structured data, free-text data (such as doctors' notes), image data (such as MRI images) and sensor data. Hence, data extraction is of great concern for further analysis. Furthermore, data cleansing is needed to remove inconsistencies and errors, and data annotation with medical experts' assistance contributes to effectiveness and efficiency of this whole process from acquisition to extraction and finally cleansing. Thirdly, data integration is employed to combine various sources of data, such as different hospitals' data for the same patient. Finally, processed EHR data is modelled and analyzed, and then analytics results are interpreted and visualized. In this section, several key steps for processing EHR data, namely, data annotation, data cleansing, data integration and data analytics/modelling are described in detail respectively.

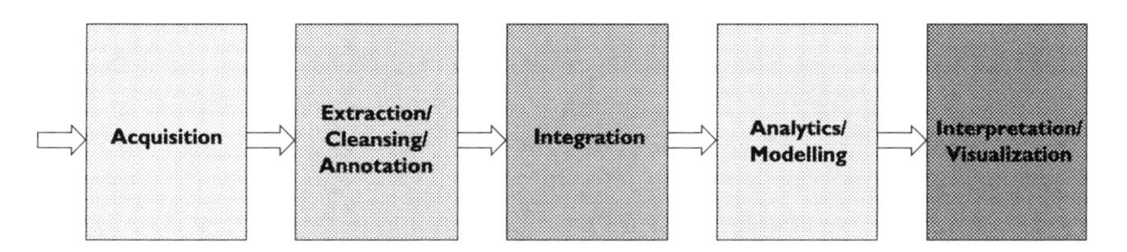

Fig. 4 The big data analysis pipeline [45]

3.1 Data Annotation

Incompleteness is the leading data quality issue when using EHR data to build a learning model [10], since many study variables have missing values to various degrees. The uncertainty of EHR data can be resolved by model inference using various learning techniques [110]. However, the rationale of most healthcare problems can be too complex to be inferred by machines simply using limited EHR data. In such cases, enriching and annotating EHR data by medical experts are the only choice to help the machine to interpret EHR data correctly.

The acquisition of supervised information requires annotations by experts, resulting in a costlier exploitation of data. To reduce the cost involved in data annotation, voluminous research works have been conducted. In general, most of the research issues belong to active learning, which aims to only annotate those important data instances while inferring others and thereby the total number of annotated data is significantly reduced. The key idea of active learning is that learning algorithms can achieve higher accuracy with fewer training labels if they can choose the data from which they learn. The general solutions of active learning include reducing the uncertainty in training models [59], differentiating hypotheses which are consistent with the current learning set (i.e. Query-By-Committee) [78, 97, 102], maximizing the expected model change after receiving a new sample [96], minimizing the expectation [90] or variance [20] of the empirical loss, maximizing the information density among the whole query space [96] and etc.

However, in current status, all these methods have limitations in real healthcare applications. The fundamental reason is that the supervised information in some complex analytics tasks may be hard to be quantified by a human. Since most easy annotating tasks can usually be well recognized by simply using machine efforts, the required tasks for expert annotation are usually complex jobs such as inference flow in a medical concept graph. These categories of supervised information can hardly be annotated via quantified labels which are well studied in the active learning community and integrated to the healthcare analytics system.

3.2 Data Cleansing

In this section, we discuss the importance of data cleansing for EHR data (including EMR data and sensor data). As mentioned in Sect. 2.4, EMR data is typically noisy due to several reasons, for example, coding inaccuracies, erroneous inputs, etc. Before raw EMR data is ready for use, we should develop data cleansing techniques. This requires us to understand the healthcare background of the dirty EMR data and work with domain experts to achieve better cleansing performance. Data cleansing is quite challenging when we consider sensor data. Data from sensor/mobile devices is inherently uncertain due to lack of precisions, failures of transmissions and instability of battery life, etc. Thus, it is essentially required to (i) identify and remove inaccurate, redundant, incomplete and irrelevant records from collected data and (ii) replace or interpolate incorrect and missing records with reasonably assigned values. These processes are expected to improve data quality assessed by its accuracy, validity and integrity, which lead to reliable analytics results.

3.3 Data Integration

Data integration is the process of combining heterogeneous data from multiple sources to provide users with a unified view. [25, 32, 36] explore the progress that has been made by the data integration community and some principles, as well as theoretical issues, are introduced in [24, 58].

Data integration techniques for EMR data and sensor data have different characteristics. For EMR data, we need to integrate heterogeneous EMR data from different sources including structured data such as diagnoses, lab tests, medications, unstructured free-text data like discharge summary, image data like MRI, etc. Different from EMR data, sensor data is generated by various types of sensor/mobile devices at different sampling rates. The heterogeneity of abundant data types brings another challenge when we integrate data streams due to a tradeoff between the data processing speed and the quality of data analytics. The high degree of multi-modality increases the reliability of analytics results, but it requires longer data processing time. The lower degree of multi-modality will improve data processing speed but degrade the interpretability of data analytics results. The efficient data integration helps reduce the size of data to be analyzed without dropping the analytics performance (e.g., accuracy).

3.4 Data Analytics and Modelling

After the three processing steps described above, we focus on EHR data analytics and modelling part. We have proposed a healthcare analytics framework as shown in Fig. 5. This framework is composed of four phases which can give a better representation of medical features, and exploit the intrinsic information in EHR data and therefore, benefit further data analytics performance. The key idea for each phase is demonstrated as follows.

EHR Regularization: In this step, we focus on transforming the EHR data into a multivariate time series, solving the problems of irregularity, missing data and data sparsity, and bias as discussed in Sect. 2. The output of this phase is an unbiased, regularly sampled EHR time series.

Medical Feature Representation: In this phase, we aim to represent the medical features to reflect their feature-time relationships. To be specific, we learn for each medical feature whether this feature has influence after a certain time period and which features it poses influence on.

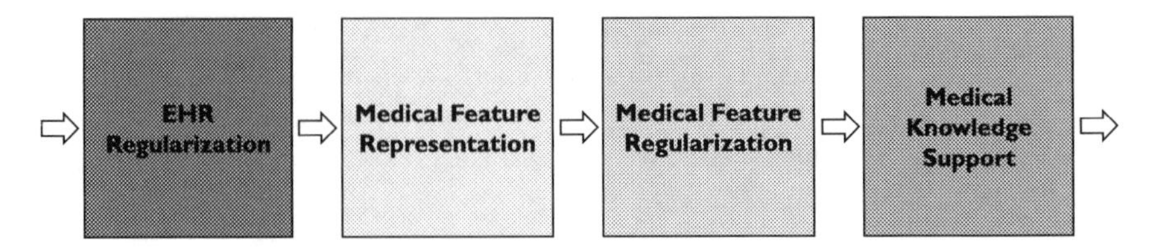

Fig. 5 Our healthcare analytics framework

Medical Feature Regularization: After regularizing EHR data into a more suitable format for analytics and representing features to reveal underlying relationships, we now turn to re-weight medical features for better analytics results. This re-weighting can be achieved by trading-off features' confidence and significance and differentiating common from rare, significant from noisy features.

Medical Knowledge Support: In this phase, we propose to instil medical knowledge into typical machine learning and deep learning models for better analytics performance. This will involve finding the best structures to represent existing medical knowledge (i.e., domain knowledge) and developing the model training scheme using such knowledge.

4 Healthcare Applications

This section presents several healthcare applications, services and systems that are supported by data analytics in EMR data and sensor data. Figure 6 illustrates some of them using EMR data.

4.1 Applications for EMR Data

4.1.1 Clustering

Clustering can help detect similar patients or diseases. Since the raw healthcare data is not clean, there are usually two kinds of approaches for researchers to derive meaningful clusters. The first approach tends to learn robust latent representations first, followed by clustering methods while the other approach adopts probabilistic clustering models which can deal with raw healthcare data effectively. In [105], diseases are first embedded into 200-dimension using a modified RBM model, eNRBM model. These latent 200-dimension hidden vectors are then projected into 2D space using t-SNE. In this 2D space, we can see several meaningful groups consisting of related diagnoses and procedures. Similar to [79, 105] embeds raw patient vectors into latent vectors using a modified RBM, then patient clustering is performed on these latent

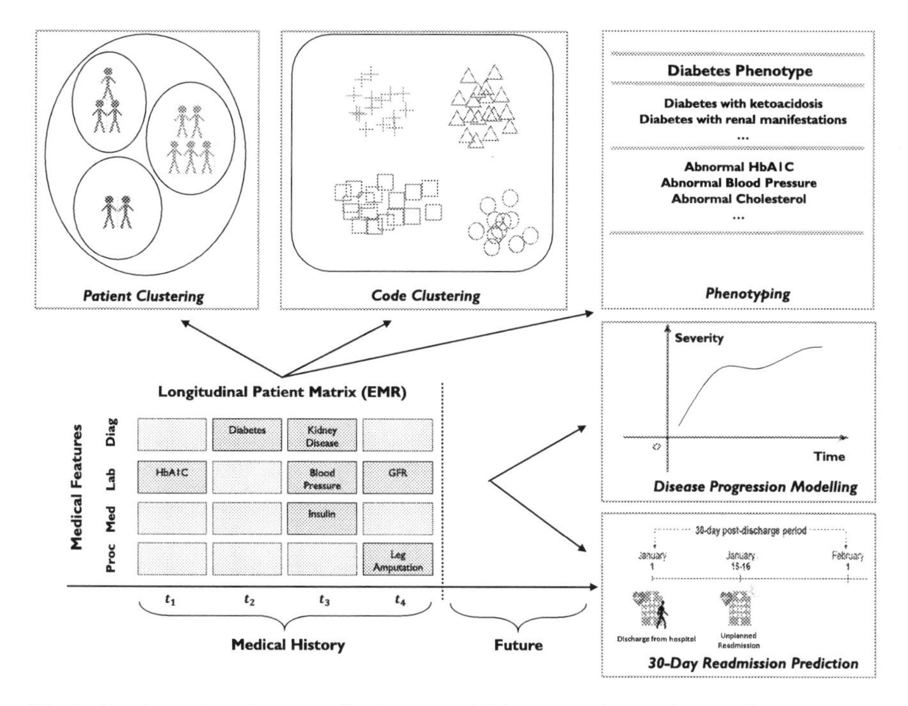

Fig. 6 An illustration of some applications using EMR data analytics. From medical history, we can perform patient clustering, code clustering and phenotyping tasks, while regarding prediction of patients' future, we can do disease progression modelling and 30-day readmission prediction [53]

vectors. Experiments show some groups of patients are closely related to a specific disease condition (say Type I diabetes). [98] identifies multivariate patterns of perceptions using cluster analysis. Five different patient clusters are finally identified and statistically significant inter-cluster differences are found. In [72], a probabilistic clustering model is applied for multi-dimensional, sparse physiological time series data. It shows that different clusters of patients have large differences in mortality rates. Moreover, this clustering model can be used to construct high-quality predictive models. Similarly, in [94], a probabilistic sub-typing model is proposed to cluster time series of clinical markers in order to identify homogeneous patient subgroups.

4.1.2 Phenotyping

Computational phenotyping has become a hot topic recently and has attracted the attention of a large number of researchers because it can help learn robust representations from sparse, high-dimensional, noisy raw EMR data. It has several kinds of forms including (i) rules/algorithms that define diagnostic inclusion criteria (ii) latent factors or latent bases for medical features [49].

Traditionally, doctors regard phenotyping as rules that define diagnostic or inclusion criteria. The task of finding phenotypes is achieved by a supervised task [73]. A number of features are first chosen by domain experts, then statistical methods such as logistic regression or chi-square test are performed to identify the significant features for developing acute kidney injury during hospital admissions. PheKB[5] is a phenotype knowledge base that shows many rules for different diseases and medical conditions. Traditional methods using statistical models are easier to be implemented and interpreted, but they may require a large amount of human intervention.

Recently, machine learning researchers are working on high-throughput methods to derive more meaningful phenotypes. These works mainly discover latent factors or bases as phenotypes. [39] first constructs a three-dimensional tensor which includes patients, diagnoses as well as procedures to represent the raw input data. Then this tensor is split into several interaction tensors and a bias tensor. Each interaction tensor is a phenotype and the non-zero features in each tensor can be regarded as the features of the corresponding phenotype. [111] is similar to [39], and it represents phenotypes in the form of interaction tensors. However, different from [39], it emphasizes on imposing knowledge into the learned phenotypes and proposes to derive distinct phenotypes. In [118], raw patient data is represented using a two-dimensional longitudinal patient matrix with one axis being time and the other being medical features. Then the algorithm decomposes this longitudinal patient matrix into a latent medical concept mapping matrix and a concept evolution matrix. Phenotypes can then be obtained from the latent medical concept mapping matrix by discovering feature groups inside the matrix. Different from traditional statistical methods, phenotyping algorithms based on high-throughput machine learning methods can generate a number of phenotypes at the same time. Moreover, some of the unsupervised algorithms can derive phenotypes which are independent of prediction tasks and are more general.

Deep learning achieves record-breaking performance in a number of image and speech recognition tasks for its distinguished ability to detect complex non-linear relations from raw data and the ability to learn robust high-level abstractions [8, 50]. Since body system itself is complex and highly non-linear, it may be potential for us to utilize deep learning methods to perform phenotyping tasks. [57] is an early work that applies deep learning models in computational phenotyping. It first applies Gaussian process regression to transform the uric acid sequence to a probability density function. Then an auto-encoder is used to learn the hidden representations of Gaussian distribution's mean vectors. The learned weights of the auto-encoder are regarded as phenotypes and the learned features are also visualized. Similar to [57, 105] utilizes a simple two-layer unsupervised deep learning model, RBM, to learn hidden representations of patients' raw input vectors (aggregated counts of medical features, such as diagnoses, procedures). Each unit of this RBM's hidden layer is regarded as a phenotype and this hidden vector is then used for clustering and classification tasks. Different from [57] and [105] which employ an unsupervised model, [16] utilizes a supervised MLP model to extract phenotypes

[5]https://phekb.org/.

from ICU time-series data. In order to visualize MLP's ability to disentangle factors of variation, the authors apply tools from causal inference to analyze the learned phenotypes quantitatively and qualitatively.

4.1.3 Disease Progression Modelling

Disease progression modelling (DPM) is to employ computational methods to model the progression of a specific disease [76]. With the help of DPM, we can detect a certain disease early and therefore, manage the disease better. For chronic diseases, using DPM can effectively delay patients' deterioration and improve patients' healthcare outcomes. Therefore, we can provide helpful reference information to doctors for their judgment and benefit patients in the long run.

Statistical Regression Methods

Traditionally, many related works employ statistical regression methods for DPM, which can model the correlation between patients' medical features and patients' condition indicators [27, 95]. Then, via such correlation, we can have access to the progression of patients with patients' features. For example, in [95], an accurate risk score model through a multivariate Cox regression model is proposed for predicting patients' probability of developing diabetes within five years. Similarly, in [27], a robust linear regression model is employed to predict clinically probable Alzheimer's disease patients' MMSE changes in one year.

Another line of research focuses on "survival analysis", which is to link patients' disease progression to the time before a certain outcome. The linking is accomplished via a survival function. For instance, in [85], a disease progression model is proposed to predict liver transplant patients' long-term survival. The objective is to stratify patients into clusters according to their survival characteristics and then assign different intervention strategies to different patient clusters. Similarly, in [107], the time of patients' progression from amnestic mild cognitive impairment to Alzheimer's disease is studied.

While statistical regression methods are shown to be efficient due to their simple models and computation, we should note that this is accomplished with an underlying assumption that the progression (i.e. medical time-series data) of a disease follows a certain distribution. However, for real-life applications, this assumption may not be true, and the performance of statistical regression methods would suffer. Therefore, it could be difficult to generalize such methods to most clinical applications where the disease progression cannot be abstracted by a certain simple distribution.

Machine Learning Methods

Existing works which employ machine learning methods to solve DPM problem are quite various, from graphical models including Markov models [44, 110], to multitask learning methods [80, 117, 119] and to artificial neural networks [101].

In [110], a Markov jump process is employed to model COPD patients' transition behaviour between disease stages. In [44], a multi-state Markov model is proposed for predicting the progression between different stages for abdominal aortic aneurysm patients considering the probability of misclassification at the same time. Due to the structure as directed graphs, these methods have the advantages of good causality and interpretability. However, medical experts need to be involved to determine the causal relationships during model construction.

Another category of methods is to employ multi-task learning. In [117, 119], the DPM problem is formalized in the multi-task learning setting as predicting patients' future severity in multiple timepoints and select informative features of progression. Also with a multi-task learning method, in [80], the consistency between multiple modalities is considered in the objective function and missing data problem is handled. The limitations of multi-task learning methods are two-fold. First, they only make use of medical features corresponding to patients' first visits to the hospital instead of time-related features. Second, they can only deal with linear relationships in the model.

Deep Learning Methods

In [101], an artificial neural network is employed to predict the recurrence of breast cancer after surgery. With a deeper neural network than this, deep learning models become more widely applicable with its great power in representation and abstraction due to its non-linear activation functions inside. For instance, in [86], a variant of LSTM is employed to model the progression of both diabetes cohort and mental health cohort. They use "Precision at K" as the metric to evaluate the performance of models. However, the lack of interpretability is a possible limitation of these deep learning methods. Furthermore, more training data is of vital importance in order to improve deep learning models' performance.

4.1.4 Image Data Analysis

MRI is widely used to form images of the body using strong magnetic fields, radio waves, and field gradients. Analyzing these images is beneficial for many medical diagnoses and a wide range of studies focus on MRI image data classification or segmentation tasks. In [52], a novel classification method that combines both fractal and GLCM features is proven to be more effective for MRI and CT Scan Medical image classification than previous models which only utilize GLCM features. A model that combines deep learning algorithms and deformable models is developed in [3] for fully automatic segmentation of the left ventricle from cardiac MRI datasets. Experiments show that by incorporating deformable models, this method can achieve better performance in terms of accuracy and robustness of the segmentation. In [4], a review of recent methods for brain MRI image segmentation is presented.

4.2 Applications for Sensor Data

4.2.1 Mobile Healthcare

Healthcare for ageing population has become a major focus, especially in developed countries. Due to the shortage of clinical manpower, there has been a drive toward using ICT (information and communication technology), called mobile healthcare or mHealth.[6] With the advanced technologies including machine learning and high-performance computing, personalized healthcare services will be provided remotely, and diagnoses, medications and treatments will be fine-tuned for individuals on the basis of spatio-temporal and/or psycho-physiological conditions.

Human activity recognition (HAR) is one of the key technologies for mHealth. HAR research is mainly classified into two groups in terms of approaches, namely the video-based and the wearable device-based. The video-based approach continuously tracks human activities through cameras deployed in rooms; however, it raises privacy issues and requires the targeted person to remain within the vicinity of the camera [56]. Moreover, the feature extraction from the captured video/images requires complex computation for further analytics [28]. Because of these limitations, there has been a shift towards the use of wearable sensors requiring less data processing.

Nowadays, the activity recognition is implemented on smart devices for online processing [13, 99, 104] while it is done offline using machine learning tools in backend machines or servers. It has enabled smart healthcare applications such as fitness assessment [64], life logging,[7] and rehabilitation [74] where the user activities can be tracked anytime and anywhere.

From the data analytics perspective, [33] discusses the feature extraction algorithm for HAR using only a single tri-axial accelerometer. Relevant and robust features are successfully selected and the data size is reduced; thereby, the processing speed increases without degrading accuracy.

Retrieved features corresponding to activities specify patterns, and the patterns are used for classification or modelling. Sliding window methods are typically used for static or periodic activities while sporadic activities can be recognized using template matching approaches [71] or Hidden Markov Modelling (HMM) [12, 84]. In [83], a deep learning model is designed using convolutional neural networks and LSTM recurrent neural networks, which captures spatio-temporal patterns of signals from wearable accelerometers and gyroscopes.

4.2.2 Environment Monitoring

Another interesting healthcare application integrates chemical sensors [6, 66, 70] for detecting the presence of specific molecules in the environment. For example, we can collect Pollutant Standards Index (PSI) data that reflects six pollutants (i.e.,

[6]http://www.mobilehealthsummit.ca.

[7]http://www.sonymobile.com/global-en/apps-services/lifelog.

sulfur dioxide (SO_2), particulate matter (PM10) and fine particulate matter (PM2.5), nitrogen dioxide (NO_2), carbon monoxide (CO) and ozone (O_3)), from individual users and construct a fine-grained pollution map together with images and location information. The environmental monitoring for haze, sewage water and smog emission etc. has become a significant worldwide problem. Combined with the cloud computing technology, a large number of smart mobile devices make a distributed data collection infrastructure possible, and the recent scalable, parallel, resource efficient, real-time data mining technologies have enabled smart device-based data analytics [65, 120].

[77] proposes the Personal Environmental Impact Report (PEIR) system that uses location information sampled from smartphones and calculates personalized estimates of environmental impact and exposure. The running PEIR system, which runs GPS data collection at mobile devices and the HMM-based activity classification at servers before computing the PEI values, is evaluated. A major contribution of their work is that this platform can be used for various targets such as traffic condition measuring, environmental pollution monitoring, and vehicle emission estimating.

4.2.3 Disease Detection

Biochemical-sensors deployed in/on the body can detect particular volatile organic compounds (VOCs). Many studies [11, 23, 92] have unveiled the relationships between VOCs and particular diseases corresponding to VOCs, as summarized in Table 1. The big potential of such sensor devices and the big data analytics of VOCs will revolutionize healthcare both at home and in hospital.

Developments of nano-sensor arrays and micro electro mechanical systems have enabled artificial olfactory sensors, called electronic noses [30, 66], as tiny, energy efficient, portable devices. [30] discusses the essential cause of obesity from overeating and an intake of high-calorie food, and presents the way to compute energy expenditure from exhaled breath.

In [51], nano-enabling electrochemical sensing technology is introduced, which rapidly detects beta-amyloid peptides, potential bio-markers to diagnose Alzheimer's disease, and a tool is developed to facilitate fast personalized healthcare for AD monitoring.

Table 1 List of volatile organic compounds related to particular diseases

Volatile organic compound	Relevant disease
Acetoin, 1-butanol	Lung cancer
Aceton	Diabetes
Etan, pentan	Asthma
Ammonia	Hepatic encephalopathy
Hydrogen, metan	Maldigestion syndrome
Toluen	Thinner addiction
Trimethylamine	Renal failure

4.3 Healthcare Systems

Instead of solving individual problems, a number of healthcare systems have been designed and built to serve as platforms for solving the problems described above. Now we shall discuss several representative healthcare systems.

HARVEST [38] is a summarizer for doctors to view patients' longitudinal EMR data at the point of care. It is composed of two key parts: a front-end for better visualization; a distributed back-end which can process patients' various types of EMR data and extract informative problem concepts from patients' free text data measuring each concept via "salience weights".

miniTUBA [113] is designed to assist clinical researchers to employ dynamic Bayesian networks (DBN) for data analytics in temporal datasets. The pipeline of miniTUBA includes logging in the website, inputting data as well as managing project, constructing DBN models, analyzing results and doing prediction in the end. Users can use miniTUBA to discover informative causal relationships for better inference or prediction.

In [43], a system which focuses on data-driven analytics for personalized healthcare is proposed. The applications supported in this system include analyzing patient similarity, constructing predictive models, stratifying patients, analyzing cohorts and modelling diseases. The target is to achieve personalized healthcare resource utilization and deliver care services at low costs.

To provide better support for Big Healthcare Analytics, we have been implementing various software systems that form an end-to-end pipeline from data acquisition and cleansing to visualization. We call the system GEMINI [61], whose software stack is depicted in Fig. 7. We are addressing various healthcare analytics problems, such as phenotyping, disease progression modelling, treatment recommendation etc. We shall introduce each component of our software stack via the example process of doing EMR data analytics in the following.

We work on the longitudinal EMR dataset from the National University Hospital. We encounter the various challenges as discussed in Sect. 2; hence, we need to process the data, through data cleansing and data integration, before we can conduct any data analytics. Even though we want to automate the processing and relieve the burden on doctors, EMR data cannot be cleaned and integrated effectively without doctors' assistance. Hence, we leverage automatic methods and doctors' participation with their expertise domain knowledge. DICE is our general data cleansing and integration platform that exploits both doctors' expertise and knowledge base. Additionally, to assist in the data cleansing and integration, CDAS [63] which is a crowdsourcing system, selects meaningful representative tasks for the clinicians to resolve so as to reduce the overall efforts and costs. Ultimately, we tap onto the clinicians who are the subject matter experts for their knowledge, without over imposing on their time, to improve the quality of the data and the analytics process [61, 81].

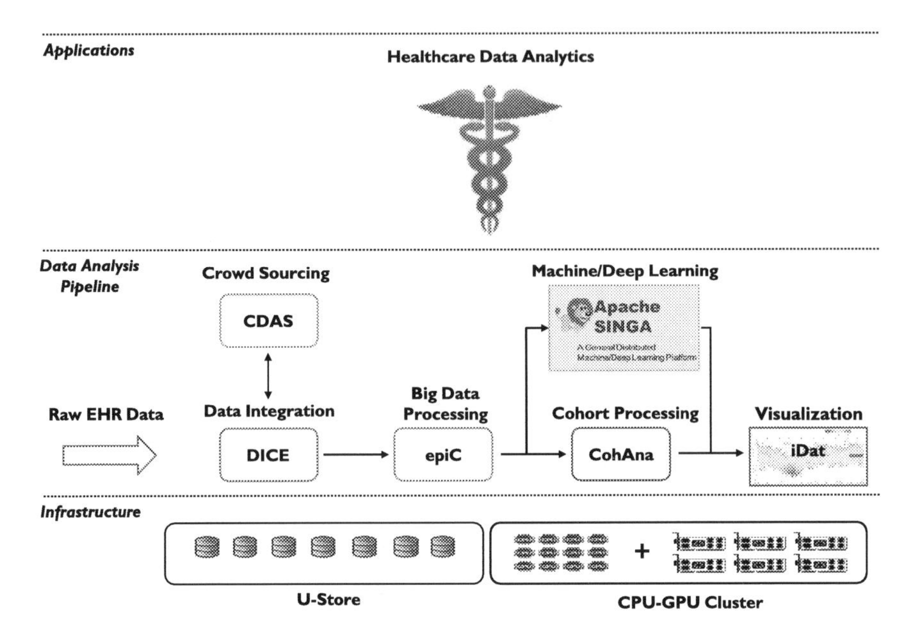

Fig. 7 GEMINI healthcare software stack

Due to the value of the data and the need to maintain it for a long period of time, we have designed and implemented UStore, which is a universal immutable storage system, to store the data. We process the data in epiC [47], which is a distributed and scalable data processing system based on Actor-like concurrent programming model. By separating computation and communication, this system can process different kinds of data (structured data, unstructured data and graph data) effectively, and also supports different computation models. However, epiC provides only database-centric processing and analytics such as aggregation and summarization. In order to provide deep analytics, we have implemented a generic distributed machine learning/deep learning platform, called Apache SINGA [82, 109]. We are implementing our deep learning models on top of Apache SINGA for analytics on various diseases.

For behavioural analysis of patients, we employ "cohort analysis" which was originally introduced in social science [31]. Cohort analysis has a wide range of healthcare applications, such as testing the hypothesis of a new treatment, seeing how similar patients in a hospital database are doing compared with the specific indexed patient, etc. For our applications, we have built CohAna [46], a column-based cohort analysis engine with an extended relation for modelling user activity data and a few new operators to support efficient cohort query processing.

To enable the clinicians to visualize the data and analytics results, we have developed iDAT, an exploratory front-end tool that allows interactive drill-down and exploration.

5 Summary and Discussions

In this chapter, we summarize the challenges of Big Healthcare Analytics and their solutions to relevant applications from both EMR data and sensor data. The challenges mainly consist of high-dimensionality, irregularity, missing data, sparsity, noise and bias. Besides the basic model construction for analytics, we discuss four necessary steps for data processing, namely data annotation, data cleansing, data integration and data analytics/modelling. Based on an examination of various types of healthcare analytics on both EMR data and sensor data, the data analytics pipeline is still the foundation for most healthcare applications. However, specific algorithms which are adopted must be adjusted by modelling the unique characteristics of medical features. With recent advancement in hardware and other technologies, smart healthcare analytics is gaining traction, and like other application domains, we are likely to experience a sharp leap in healthcare technologies and systems in the near future.

Next-generation healthcare systems are expected to integrate various types of EHR data and provide a holistic data-driven approach to predict and pre-empt illnesses, improve patient care and treatment, and ease the burden of clinicians by providing timely and assistive recommendations. Below, we discuss several applications that are likely to attract attention and interest in the near future.

Treatment recommendation system for doctors: Through various levels of automation in diagnosis model and prognosis prediction, the system may improve the medical treatment process in different degrees from helping doctors to make decisions (e.g. visualize cohort information) to outperforming doctors in treatment planning and recommendation.

Treatment explanation system for patients: Doctors may not have sufficient time to explain treatment plans to the patients in detail or may not be able to express clearly to the patients. An automatic treatment explanation system may be able to improve patient treatment compliance as well as the transparency of healthcare. Further, patients can review the plans anytime, anywhere.

Real-time surgical operation suggestion: Lots of emergency situations may happen during surgical operations. Armed with real-time sensors and reinforcement learning models, the machine may be able to deliver a better contingency plan in a much shorter time and with more accurate decision making.

Data-driven drug combination study: Drug combination discovery used to be considered as a hard problem due to the insufficiency of clinical data. An integrated system with better EHR data analytics may be able to quantify the effect of drug combinations and also discover more valuable drug combination patterns. This study can be very useful for personalized medicine recommendations, which can further help to provide a more effective healthcare.

We are looking forward to more clinical advances and healthcare products being brought to the table by both the data science and medical communities. After all, with more data and higher computational capacity, deep analytics can lead to deeper insights and hence better decisions.

Acknowledgements This work is supported by National Research Foundation, Prime Ministers Office, Singapore under its Competitive Research Programme (CRP Award No. NRF-CRP8-2011-08). Gang Chen's work is supported by National Natural Science Foundation of China (NSFC) Grant No. 61472348. Meihui Zhang is supported by SUTD Start-up Research Grant under Project No. SRG ISTD 2014 084. We would like to thank Jinyang Gao and Gerald Koh for the discussion and useful suggestions that help to improve the chapter.

References

1. Apache storm. http://storm.apache.org.
2. H. Alemdar and C. Ersoy. Wireless sensor networks for healthcare: A survey. *Computer Networks*, 54(15):2688–2710, 2010.
3. M. R. Avendi, A. Kheradvar, and H. Jafarkhani. A combined deep-learning and deformable-model approach to fully automatic segmentation of the left ventricle in cardiac mri. *Medical image analysis*, 30:108–119, 2016.
4. M. A. Balafar, A. R. Ramli, M. I. Saripan, and S. Mashohor. Review of brain MRI image segmentation methods. *Artificial Intelligence Review*, 33(3):261–274, 2010.
5. H. Banaee, M. U. Ahmed, and A. Lout. Data mining for wearable sensors in health monitoring systems: A review of recent trends and challenges. *Sensors*, 13(12), 2013.
6. A. J. Bandodkar, I. Jeerapan, and J. Wang. Wearable chemical sensors: Present challenges and future prospects. *ACS Sensors*, 1:464–482, 2016.
7. I. M. Baytas, K. Lin, F. Wang, et al. Stochastic convex sparse principal component analysis. *EURASIP Journal on Bioinformatics and Systems Biology*, 2016(1):1–11, 2016.
8. Y. Bengio, A. Courville, and P. Vincent. Representation learning: A review and new perspectives. *IEEE Transactions on Pattern Analysis and Machine Intelligence*, 35(8):1798–1828, 2013.
9. J. Bian, B. Gao, and T.-Y. Liu. Knowledge-powered deep learning for word embedding. In *Joint European Conference on Machine Learning and Knowledge Discovery in Databases*, pages 132–148, 2014.
10. T. Botsis, G. Hartvigsen, F. Chen, and C. Weng. Secondary use of ehr: data quality issues and informatics opportunities. *AMIA Summits Transl Sci Proc*, 2010:1–5, 2010.
11. Y. Y. Broza and H. Haick. Nanomaterial-based sensors for detection of disease by volatile organic compounds. *Nanomedicine (Lond)*, 8(5):785–806, 2013.
12. A. Bulling, U. Blanke, and B. Schiele. A tutorial on human activity recognition using body-worn inertial sensors. *ACM Computing Survey*, 46(3):1–33, 2014.
13. N. A. Capela, E. D. Lemaire, N. Baddour, et al. Evaluation of a smartphone human activity recognition application with able-bodied and stroke participants. *NeuroEngineering and Rehabilitation*, 13(5), 2016.
14. R. Caruana. Multitask learning. *Machine learning*, 28(1):41–75, 1997.
15. R. D. Caytiles and S. Park. A study of the design of wireless medical sensor netork based u-healthcare system. *International Journal of Bio-Science and Bio-Technology*, 6(3):91–96, 2014.
16. Z. Che, D. C. Kale, W. Li, et al. Deep computational phenotyping. In *Proceedings of the 21th ACM SIGKDD International Conference on Knowledge Discovery and Data Mining*, pages 507–516, 2015.

17. Z. Che, S. Purushotham, K. Cho, et al. Recurrent neural networks for multivariate time series with missing values. *arXiv preprint* arXiv: 1606.01865, 2016.
18. Z. Che, S. Purushotham, R. Khemani, et al. Distilling knowledge from deep networks with applications to healthcare domain. *arXiv preprint* arXiv: 1512.03542, 2015.
19. K. Cho, B. Van Merriënboer, C. Gulcehre, et al. Learning phrase representations using rnn encoder-decoder for statistical machine translation. *arXiv preprint* arXiv: 1406.1078, 2014.
20. D. A. Cohn. Neural network exploration using optimal experiment design. In *NIPS*, 1994.
21. R. Cort, X. Bonnaire, O. Marin, et al. Stream processing of healthcare sensor data: studying user traces to identify challenges from a big data perspective. In *Proceedings of the 4th International Workshop on Body Area Sensor Networks*, 2015.
22. B. Cui, H. Mei, and B. C. Ooi. Big data: the driver for innovation in databases. *National Science Review*, 1(1):27–30, 2014.
23. A. G. Dent, T. G. Sutedja, and P. V. Zimmerman. Exhaled breath analysis for lung cancer. *Journal of thoracic disease*, 5:S540, 2013.
24. A. Doan, A. Halevy, and Z. Ives. *Principles of data integration*. Elsevier, 2012.
25. X. L. Dong and D. Srivastava. Big data integration. In *Data Engineering (ICDE), 2013 IEEE 29th International Conference on*, pages 1245–1248, 2013.
26. O. M. Doyle, E. Westman, A. F. Marquand, et al. Predicting progression of alzheimers disease using ordinal regression. *PloS one*, 9(8):e105542, 2014.
27. S. Duchesne, A. Caroli, C. Geroldi, et al. Relating one-year cognitive change in mild cognitive impairment to baseline MRI features. *Neuroimage*, 47(4):1363–1370, 2009.
28. A. S. Evani, B. Sreenivasan, J. S. Sudesh, et al. Activity recognition using wearable sensors for healthcare. In *Proceedings of the 7th International Conference on Sensor Technologies and Appplications*, 2013.
29. L. Filipe, F. Fdez-Riverola, N. Costa, et al. Wireless body area networks for healthcare applications: Protocol stack review. *International Journal of Distributed Sensor Networks*, 2015:1:1–1:1, 2015.
30. J. W. Gardner and T. A. Vincent. Electronic noses for well-being: Breath analysis and energy expenditure. *Sensors*, 16(7):947, 2016.
31. N. D. Glenn. *Cohort analysis*. Sage, 2005.
32. D. Gomez-Cabrero, I. Abugessaisa, D. Maier, A. Teschendorff, M. Merkenschlager, A. Gisel, E. Ballestar, E. Bongcam-Rudloff, A. Conesa, and J. Tegnér. Data integration in the era of omics: current and future challenges. *BMC Systems Biology*, 8(2):1–10, 2014.
33. P. Gupta and T. Dallas. Feature selection and activity recognition system using a single triaxial accelerometer. *IEEE Transactions on Biomedical Engineering*, 61(6):1780–1786, 2014.
34. I. Guyon and A. Elisseeff. An introduction to variable and feature selection. *Journal of machine learning research*, 3:1157–1182, 2003.
35. M. Haghighi, P. Woznowski, N. Zhu, et al. Agent-based decentralised data-acquisition and time-synchronisation in critical healthcare applications. In *Proceedings of the IEEE 2nd World Forum on Inernet of Things*, 2015.
36. A. Halevy, A. Rajaraman, and J. Ordille. Data integration: The teenage years. In *Proceedings of the 32nd International Conference on Very Large Data Bases*, pages 9–16, 2006.
37. W. R. Hersh, M. G. Weiner, P. J. Embi, et al. Caveats for the use of operational electronic health record data in comparative effectiveness research. *Medical care*, 51:S30–S37, 2013.
38. J. S. Hirsch, J. S. Tanenbaum, S. Lipsky Gorman, et al. Harvest, a longitudinal patient record summarizer. *Journal of the American Medical Informatics Association*, 22(2):263–274, 2014.
39. J. C. Ho, J. Ghosh, and J. Sun. Marble: high-throughput phenotyping from electronic health records via sparse nonnegative tensor factorization. In *Proceedings of the 20th ACM SIGKDD international conference on Knowledge discovery and data mining*, pages 115–124, 2014.
40. S. Hochreiter and J. Schmidhuber. Long short-term memory. *Neural computation*, 9(8):1735–1780, 1997.
41. G. Hripcsak and D. J. Albers. Next-generation phenotyping of electronic health records. *Journal of the American Medical Informatics Association*, 20(1):117–121, 2013.

42. G. Hripcsak, D. J. Albers, and A. Perotte. Parameterizing time in electronic health record studies. *Journal of the American Medical Informatics Association*, 22(4):794–804, 2015.
43. J. Hu, A. Perer, and F. Wang. Data driven analytics for personalized healthcare. In *Healthcare Information Management Systems*, pages 529–554. Springer, 2016.
44. C. H. Jackson, L. D. Sharples, S. G. Thompson, et al. Multistate markov models for disease progression with classification error. *Journal of the Royal Statistical Society: Series D (The Statistician)*, 52(2):193–209, 2003.
45. H. Jagadish. Challenges and opportunities with big data, 2012.
46. D. Jiang, Q. Cai, G. Chen, et al. Cohort query processing. *Proceedings of the VLDB Endowment*, 10(1), 2017.
47. D. Jiang, G. Chen, B. C. Ooi, et al. epic: an extensible and scalable system for processing big data. *Proceedings of the VLDB Endowment*, 7(7):541–552, 2014.
48. K. Kalantar-Zadeh, C. K. Yao, K. J. Berean, et al. Intestinal gas capsules: A proof-of-concept demonstration. *Gastroenterology*, 150(1):37–39, 2016.
49. D. C. Kale, Z. Che, M. T. Bahadori, et al. Causal phenotype discovery via deep networks. In *AMIA Annual Symposium Proceedings*, pages 677–686, 2015.
50. A. Karpathy and L. Fei-Fei. Deep visual-semantic alignments for generating image descriptions. *arXiv preprint* arXiv: 1412.2306, 2014.
51. A. Kaushik, R. D. Jayant, S. Tiwari, et al. Nano-biosensors to detect beta-amyloid for alzheimer's disease management. *Biosensors and Bioelectronics*, 80(15):273–287, 2016.
52. R. Korchiyne, S. M. Farssi, A. Sbihi, R. Touahni, and M. T. Alaoui. A combined method of fractal and GLCM features for MRI and CT scan images classification. *arXiv preprint* arXiv: 1409.4559, 2014.
53. H. Krumholz, S.-L. Normand, P. Keenan, et al. 30-day heart failure readmission measure methodology. Technical report, Yale University/Yale-New Haven Hospital Center for Outcomes Research And Evaluation (YNHH-CORE), 2008.
54. Z. Kuang, J. Thomson, M. Caldwell, et al. Computational drug repositioning using continuous self-controlled case series. *arXiv preprint* arXiv: 1604.05976, 2016.
55. S. Kumar, M. Willander, J. G. Sharma, et al. A solution processed carbon nanotube modified conducting paper sensor for cancer detection. *Journal of Materials Chemistry B*, 3:9305–9314, 2015.
56. O. D. Lara and M. A. Labrador. A survey on human activity recognition using wearable sensors. *IEEE Communications Surveys and Tutorials*, 15(3):1192–1209, 2013.
57. T. A. Lasko, J. C. Denny, and M. A. Levy. Computational phenotype discovery using unsupervised feature learning over noisy, sparse, and irregular clinical data. *PloS one*, 8(6):1–13, 2013.
58. M. Lenzerini. Data integration: A theoretical perspective. In *Proceedings of the 21st ACM SIGMOD-SIGACT-SIGART Symposium on Principles of Database Systems*, PODS '02, pages 233–246. ACM, 2002.
59. D. D. Lewis and W. A. Gale. A sequential algorithm for training text classifiers. In *Proceedings of the 17th Annual International ACM SIGIR Conference on Research and Development in Information Retrieval*, SIGIR '94, pages 3–12, New York, NY, USA, 1994. Springer-Verlag New York, Inc.
60. Q. Lin, B. C. Ooi, Z. Wang, et al. Scalable distributed stream join processing. In *Proceedings of the 2015 ACM SIGMOD International Conference on Management of Data*, pages 811–825, 2015.
61. Z. J. Ling, Q. T. Tran, J. Fan, et al. GEMINI: An integrative healthcare analytics system. *Proceedings of the VLDB Endowment*, 7(13):1766–1771, 2014.
62. Z. C. Lipton, D. C. Kale, C. Elkan, et al. Learning to diagnose with lstm recurrent neural networks. *arXiv preprint* arXiv: 1511.03677, 2015.
63. X. Liu, M. Lu, B. C. Ooi, et al. CDAS: a crowdsourcing data analytics system. *Proceedings of the VLDB Endowment*, 5(10):1040–1051, 2012.
64. J. W. Lockhart, T. Pulickal, and G. M. Weiss. Applications of mobile activity recognition. In *ACM Conference on Ubiquitous Computing*, pages 1054–1058, 2012.

65. J. W. Lockhart, G. M. Weiss, J. C. Xue, et al. Design considerations for the wisdm smart phone-based sensor mining architecture. In *Proceedings of the 5th International Workshop on Knowledge Discovery from Sensor Data*, pages 25–33, 2011.
66. P. Lorwongtragool, E. Sowade, N. Watthanawisuth, et al. A novel wearable electronic nose for healthcare based on flexible printed chemical sensor array. *Sensors*, 14(10):19700, 2014.
67. V. Loscrí, L. Matekovits, I. Peter, et al. In-body network biomedical applications: From modeling to experimentation. *IEEE Transactions on Nanobioscience*, 15(1):53–61, 2016.
68. L. L. Low, K. H. Lee, M. E. Hock Ong, et al. Predicting 30-day readmissions: performance of the lace index compared with a regression model among general medicine patients in singapore. *BioMed research international*, 2015.
69. D. Malak and O. B. Akan. Molecular communication nanonetworks inside human body. *Nano Communication Networks*, 3(1):19–35, 2012.
70. C. Manjarrs, D. Garizado, M. Obregon, et al. Chemical sensor network for ph monitoring. *Journal of Applied Research and Technology*, 14(1):1–8, 2016.
71. J. Margarito, R. Helaoui, A. M. Bianchi, et al. User-independent recognition of sports activities from a single wrist-worn accelerometer: A template-matching-based approach. *IEEE Transactions on Biomedical Engineering*, 63(4):788–796, 2016.
72. B. M. Marlin, D. C. Kale, R. G. Khemani, et al. Unsupervised pattern discovery in electronic health care data using probabilistic clustering models. In *Proceedings of the 2nd ACM SIGHIT International Health Informatics Symposium*, pages 389–398, 2012.
73. M. E. Matheny, R. A. Miller, T. A. Ikizler, et al. Development of inpatient risk stratification models of acute kidney injury for use in electronic health records. *Medical Decision Making*, 30(6):639–650, 2010.
74. A. McLeod, E. M. Bochniewicz, P. S. Lum, et al. Using wearable sensors and machine learning models to separate functional upper extremity use from walking-associated arm movements. *Physical Medicine and Rehabilitation.*, 97(2):224–231, 2016.
75. N. Q. Mehmood, R. Culmone, and L. Mostarda. A flexible and scalable architecture for real-time ANT+ sensor data acquisition and nosql storage. *International Journal of Distributed Sensor Networks*, 12(5), 2016.
76. D. Mould. Models for disease progression: new approaches and uses. *Clinical Pharmacology & Therapeutics*, 92(1):125–131, 2012.
77. M. Mun, S. Reddy, K. Shilton, et al. Peir, the personal environmental impact report, as a platform for participatory sensing systems research. In *Proceedings of the 7th International Conference on Mobile Systems, Applications, and Services*, pages 55–68, 2009.
78. I. Muslea, S. Minton, and C. A. Knoblock. Selective sampling with redundant views. In *AAAI/IAAI*, pages 621–626, 2000.
79. T. D. Nguyen, T. Tran, D. Phung, et al. Latent patient profile modelling and applications with mixed-variate restricted boltzmann machine. In *Pacific-Asia Conference on Knowledge Discovery and Data Mining*, pages 123–135, 2013.
80. L. Nie, L. Zhang, Y. Yang, et al. Beyond doctors: Future health prediction from multimedia and multimodal observations. In *Proceedings of the 23rd ACM international conference on Multimedia*, pages 591–600, 2015.
81. B. C. Ooi, K. L. Tan, Q. T. Tran, et al. Contextual crowd intelligence. *ACM SIGKDD Explorations Newsletter*, 16(1):39–46, 2014.
82. B. C. Ooi, K.-L. Tan, S. Wang, et al. SINGA: A distributed deep learning platform. In *Proceedings of the 23rd ACM International Conference on Multimedia*, pages 685–688, 2015.
83. F. J. Ordez and D. Roggen. Deep convolutional and lstm recurrent neural networks for multimodal wearable activity recognition. *Sensors (Basel, Switzerland)*, 16(1):115, 2016.
84. F. J. Ordonez, G. Englebienne, P. de Toledo, et al. In-home activity recognition: Bayesian inference for hidden markov models. *IEEE Pervasive Computing*, 13(3):67–75, 2014.
85. R. K. Pearson, R. J. Kingan, and A. Hochberg. Disease progression modeling from historical clinical databases. In *Proceedings of the eleventh ACM SIGKDD international conference on Knowledge discovery in data mining*, pages 788–793, 2005.

86. T. Pham, T. Tran, D. Phung, et al. Deepcare: A deep dynamic memory model for predictive medicine. In *Pacific-Asia Conference on Knowledge Discovery and Data Mining*, pages 30–41, 2016.
87. R. Pivovarov, D. J. Albers, J. L. Sepulveda, et al. Identifying and mitigating biases in ehr laboratory tests. *Journal of biomedical informatics*, 51:24–34, 2014.
88. R. Pivovarov, A. J. Perotte, E. Grave, et al. Learning probabilistic phenotypes from heterogeneous ehr data. *Journal of biomedical informatics*, 58:156–165, 2015.
89. S. R. and C. L. Stress detection using physiological sensors. *IEEE Computer*, 48(10):26–33, 2015.
90. N. Roy and A. McCallum. Toward optimal active learning through monte carlo estimation of error reduction. *ICML, Williamstown*, pages 441–448, 2001.
91. M. Salai, I. Vassnyi, and I. Ksa. Stress detection using low cost heart rate sensors. *Journal of Healthcare Engineering*, 2, 2016.
92. Y. Sasaya and T. Nakamoto. Study of halitosis-substance sensing at low concentration using an electrochemical sensor array combined with a preconcentrator. *IEEE Journal of Transactions on Sensors and Micromachines*, 126, 2006.
93. J. L. Schafer and J. W. Graham. Missing data: our view of the state of the art. *Psychological methods*, 7(2):147, 2002.
94. P. Schulam, F. Wigley, and S. Saria. Clustering longitudinal clinical marker trajectories from electronic health data: Applications to phenotyping and endotype discovery. In *Proceedings of the 29th AAAI Conference on Artificial Intelligence*, pages 2956–2964, 2015.
95. M. B. Schulze, K. Hoffmann, H. Boeing, et al. An accurate risk score based on anthropometric, dietary, and lifestyle factors to predict the development of type 2 diabetes. *Diabetes care*, 30(3):510–515, 2007.
96. B. Settles and M. Craven. An analysis of active learning strategies for sequence labeling tasks. In *Proceedings of the Conference on Empirical Methods in Natural Language Processing*, EMNLP '08, pages 1070–1079, Stroudsburg, PA, USA, 2008. Association for Computational Linguistics.
97. H. S. Seung, M. Opper, and H. Sompolinsky. Query by committee. In *Proceedings of the Fifth Annual Workshop on Computational Learning Theory*, COLT '92, pages 287–294, New York, NY, USA, 1992. ACM.
98. M. J. Sewitch, K. Leffondré, and P. L. Dobkin. Clustering patients according to health perceptions: relationships to psychosocial characteristics and medication nonadherence. *Journal of psychosomatic research*, 56(3):323–332, 2004.
99. M. Shoaib, S. Bosch, O. D. Incel, et al. A survey of online activity recognition using mobile phones. *Sensors*, 15(1):2059–2085, 2015.
100. C. M. Stonnington, C. Chu, S. Klöppel, et al. Predicting clinical scores from magnetic resonance scans in alzheimer's disease. *Neuroimage*, 51(4):1405–1413, 2010.
101. N. Street. A neural network model for prognostic prediction. In *Proceedings of the 15th International Conference on Machine Learning*, pages 540–546, 1998.
102. S. Tong and D. Koller. Support vector machine active learning with applications to text classification. *J. Mach. Learn. Res.*, 2:45–66, Mar. 2002.
103. S. N. Topkaya and D. Ozkan-Ariksoysal. Prostate cancer biomarker detection with carbon nanotubes modified screen printed electrodes. *Electroanalysis*, 28(5), 2016.
104. C. Torres-Huitzil and A. Alvarez-Landero. *Accelerometer-Based Human Activity Recognition in Smartphones for Healthcare Services*, pages 147–169. Springer, 2015.
105. T. Tran, T. D. Nguyen, D. Phung, et al. Learning vector representation of medical objects via emr-driven nonnegative restricted boltzmann machines (enrbm). *Journal of biomedical informatics*, pages 96–105, 2015.
106. C. van Walraven, I. A. Dhalla, C. Bell, et al. Derivation and validation of an index to predict early death or unplanned readmission after discharge from hospital to the community. *Canadian Medical Association Journal*, 182(6):551–557, 2010.
107. P. Vemuri, H. Wiste, S. Weigand, et al. MRI and CSF biomarkers in normal, MCI, and AD subjects predicting future clinical change. *Neurology*, 73(4):294–301, 2009.

108. F. Wang, N. Lee, J. Hu, et al. Towards heterogeneous temporal clinical event pattern discovery: a convolutional approach. In *Proceedings of the 18th ACM SIGKDD international conference on Knowledge discovery and data mining*, pages 453–461, 2012.
109. W. Wang, G. Chen, A. T. T. Dinh, et al. SINGA: Putting deep learning in the hands of multimedia users. In *Proceedings of the 23rd ACM International Conference on Multimedia*, pages 25–34, 2015.
110. X. Wang, D. Sontag, and F. Wang. Unsupervised learning of disease progression models. In *Proceedings of the 20th ACM SIGKDD international conference on Knowledge discovery and data mining*, pages 85–94, 2014.
111. Y. Wang, R. Chen, J. Ghosh, et al. Rubik: Knowledge guided tensor factorization and completion for health data analytics. In *Proceedings of the 21th ACM SIGKDD International Conference on Knowledge Discovery and Data Mining*, pages 1265–1274, 2015.
112. B. J. Wells, A. S. Nowacki, K. Chagin, et al. Strategies for handling missing data in electronic health record derived data. *eGEMs (Generating Evidence & Methods to improve patient outcomes)*, 1(3):7, 2013.
113. Z. Xiang, R. M. Minter, X. Bi, et al. minituba: medical inference by network integration of temporal data using bayesian analysis. *Bioinformatics*, 23(18):2423–2432, 2007.
114. T. Yokota, P. Zalar, M. Kaltenbrunner, et al. Ultraflexible organic photonic skin. *Science Advances Online Edition*, 2(4), 2016.
115. H. Zhang, G. Chen, B. C. Ooi, et al. In-memory big data management and processing: A survey. *IEEE Transactions on Knowledge and Data Engineering*, 27(7):1920–1948, 2015.
116. X. Zhang, B. Hu, L. Zhou, et al. An eeg based pervasive depression detection for females. In *Proceedings of the 2012 International Conference on Pervasive Computing and the Networked World*, pages 848–861, 2013.
117. J. Zhou, J. Liu, V. A. Narayan, et al. Modeling disease progression via fused sparse group lasso. In *Proceedings of the 18th ACM SIGKDD international conference on Knowledge discovery and data mining*, pages 1095–1103, 2012.
118. J. Zhou, F. Wang, J. Hu, et al. From micro to macro: data driven phenotyping by densification of longitudinal electronic medical records. In *Proceedings of the 20th ACM SIGKDD international conference on Knowledge discovery and data mining*, pages 135–144, 2014.
119. J. Zhou, L. Yuan, J. Liu, et al. A multi-task learning formulation for predicting disease progression. In *Proceedings of the 17th ACM SIGKDD international conference on Knowledge discovery and data mining*, pages 814–822, 2011.
120. T. Zhu, S. Xiao, Q. Zhang, et al. Emergent technologies in big data sensing: A survey. *International Journal of Distributed Sensor Networks*, 2015(8):1–13, 2015.

Process Streaming Healthcare Data with Adaptive MapReduce Framework

Fan Zhang, Junwei Cao, Samee U. Khan, Keqin Li and Kai Hwang

Abstract As one of the most widely used healthcare scientific applications, body area network with hundreds of interconnected sensors need to be used to monitor the health status of a physical body. It is very challenging to process, analyze and monitor the streaming data in real time. Therefore, an efficient cloud platform with very elastic scaling capacity is needed to support such kind of real-time streaming data applications. The state-of-art cloud platform either lacks of such capability to process highly concurrent streaming data, or scales in regards to coarse-grained compute nodes. In this chapter, we propose a task-level adaptive MapReduce framework. This framework extends the generic MapReduce architecture by designing each Map and Reduce task as a scalable daemon process. The beauty of this new framework is the scaling capability being designed at the Map and Reduce task level, rather than being scaled at the compute-node level, as traditional MapReduce does. This design is capable of not only scaling up and down in real time, but also leading to effective use of compute resources in cloud data center. As

F. Zhang (✉)
IBM Massachusetts Laboratory, Littleton, MA 01460, USA
e-mail: fzhang@us.ibm.com

J. Cao
Research Institute of Information Technology, Tsinghua University, Beijing 100084, China
e-mail: jcao@tsinghua.edu.cn

S.U. Khan
Department of Electrical and Computer Engineering, North Dakota State University, Fargo, ND 58108-6050, USA
e-mail: samee.khan@ndsu.edu

K. Li
Department of Computer Science, State University of New York, New Paltz, New York 12561, USA
e-mail: lik@newpaltz.edu

K. Hwang
Department of Electrical Engineering and Computer Science, University of Southern California, Los Angeles, CA 90089, USA
e-mail: kaihwang@usc.edu

© Springer International Publishing AG 2017

S.U. Khan et al. (eds.), *Handbook of Large-Scale Distributed Computing in Smart Healthcare*, Scalable Computing and Communications,
DOI 10.1007/978-3-319-58280-1_3

a first step towards implementing this framework in real cloud, we have developed a simulator that captures workload strength, and provisions the just-in-need amount of Map and Reduce tasks in realtime. To further enhance the framework, we applied two streaming data workload prediction methods, smoothing and Kalman filter, to estimate the workload characteristics. We see 63.1% performance improvement by using the Kalman filter method to predict the workload. We also use real streaming data workload trace to test the framework. Experimental results show that this framework schedules the Map and Reduce tasks very efficiently, as the streaming data changes its arrival rate.

Keywords Adaptive Mapreduce · Big data · Healthcare scientific applications · Kalman filter · Parallel processing

1 Introduction

Big-data technology has been a driving force for the state-of-art healthcare science. Most of the healthcare applications are composed of processes that need to manage Gigabytes of real-time and streaming data. For example, the Body Area Network [1] that is widely recognized as a medium to access, monitor, and evaluate the real-time health status of a person, has long been notorious for its computing intensiveness to process Gigabytes of data [2, 3] in real-time. Such data are collected from well-configured sensors to sample the real-time signals of body temperature, blood pressure, respiratory and heart rate, chest sound, and cardiovascular status, to name a few among others.

To process stream big-data in real-time, traditional parallelized processing frameworks, such as Hadoop MapReduce [4], Pregel [5], and Graphlab [6, 7], are structurally constrained and functionally limited. The major difficulty lies in their designs, which are primarily contrived to access and process the static input data. No built-in iterative module can be used when the input data arrives in a stream flow. Moreover, the existing frameworks are unable to handle the scenarios when the streaming input datasets are from various sources and have different arrival rates. Streaming data sample rates are consistently changed while the healthcare scientific applications are running. For example, the data collected when a person is sleeping is usually far less than the data collected when the person is running or swimming.

Cloud computing, with most of its few open-source tools and programming models, have provided a great opportunity to process such time-varied streaming data healthcare applications. Amazon Elastic MapReduce (EMR) framework [8], as an example, is typically represented by its compute instances being automatically scaled up or down and scaled in or out when workload changes. However, the granularity of the scaling is too coarse for most of the healthcare applications, meaning we need more fined-grained scaling objects, such as CPU core, memory size or active processing tasks, to be used in order to be able to scale in real time. In our early research paper [9], we have discovered and identified an issue when scaling large number of compute instance, named the large-scale limitation issue. This issue demonstrates the most MapReduce applications fail to promise its scaling capability when the number of the compute instances exceeds the actual need. Therefore, the scalability would find itself more tractable when one the MapReduce application scales at a task level—increasing or reducing the Map and Reduce task number when a variation of the workload is predicted.

Tools with such fined-grained scaling capability are really rare to find. For example, the number of the Map tasks and Reduce tasks in a launched MapReduce job is fixed and can never be changed over time. However, such a fined-grained processing is widely needed. It is also very possible to do so since the number of the Map tasks are usually related the number of chunks of the input dataset sizes, and the number of the Reduce tasks is related to the hashing algorithm used for the intermediate keys. There is no strong constraint between the number of the Map Tasks and Reduce Tasks. All these make the scaling of the Map and Reduce tasks possible. In the next section, we will survey a few commercial tools that have been widely used in business for similar purposes.

Towards that end, we propose a full-fledged MapReduce framework that is tailored for processing streaming data in healthcare scientific applications. The framework goes beyond the traditional Hadoop MapReduce design, while also providing a much more generic framework in order to cover a wider group of real-time applications. Traditional Hadoop MapReduce requires the Map and Reduce number to be fixed, while this new MapReduce framework doesn't require so. Furthermore, Each Map and/or Reduce task is mandatory to reside on its own JVM in traditional Hadoop MapReduce. In the new framework, one such a Map and/or Reduce task can be specified much differently, whether it be in a JVM, a local thread or process, or even an entire compute node, to name a few among others. In other words, this framework absorbs the MapReduce design primitive, that the Map tasks outputting data to all the Reduce tasks, but in a way that requires much less constraint. It's our expectation that this new framework is supposed to streamline the streaming data processing, which has never been implemented in traditional Hadoop MapReduce at all. The major contribution of this chapter is summarized below.

(1) A unique task-level and adaptive MapReduce framework is proposed in order to process rich and varied arrival rate streaming data in healthcare applications. This framework enriches the traditional Hadoop MapReduce design in a way that specifically addresses the varied arrival rate of streaming data chunks. The framework is mathematically grounded on quite a few theorems and corollaries, in order to demonstrate its scaling capability. A full stack simulator is also developed with extensive experiments to validate the effectiveness.

(2) In order to better process streaming data and better use compute resources in a scaling process, a workload arrival rate prediction mechanism is therefore needed. This chapter covers two innovative workload prediction algorithms. Real-life healthcare experiments are used to compare the performance of them.
(3) Finally, we demonstrate more experiment results by showing the close relationship between the active numbers of the Map/Reduce tasks with the number of the streamed workload tasks. This reveals the adaptively of framework, as well as the correctness of the mathematical foundation.

This chapter is organized as follows. The first section introduces a real model of healthcare scientific applications, and necessitates the requirement of processing stream-style big-data. In the second section, we report the related work, and also introduce our unique approach. A real-life healthcare application study is followed in section three. After that, we reveal the methodology of the proposed task-level adaptive MapReduce framework. Two innovative methods for predicting the streaming data workload are proposed in the next section. Experiment settings and the results are introduced in the fifth section. Finally, we conclude the work and summarize a few aspects of directions to continue the work.

2 Related Work and Our Unique Approach

There is an escalating interest on leveraging the state-of-art big-data platform to process stream data in real-time. In this section, we investigate previous publications in this area. Thereafter, we briefly describe our unique approach to show the advantage among other solutions.

2.1 Related Work

Health Information System [10] was originated and further extended from the hospital information system [11] that addresses what is called the health informatics issues. The major challenge involves the shift from paper-based to computer-based, and further to the Internet-based data storage processing. Patients, healthcare consumers, and professionals are more involved into a collaboration phase from a traditional in- or out-patient medication, to a widely acceptable online on-demand treatment. Such a shift requires a significantly powerful interconnection compute network and highly scalable compute nodes for both computing and big-data processing.

MapReduce is a simple programming model for developing distributed data intensive application in cloud platforms. Ever since Google initially proposed it on a cluster of commodity machines, there have been many follow-up projects. For instance, Hadoop [12] is a Mapreduce framework developed by Apache, and Phoenix [13] is another framework designed for shared memory architecture by Stanford University. Pregel [5] is a message-based programming model to work on real-life applications that can be distributed as an interdependent graph. It uses vertex, messages, and multiple iterations to provide a completely new programming mechanism. GraphLab [6, 7] is proposed to deal with scalable algorithms in data mining and machine learning that run on multicore clusters.

The above-mentioned tools have a wide impact on the big-data community and have been extensively used in real-life applications. Along those lines, other research efforts addressing streaming data have been proposed. Nova [14], due to its support for stateful incremental processing leveraging Pig Latin [15], deals with continuous arrival of streaming data. Incoop [16] is proposed as an incremental computation to improve the performance of the MR framework. Simple Scalable Streaming System (S4) [17], introduced by Yahoo!, is universally used, distributed, and scalable streaming data processing system. As one of its major competitor, Twitter is using Storm [18] that has also gained momentum in real-time data analytics, online machine learning, distributed remote procedure call, ETL (Extract, Transform and Load) processing, etc. Other companies, such as Facebook, Linkedin and Cloudrera, are also developing tools for real-time data processing, such as Scribe [19], Kafka [20], and Flume [21]. Even though the programming languages are different, they all provide highly efficient and scalable structure to collect and analyze real-time log files. Complex Event Processing systems (CEP) are also gaining interest recently. Popular CEP systems include StreamBase [22], HStreaming [23], and Esper&NEsper [24]. Essentially the CEP systems are primary used in processing inter-arrival messages and events.

Different from these research and commercial products, our work goes beyond a programming model framework, but also serves as a simulator to help users identify how their compute resources can be effectively used. Secondly, the framework is still based on a generic MapReduce, but not entirely a Hadoop MapReduce framework. We do not intend to design a completely new framework, but we aim to extend a widely acceptable model to allow it to seamlessly process streaming data. Our work may aid the programmers to manipulate the streaming data applications to process such kinds of flow data in a more scalable fashion.

2.2 *Our Unique Approach*

In a nutshell, our approach implements each Map and Reduce task as a running daemon. Instead of processing local data in Hadoop Distributed File System

(HDFS) as what traditional Hadoop usually does, the new Map tasks repeatedly pull the cached stream data in the HDFS, generate the Map-stage intermediate key-value pairs and push them to the corresponding Reduce tasks. These Reduce tasks, quite similar to what the Map tasks, are also implemented in such a way. These Reduce tasks repeatedly pull the corresponding data partitions from the entire Map task output, generate the Reduce-stage intermediate key-value pairs and push them to the local disk cache. In this way, each Reduce task has to cache the intermediate status of all the output key-value pairs when the application is on going.

Take a simple example to illustrate the scenario. Multiple users are collaborating by adding/removing/updating words, sentences and files to HDFS as data streams. An enhanced WordCount application requires obtain the real-time count of each word when the texts are consistently updated. Map tasks are implemented in a stateless manner, meaning that they just simply process the corresponding input data and produce output without having to worry about previous data that they have processed. However, the Reduce tasks must be implemented in a stateful way. This means that each of the Reduce task has to save the real-time count of each word and adaptively add or reduce the count whenever there is a change in the HDFS.

The essence of our approach, as we can see from the analysis, lies in the seamless connection to the MapReduce implementation. Users write data streaming applications as they did in writing traditional MapReduce applications. The only difference, however, is that they need to write such a Map and Reduce daemon function. Secondly, our approach can be implemented to scale the Map and Reduce task number separately. Traditional MapReduce framework which scales compute nodes usually leads to low compute resource usage when the active running tasks cannot utilize these compute nodes effectively.

An example is used here to illustrate the adaptive MapReduce application that calculates the real-time occurrence of each word in a set of documents. Multiple people consistently update these documents, and therefore the statistics of each word count differ from time to time.

The Map tasks below are continuously fed by input data stream, and enter into a loop that would not stop until the data stream update ends. For each of the loop, all the words are extracted and emitted key value pairs as tradition WordCount does. The Reduce tasks, also being launched in a loop, are fed continuously by the intermediate data produced by all of the Map tasks. The only difference here is the result, which needs to be fetched from HDFS. Because for each result that has been calculated, it needs repeatedly updating. Therefore, Reduce tasks should be able to not only write data back to the HDFS, but also retrieve data back from HDFS for updating.

```
Map Function: map(String k, String v):
// k: doc name in a streaming data
// v: doc contents
While(HasMoreData)
    value = GetStreamDataContent();
    for each word w in value:
        EmitIntermediate(w, "1");
```

```
Reduce Function: reduce(String k, Iterator vs):
// k: a word
// vs: a list of counts
While(HasMoreIntermediateData)
    int result = getResultFromHDFS;
    for each v in vs:
        result += ParseInt(v);
        Emit(AsString(result));
```

3 Problem Formulation of a Real-Life Healthcare Application

In Fig. 1, we illustrate a case study of the body area network as a real-life healthcare application. Health status regarding the respiration, breath, cardiovascular, insulin, blood, glucose and body temperature, which are consistently collected by sensors deployed all over the human body. This is wearable computing, which sends data periodically to a mobile phone via local network. The sample frequency is determined by the capacity of the sensors as well as the processing rate of the mobile device.

Because most of the mobile devices nowadays are equipped with advanced processing unit and large memory space, data can be continuously transferred to a mobile device and even processed within the mobile device. Therefore, the various sources of input data can be even locally analyzed before moving to the remote data center. The data center has information on various disease symptoms and the corresponding value threshold in regards to the insulin pump and glucose level, etc. The purpose of the follow-up data transferring is to compare the collected data with those in the database, and quickly alert the user the potential symptom he/she is supposed to see, and provide a smart medical suggestion in real-time.

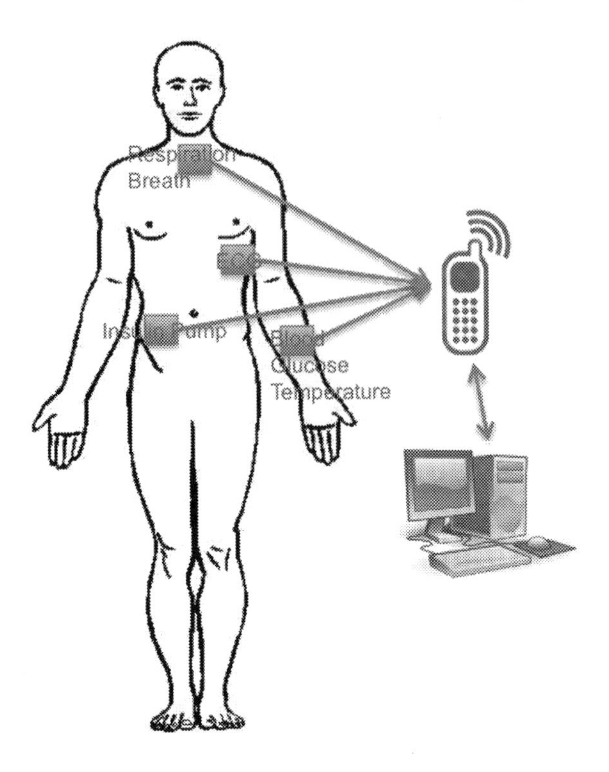

Fig. 1 As a case study of the body area network, data streams collected from various sensors are pushed to a mobile device and backend data center for real-time medical treatment

Data sampled within a wearable computing can usually go up to GB per minutes. With a high sample rate, more accurate data can therefore be used, and the diagnosis can be more in real time, and the alert can be better in use. Therefore, it is strongly needed that the data center can support thousands of users' real-time data access, as well as computing across multiple dimensions of syndromes and features to be collected.

4 Task-Level Adaptive MapReduce Framework

In this section, we brief an overview of the Hadoop MapReduce framework as a start. Thereafter, the task-level provisioning framework is introduced in the subsequent text.

4.1 Preliminary of Hadoop MapReduce Framework

The standard Hadoop MapReduce framework is depicted in Fig. 2. There are *4* parallel Map tasks and *3* parallel Reduce tasks, respectively. Because the total

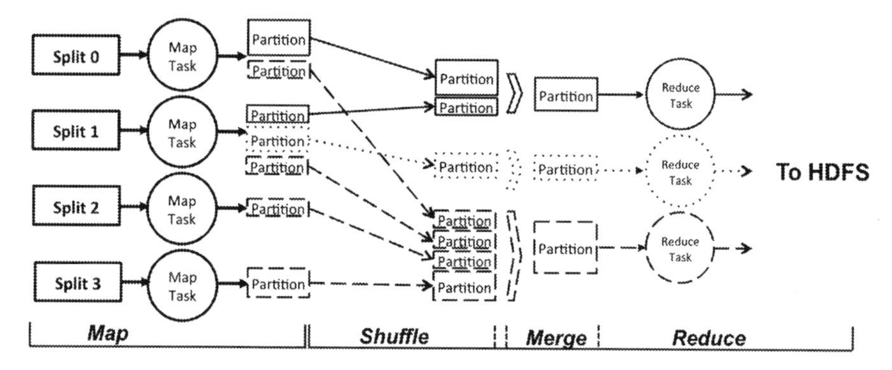

Fig. 2 A MapReduce framework splits the input file into 4 segments, and each segment corresponds to one Map task. Map Tasks output data partitions, which are further shuffled to the corresponding Reduce tasks. There are *3* reduce tasks which generate *3* separate outputs

number of the Map tasks normally equals to the number of the input data splits, there are four data splits as well. Each Map task performs a user-defined Map function on the input data that resides in the HDFS and generates the intermediate key-value pair data. These intermediate data are organized on the *partition* basis. Each of the partition consists of certain key-value data pairs, whose keys can be classified into one group. The simplest classification method is a hash function. Within such a hash capability, data partition belonging to the same group are shuffled across all the compute nodes and merged together locally. There are three data partitions shown in the figure. These merged data partitions, as indicated by three different framed rectangular boxes, are consumed by three Reduce tasks separately. The output data generated by all the Reduce tasks are written back to the HDFS.

Each Map task resides in a Map slot of a compute node. Usually Two Map slots reside in one compute node. The slot number per node can be adjusted in the configuration file. The total number of the Map slots determines the degree of parallelism that indicates the total number of Map tasks that can be concurrently launched. The rational for the Reduce task and Reduce slot is the same. The whole Hadoop MapReduce workflow is controlled in a JobTracker located in the main computer node, or what is called the NameNode. The Map and Reduce tasks are launched at the TaskNodes, with each task corresponding to one TaskTracker to communicate with the JobTracker. The communication includes heart-beat message to report the progress and status of the current task. If detecting a task failure or task straggler, the JobTracker will reschedule the TaskTracker on another Task slot.

As we can see from Fig. 2 above, the Hadoop MapReduce is essentially a scheduling framework that processes data that can be sliced into different splits. Each Map task is isolated to process its input data split and no inter-Map communication is needed. The Hadoop MapReduce framework can only be applied to process input data that already exist. However, real-life big-data applications typically require the input data be provisioned in streaming and be processed in real-time. Therefore, an enhanced MapReduce framework is required to cater for such a need. That is the motivation behind out design of the task-level adaptive MapReduce framework.

4.2 Task-Level Adaptive MapReduce Framework

An adaptive MapReduce framework is proposed to process the streaming data in real-time. One of the most significant challenges here is how to process the streaming data with varied arrival rate. Real-life applications entail workloads of a variety of many patterns. Some of the workloads show a typical pattern of periodical and unpredictable spikes, while others are more stable and predictable. There are four technical issues that we should consider when designing the adaptive framework.

First, the framework should be both horizontally and vertically scalable to process a mixture of such varied workloads. In other words, the scheduling system should either be able to manage compute node count, but also types. For some Hadoop MapReduce applications, merely managing the number of compute nodes is not necessarily sufficient. Certain kinds of workloads require large CPU-core instances while others need large-memory instances. In a nutshell, scaling in a heterogonous system is one of the primary principles.

Second, the number of the active Map and Reduce tasks should be in accordance with the cluster size. Even though the Map and Reduce count determines the overall performance of the whole system, it still doesn't perform that desirable if the cluster is either over provisioned or under provisioned.

Third, scaling the Reduce tasks is very tedious. This is determined by the design of the Reduce phase. If the number of the Reduce task increases, the hash function that maps a particular Map output partition data to a Reduce function will change. Take modular operation as a hash function as an example. Increasing the Reduce count from r to r' leads to *key mod r* to *key mod r'* as the corresponding new hash function. A reorganization of the Reduce output will be added to the Reduce phase when the number of the Reduce task has changed.

Fourth, we also need to consider the heterogeneity of the processing capabilities of different Map tasks. Some of the Map tasks may be scheduled on a slow node while others are on much faster nodes. An appropriate load balancing mechanism can further improve the rescheduling philosophy implemented in the traditional Hadoop MapReduce. The purpose is to coordinate the progress of the entire task without leading to skew task execution time.

Fifth, the optimal runtime of Map and Reduce task count should be specified. Traditionally, the initial Map task number depends on the input dataset size and the HDFS block size. The Reduce task count is determined by the hash function. The new framework requires a redesign of the Map and Reduce Task scheduling policy by considering the input data arrival rate instead of their sizes instead.

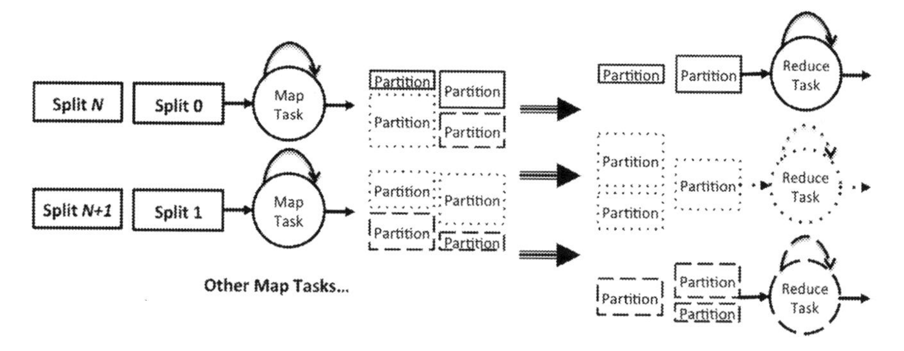

Fig. 3 A demonstration of task-level adaptive MapReduce framework which processes streaming data. Each Map and Reduce task has a non-stop running daemon function which continuously processes the input data

To satisfy all the purposes above, we demonstrate a task-level adaptive MapReduce framework in Fig. 3. Two Map tasks are used as representatives of the Map stage. Each Map task, different from the Map task of the traditional Hadoop MapReduce, defines a loop function as shown in the loop-back arrow. The two Map tasks are launched as special runtime daemons to repeatedly process the streaming data. Each of the Map task produces two continual batches of output data partitions. Similarly, the Reduce tasks are also scheduled in such a loop-like daemon that continuously processes their corresponding intermediate data produced by all the Map tasks.

In this new task-level adaptive MapReduce framework, the JobTrackers need to be redesigned to maintain a pool of TaskTrackers, and the TaskTracker count may change as the workload changes.

There are two ways to feed data streams into the Map tasks. A proactive strategy caches streaming data locally first and pushes them every fixing period of time, say 1 min. As an alternative option, data splits can also be pushed in a reactive way. In other words, a cache size is defined in HDFS before the input data starts to move in, whenever the cache usage hits a ratio, say 85%, the data splits begin to be pushed to the Map tasks.

4.3 Adaptive Input Data Split Feeding

The adaptive MapReduce framework starts from a novel runtime scheduler that feeds different Map tasks with different number of data splits. In Fig. 4a, we show a study case of the adaptive input data split feeding. As a start, six splits of input data arrive. The scheduler, without knowing the processing capability of each Map task, distributes the data splits evenly to the two Map tasks, which results to each Map task having three data splits. Suppose the first Map task is executed on a faster

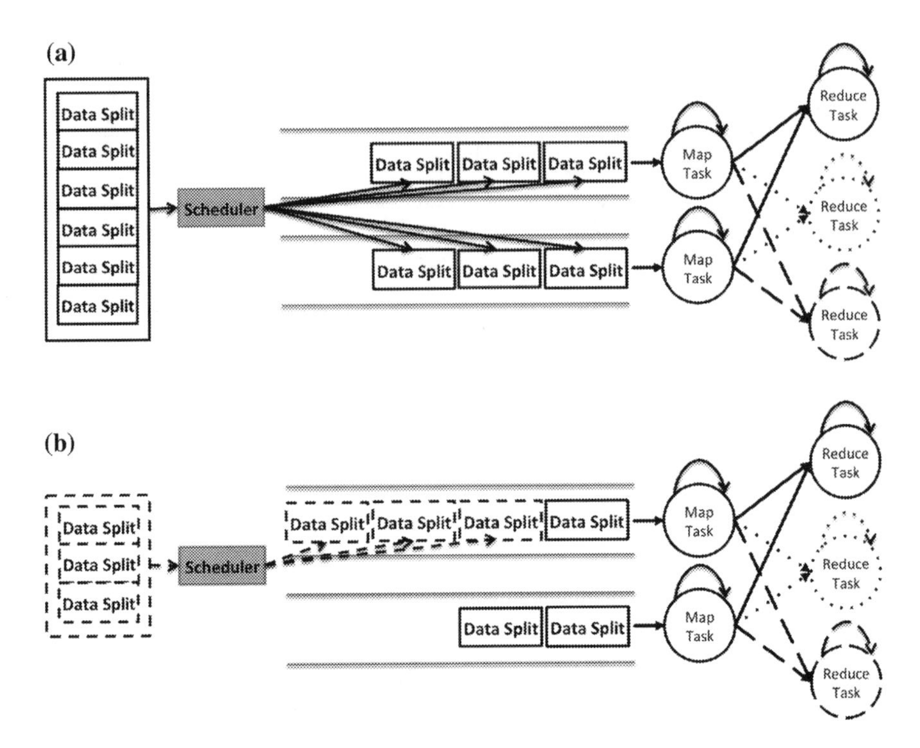

Fig. 4 A demonstration of the adaptive input data split feeding. **a** Initially six data splits arrive. Without knowing the compute capacity of each Map task, scheduler divides the workload evenly between the two queues, each one having three data splits. **b** After being aware of the processing capacity of each Map task, the scheduler sends three data splits to Map task one which shows twice the processing capacity at the consecutive scheduling period

compute node and has processed two splits of the input data while the second Map task has processed only one. Being aware of such a skewed processing capability, the scheduler sends the newly arrival three data splits adaptively to balance the workload in Fig. 4b. This leads to Map task one has four data splits while Map task two has two, and the total execution time of the Map stage is minimized.

In this case, processing the three newly arrival data splits doesn't result in an increase of Map task count, but trigger the scheduler to dispatch them fairly to all the Map tasks. Scheduler caches the input data locally in HDFS and regularly sends them to different Map tasks. The time interval is also adaptively determined by the arrival rate of the data splits.

To refresh readers' memory and ease difficulty in understanding all the mathematics below, we plot table one below, which summarizes all the symbols and explain their meanings (Table 1).

Suppose there are m Map tasks and the task queue length of each Map task be Q. In the Fig. 4, we set m equal to 2 while Q equal to 4. Suppose as a start the input data has n_0 data splits. As long as n_0 be less than $m * Q$, each Map task gets approximately n_0/m data splits (Fig. 5).

Table 1 Symbols, notations and abbreviations with brief introduction

Notation	Brief definitions with representative units or probabilities
m	The total number of available Map tasks
Q	The total number of data splits that can be accommodated in each Map task
n_0	The total number of data splits arrives at the start time
t	The scheduling period, denoting the data feeding frequency from the scheduler to all Map tasks
dMapTaskN(j)	The number of data splits that remained in the queue of Map task j at time t_i
dMapTaskN'(j)	The number of data splits that remained in the queue of Map task j at time t_{i+1}
eMapTaskC(j)	The estimated data processing capacity for Map task j
addedDataSplit (j)	The number of data splits that needs to be added to Map task j after new stream data arrives
TT	Estimated finish time of all the Map tasks
α	Upper bound percentage threshold used when Map task number above $\alpha * Q$ in a queue, Map tasks are over provisioned
β	Lower bound percentage threshold used when Map task number below $\beta * Q$ in a queue, Map tasks are under provisioned

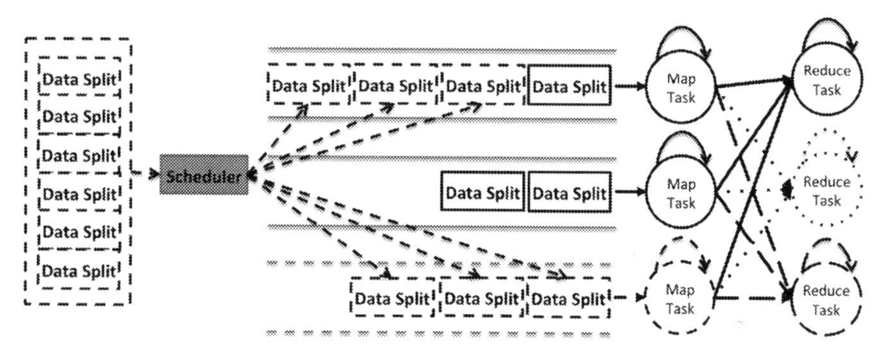

Fig. 5 Demonstrates of adding an adaptive Map task. Continued from the previous example, if the input data split count is six, the scheduler adaptively launches one Map task instead of feeding all the data splits to the queues. The other three data splits are moved to the newly added Map task

The scheduling period, namely the time interval between two data feeding periods is t. In other words, every t units (seconds or minutes) of time, scheduler feeds one batch of the cached data into the Map queues. Suppose at time t_i, the data splits count of each Map task queue equals to [*dMapTaskN(0), dMapTaskN(1), …, dMapTaskN(m − 1)*] after the newly arrived data splits have been pushed into the queues. After time t at t_{i+1}, the remaining task count becomes [*dMapTaskN'(0), dMapTaskN'(1), …, dMapTaskN'(m − 1)*]. The estimated processing capacity of each Map task is estimated as [*(dMapTaskN'(0) − dMapTaskN(0))/t, (dMapTaskN'(1) – dMapTaskN(1))/t,…, (dMapTaskN'(m − 1) – dMapTaskN(m − 1))/t*].

Suppose n_{i+1} data splits arrive at time t_{i+1}. We consider a scheduling algorithm that effectively distributes all these data splits to all the Map tasks in Theorem 1. Second, we consider in Corollary 1 that whether the Map task number should remain the same or need to change. Third, if the Map task number needs to change, we calculate the variation of the Map tasks in Theorem 2. We separate the analysis into two different sections. In this section we discuss a scenario that workload doesn't have to trigger the change of the Map tasks. In the following section, we continue to discuss scenarios that Map task number needs to change.

Theorem 1 ***Condition***: *Suppose there are m_i Map tasks being actively used at time $t + 1$. As a new stage, N_{i+1} new data splits arrive. For any Map task j, dMapTaskN (j) data splits are in its queue. Its estimated data processing capacity is eMapTaskC (j).*

Conclusion: *The new data split count to be added to its queue is represented by:*

$$\begin{aligned} addedDataSplit(j) = {} & eMapTaskC(j) \\ & * (N_{i+1} + SUM(dMapTaskN(:))) \\ & / SUM(eMapTaskC(:)) \\ & - dMapTaskN(j) \end{aligned} \tag{1}$$

SUM(dMapTaskN(:)) denotes the total number of data splits across all the queues. SUM(eMapTaskC(:)) denotes the aggregated processing capacity of all the Map tasks.

Proof The scheduling target is to make sure all the tasks of the Map queues be finished almost at the same time, and let that task time be an unknown value *TT*. For any Map task *j*, $TT = (dMapTaskN(j) + addedDataSplit(j))/eMapTaskC(j)$, $j \in [0, m_i - 1]$. Note that $\Sigma\ dMapTaskN(j) = N_{i+1}$. Solving a total of $m_i - 1$ equations leads to the proof of theorem 1. **Q.E.D**

Corollary 1 *Let Q be the queue length of each Map task, namely the total number of data splits that can be accommodated in one Map task queue. Other conditions are the same as in the Theorem 1. Then new Map tasks need to be added if $\exists\, j \in [0, m_i - 1]$, $dMapTaskN(j)) + addedDataSplit(j) > \alpha * Q$. Similarly, Map task number needs to be reduced if $\forall\, j \in [0, m_i - 1]$, $dMapTaskN(:) + addedDataSplit(j) < \beta * Q$. Symbol $\alpha \in [0, 1]$ is a preset threshold to determine how full the Map task queues are allowed. Similarly, $\beta \in [0, 1]$ is preset to determine how empty the Map task queues are allowed.*

Proof If $\exists\, j \in [0, m_i-1]$, $dMapTaskN(j)) + addedDataSplit(j) > \alpha * Q$, this means the Map task number of one Map task queue will be above threshold if the new data splits were added. It automatically triggers a Map task increase request to the scheduler. Similarly, if $\forall\, j \in [0, m_i-1]$, $dMapTaskN(j) + addedDataSplit(j) < \beta * Q$ holds, this indicates the Map task count of each Map queue is less than a preset value, which means sufficient resources have been provided. A request is therefore sent out to reduce the Map task count. **Q.E.D**

In a nutshell, the purpose of designing such an adaptive scheduler is to leverage the processing capability of all the Map tasks and balance the start time of all the Reduce tasks.

4.4 Adaptive Map Task Provisioning

In the previous section, we focus on discussing the Map task provisioning mechanism that determines the time Map task needs to be updated. A natural extension along that line requires answer a provisioning mechanism—how many Map tasks need to be added or reduced in order to efficiently process the new stream data splits. If adding Map task is required, how to distribute the stream data splits across all the Map tasks, including the new ones. On the contrary, if reducing Map task is required, how to distribute the stream data splits, as well as the data splits in the queues that are supposed to remove, to all the remaining Map task queues.

Theorem 2 *Given the condition in Theorem* 1 *and* $\exists j \in [0, m_i - 1]$, *dMapTaskN(j)) + addedDataSplit(j)* $> \alpha * Q$, *the number of the new Map tasks that is needed is given below:*

$$\lfloor (N_{i+1} - aQ\ SUM(eMapTaskC(:))\ /\ eMapTaskC(j^*) + SUM(dMapTaskN(j))) * eMapTaskC(j^*)\ /\ aQ \rfloor + 1 \quad (2)$$

For the Map task j, the new data splits count added to its queue equals to the formula below when $j \in [0, m_i - 1]$.

$$aQ\ eMapTaskC(j)\ /\ eMapTaskC(j^*) - dMapTaskN(j)) \quad (3)$$

Suppose the default estimated computing capacity of each new Map task is eMapTaskC. For the new added Map task, each is allocated an initial number of data splits in their queues. The data split number is given below:

$$aQ\ eMapTaskC\ /\ eMapTaskC\left(j^*\right) \quad (4)$$

Proof Suppose Map task j^* has the maximum computing capacity across all the Map tasks: *eMapTaskC(j*) > eMapTaskC(j)* for all $j \in [0, m_i - 1]$. Then the maximum data splits count allowed to be added to its queue equals to αQ − *dMapTaskN(j*))*. Proportionally compared, the maximum data split count of the *j*th Map task queue equals to αQ *eMapTaskC(j)/eMapTaskC(j*) − dMapTaskN(j))* and Eq. (3) is proven. Therefore, aggregating all the data splits that are allocated to Map task *j* equals to αQ *SUM(eMapTaskC(:))/eMapTaskC(j*) − SUM(dMapTaskN(:))*. Since we assume that all the Map tasks can be finished within αQ*/eMapTaskC(j*)*, then given the default processing capacity of all the new Map tasks for the remaining data splits, the needed Map tasks count is calculated by dividing the remaining data split count over the expected Map task finish time and Eq. (2) is therefore proven. Equation (4) is calculated by multiplying the predicted Map task execution time with the default processing capacity of each Map task. **Q.E.D**

Theorem 3 *Given the condition in Theorem* 1 *and* $\forall j \in [0, m_i - 1]$, *dMapTaskN(j) + addedDataSplit(j)* $< \beta * Q$ *and Suppose dMapTaskN(0) > dMapTaskN(1) > … > dMapTaskN*$(m_i - 1)$, *the Map Task set {MapTask_0, MapTask_1, …, MapTask_k} needs to be removed if:* $\forall j \in [k, m_i - 1]$, *dMapTaskN(j) + addedDataSplit(j, k)* $< \beta * Q$ *and* $\exists j \in [k + 1, m_i - 1]$, *dMapTaskN(j)) + addedDataSplit(j, k + 1)* $> \alpha * Q$. *After removing the Map tasks, the remaining Map task j* ($j \in [k + 1, m_i - 1]$) *adds data split count: addedDataSplit (j, k + 1) A more general term is defined as follows.*

$$
\begin{aligned}
addedDataSplit(j, p) = {} & eMapTaskC(j) \\
& * (N_{i+1} + SUM(dMapTaskN(:))) \\
& / SUM(eMapTaskC(p{:}\, m_i - 1)) \\
& - dMapTaskN(j)
\end{aligned} \tag{5}
$$

Proof A descending order of the remaining data splits leads to removing the Map task starting from the slowest one. The slower one Map task is, the slower that Map queue tasks to finish. We start to remove *MapTask_0* and add its queued data splits to N_{i+1}. Reallocating the total N_{i+1} + *dMapTaskN(0)* data splits to the remaining $m_i - 1$ Map tasks. If the data split count of each these remaining Map task still lower than $\beta * Q$, the procedure moves on. This procedure stops until when at least there is one Map task has its queued data split count larger than $\alpha * Q$. **Q.E.D**

4.5 Adaptive Reduce Task Provisioning

Adaptive provisioning of the Reduce tasks is far less straightforward than provisioning the Map tasks. Since Hadoop MapReduce is a framework primarily designed to scale the Map stage by involving embarrassingly parallel Map tasks, the Reduce tasks require network resource and an *m* to *r* data shuffling stage. In Fig. 6, we identify a scaling scenario of adding a new Reduce task to the original three tasks. The new added Reduce task should have no impact on saving the network usage since all the intermediate data still have to be moved among all the compute nodes. The only difference is the degree of parallelism in the Reduce stage, that each Reduce task can process less data partitions as well as move less output data back to HDFS.

As aforementioned, the Map tasks can be added incrementally one by one. However, this doesn't necessarily guarantee the best scheduling performance if

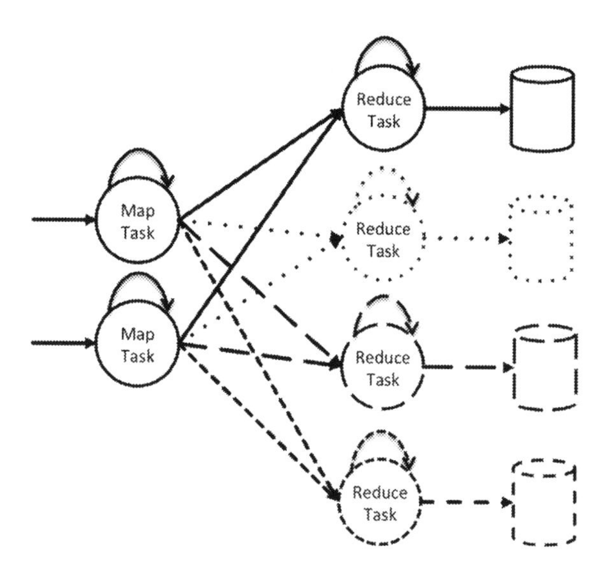

Fig. 6 A graphical illustration shows one parallel Reduce task being added. This added Reduce task brings no benefit in the data shuffling stage but results to a reduced data volume to be processed/outputted for each Reduce task

Reduce tasks were to be added in the same way. This is because there is no strict demand that one input data split should go to a particular Map task. The Reduce tasks, however, only accepts their partition data in need. Adding one Reduce task would inevitable change the hash function, which accordingly leads to the data partition changed, and mess the shuffling process.

Take an example here. Suppose the key set of the dataset is an nine-number set [0, 1, 2, …, 8]. There are three Reduce tasks R1, R2 and R3 as shown in Fig. 6. The hash function is a simple modular operation, e.g. key mod 3. Therefore, R1 gets partition data whose keys are [0, 3, 6]; R2 gets partition data whose keys are [1, 4, 7]; R3 gets partition data whose keys are [2, 5, 8]. Adding one Reduce task leads to the partition be [0, 4, 8] for R1, [1, 5] for R2, [2, 6] for R3 and [3, 7] for R4. In all, there are six keys that are either moved to R4 or being exchanged among inside R1, R2, and R3. Similar conclusion applies to the case that five Reduce tasks are used. However, if the Reduce task number doubled to 6, then [0, 6] will be for R1; [1, 7], [2, 8], [3], [4], [5] are keys for R2 to R6 respectively. Then there are data associated with only three keys, [3, 4] and [5], that needs to moved.

In such a case, a workaround would be replacing the hash function with an enumerated list of the keys as a lookup table. For each intermediate key-value pair needs to be shuffled, the corresponding Reduce task number is searched through the list. For example, the list can be like this [R1, 0, 1, 2], [R2, 3, 4, 5], [R3, 6, 7, 8]. If a new Reduce task R4 is added, we can simply create a new entry as [R4, 2, 8], and remove the keys [2] and [8] from their corresponding list.

The downside of the workaround approach can be easily identified. The search operation might involve I/O data accessing, which is far less efficient than calculating the hash function. We can put the mapping list in memory instead if the total number of the keys is not very large.

5 Experimental Studies

In this section, we first propose two methods for stream data workload prediction. After that, we show our experimental results of the prediction performance of the methods and the makespan of using these methods. Last, we report our task-level adaptive experimental results in terms of the Map and Reduce count in runtime when workload changes.

5.1 *Workload Prediction Methods*

For stream data applications, adaptive MapReduce task provisioning strategy should align with the workload variation. However, workloads are normally unknown in advance. In this section, we investigate two widely used prediction methods first and compare them prediction performance using real workload in the next section.

Stochastic control, or learning-based control method, is a dynamic control strategy to predict workload characteristics. There are numerous filters that can be applied. For example, smooth filter, or what we normally call as smoothing technique, predicts real-time workload by averaging the workload of a previous time span. The basic assumption here is that workload behaves reactively and not subject to significant variation in a short period of time. The average of the past one period would best represents the future workload.

There are many further improvements on the smoothing technique. For example, weighted smoothing gives higher weights to more recent workload than those that are old. The assumption here is that more recent workload would show higher impact on the real-time workload than older ones. Other prediction methods include AR method, which applies polynomial functions to approximate the workload. Among others, we want to bring forward the Kalman filter [25], also named as linear quadratic estimation, which is also widely used in workload prediction. Kalman filter works on a series of historical data stream of noise, updates and predicts future trend with statistically optimal estimations.

5.2 *Experimental Settings*

We use SimEvent [26] to simulate the experiments. This is a toolkit component included in Matlab. Each map/reduce task is simulated as a queue. During the runtime, the Map and Reduce tasks serve workload at different capacity, therefore the proposed task-level scheduling framework fits into such a need.

Both the Kalman Filter and the Smooth Filter are used to predict the workload. Two metrics, workload prediction accuracy and makespan, are both used for the three methods. The workloads we use were primary produced from real body area network data trace [27, 28]. The workload fluctuation amplitude, on the other hand, applies the web data trace from the 1998 Soccer World Cup site [29]. This workload trace has the average arrival rate data on each single minute over a 60-min duration as shown in Fig. 7a, d and g. We carefully choose three typical and varied stream data workload types: small, intermediate and strong, for the purpose of simulation. Small workload typically generates 20–60 data splits per minute. Intermediate workload generates 30–150 data splits per minute while strong workload generates 160–1180 data splits per minute.

5.3 Experimental Results

In Fig. 7b, e and h, the Kalman filter shows no more than to 19.97% prediction error compared to 50% of that when using the Smooth filter method in the light workload

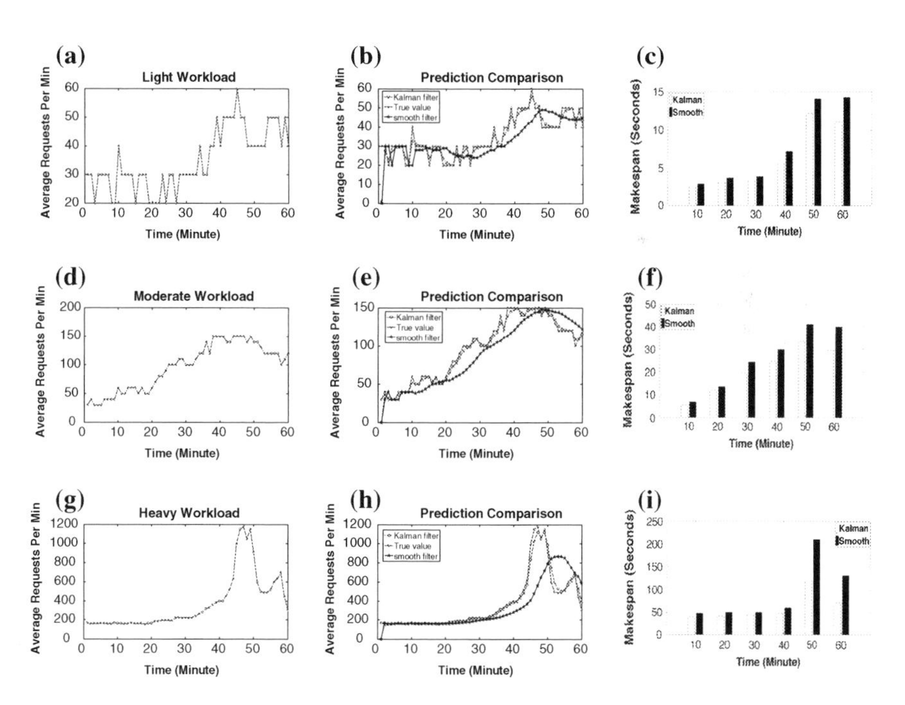

Fig. 7 Comparison under three types of workloads. Figure **a**, **d** and **g** are light, moderate and heavy workload respectively; Figure **b**, **e** and **h** demonstrate the workload prediction accuracy of the two method: Smooth filter and Kalman filter; Figure **c**, **f** and **i** report the makespan of using the two prediction methods. Kalman filter based workload prediction performs better than the Smooth filter based prediction method

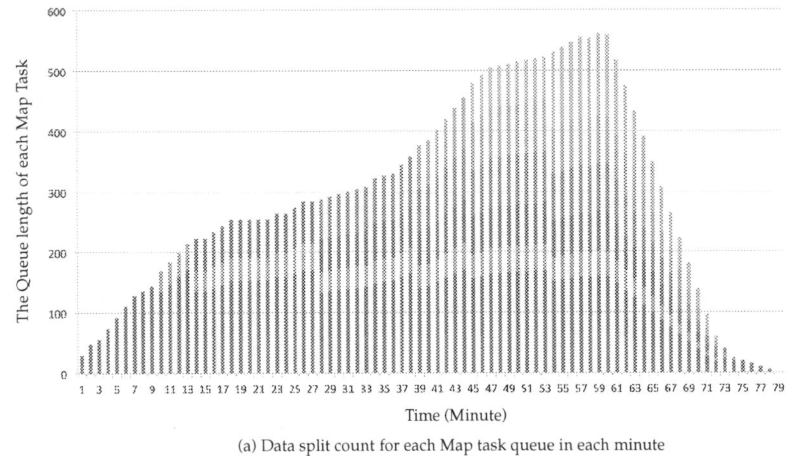

(a) Data split count for each Map task queue in each minute

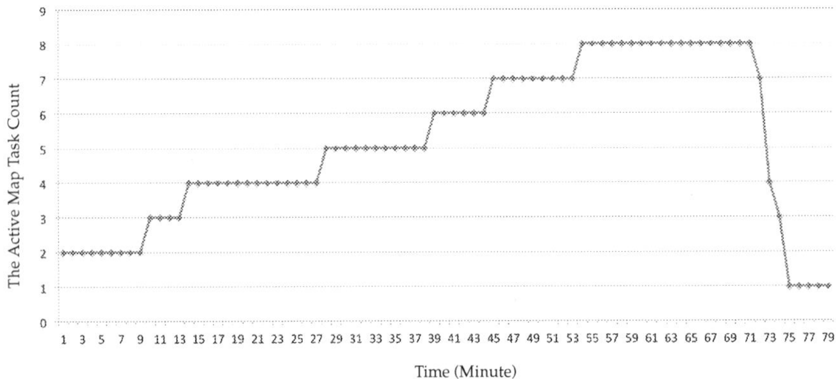

(b) Map task count in each minute

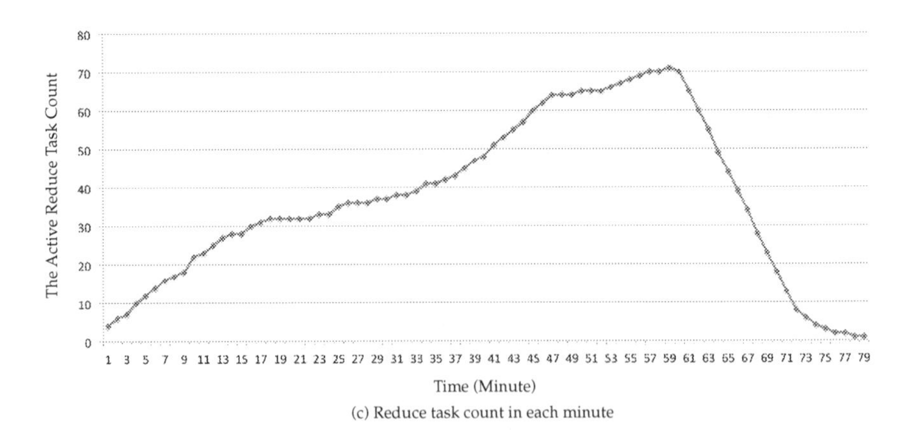

(c) Reduce task count in each minute

Fig. 8 Demonstration of the Map task queue, Map task number and Reduce task number in each minute of the light workload case. The Map and Reduce count adaptively follow the workload trend firmly

case. Under the intermediate workload, the prediction errors of these two filters are constrained to 14.1% and 35% respectively. For the strong workload scenario, these values turned to 27.2% and 90.3% for the two methods. Comparing the prediction error of the two methods across all the workload cases, the maximum margin is the strong workload case, which is typically 63.1% less by using the Kalman filter method.

From Figure 7c, f and i, we can see that under the three types of workloads, the Kalman based workload prediction based method outperforms the smooth filter based method over up to 28, 34 and 85%. All these results indicate that a good prediction method only gives a satisfactory estimation of the workload trend, but also improves the scheduling performance.

In Fig. 8, we demonstrate the scheduling effect of the proposed framework. Figure 8a illustrates the data split count of each Map task queue every minute. Figure 8b demonstrates the Map task count that are actively running. Theorems 2 and 3 calculate these Map task count. The count of each Reduced task every minute is reported in Fig. 8c. The Reduce task counts are calculated by the total data partition for all the Reduce tasks over the processing capacity.

We can see that as the workload increases, the Map task count also increases accordingly. As a result, each Map task has more data splits waiting in its queue, and so do the Reduce tasks. In Fig. 8a, the rising trend becomes less significant when hitting the 61th minute since no more follow-up stream data splits arrived. However, it is not until the 71th minute when the Map task number starts to noticeably reduce as reported in Fig. 8b. The reason is that the data splits in each Map task is accumulating in the previous 61 min. Until the 71th minute the data splits of each Map task queue are sufficiently short and the Theorem 3 starts to reduce the total Map tasks.

6 Conclusions and Future Work

We proposed a task-level adaptive MapReduce framework in this chapter. We conclude three major aspects of contribution, and then illustrate the future work that should extend the work.

6.1 Conclusions

A significant amount of scientific applications require effective processing of streaming data. However, there's a gap between the state-of-art big data processing frameworks Hadoop MapReduce for such a need. Since Hadoop MapReduce has gained its dominance in big-data processing domain for years, even though we have seen many existing streaming data processing toolkits, such as Storm, Spark Streaming, we still believe that, it would benefit the whole MapReduce community if the framework could be adapted for the need of processing the streaming data, without having to move to a new framework. Therefore we propose such an adaptive Hadoop MapReduce framework, which is built on top of MapReduce, but could also be easily implemented in a virtualized cloud platform. We conclude the contribution of this work in the following three aspects.

(1) **Proposed a task-level adaptive MapReduce framework**. Traditional Hadoop MapReduce fixes the number of the Map and Reduce tasks. In this new framework, we suggest a framework that removes such a constraint, which allows the Map and Reduce task number to be adaptive given the runtime workload. Users don't have to change their programming habit in traditional MapReduce, and this framework allows such a transition from processing fixed dataset to streaming data seamlessly.
(2) **Runtime Map and Reduce task estimation**. The workload, as well as the queuing length of each task determines the runtime Map/Reduce task count. We have created a full-fledged mathematical model to estimate the real time task number, in order to optimize the streaming data processing rate, as well as keeping the cost of using compute resource at an acceptable level.
(3) **Adaptive task simulator**: With a simulator being used not only as a workload prediction toolkit, but also mathematically calculates the active number of Map/Reduce tasks in real time as the workload changes. This simulator implements the mathematically model we propose in this chapter, and estimates the workload in a way we proposed in the subsequent sections.

6.2 Future Work

We suggest extending this work in the following two directions:

(1) **Coherent scaling of Map/Reduce tasks and compute resources.** Scaling Map or Reduce task only is mainly investigated in this chapter. However, the scaling needs to be multi-tier, meaning the number of compute nodes also needs to align with the existing number of Map or Reduce tasks. It would be significantly useful if the framework supports the coherent scaling of compute resources, as well as the Map and Reduce tasks, from both theoretical aspect and implementation.
(2) **Continue the framework in large-scale heterogeneous cloud systems.** In a large cloud platform, the framework can be way complicated than our experimental scale. Lots of runtime issues, such as resource contention, virtual resource scaling cost etc., would happen during the course of scaling. This will bring other concerning issues that go beyond the description of the mathematical framework we propose above.
(3) **Release the simulation toolkit**. The simulation toolkit should be packaged into a software library in Hadoop MapReduce online in order to make sure the

service be available for such adaptive MapReduce applications online. For larger-size virtualized cloud platform, it can be deployed online and expose its API for public use. Furthermore, we plan to implement the adaptive scaling framework in Spark, in order to see the effectiveness within in-memory computing.

Acknowledgements This work was supported in part by the National Nature Science Foundation of China under grant No. 61233016, by the Ministry of Science and Technology of China under National 973 Basic Research Grants No. 2011CB302505, No. 2013CB228206, Guangdong Innovation Team Grant 201001D0104726115 and National Science Foundation under grant CCF-1016966. The work was also partially supported by an IBM Fellowship for Fan Zhang, and by the Intellectual Ventures endowment to Tsinghua University.

References

1. S. Ullah, H. Higgins, B. Braem, et al. A Comprehensive Survey of Wireless Body Area Networks. Journal of Medical Systems 36(3)(2010) 1065–1094.
2. M. Chen, S. Gonzalez, A. Vasilakos, et al. Body Area Networks: A Survey. ACM/Springer Mobile Networks and Applications. 16(2)(2011) 171–193.
3. R. Schmidt, T. Norgall, J. Mörsdorf, et al. Body Area Network BAN–a key infrastructure element for patient-centered medical applications. Biomed Tech 47(1)(2002)365–8.
4. J. Dean and S. Ghemawat, Mapreduce: Simplified Data Processing On Large Clusters, in: Proc. of 19th ACM symp. on Operating Systems Principles, OSDI 2004, pp. 137–150.
5. G. Malewicz, M. H. Austern, A. J. C. Bik, et al. Pregel: A System for Large-Scale Graph Processing, in: Proc. of the 2008 ACM SIGMOD international conference on Management of data, SIGMOD 2010, pp. 135–146.
6. Y. Low, J. Gonzalez, A. Kyrola, et al, GraphLab: A New Framework for Parallel Machine Learning, in: Proc. of the 26th Conference on Uncertainty in Artificial Intelligence, UAI 2010.
7. Y. Low, J. Gonzalez, A. Kyrola, et al, Distributed GraphLab: A Framework for Machine Learning and Data Mining in the Cloud, Journal Proceedings of the VLDB Endowment, 5(8) (2012), pp. 716–727.
8. http://aws.amazon.com/elasticmapreduce/.
9. F. Zhang, M. F. Sakr, Cluster-size Scaling and MapReduce Execution Times, in: Proc. of The International Conference on Cloud Computing and Science, CloudCom 2013.
10. R. Haux, Health information systems–past, present, future, International Journal of Medical Informatics, 75(3–4)(2006), pp. 268–281.
11. P. L. Reichertz, Hospital information systems—Past, present, future, International Journal of Medical Informatics, 75(3–4)(2006), pp. 282–299.
12. http://hadoop.apache.org/.
13. J. Talbot, R. M. Yoo and C. Kozyrakis, Phoenix++: modular MapReduce for shared-memory systems, in: Proc. of the second international workshop on MapReduce and its applications, MapReduce 2011, pp. 9–16.
14. O. Christopher, C. Greg and C. Laukik, et al, Nova: Continuous Pig/Hadoop Workfows, in: Proc. of the 2011 ACM SIGMOD international conference on Management of data, SIGMOD 2011, pp. 1081–1090.
15. C. Olston, B. Reed, U. Srivastava, et al, Pig latin: a not-so-foreign language for data processing, in: Proc. of the 2008 ACM SIGMOD international conference on Management of data, SIGMOD 2008, pp. 1099–1110.

16. P. Bhatotia, A. Wieder and R. Rodrigues, et al, Incoop: MapReduce for incremental computations, in: Proc. of the 2nd ACM Symposium on Cloud Computing, SoCC 2011.
17. L. Neumeyer, B. Robbins and A. Nair, et al, S4: Distributed Stream Computing Platform, in: Proc. of the International Workshop on Knowledge Discovery Using Cloud and Distributed Computing Platforms, KDCloud 10, pp. 170–177.
18. http://storm.incubator.apache.org/.
19. http://www.scribesoft.com/.
20. J. Kreps, N. Narkhede, J. Rao et al. Kafka: A Distributed Messaging System for Log Processing. in: Proc. of 6th International Workshop on Networking Meets Databases NetDB 2011.
21. http://flume.apache.org/index.html.
22. http://www.streambase.com/.
23. http://www.hstreaming.com/.
24. http://esper.codehaus.org/.
25. R. E. Kalman, A new approach to linear filtering and prediction problems, Journal of Basic Engineering 82(1)(1960), pp. 35–45.
26. http://www.mathworks.com/products/simevents/.
27. C. Otto, A. Milenković, C. Sanders and E. Jovanov, System architecture of a wireless body area sensor network for ubiquitous health monitoring, 1(4)(2005), pp. 307–326.
28. E. Jovanov, A. Milenkovic, C. Otto1 and P. C de Groen, A wireless body area network of intelligent motion sensors for computer assisted physical rehabilitation, Journal of NeuroEngineering and Rehabilitation, 2(6)(2005), pp. 1–10.
29. M. Arlitt, T. Jin, Workload characterization of the 1998 World Cup Web Site (Tech. Rep. No. HPL-1999-35R1). Palo Alto, CA: HP Labs.

High-Performance Monte Carlo Simulations for Photon Migration and Applications in Optical Brain Functional Imaging

Fanny Nina-Paravecino, Leiming Yu, Qianqian Fang and David Kaeli

The human brain is unarguably one of the most complex biological organs known to-date. After decades of study, our knowledge on how our brains work remains very limited. Non-invasive optical brain imaging using non-ionizing near-infrared light has attracted worldwide research attention over the past decades, and has shown increasing utility in exploring brain functions and diagnosing brain diseases. However, due to the complex nature of the human brain anatomy, especially the presence of low-scattering cerebrospinal fluid (CSF), quantitative analysis of optical brain imaging data has been challenging due to the extensive computation needed to solve the generalized models. Drastic simplifications of complex brain anatomy using layered slabs or spheres have been widely used by the research community. However, these simplified models are believed to lead to inaccurate quantification of brain physiology. Here we discuss a computationally efficient and numerically accurate Monte Carlo photon simulation package—Monte Carlo eXtreme (MCX) —by incorporating GPU-based parallel computing. MCX allows researchers to use 3D anatomical scans from MRI or CT to perform accurate photon transport simulations. Compared to conventional Monte Carlo (MC) methods, MCX provides a dramatic speed improvement of two to three orders of magnitude, thanks largely to the massively parallel threads enabled by modern GPU architectures.

F. Nina-Paravecino · L. Yu · D. Kaeli (✉)
Department of Electrical and Computer Engineering, Northeastern University, Boston, USA
e-mail: kaeli@ece.neu.edu

F. Nina-Paravecino
e-mail: fninaparavecino@ece.neu.edu

L. Yu
e-mail: ylm@ece.neu.edu

Q. Fang
Department of Bioengineering, Northeastern University, Boston, USA
e-mail: q.fang@neu.edu

© Springer International Publishing AG 2017

S.U. Khan et al. (eds.), *Handbook of Large-Scale Distributed Computing in Smart Healthcare*, Scalable Computing and Communications,
DOI 10.1007/978-3-319-58280-1_4

In this chapter, we provide a brief introduction to optical brain imaging techniques, their challenges, and our parallel MC simulation framework. We focus on a number of optimization techniques we have explored to improve computational efficiency, leveraging knowledge of new features offered in new generations of GPU architectures. The current and potential applications of this technique in biomedical imaging are discussed.

1 Introduction

Human brain functions have been conventionally studied using functional MRI (fMRI), electroencephalogram (EEG), or magnetoencephalography (MEG), among others [5]. In recent years, a new method that uses non-ionizing near-infrared light, functional near-infrared spectroscopy (fNIRS) [14, 27], has attracted significant attention from the global engineering and clinical communities. By shining only low-power near-infrared light and measuring the absorbed and scattered light in brain tissue, scientists are able to recover the transient dynamics of oxy-/deoxy-hemoglobins and blood oxygen level. Such measurements were found correlated with various neurological disorders (Alzheimer's disease, Parkinson's disease, epilepsy, stroke, etc.).

Compared to fMRI, the fNIRS technique has become a more accessible neuroimaging modality that offers non-invasive, safe, and relatively low-cost means for indirect and direct monitoring of brain activities. fNIRS also offers insights into the etiology and treatment of various brain disorders, and is well positioned to complement fMRI, EEG and MEG. However, as an emerging technology, fNIRS is still limited in several ways. These limitations include low spatial resolution in optical images, diminished sensitivity to deep brain structures, and challenges in removing the physiological noise coupled from the extra-cerebral tissue layers.

Furthermore, fNIRS is a model-based imaging modality. That means the output in fNIRS requires quantitatively solving a mathematical model that governs the photon-tissue interactions in the brain. Unlike most other parts of the human body where scattering effects are significantly greater than the absorption; human brains are surrounded by a layer of low-scattering liquid called the cerebrospinal fluid (CSF). Photons traveling inside the CSF experience much lower scattering than in other layers of the brain—scalp, skull, gray and white matter tissues. Because of the presence of CSF, modeling photon transport inside human brains requires solving the radiative transport equation, or RTE—an integro-differential equation that is defined in a 6-dimensional space ($x/y/z$ in space, two angular dimensions and one temporal dimension). The widely used diffusion approximation (DA) to the RTE is unfortunately unsuitable in the CSF and was shown to generate erroneous solutions when modeling the brain.

Several approaches have been studied to solve the RTE more efficiently in order to handle general media such as the CSF in the brain. Deterministic algorithms based on the variational principal, such as the finite volume (FV) method, were proposed. However, the requirement of discretizing a high dimensional space results in high memory demands and low computational speed. A multi-grid approach was proposed [10] to accelerate the solution process. However, the high dimensionality of the data prevents it from performing time-resolved MC simulations.

On the other hand, one can use the Monte Carlo (MC) method—a stochastic approach by random sampling—to solve the RTE. In an MC-based photon transport simulation, a large number of "photon packets" are simulated by treating each photon packet as a "particle" and traversing it through the media using a random walk. As the photon packet travels through the tissue structures, photon energy losses are recorded along its trajectory, the summation of which eventually forms a photon fluence distribution map. Because the MC approach directly solves the RTE, it has been widely accepted as the gold standard for modeling light transport inside arbitrarily complex media because of its accuracy and generality. However, similar to the variational RTE solvers, MC photon transport simulation suffers from low computational efficiency; a traditional MC light transport simulator takes hours or even days to solve a moderate-sized problem [2]. Nonetheless, MC has gained great popularity in the biophotonics community, primarily because of the simplicity of the method and straightforward implementation.

A major advantage of the MC RTE solver, as compared to a variational RTE solver, is the ease of parallel programming. This is because the simulation of each photon packet is nearly independent of the simulation of any other packet. In other words, the MC photon transport simulation can be categorized as an "embarrassingly parallel" problem. Over the past decade, there have been a number of efforts devoted to developing efficient parallel MC RTE solvers.

Shortly after a proof-of-concept study published by Alerstam et al. in 2008 [1], Fang and Boas reported the first GPU accelerated general-purpose MC photon transport simulation algorithm and the associated software package in 2009 [9]. They achieved a more than 300-fold speedup using an early generation GPU processor (NVIDIA 8800GT). An open source cross-platform software package based on this research—Monte Carlo eXtreme (MCX)—has been developed and disseminated to the research community. MCX is capable of simulating arbitrarily complex 3D tissue structures by using a rasterized 3D domain. The user can initialize a simulation using an anatomical image derived from an MRI or CT scan.

Over the past 7 years, this work has generated over 320 citations, and more than 9,000 downloads across the world. The diverse applications of MCX range from the investigation of multi-modal neuroimaging to pre-clinical studies using small animal models, from breast imaging to fundamental particle physics research, from developing innovative photoacoustic instrumentation to prototyping portable devices for blood glucose monitoring. A large number of the published papers using MCX focus on optical brain functional imaging applications, due primarily to the suitability and accuracy of this approach. MCX not only benefits researchers in the biophotonics community, but also provides valuable insights when designing modern general-purpose GPU architectures [7, 32].

The accelerated development of new GPU architectures presents both opportunities and challenges to the further development of the MCX simulation platform. On one hand, the computational throughput of new generations of GPUs has been improved at a consistently faster pace than the CPU hardware. This means that, even we do not modify our GPU simulation code, MCX will execute faster on the newer GPU hardware. On the other hand, new GPU architectures are packaged with new and more complex hardware features—additional compute units, larger high-speed memory, and new thread/block scheduling mechanisms. In order to fully utilize the new features available in the latest GPU hardware, we need to continually adapt of our MCX implementation. These improvements will enable researchers to better understand brain functions and diagnose diseases by providing more accurate and high-resolution optical images.

In this chapter, we provide an introduction to our GPU-accelerated Monte Carlo photon transport simulation platform, summarizing the range of optimization techniques we have explored. By leveraging new features introduced in each generation of GPU architecture, we can further improve the throughput of our photon-modeling framework. MCX is able to model photon transport, working at a reasonable resolution, in just a few seconds. This suggests that MC basedphoton migration can be used for other applications beyond forward modeling, such as tomographic imaging data analysis and fNIRS image reconstruction, where tens to hundreds of optical sources and detectors are used.

The remainder of this chapter is organized as follows. Section 2 presents background on GPU architecture. In Sect. 3, we describe our MCX simulation framework for 3D turbid media, and related techniques that we have developed to better leverage the computing resources present on the modern parallel architectures (e.g., NVIDIA and AMD GPUs). Section 4 focuses on specific applications, including sensitivity of the cerebral cortex, validation of the anatomical brain atlas, and brain cancer. Section 5 covers final evaluation and discusses future directions.

2 Background

As we enter the era of GPU computing, demanding applications with substantial parallelism can leverage the massive parallelism of GPUs to achieve superior performance and efficiency. Today, GPU computing has enabled applications that were previously thought to be infeasible because of long execution times. There are two well-known frameworks that allow general purpose programming in GPUs: Compute Unified Device Architecture (CUDA), and Open Compute Language (OpenCL).

The CUDA framework was introduced by NVIDIA [24], with the intention of following Single Instruction Multiple Thread (SIMT) execution model. In that sense, a kernel executes a program in a group of parallel threads; each thread-block is formed by group of threads, and a grid if formed by a group of thread-blocks. Following the SIMT execution model, all threads execute the same instructions independently. Each thread has its registers and private local memory. Each thread-block allows communication among its threads through shared memory. Thread-blocks communicate between themselves using global memory

OpenCL was introduced in 2009 by the Khronos group to execute parallel software across vendor-independent heterogeneous platforms (CPU, GPU, DSP, and FPGA) [11, 15, 18]. OpenCL provides a standard interface to run task parallel and data parallel codes. The OpenCL framework follows a similar scheme as the CUDA framework: "work-items" represent threads, "work-groups" represent thread-blocks (or blocks), and "ND-ranges" represent grid configurations.

GPUs have been rapidly evolving over the past few years. In the following section, we describe in detail some of the new features delivered on recent GPU generations from two major GPU manufacturers—NVIDIA and Advanced Micro Devices (AMD).

2.1 NVIDIA GPUs

A Stream Multiprocessor (SM) is the architectural centerpiece of an NVIDIA GPU. It can execute more than one thread-block at the same time, and is comprised of hundreds of CUDA cores. A number of resources are shared at different levels of concurrency. For instance, registers and shared memory have the highest access speed but are also scarce resources in the SM, while global memory represents the slowest memory access but provides enough space for storing large data sets. Over the past few years, we have seen a steady increase in the number of SMs and CUDA cores, supporting the evolution of the NVIDIA GPUs with the goal of providing better performance with each generation.

NVIDIA typically names each new generation of GPU microarchitecture by a code name (Fermi, Kepler, Pascal, etc.). For each architecture generation, NVIDIA also gives a code name for each specific GPU chip design, typically in the format of "G?" followed by 3 digits, where "?" denotes the first letter of the corresponding architecture's code name (for example, "F" for Fermi).

The NVIDIA Fermi (the first chip was GF110) GPU was released in 2009. Compared to its predecessors, Fermi has a larger number of CUDA cores per SM, more space for shared memory, configurable-shared memory, and Error Correcting Codes (ECC) to protect main memory and caches from bit flips. Each SM in a Fermi processor contains 32 CUDA cores, 16 load/store units, and four special function units (SFUs) [25]. The Fermi family has been used in a number of applications, promising peak single-precision floating performance of up to 1.5 TFLOPS.

In the last 4 years, three new NVIDIA GPU architectures have been released: Kepler, Maxwell and Pascal. A number of new features were introduced in each GPU generation. For instance, the Kepler GK110 processor comprises up to 15 Kepler SM units. Each SMX has 192 single-precision CUDA cores, 64 double-precision units, 32 load/store units, and 32 special function units, which can

Table 1 A comparative feature analysis between four generations of NVIDIA GPUs

GPU	GTX 590	GTX Titan	GTX 980 Ti	GTX 1080
Family	Fermi	Kepler	Maxwell	Pascal
Chip	GF110	GK110	GM200	GP104
Compute capability	2.0	3.5	5.2	6.1
SM	16	14	22	20
CUDA cores	32	192	128	128
Total cores	512	2688	2816	2560
Global Mem. (MB)	1474	6083	6083	8113
Shared Mem. (KB)	48	48	48	48
Threads/SM	1536	2048	2048	2048
Threads/block	1024	1024	1024	1024
Clock rate (GHz)	1.26	0.88	1.29	1.84
TFLOPS	1.50	4.29	6.50	9.00

execute a sine, cosine, reciprocal or square root operation in each thread per clock [20]. A Kepler GK110 processor can provide up to 4.29 TFLOPS single-precision and 1.43 TFLOPS double-precision floating-point performance.

NVIDIA's Maxwell GPU architecture provides only a few enhancements to previous GPU generations. It provides significant power efficiency [23]. The Maxwell GM200 chip consists of 22 Maxwell SMs, where each SM includes 128 CUDA cores.

NVIDIA introduced the Pascal architecture in 2016. For example, the GP104 chip comprises 7.2 billion transistors and 2,560 single-precision CUDA cores. The GP104 chip introduced the use of GDDR5x GPU memory [23], with a 256-bit memory interface, which provides 43% more memory bandwidth than NVIDIA's prior GeForce GTX 980 GPUs. The GP104 GPU consists of four Graphic Processing Clusters (GPC), 20 Pa SMs, and each SM contains 128 CUDA cores [22] (Table 1).

2.2 AMD GPUs

AMD, the second leading GPU manufacturer in the world, presents a different design for its GPUs. AMD integrates a scalar unit into its Graphics Core Next (GCN) compute unit architecture [16]. The heart of the GCN is the Compute Unit (CU) design that is used in the shader array. The GPU consists of many CUs, where each CU includes 4 separate Single Instruction Multiple Data (SIMD) units for vector processing.

In the AMD SIMD execution model, each unit executes single operations across 16 work-items (equivalent to threads in NVIDIA architectures), but each can be working on a separate wavefront (equivalent to the concept of a "warp", or "thread

Table 2 Radeon HD 7970 specification

GPU	Radeon HD 7970
Codename	Tahiti XT
Cores	2048
Global Mem.	3072 MB
Clock rate	0.9 GHz
TFLOPS	3.7

group in lock-steps", on NVIDIA architectures). The SIMD units in each GCN compute unit have a combination of private and shared resources. The instruction buffering, registers and vector Arithmetic Logic Units (ALUs) are private for each of the 4 SIMD units to sustain high performance and utilization (Table 2).

3 GPU-Accelerated Monte Carlo Photon Transport Simulator for 3D Turbid Media

We have developed two parallel implementations of Monte Carlo simulation for photon migration in 3D turbid media: (1) Monte Carlo eXtreme for CUDA (MCX) and (2) Monte Carlo eXtreme for OpenCL (MCXCL).

Our GPU-accelerated Monte Carlo photon simulator was initially published in 2009 [9]. In this original paper, we reported an over 300× speedup when running on a first-generation CUDA GPU (G92) comparing to a single-threaded CPU code [2] running on an Intel Xeon 5120 CPU. In the remainder of this section, we will discuss our implementation of MCX targeting different GPUs, and then discuss our recent efforts on improving the computational efficiency of this code using knowledge of the underlying GPU architecture.

3.1 Optimization of GPU-Accelerated Monte Carlo Simulations for NVIDIA GPUs

Based on the evolution of GPU architectures, we have extended and improved MCX to take advantage of the new features and resources added in each GPU generation. As a result, we have significantly improved the simulation speed and accuracy of our MCX software. Improvements include development of highly efficient ray-tracing algorithms, more efficient random number generation, and more effective thread/block configurations, among others.

Figure 1 illustrates the thread execution flow in MCX. Each thread simulates the lifetime of a photon, and repeats the process until there are no more photons to simulate.

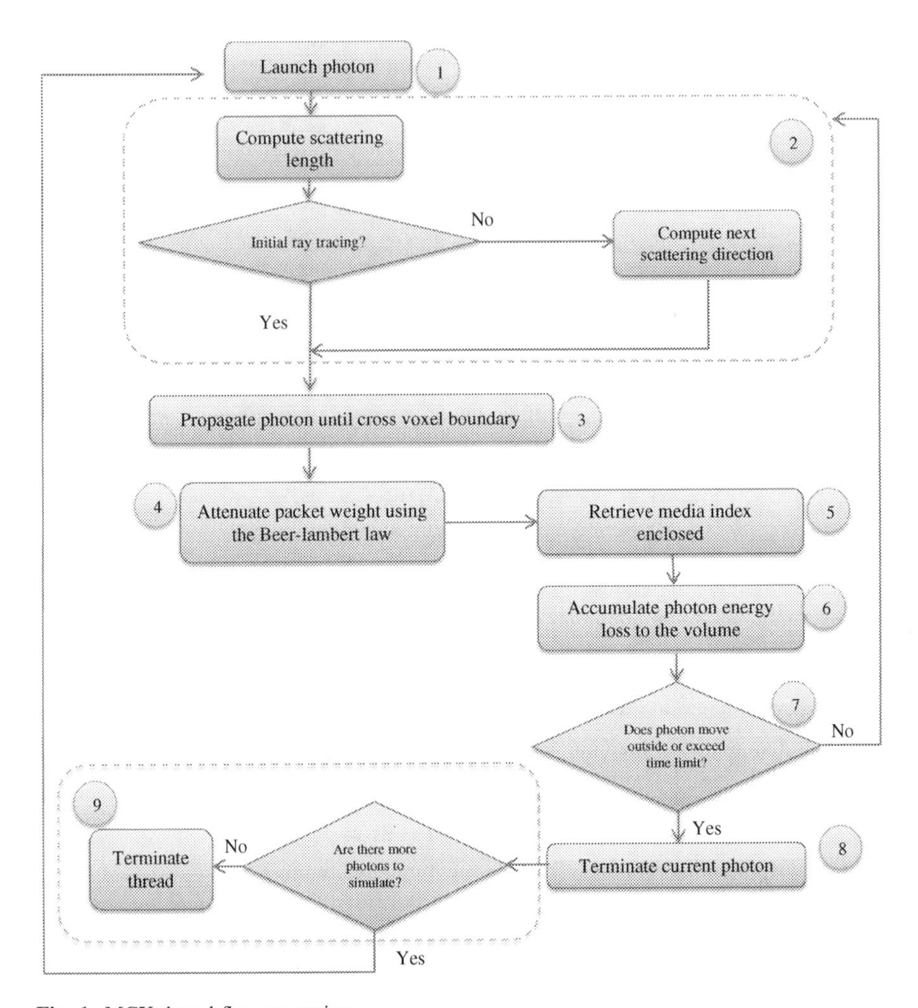

Fig. 1 MCX thread flow execution

In each MCX GPU thread, we simulate a specified number of photon packets, determined by the total number of photons to be simulated and the total number of threads. As each photon packet traverses through the domain, we accumulate photon energy-loss to the volume. The final output of the simulation is a 3D fluence distribution accumulated by all GPU threads. The simulation algorithm can be divided into nine key steps, as illustrated in Fig. 1. In Step ①, we launch photons from a source (the user can specific a pencil beam, Gaussian beam, pattern source, etc.). Step ② simulates a scattering event, including determination of a random scattering length, a random azimuthal angle and a zenith angle using the scattering coefficient of the current voxel. Step ③ is the core of our implementation. It performs a ray-voxel ray-tracing calculation, and propagates the photon packet to the end of the current scattering path (if the end-point is within the current voxel), or to the entry point of the next voxel (if the scattering path goes beyond the current voxel); the two branches in this step may generate a divergence in the program flow. Step ④ computes the photon energy loss based on the Beer-Lambert law. Step ⑤ retrieves the next voxel's optical properties by reading from global memory. Step ⑥ accumulates the photon energy loss calculated in Step ④ to the volume. Step ⑦ verifies if a photon exits the boundary or if the maximum time gate has been reached; if the conditions are not satisfied, it continues to propagate the photon by repeating Step ②, otherwise it continues to Step ⑧. Step ⑧ terminates the current photon. Step ⑨ determines whether the desired photons have been simulated; if not, the framework begins again from Step ①; otherwise the GPU thread terminates.

Over the past year, we have extensively optimized MCX, guided by insights about GPU architectural characteristics. A number of enhancements have been added to MCX in order to improve performance. We have implemented an automatic thread/block/grid configuration strategy that increases simulation speed of MCX across all existing generations of GPUs. We also optimize the utility of the registers and shared-memory; this allows us to launch more blocks per SM on NVIDIA hardware, leading to reduced simulation times. Furthermore, we have implemented a custom math intrinsic function—*nextafter* [19], which was identified as a performance bottleneck by a profiling analysis. In addition, we have also implemented a more efficient GPU random generator using the *xorshift128+* algorithm [17]. Combining all the above optimization strategies, we were able to improve MCX's simulation speed by a factor from 1.6× to 2.8×, depending on the GPU architecture targeted.

The improved MCX has been carefully benchmarked across the four latest generations of NVIDIA GPUs: Fermi, Kepler, Maxwell and Pascal. In the following sections, we discuss performance of our implementation. All results presented use CUDA 7.5, the NVIDIA driver version 367.44, and are run on Ubuntu 14.04.

To demonstrate the performance benefits of each optimization technique considered, we first characterize the "baseline" performance by running MCX with all of the above enhancements enabled. The baseline was characterized by running a standard benchmark problem [9], where 10^8 photon packets are simulated over a uniform 60 × 60 × 60 mm^3 domain filled with homogeneous media (absorption coefficient $\mu_a = 0.005$ (mm^{-1}), scattering coefficient $\mu_s = 1$ (mm^{-1}), anisotropy $g = 0.01$ and reflective index $n = 1$). A "pencil" beam source is used to launch photons at the center of the bottom face of the cubic domain, with a photon initial direction pointing to the $+z$-axis. The baseline performance of MCX across our 4 NVIDIA architectures is shown in Fig. 2. Here, the MCX performance is quantified by reporting the simulation speed in terms of photon/ms. The specific graphics cards used in these benchmarks are noted on the y-axis.

In Fig. 3, we plot the speedup ratios comparing the fully optimized MCX versus running with all optimizations disabled. From this plot, we see an impressive 2.8-fold acceleration was observed for the Kepler architecture; for Fermi, Maxwell and Pascal, a 60–80% speedup was achieved. We believe that the higher speedup

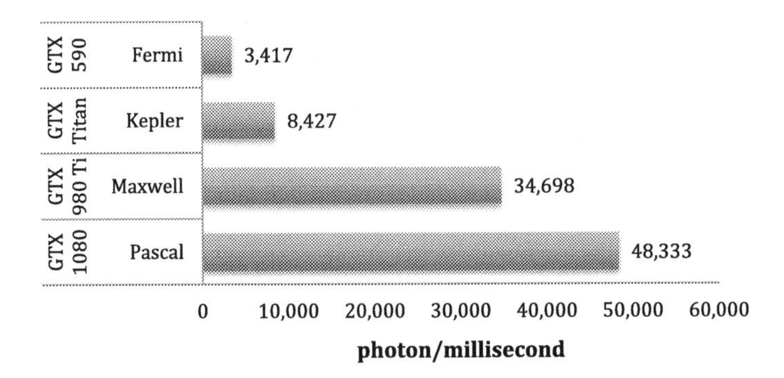

Fig. 2 MCX performance (measured in photon/ms) across Fermi, Kepler, Maxwell, and Pascal GPUs characterized by simulating 10^8 photons in a homogeneous cubic domain

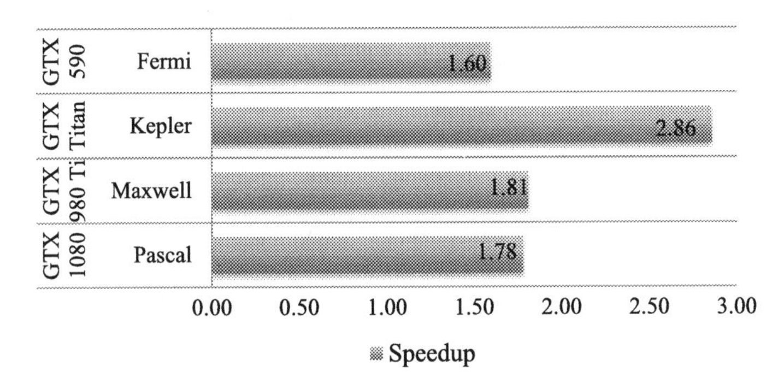

Fig. 3 Speedup factors for Fermi, Kepler, Maxwell and Pascal GPUs

ratio observed on the Kepler GPU was due to a higher number of CUDA cores per SM comparing to the other GPU generations.

To assess the scalability of our algorithm and implementation, we compare the theoretical throughput (measured in tera-floating-point operations per second, or TFLOPS) differences between different GPUs with the speed ratios of MCX achieved on the respective GPUs. In Fig. 4, we particularly characterized the scalability of MCX for two GPU families: Kepler and Maxwell. The normalized throughput (GT 730 and GTX 980 are used as the references for Kepler and Maxwell, respectively) are plotted against the normalized MCX simulation speed.

For the Kepler family, four GPUs are analyzed: (i) GT 730, (ii) Tesla K20c, (iii) Tesla K40c, and (iv) GTX Titan. The GT 730 is used as a baseline for all Kepler GPUs. The normalized MCX speed shows a strong correlation to the normalized theoretic throughput in all tested devices.

For the Maxwell family, three GPUs are analyzed: (i) GTX 980, (ii) GTX 980 Ti, and (iii) GTX Titan X. The GTX 980 is used as the baseline in this case. Similarly, we can observe a strong correlation between the speed improvements of

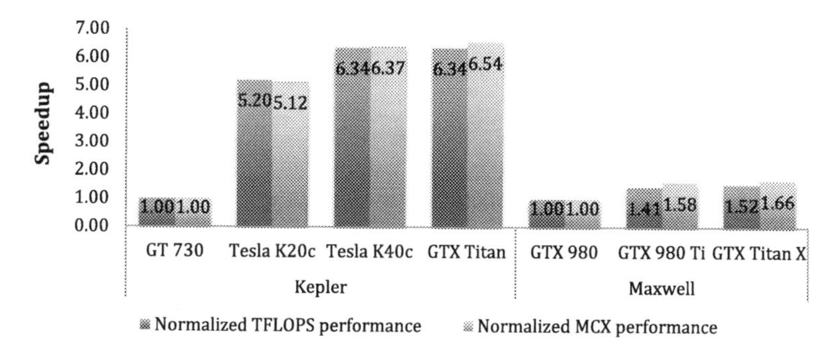

Fig. 4 Speedup comparison between theoretical throughput and MCX performance speed across different Kepler and Maxwell GPUs

MCX and the theoretical throughput of the GPU. Based on these plots, we can conclude that MCX's performance scales nicely across a variety of GPUs.

In the rest of this section, we characterize the speed enhancement resulted from each individual optimization technique. Here, four optimization techniques are considered: (i) optimization of threads and block configurations, (ii) reduction of shared memory usage, (iii) customized NVIDIA math library function and pre-compute reciprocal vector, and (iv) an improved random generation algorithm (*xorshift128+*). Although these improvements were incorporated into MCX in a chronological order, to simplify this analysis, we use a "take-one-out" approach to identify the impact of each individual optimization strategy. The baseline here is the latest software (checked out on Sept. 22, 2016) with all enhancements enabled. Then, as we remove one enhancement at a time, we report to the drop in performance; this is equivalent to the speedup when a feature is enabled. This approach ensures that the software has applied all the updates accumulated during over the multiple years of development.

As indicated in Fig. 3, the performance change due to each software enhancement is GPU architecture dependent. For this reason, we benchmarked MCX and obtained simulation speed (measured in the unit of photon/ms) on a variety of NVIDIA GPU cards, spanning between 4 different generations.

3.1.1 Optimization of Thread and Block Configurations

The number of threads per block (B) and total thread number (T) are important parameters when running a CUDA kernel on the GPU. On one hand, we need to launch a sufficient number of threads, i.e. large T, in order to maximize the utility of GPU resources; on the other hand, the block size (B) determines how many blocks can be simultaneously executed in an SM because an SM has limited resources. Both parameters are directly related to the SM and the core count on a particular GPU.

By taking advantage of the "persistent" nature of the MCX kernel, i.e. a persistent thread (PT), we can dynamically compute the best B and T values according to the resources presented in different architectures. We consider the maximum number of blocks supported per SM, and the maximum number of threads per SM, to determine B. We try to launch as many threads as possible to each block, without generating inactive threads. We consider the number of SMs in the GPU (B) and then use this value to determine the best value of T. By doing this, we launch as many blocks on an SM without increasing the queue of blocks waiting to be executed.

Figure 5 shows the improvement in performance for the best values of B and T. A speedup of over 27% was observed on the Kepler architecture; an over 10% improvement on Maxwell, and a 2% improvement on Pascal. On Fermi we observed a 2% performance decrease when using this feature; we believe this is related to the limited resources on Fermi GPUs and will perform further analysis.

3.1.2 Optimizing Register and Shared-Memory Utility

The MCX kernel requires a large number of registers (over 60). This restricts the number of simultaneous blocks that can be executed in an SM. In the meantime, MCX utilizes shared memory to allow each thread to store the partial-path-length data before a photon is terminated. We also use the shared memory to store thread-specific variables to reduce register pressure. However, we recognize that there is an "optimal" size of the requested shared memory in the MCX simulation. Requesting a large-sized shared memory can restrict the number of blocks that can be simultaneously executed in an SM, thus decreasing performance. Apparently, the optimal shared memory size is related to the total available shared memory space, which is GPU architecture dependent. We have experimented different strategies to transfer variables between the register and shared memory space and identified a "sweet-spot" for the performance.

Our automatic configuration also cuts shared memory demand by half as compared to previous versions of MCX. Figure 6 shows the performance improvement achieved with and without this enhancement. The speed of MCX improves by 51% on the Kepler, 30% on the Maxwell, and 2% on the Pascal. Performance on the Fermi is not impacted by this technique.

3.1.3 Customized NVIDIA Math Library Function and Reduction of Division Operations

Continuing our analysis of the MCX kernel, we identify as bottleneck the executing of the NVIDIA math intrinsic *nextafter*. Specifically, in Step ③ when a photon reaches the voxel boundary and the *hitgrid* function is executed. We implemented a specialized math function to replace an intrinsic math function *nextafter* in the CUDA library, and reduced the number of division operations—one of the most

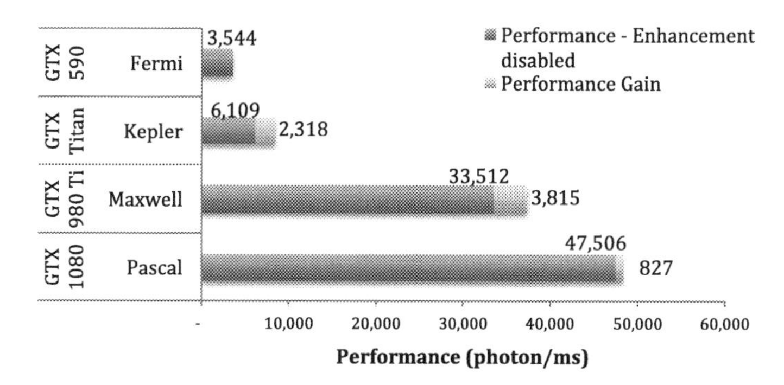

Fig. 5 Performance impact by optimization of threads and block configuration

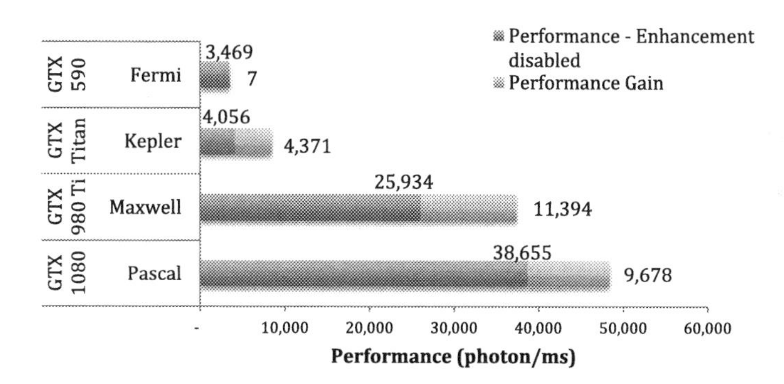

Fig. 6 Performance impact by optimizing shared-memory and register utility

expensive math operations in the GPU [19]—by storing the computed division output and reuse as much as possible. In MCX, since photons traverse a grid-structure with finite dimensions, we simplified the *nextafter* implementation by removing the branches related to handling extreme cases (e.g., encountering NaN or infinity).

With these changes, we observed a speed improvement of 2% for Fermi, 17% for Kepler, 29% for Maxwell, and 18% for Pascal. Figure 7 shows the performance improvements provided by enabling this feature on the four NVIDIA GPUs.

3.1.4 More Efficient Random Number Generation

In our original implementation of MCX, we implemented a GPU-friendly Logistic-lattice-based random number generator [9] (RNG). By utilizing performance profiling, we identified that the RNG is producing another hotspot of the code. To accelerate the RNG computation, we implemented a new random number generator based on the *xorshift128+* algorithm [17]. The new RNG involves only

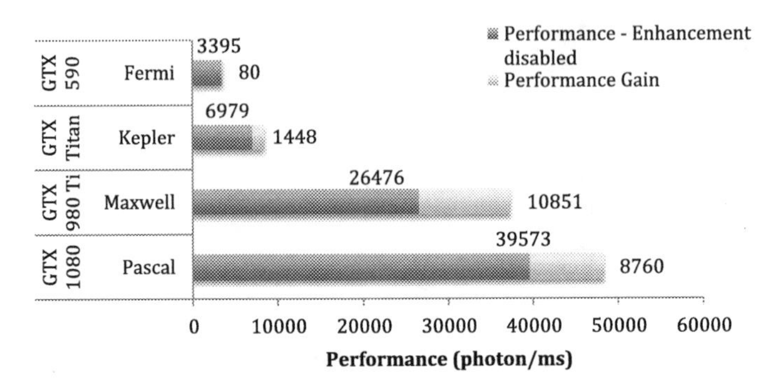

Fig. 7 Performance impact of customized *nextafter* function and reduction of division operations

integer operations and a 64-bit state. In comparison, the Logistic-lattice RNG involves floating-point operations and a 128-bit state.

Figure 8 shows the performance impact of using this new random generation algorithm for each of the NVIDIA GPU architectures. We observed a speedup enhancement of 3% for Fermi, over 14% for Kepler, over 31% for Maxwell and over 21% for Pascal.

3.2 MCXCL

In order to provide a portable, scalable and hardware-independent Monte Carlo simulation for photon migration in a 3D turbid media targeting heterogeneous computing, we developed MCXCL—our OpenCL implementation of the MCX algorithm. OpenCL provides two methods of compilation: (i) off-line compilation, and (ii) online compilation. We focus on the second method. OpenCL for online compilation uses a just-in-time compilation (JIT) method, with the main advantage that it provides adaptive compilation of the kernel. To support JIT compilation, the kernel is built from source during runtime using the OpenCL runtime library.

MCXCL shares a similar algorithm workflow as MCX, as illustrated in Fig. 1, with compilation enhancements such as fast-math and macros. Furthermore, MCXCL adaptively adjusts its thread/block/grid configurations for different computing devices, such as NVIDIA GPUs, AMD GPUs, and Intel CPUs. Figure 9 shows the simulation speed of MCXCL across various computing processors from different hardware vendors.

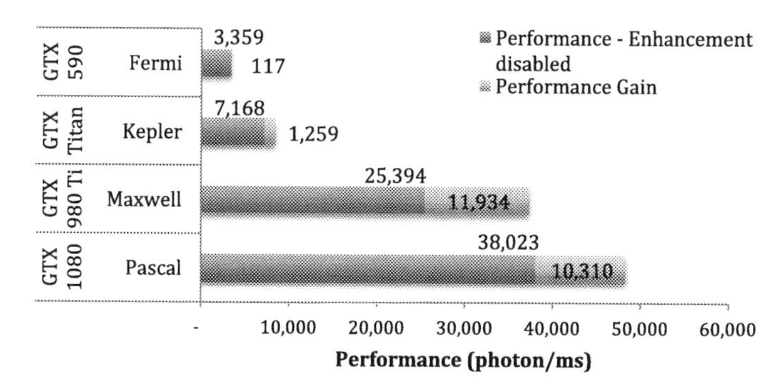

Fig. 8 Performance improvements from a new random number

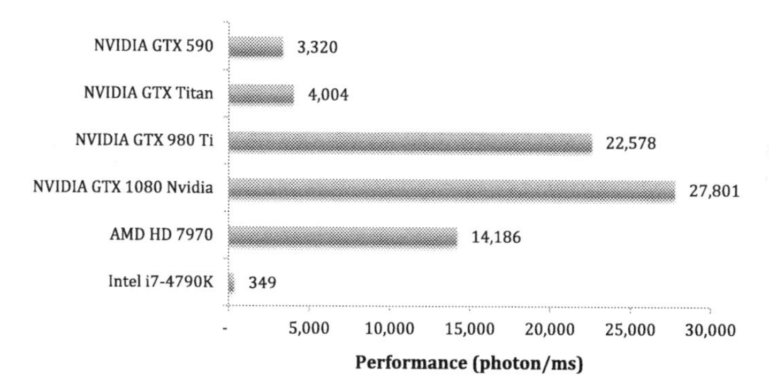

Fig. 9 Simulation speed of MCXCL benchmarked across various NVIDIA GPUs, AMD GPUs, and Intel CPUs

4 Applications

Monte Carlo simulation of photon migration in turbid media—and specifically MCX—has been widely used in the study of sensitivity of cerebral cortex [12, 13, 26, 27], anatomical brain atlases [3, 4, 30], and brain cancer [28, 29].

4.1 Quantification of Sensitivity of Cerebral Cortex

Gorshkov et al. [12] proposed a CPU-based Monte Carlo simulation for photon migration in brain tissue. Their approach did not utilize GPUs because of the lack of advanced global memory in earlier GPU generations. Despite that, they have demonstrated that a Monte Carlo simulation for photon migration in 3D media is a valuable source for non-invasive brain analysis. Their main analysis is on the planar and spherical source light injections.

Perdue et al. [26] quantified the variability in diffuse optical tomography (DOT)—a multichannel NIRS—and the effect of cerebral vasculature on the forward model in young adult subjects. They used a mesh-based Monte Carlo (MMC) method [8] to create the forward models for a set of eight MRI-derived head geometries. Their study demonstrated the variability in terms of DOT sensitivity over the cortex due to anatomical variations.

Guo et al. [13] described a four-layered model of NIR light propagation in a human head using Monte Carlo simulation. Following the same scheme as MCX, they have addressed the impact of both a source and a detector through the experiments with source-detector spacing at wavelengths of 690, 800, and 1300 nm. They demonstrated that 1300 nm is more appropriate to measure brain activity, achieving better sensitivity and spatial resolution.

Perlman et al. [27] have studied brain activity in younger subjects using optical techniques. Their study focused on the development of prefrontal cortex function for children (i.e., patients 3–7 years old). They used MCX to simulate the optical forward model in order to describe the sensitivity of the underlying brain. Their study successfully captured both typical and atypical brain executive function during childhood.

4.2 *Atlas-Based Brain Functional Imaging*

Caffini et al. [3] validated the use of a brain atlas for analyzing NIRS data obtained from brain activation when the subject-specific head anatomy is not available. They used MCX to solve the forward problem and designed a probe to measure the image error introduced by using a brain atlas instead of the human-subject head anatomy. With the help of MCX simulations, they have identified an error of 2 ± 2 cm in activation localization. Such findings quantified limitations in the current atlas-based brain analysis and suggested spatial variations of localization errors among different brain regions.

Cooper et al. [4] validated the atlas-guided DOT methods described by Custo et al. [6] and quantified the corresponding error in the localization of the cortical activation. They used 32 subjects and simulated DOT measurements on brain activation using MCX in the subject space and then reconstruct them in both environments: the atlas registered to the subject and the subject's true anatomy.

Selb et al. [30] implemented a flexible fitting routine on time-domain NIRS data using MCX to address the NIRS estimations of the adult brain considering the contamination of extra-cerebral layers. They compared the results for two different geometries: a two-layer slab with variable thickness of the first layer, and a template atlas head registered to the subject's head surface. They demonstrated that both geometries provided better results than the commonly used homogeneous model, which does not consider the contamination of the extra-cerebral layers.

4.3 Brain Cancer Imaging

Prabu Verleker et al. [28, 29] have been working on the study of cancer and metastasis treatment through the activation of NIR-induced drug release. In 2014, they developed an optically targeted therapeutic treatment for metastatic breast cancer in the brain by optical simulating—using MCX—the photon distribution and subsequent drug activation in the brain.

In 2015, Prabu Verleker et al. [28] introduced a key study to treat cancer and metastasis by delivering lapatinib-drug-nanocomplexes and activating NIR-induced drug release. They presented an alternate empirical approach to estimate NIR photon propagation in brain tissues and tested against MCX. They were able to achieve a 700× speedup compared to the CPU based models.

5 Conclusions and Future Works

MCX has been used to explore a wide range of biological tissue studies, including the cerebral cortex analysis, brain analysis and brain cancer. MCX has been tested in different scenarios, and validated with real experiments. We plan to continue to improve the simulation speed, portability, stability and robustness of MCX, especially since our work will continue to impact the growing user community. Our work is presently impact a broad range of applications. By specifically addressing compute bottlenecks in MCX, we can significantly improve the simulation speed when run on current and future GPU architectures. These enhancements are critical for enabling new classes of performant imaging applications, such as real-time data analysis and instrument optimization.

We have implemented MCX targeting two parallel processing frameworks: CUDA and OpenCL. We optimized our MCX implementation targeting a number of enhancement areas: (i) the thread and block configuration, (ii) usage of shared memory, (iii) customized *nextafter* and pre-compute reciprocal vector, and (iv) introducing new algorithms (e.g., a random generation algorithm). We can achieve more than a nearly 3× speedup for Kepler GPUs, and more than a 1.6× for Fermi, Maxwell and Pascal. Our best performing GPU platform can achieve simulation throughput of over 48,000 photons/ms.

MCXCL is our OpenCL implementation of the MCX algorithm. The code is highly portable across a wide range of devices (including both CPUs and GPUs). Running MCXCL, we had achieved run-time code optimization by dynamically defining just-in-time compilation flags based on user's input. This resulted in 40% increase in simulation speed.

The current implementation of our MCX modeling framework provides solid performance when run on a single GPU. However, it is very common these days to have access to multiple GPUs simultaneously. One main path for the future of MCX is to explore CUDA Multi Process Service (CUDA-MPS), where we can leverage many GPUs simultaneously. We have already proposed a partitioning mechanism to achieve better workload balance when running MCX across multiple GPUs simultaneously, and we are planning to extend this work with CUDA-MPS [21]. We are also considering to utilize GPU virtualization in future work [31].

Furthermore, we have been working on the implementation of C++ templates for code specialization and constant propagation. Code specialization is an efficient mechanism to reduce code branching in a complex GPU kernel such as MCX, while constant propagation avoids dynamic code generation. We anticipate that additional acceleration can be obtained once we complete this implementation.

References

1. Alerstam, E., Svensson, T. & Andersson-Engels, S., 2008. Parallel computing with graphics processing units for high-speed Monte Carlo simulation of photon migration. *Journal of Biomedical Optics*, 13(6), p. 60504.
2. Boas, D. et al., 2002. Three dimensional Monte Carlo code for photon migration through complex heterogeneous media including the adult human head. *Optics express*, 10(3), pp. 159–170.
3. Caffini, M. et al., 2010. Validating an Anatomical Brain Atlas for Analyzing NIRS Measurements of Brain Activation. *Biomedical Optics and 3-D Imaging*, p. JMA87.
4. Cooper, R.J. et al., 2012. Validating atlas-guided DOT: A comparison of diffuse optical tomography informed by atlas and subject-specific anatomies. *NeuroImage*, 62(3), pp. 1999–2006.
5. Cox, D.D. & Savoy, R.L., 2003. Functional magnetic resonance imaging (fMRI) "brain reading": detecting and classifying distributed patterns of fMRI activity in human visual cortex. *Neuroimage*, 19(2), pp. 261–270.
6. Custo, A. et al., 2010. Anatomical atlas-guided diffuse optical tomography of brain activation. *NeuroImage*, 49(1), pp. 561–567.
7. Diamos, G. et al., 2011. SIMD re-convergence at thread frontiers. *Proceedings of the 44th Annual IEEE/ACM International Symposium on Microarchitecture - MICRO-44 '11*, p. 477.
8. Fang, Q., 2010. Mesh-based Monte Carlo method using fast ray-tracing in Plücker coordinates. *Biomedical optics express*, 1(1), pp. 165–75.
9. Fang, Q. & Boas, D.A., 2009. Monte Carlo simulation of photon migration in 3D turbid media accelerated by graphics processing units. *Optics express*, 17(22), pp. 20178–20190.
10. Gao, H., Phan, L. & Lin, Y., 2012. Parallel multigrid solver of radiative transfer equation for photon transport via graphics processing unit. *Journal of Biomedical Optics*, 17(9), pp. 96004–1.
11. Gaster, B. et al., 2012. *Heterogeneous Computing with OpenCL: Revised OpenCL 1.2*, Newnes.
12. Gorshkov, A. V. & Kirillin, M.Y., 2012. Monte Carlo simulation of brain sensing by optical diffuse spectroscopy. *Journal of Computational Science*, 3(6), pp. 498–503.
13. Guo, Z., Cai, F. & He, S., 2013. Optimization for Brain Activity Monitoring With Near Infrared Light in a Four-Layered Model of the Human Head. *Progress In Electromagnetics Research*, 140(April), pp. 277–295.
14. Irani, F. et al., 2007. Functional near infrared spectroscopy (fNIRS): an emerging neuroimaging technology with important applications for the study of brain disorders. *The Clinical neuropsychologist*, 21(1), pp. 9–37.
15. Kaeli, D.R. et al., 2015. *Heterogeneous Computing with OpenCL 2.0*, Morgan Kaufmann.

16. Mantor, M. & Houston, M., 2011. AMD Graphics Core Next. *AMD Fusion Developer Summit.*
17. Marsaglia, G., 2003. Xorshift RNGs. *Journal of Statistical Software*, 8(14), pp. 1–6.
18. Munshi, A., 2009. The opencl specification. In *2009 IEEE Hot Chips 21 Symposium (HCS)*. pp. 1–314.
19. NVIDIA, 2013. CUDA Math API., p. 23.
20. NVIDIA, 2012. Kepler GK110. *Whitepaper*.
21. NVIDIA, 2015. Multi Processing Service.
22. NVIDIA, 2016. NVIDIA GeForce GTX 1080. *Whitepaper*, pp. 1–52.
23. NVIDIA, 2014. NVIDIA GeForce GTX 980 Featuring Maxwell, The Most Advanced GPU Ever Made., pp. 1–32.
24. NVIDIA, 2008. Programming guide.
25. Patterson, D., 2009. The top 10 innovations in the new NVIDIA Fermi architecture, and the top 3 next challenges. *NVIDIA Whitepaper*, pp. 3–10.
26. Perdue, K.L., Fang, Q. & Diamond, S.G., 2012. Quantitative assessment of diffuse optical tomography sensitivity to the cerebral cortex using a whole-head probe. *Physics in Medicine and Biology*, 57(10), pp. 2857–2872.
27. Perlman, S.B., Huppert, T.J. & Luna, B., 2015. Functional Near-Infrared Spectroscopy Evidence for Development of Prefrontal Engagement in Working Memory in Early Through Middle Childhood. *Cerebral cortex (New York, N.Y.: 1991)*, p. bhv139.
28. Prabhu Verleker, A. et al., 2015. An empirical approach to estimate near-infra-red photon propagation and optically induced drug release in brain tissues., 9308, p. 93080T.
29. Prabhu Verleker, A. et al., 2014. An Optical Therapeutic Protocol to treat brain metastasis by mapping NIR activated drug release: A Pilot Study., pp. 14–16.
30. Selb, J. et al., 2014. Comparison of a layered slab and an atlas head model for Monte Carlo fitting of time-domain near-infrared spectroscopy data of the adult head. *Journal of biomedical optics*, 19(1), p. 16010.
31. Ukidave, Y., Li, X. & Kaeli, D., 2016. Mystic: Predictive Scheduling for GPU Based Cloud Servers Using Machine Learning. *Proceedings - 2016 IEEE 30th International Parallel and Distributed Processing Symposium, IPDPS 2016*, pp. 353–362.
32. Wu, H. et al., 2012. Characterization and transformation of unstructured control flow in bulk synchronous GPU applications. *International Journal of High Performance Computing Applications*, 26(2), pp. 170–185.

Building Automation and Control Systems for Healthcare in Smart Homes

M. Frenken, J. Flessner and J. Hurka

Abstract The chapter presents an overview of building control systems addressing healthcare issues in home environments. Main goal of a building control installation is to ensure energy efficiency and comfort in home or functional buildings. Nevertheless, recent scientific work on the design of building control systems focuses on the inhabitants' state of health. The chapter starts with a definition and distinction of several synonymously used terms in the field of building automation and control systems (BACS) and a general architectural design. Section 2 introduces a classification of health related applications using BACS while Sect. 3 gives selected examples for each class to give an overview about possibilities, limits and efforts on the creation of building environments with positive health effects using building control systems. Those example applications will range from adaptive lighting control for health treatment (e.g. in dementia, or depression) to smart home automation networks for activity recognition. Each mentioned system is aiming to create an improved environment, support healthy living, or to detect emergencies and to react adequately. Finally, the achievements of recent scientific works are summarized and recommendations for the development of even more adaptive and healthier building environments through distributed building system technologies are discussed.

M. Frenken (✉) · J. Flessner · J. Hurka
ITAS - Institute for Technical Assistance Systems, Jade University of Applied Sciences Oldenburg, 26121 Oldenburg, Germany
e-mail: Melina.frenken@jade-hs.de

J. Flessner
e-mail: Jannik.flessner@jade-hs.de

J. Hurka
e-mail: Johannes.hurka@jade-hs.de

© Springer International Publishing AG 2017

S.U. Khan et al. (eds.), *Handbook of Large-Scale Distributed Computing in Smart Healthcare*, Scalable Computing and Communications,
DOI 10.1007/978-3-319-58280-1_5

1 Introduction

Traditionally, building services and technical building management have been established to guarantee optimal comfort criteria (temperature, humidity, and air movement) inside of buildings. Nevertheless, building automation and control systems (BACS) have been discussed mainly under the aspects of energy efficiency, security, comfort, and multimedia for the last years. Only recently, the influence of BACS on well-being and health came back into focus. Huisman et al. show and analyze in [38] a growing body of literature that examines the effect of the physical environment on the healing process and the well-being.

The physical environment may contain a BACS with a specific set of functions. Regarding to Huisman et al. [38], an intelligent implementation of these functions can contribute to the optimization of the physical environment toward particular users need, health, and well-being. The intelligence of this implementation is the key factor for a successful final system. Therefore, a closer inspection of the BACSs components and functions is crucial.

The chapter is organized as follows. The introduction goes on with a definition and distinction of several, synonymously used terms in the field of BACS and a general architectural design. Section two introduces the classification of health related applications using BACS while section three uses this classification to give selected examples for each class. Section four will sum up the opportunities and limitations. The chapter will close with conclusive recommendations.

1.1 Large-Scale Distributed Computing and Building Control Systems

Building automation and control systems, smart home systems, home automation, and even building services and technical building management are terms among others which are often used synonymously to describe an intelligent building environment. To prevent confusion, the chapter will introduce and use such terms as defined in the international standard DIN EN ISO 16484-2:2016-08 [16] and the VDI guideline 3814:2009-11 [77] that are closely linked to each other.

Building services (BS) comprise all utilities and installations supplied and distributed within a building. Such installations are not only regarding electricity but rather include gas, heating, water, and communications [16]. For smooth operation of these installations, management is needed. On a very high level *building management (BM)* combines all services related to the operation and management of a building. This is including structural and technical properties based on integral strategies [16]. BM can be subdivided. The subdivision of *technical building management (TBM)* clusters all services related to operation, documentation, energy management and optimization, information management, and monitoring technical warranties. This includes structural and technical properties as well [16].

Within TBM specific tools are applied. To achieve an energy-efficient, economical, and safe operation of all building services, systems are implemented which are summarized under the term *building automation and control system* (*BACS*). They cover both the products and engineering services for automatic controls, monitoring, operation and optimization, management, and all human interventions to the building services [16]. BACS are essential tools for TBM.

Referring to [50] BACS is a rather generic term and can be distinguished in *building automation* and *building control systems*. While building automation covers the whole measurement, control and management of building services on a higher level [77], building control is a specialized sub-group of BACS not requiring a central control unit. The individual components have their own, independent intelligence and exchange information directly with each other in a system-specific network [50]. Building control refers to the use of an installation bus. The bus connects the single system components and external devices to the system and allows communication. Such systems are mostly designed for a specific electrical installation that controls and connects all the functions and processes in a building [88]. Building control can be therefore considered as a specialization of autonomic computing systems, which comprise large numbers of interacting, independent components [40]. The components adapt and reconfigure themselves through a specialized feedback loop [34]. The topology of such a system is a network of autonomic elements building a distributed, service-oriented infrastructure where all components manage their internal behavior and their relationships with other autonomic elements [40].

BACS or rather building control systems are specialized for *individual room/zone control* which means the control of a physical environment in an area of a building (e.g. a specific zone or an individual room). A zone is thereby a defined area in a building, where a form of control can be executed. *Room control or integrated room automation* covers all application-specific devices and functions for single zone or individual room control. This includes a wide range of intelligence like integrated monitoring, interlocks, open and closed-loop control, and optimization of combined building services. Such building services always refer to a room/zone like heating, ventilating, air-conditioning and refrigeration (HVAC&R), lighting, window blinds/shades control, electrical power distribution, and other trades, by communication functions [16]. As a result, a BACS can contribute to the optimization of the physical environment toward individual user's needs, health, and well-being.

The terms smart home system, home automation, and others are neither explicitly defined in the standard documentation of the DIN EN ISO 16484-2:2016-08 nor in the VDI guideline 3814:2009-11. They are mostly used synonymously to one of the defined terms as BACS, building automation, building control, or room automation. Which system is meant in a particular situation has to be deduced from the context. To describe and control an intelligent building environment the chapter will always refer to BACS or rather to building control only.

In short, a building control system can be considered as a large-scale network of distributed, interacting, autonomous components where the size (scale) of the network is depending on the number of components. If the functions of the building control systems are used to optimize the physical environment toward a user's health the overall system uses a paradigm of large-scale distributed computing for healthcare.

1.2 Architecture of Building Control Systems

In principle, there is a difference between the topology and the architecture of a system. While a topology is mostly about the arrangement of the elements of a network in space (thus a map) [14], a system architecture is a conceptual model and therefore a representation of a system [35]. Topologies can be distinguished in two categories: physical and logical topologies. The physical topology of a network describes the components, the media, and the way the media connects the components. The logical topology is the way in which the signals act on the networks media without regard to the physical interconnection of the components [14]. A network's logical topology is not implicitly the same as its physical topology. A logical bus topology of BACS for example might have a physical star topology layout. Possible network topology forms for BACS are line, ring, star, tree, and mesh [16]. When reading the example applications of health related building control systems, it is important to keep in mind that the term bus can refer to a physical as well as a logical topology and must be therefore carefully distinguished in each example. A system architecture or system model defines the structure and the behavior of a system. Jaakkola and Thalheim distinguish five different views in a system architecture: 1. information or data view answering the "what information is being processed" question, 2. domain view answering the "what business activities must be supported" question, 3. integration view answering the "which business activities require the information" question, 4. deployment or technology view answering the "where is the information located" question, and 5. infrastructure or embedment view concentrating on the embedding of the system into other systems [35]. In the standard 16484-2 three different views for network architecture are introduced: i. the point-of-view of its functions (e.g. client-server architecture, allocated and distributed), ii. the point-of-view of its dimensions (e.g. LAN, MAN, or WAN), and iii. the point-of-view of the arrangement of its components (e.g. shape of a star, ring, line/bus, hierarchical, matrix, and free topology) [16]. Referring to Groth and Skandier the last one seems to be more conform to the definition of topology than architecture [14]. Because a topology is more or less fundamental knowledge about networks, the chapter will rather focus on possible architecture of BACS in the particular example applications. With respect to the standard 16484-2 the authors have chosen the perspective of its functions.

The conceptual architecture of BACS follows in general the scheme shown in Fig. 1. The architecture bases on the work of [21, 41, 49, 51, 68, 79]. Thereby, the

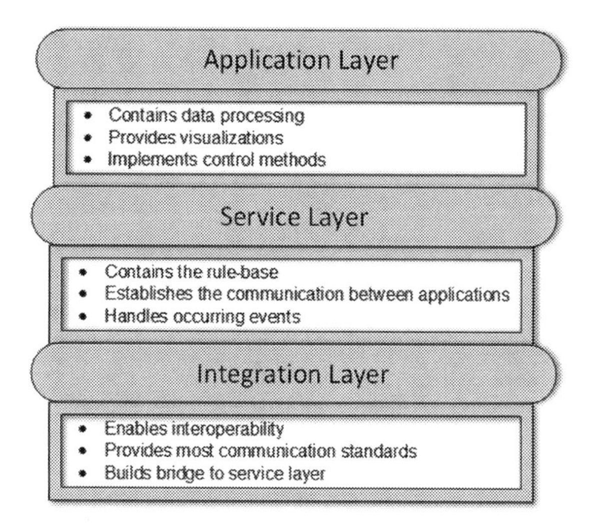

Fig. 1 General architecture of building automation networks

integration layer represents the lowest level of the architecture. Its objective is to integrate various devices of different manufacturers, which possibly use different communication standards. Furthermore, the addition of further devices should be possible through the integration of the most common communication standards. The integration layer moreover builds the bridge to the service layer by providing the communication with the integrated devices.

The objective of the service layer is the handling of occurring events, which are captured by the used devices. These events can be of importance for multiple applications at the same time. Therefore, the service layer transmits the information to all appropriate applications. Moreover, the service layer provides a rule base framework to react adequately on specific events.

The development and implementation of the desired applications is made within the application layer. This layer contains every requirement needed to process the acquired data and to implement control functions. Furthermore, visualizations and services for mobile applications are content of the application layer. This layer is at the highest level and requires the integration and service layer. The advantage of the implementation of a building automation network based on an architecture like this is the clear overview of the particular network components. Specifically for healthcare applications with building automation networks, which combine multiple sub-applications like patient identification and monitoring, a modular implementation is of importance.

In addition, the computation and communication becomes even more complex with increasing network size. Regarding healthcare applications for people in hospitals or nursing homes, a huge amount of sensors and actuators have to be integrated. Hence, health related building automation applications have increased requirements on computation and communication issues.

1.3 Computation and Communication Methods

Raynal said that "distributed computing is about mastering uncertainty" [58]. Building control systems are normally composed of distributed and mostly dynamical components such as lights, shades, etc. Those components have several execution modes like on, off, open, closed, and many other. The state of each component can be monitored within the network. The execution of the components can occur independently and simultaneously. Trigger for the execution can be the reception of internal (e.g. state change of one component) or external events (e.g. human system interaction). The distributed components of building control systems should contribute to the optimization of the physical environment toward the user's health and well-being in ensemble acting but each entity has only a partial knowledge of the involved parameters and execution modes of the other components [58]. The complexity results from the need of a proper and safe running system towards this overarching goal for each accessible combination of execution modes [34]. Uncertainty is usually given by not plannable or even not reliable human system interaction.

Hence, it is easy to see why large scale BACS are diverse. It is hard for system architects to anticipate and design all possible interactions among components or with external entities (like other systems or humans). BACS need to be computing systems that can manage themselves given only high-level objectives from the particular application (which means to perform autonomic computing [40]). That means that the system has to be capable of dealing with many issues at runtime. The design of and the (autonomic) computation within building control systems may be therefore critical in terms of correctness, reliability, safety, and security, especially when they are designed for healthcare. Modeling approaches used to consider such conditions already during the design process vary from ontology and state charts [75] through formal methods [13, 34] to evolutionary algorithms [30] or multi agent systems [61]. Corno and Sanaullah give a broad overview of modeling and verification techniques putting them into the perspective of ambient intelligence [12]. Summed up, it is not possible to give the one approach to design the perfect matching BACS, and it is even not possible to describe the one and only computing strategy for BACS in healthcare. Distributed computing may be about mastering uncertainty, but modelling a BACS for healthcare is about mastering a broad variety of multi-disciplinary approaches and choosing the one best matching to the application requirements. Thus, it is not possible to describe computation or communication strategies independent from the application.

However, one does not necessarily need to dive into BACS specific literature first to get an idea on how to solve such issues. Literature about autonomic computing will give a very good point of entry. Kephart and Chess for example summarize the Self-Challenges (Self-Management, Self-Configuration, Self-Optimization, Self-Healing, and Self-Protection) of autonomic computing [40], each of them easily applicable to BACS. They also give considerations regarding architecture, engineering and science theory.

Existing architectures, communication methods and computation approaches are essential for the design process of building applications. In the following, the classification of healthcare related building automation applications is described.

2 Classification of Health Related Applications Using Building Automation Networks

The building automation networks address a large field of different health related applications, even though the main scientific effort is focused on energy efficiency. The design of building automation networks with the aim to improve the energy efficiency often leaves the requirements of the inhabitant out and has potentially a negative effect on the inhabitant's state of health [48, 81]. Therefore, the interest in approaches to improve the healthcare via building automation applications awakened in recent years.

Healthcare applications using building automation involve heating networks, ventilation networks, lighting networks, activity recognition and inhabitant monitoring systems, and safety applications. The heating, ventilation and lighting systems are supposed to effect the inhabitant's state of health positively through the adequate regulation of environmental factors, like temperature, indoor air quality and illumination. Apart from the usual usage of light, it effects the inhabitant's mood and is able to support the therapy of mental diseases. Another application topic is the recognition of activities and the monitoring of the inhabitant via building automation networks. The goals of activity recognition and patient monitoring are the detection of anomalies. Safety applications are supposed to protect the inhabitant from accidents and to initiate adequate reactions.

To further classify these applications, they will be grouped into passive and active support applications. In addition, a hybrid form of passive and active support is defined as adaptive support. An overview of the classification is shown in Fig. 2. Passive healthcare applications include building automation networks with the

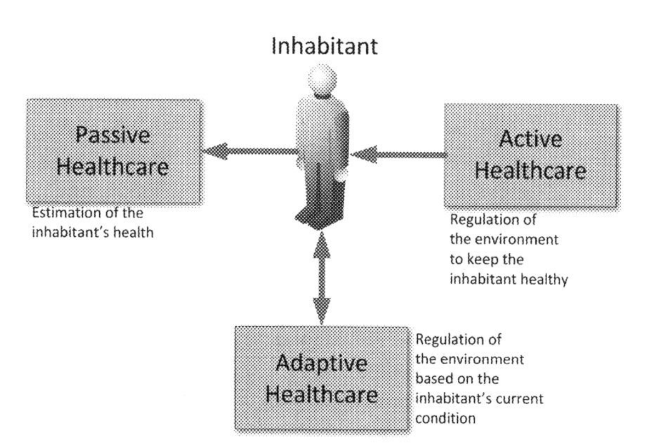

Fig. 2 Overview of the classification of health related applications for building automation

focus on the estimation of the inhabitant's condition and the detection of critical situations. These applications do not influence the inhabitant directly. They are supposed to determine the inhabitant's condition via the interpretation of received sensor data. The determined condition of the inhabitant is afterwards used to make emergency calls if needed or to propose the consultation of a medic.

On the other hand, active applications influence the inhabitant directly via the operation of adequate actuators within the building automation network. The purpose of these active applications is the improvement of the environment concerning the inhabitant's health. The current condition of the inhabitant is not involved in the regulation of the environment. Hence, these systems regulate the environment based on recent studies on adequate environmental factors, but do not dynamically react on the inhabitant's condition. Applications merging the passive determination of the inhabitant's condition and the active regulation of the environment are described as adaptive applications. They regulate the environment via different actuators after the determination of the inhabitant's condition. In this way the adaptive applications are able to react to suddenly occurring changes.

In the following, the classes of building automation applications will be described in detail with the focus on health and comfort issues.

2.1 *Passive Healthcare Applications*

The objective of passive healthcare applications is the interpretation of sensor data in order to determine the inhabitant's condition. A central aspect is hence the recognition of activities and thereby the monitoring of the inhabitant. Another field of applications concerns safety issues and the ability to react adequately on emergencies and the deteriorating of the inhabitant's state of health.

2.1.1 Activity Recognition and Inhabitant Monitoring

Activity recognition and inhabitant monitoring in conjunction with building automation networks are highly regarded topics of current scientific efforts. Such networks aim to recognize *Activities of Daily Living* (*ADL*) in order to enable the assessment of the inhabitant's condition. The ability to master ADLs like eating, cooking and drinking decreases with advancing age and after occurring impairments. Therefore, the recognition of ADLs is a first step to estimate the inhabitant's state of health and his ability to live independently.

Accordingly, a main objective of the topic is the design of unobtrusive building automation networks to recognize the executed activities and monitor the condition of the inhabitant. A possibility to implement the activity recognition is the integration of usual domestic appliances in the building automation network to analyze their particular use. To estimate the particular use of a domestic appliance the measurement of the energy consumption is a common method.

Another way to implement the activity recognition is the interpretation of data from additional sensors like contact sensors or motion detectors. Force sensors, for example, are useful to determine whether and how long the inhabitant used a particular seat. The sensor information is necessary for the estimation of the inhabitant's state of health and for predicting the following activities. Moreover, intelligent algorithms are implemented to identify daily routine patterns. The analysis of these patterns and of anomalies within the routine are useful for the monitoring of the inhabitant.

The monitoring of the inhabitant's activity level is helpful to draw conclusions about the inhabitant's condition. In the case of a decreasing activity level examinations can be made to assess changes in the inhabitant's state of health. This approach aims to identify an impairment in an early stage in order to intervene immediately and to prevent the worsening of the impairment.

In general, a single computation unit is used to gather all information acquired from the sensors. This architecture easily provides the possibility to use the complete information of all sensors for the detection of activity patterns. Therefore, a major challenge for the creation of these large-scale distributed sensors networks is to implement a fast and robust communication method to avoid the loss of information. A working communication is a requirement to establish an activity recognition and patient monitoring network for real-life applications.

2.1.2 Safety

Healthcare applications which deal with the recognition of critical situations and trigger any kind of reaction belong to the safety topic. Passive safety applications within the building automation network are thereby defined as applications without direct support ability. In fact, these applications are focused on the detection of emergencies and the preparation of an interface to the outer world in order to request appropriate aid.

Consequently, the ability to recognize anomalies in the behavior has to be implemented. This is achievable with building automation sensors itself or for instance with wearable devices. Therefore, in the case of an appearing anomaly, like the detection of a fall or an abrupt interruption of the daily routine, a check of the inhabitant's condition via telephone call or another application can be executed. In the event that the inhabitant is not contactable, the neighbor gets informed or an emergency call is made. The building automation network in conjunction with a gateway to the mobile communications network and internet provides an ideal architecture to establish automatic emergency notifications. In order to decrease the time between the emergency call and the arrival of helpers a large network connecting the neighborhood is supposable.

Specifically the building automation systems within hospitals can be a benefit during emergency situations. In the case of an occurring emergency, an implemented localization ability within the building automation network could accelerate the notification of the nearest expert [28]. Such a system would minimize the arrival time of emergency aid. In addition, the localization of patients with building automation technology can support the hospital nurses during the search for missing patients. To create a building automation system with patient monitoring within hospitals, a large area and multiple patients, nurses, and doctors have to be covered. Hence, several sensors are needed to record the people's location and measure the patient's physical parameter, which results in a major challenge for the network design concerning the analysis and communication. In order to reduce the communication load within the building network, splitting the whole network into sub-networks with multiple distributed computation units can be a solution.

2.2 Active Healthcare Applications

In contrast to passive healthcare applications, active applications influence the inhabitant directly. The building automation networks use their actuators to regulate the environmental factors in order to create a healthy environment. The control methods for the regulation of the environment are not influenced by short-time or daily variations of the inhabitant's condition. Hence, sensors for the monitoring of the inhabitant have minor priority within active healthcare applications. The applications are in fact focused on the monitoring of the environmental factors, which is used to improve the environmental control.

The particular applications are thereby organized in subsections like ventilation control, heating control and lighting.

2.2.1 Active Ventilation Control

Within building environments the inhabitants are exposed to various air pollutants. The concentrations of these air pollutants define the indoor air quality. One aim of the ventilation control is to substitute the polluted with fresh or filtered air. The amount of exchanged air within a certain time interval is described by the parameter air change rate.

There exist concentration limits for air pollutants in the indoor air in current standards as well. The objective of these standards is to suggest air change rates in order to keep air pollutant concentrations below a certain level. Intelligent ventilation systems use sensors to measure particular pollutant concentrations to adapt the air change rate according to the current concentrations. A common way to design an intelligent ventilation control is to use the CO_2 concentration as an indicator for the indoor air quality. Less adaptive systems are based on room size and mean occupancy, following the instructions of current national or international standards, like the WHO guidelines [83] and the DIN ISO EN 13779 [15].

One approach to estimate an adequate and healthy air change rate is to involve the perceived indoor air quality. Fanger [24] conducted studies about the perception of the indoor air quality and interpreted the results to determine a model to calculate an adequate air change rate based on the desired quality and existing pollution sources. This approach does not differentiate between particular conditions of the inhabitant. Parts of this approach influenced the instructed air change rates in current regulation standards. A further study by Fang et al. [23] proved that the perception of the indoor air quality is not solely dependent on air pollutants. The perception is as well influenced by other environmental factors like temperature and humidity.

Except for the perception in order to identify comfortable air change rates, the human and his condition is not involved within the common ventilation control process. In conclusion, active ventilation control applications disregard the inhabitant's state of health and adapt their performance based solely on environmental factors and building information. Thereby, the complex relations between the environmental factors have to be regarded during the design of health supportive ventilation systems.

2.2.2 Active Heating Control

The objective of heating control is to satisfy the inhabitant's thermal sensation and to avoid negative health effects through inadequate indoor temperatures [31]. The thermal sensation is amongst others described in international and national standards [17]. The determination of the predicted mean vote (PMV) is an indicator for the probable thermal sensation. The thermal sensation depends on the relation between body temperature and indoor temperature. According to this, the analysis of the environmental parameters can lead to the estimation of the probable thermal sensation, which is useful for the temperature regulation. Therefore, the monitoring of adequate environmental factors is a major challenge for active heating control via building automation networks.

The heating system measures the temperature in every regulated room and reacts to occurring differences between the current temperature and the target value. The time needed to compensate these differences is a quality characteristic of heating systems. The target value is set directly by the inhabitant.

Usually, systems for temperature control measure solely local environmental factors. The measurement of the environmental condition in just one spot is not sufficient to make a precise assumption for the whole building environment. Because of this, recent scientific works develop distributed building automation systems in order to reach a more detailed representation of the environmental factors. The awareness of the health effects of temperature led to the introduction of specifications for temperature and humidity limits [17]. The temperatures must not exceed or fall below a certain interval to avoid mold formation and an unhealthy environment. Therefore, the design of the heating systems has to respect the health related findings about the indoor temperature.

Nevertheless, active temperature control systems leave out the activities and condition of the inhabitant. Differences relating to the mobility or activity of different inhabitants are not considered automatically. In the event of discomfort concerning the indoor temperature, the inhabitant has to adjust the target value himself.

2.2.3 Active Lighting Control

Active lighting applications aim to support the inhabitant amongst others by highlighting possible barriers to prevent falls or escape routes in critical situations.

Moreover, another approach for active lighting control focuses on the direct effects of light on the inhabitant's health. Several studies proved that light has a significant effect on the inhabitant's state of health, in particular on mental issues [60, 62]. As a result, these studies suggest a positive health effect of the simulation of the circadian rhythm via light illuminance and color. To achieve a positive effect on the melatonin production, 6 h of bright light in the morning followed by 10 h of normal lighting is recommended by Barroso and Den Brinker [6].

Furthermore, light represents an ambient output possibility for memory applications or other notification systems.

2.3 Adaptive Healthcare Applications

Applications which regulate environmental factors based on information from inhabitant monitoring and activity recognition are classified as adaptive ones. The diverse recognizable activities and conditions of the inhabitant are related to different physical and mental loads. These different loads result in differing requirements regarding the environmental factors. This knowledge enables the building automation applications to influence the inhabitant positively with respect on his requirements.

Moreover, wearable devices for the inhabitant monitoring can be integrated in the building automation network. A possible concept to include the patient monitoring via wearable devices within a building automation system is shown in Fig. 3. The wearable device measures parameters like heart rate, skin conductance and body temperature for the estimation of the inhabitant's condition and activity level. Afterwards, these information are analyzed by a centralized computation unit. As result, the requirements of the inhabitant will be used to regulate the components of the building automation network. A possible scenario is the increase of the air change rate to an adequate level, if a high activity level was measured. A high activity level is associated with an increased breathing frequency, which results in an increased demand on the amount of fresh air.

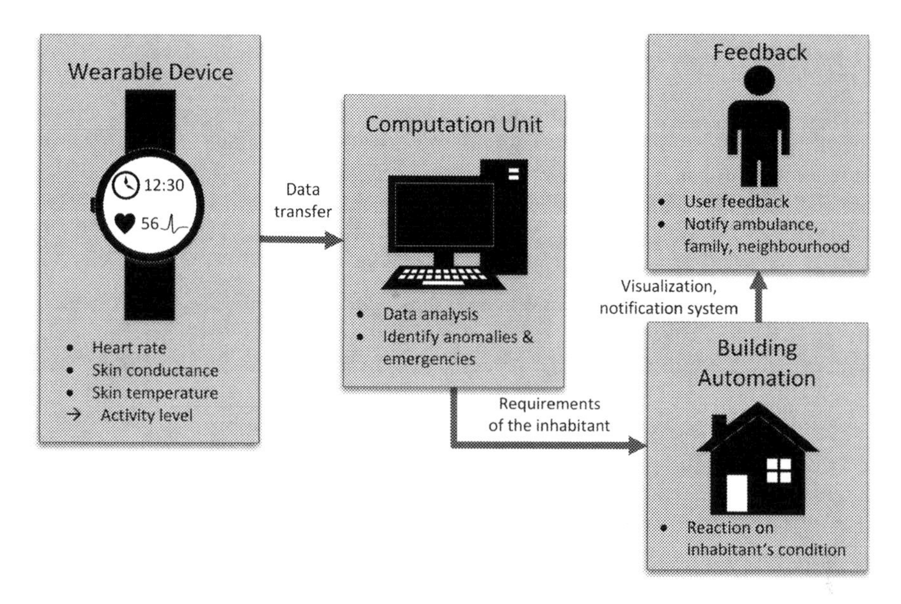

Fig. 3 Components and connections of a possible adaptive patient monitoring system within a building automation network

2.3.1 Adaptive Ventilation Control

The objective of an adaptive ventilation system is to provide the adequate amount of unpolluted air dependent on the inhabitant's requirements. Adaptive ventilation systems adjust the air change rate with respect to the inhabitant's condition. Recent scientific research suggests that the common air change rates, which are instructed by current international standards, are not high enough to establish a healthy environment. One reason for these insufficient recommendations could be the high priority on energy efficiency. Specifically, the effect of the air quality on various diseases is proved by several studies [7, 9, 36, 81]. These studies suggest that the regulation of environmental factors based on the particular state of health of the inhabitant is beneficial. Therefore, new approaches have to be implemented to include all required information within the ventilation control system.

These facts suggest the assumption that a human-centered design of the ventilation control, apart from energy efficiency issues, is a promising approach for the development of health related ventilation applications. The involvement of the current requirements of the inhabitant towards the indoor air quality is a crucial aspect for the design process.

2.3.2 Adaptive Heating Control

Dependent on the inhabitant's condition and activity level the requirement on the indoor temperature differs. One possibility to take advantage of the activity recognition is to adapt the indoor temperature concerning the current physical load of the inhabitant. High physical activity results in increasing body heat. The adaptive building automation network is able to detect this condition and reacts by lowering the indoor temperature to compensate the increased body heat. Such a feature secures the thermal sensation and reduces the needed effort to keep the body heat in balance, which results in an avoidance of physical overstraining. The adjustment of the temperature in relation to the physical load of the inhabitant is an example of an adaptive heating control.

Moreover, several studies proved that there exists a relation between thermal sensation and physiological values, like the heart rate variability [29, 45, 85]. An increased heart rate variability is thereby associated with thermal discomfort if the inhabitant is at rest. Hence, the involvement of a real-time heart rate variability monitoring within an adaptive heating system is a promising approach for adaptive heating control. In addition, Lloyd et al. [46] found a significant effect of adequate thermal condition on the inhabitant's state of health and blood pressure. These findings underline the relation between heating, health and comfort.

In conclusion, temperature has an effect on the inhabitant's state of health. Therefore, adaptive heating systems have to be designed in order to provide an adequate and healthy environment for the particular inhabitant. To achieve this, the system needs to acquire the relevant and necessary information about the inhabitant. As described before, adaptive building applications are based on activity recognition or inhabitant monitoring. This applies for adaptive heating systems too.

2.3.3 Adaptive Lighting Control

Adaptive lighting deals with the control of light sources to support the inhabitant adequately. An important information for light control is the current activity executed by the inhabitant. With this information, for example, a nightly visit to the bathroom is supported by the adequate illumination of the path.

It was shown that light is able to impact the therapy of mental diseases [62, 78]. Consequently, the adjustment of the light intensity and the luminous color based on the current mood of the inhabitant is another possibility to influence the inhabitant positively. Adaptive light therapy applications have thereby the ability to react on daily changes and occurring relapses.

3 Examples of Healthcare Applications Based on Building Automation Networks

The intention of the following chapter is to outline recent scientific efforts concerning building automation networks with health related applications. These examples cover passive, active and adaptive healthcare applications. Only implemented systems composed of unobtrusive environmental or wearable sensors are regarded. Hence, cameras and other approaches, which require the analysis of video data are neglected.

3.1 Passive Healthcare Applications

In the following, implemented healthcare applications without direct influence on the inhabitant are described. Therefore, approaches for activity recognition and safety issues are presented.

3.1.1 Systems for Activity Recognition and Inhabitant Monitoring

Suryadevara and Mukhopadhyay [69] equipped an experimental environment with electrical monitoring sensors, force sensors, water flow sensor, and additional panic buttons to create an activity recognition system (Fig. 4). To secure a trouble-free communication the ZigBee protocol was used by the scientists. Storage problems resulting from continuous sensor data streams can be avoided through the filtering of the data for changes of the particular sensor status. The adequately positioned sensors enable the system to record the time spent on different activities. These periods are analyzed to determine an indication of the inhabitant's state of health. Particularly, the time of inactivity between the uses of appliances is observed and used to calculate a wellness indication. As second wellness parameter, the current usage duration is compared with the estimated common usage duration. This approach solely contains activities which are simple to recognize via a single sensor.

More complex activities, containing several different operations, are not considered. A complex activity consists thereby of a specific sequence of sensor events. The determination of these activities, even with varying time intervals between the particular sensor events, is a major task for computation. In particular the processing of the multidimensional data from the various sensors is a main challenge for complex activity recognition.

Thereby, the first computation step contains the segmentation of sensor events. The segmentation method defines which sensor events of a recorded sequence are used for the recognition process [43]. A common method is the analysis of the sensor events within a defined time interval. This approach results in a varying

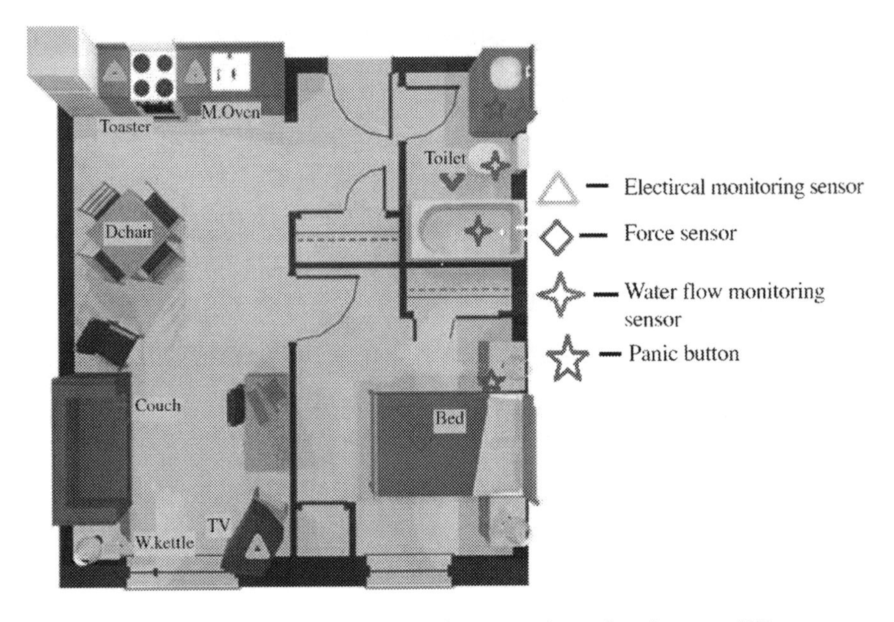

Fig. 4 Spatial arrangement of different sensors in an experimental environment [69]

number of analyzed sensors events. In addition to this, another approach uses the number of sensor events to segment the sensor information, which leads to segments with varying time intervals. These approaches are not sufficient for real environments because of the diversity of the duration and number of sensor events within the various activities [86]. To solve this problem the consideration of further information about the regarded activities is beneficial. For this purpose information like time, duration, location, needed resources and previous activities are consulted to gain a detailed overview about the activities [80]. The increase of required data results in an increase of communication and computation complexity.

Furthermore, Cook et al. [11] dealt with the appearance of unknown patterns during the online activity recognition. Unknown patterns are sequences of sensor events which were not learned before the start of the system. The scientists developed a method to learn and recognize these patterns during runtime and use them to increase the recognition rate of the learned activities. In order to learn the unknown patterns, a support vector machine was implemented. Support vector machines are machine learning models which are able to process multidimensional data. Specifically, building automation networks provide multidimensional data acquired from different sensor types. Therefore, support vector machines are an appropriate solution for particular computation challenges.

This approach was subsequently used for experiments to determine health events via changes in the daily routine of the inhabitant [65]. The results of the long-term study with two elderly inhabitants indicate a notable relation between occurring health events and the detection of changes within the daily routine patterns.

The distributed building automation networks for health monitoring are mostly designed to observe just a single inhabitant. Tunca et al. [73] created a building automation network for activity recognition and health monitoring in order to recognize the activities of two inhabitants. For this purpose, two apartments were equipped with multiple sensors for the recognition of 27 different activities. The communication between the sensors and a central computation unit is based on the ZigBee protocol. An experiment within the two apartments was done and multiple machine learning algorithms for the activity recognition were tested. As a result, an artificial neural network achieved the best overall performance. In conclusion, the authors described a system which is able to recognize the activities of two inhabitants living in the same apartment. Moreover, they pointed out that the analysis of the time, duration and frequency of specific activities is a sufficient indication for the estimation of the inhabitant's health.

In particular activity recognition applications have to process a huge amount of multidimensional data received from the large-scale building automation networks. A promising approach for data processing within building automation networks are thereby machine learning algorithms which satisfy the computation requirements.

3.1.2 Safety Applications

There exist various approaches and gateways for the connection of large-scale building automation networks with the outer world [56, 71, 74]. Safety applications require an architecture which includes such gateways to provide the ability to call for adequate aid.

A possible reason for the activation of an emergency alarm is the measurement of unusual environmental factors. Ransing and Rajput [57] developed a building automation network based on the ZigBee protocol for temperature monitoring. The network is designed to detect fires and gas leakages and is connected with the mobile communication network in order to notify the inhabitant via mobile phone.

Moreover, safety applications concerning the inhabitant's state of health are focused by recent scientific research. According to this, the approach from Skubic et al. [63] contains a building automation network which is connected with clinical caregivers via a web portal. The data from the building automation network, providing door, motion, and bed sensors, is analyzed within a central computation unit. In the case of the detection of an anomaly in the inhabitant's behavior, an e-mail is sent to clinical experts to assess the provided data and to react adequately.

A direct way to monitor the inhabitant is followed by Aguirre et al. [2] within the NASISTIC system. The presented system contains, in addition to environmental sensors, a selection of medical sensors, including devices for the measurement of blood pressure, weight, medicine taking, and electrocardiogram. Combined with the information of water sensors, light sensors, presence sensors, and gas sensors the medical information are transmitted to gateways via Bluetooth. These gateways represent a possibility to inform medics or family members about the inhabitant's state of health and behavior via an internet server. Therefore, the medics and family members are enabled to react if abnormalities occur.

Not every detected anomaly necessarily requires the notification of experts. Therefore, Arcelus et al. [5] introduced the classification of anomalies in four different categories with increasing importance: mild abnormality, caution, high alert, emergency. While a phone call is sufficient for occurring mild abnormality or caution alerts, a high alert or emergency should have a visit of a caregiver or medic as consequence. These examples show that safety applications benefit from the proceedings in the Internet of Things and appropriate system architecture design.

3.2 Active Healthcare Applications

In the following, active healthcare applications concerning the ventilation, heating and lighting control will be presented.

3.2.1 Active Ventilation Systems

As an essential part of many buildings, the ventilation control is a highly regarded scientific topic. The possible negative effects of insufficient air quality are well reviewed [7, 8, 36, 67, 81, 83].

Accordingly, several applications were developed to detect harmful pollutants within the indoor air and to react adequately. These pollutants are emitted by the different building materials and inhabitants. Several different national and international guidelines recommend concentration limits for the various pollutants.

In this context, Kumar and Hancke [44] developed a wireless sensor network to monitor the CO_2 and CO concentration within the air at different locations. These information are afterwards used to determine the probable comfort level, which enables the adjustment of the air change rate according to the current condition.

Specifically, healthcare environments which nurse impaired and weakened patients have an increased demand on the indoor air quality. Therefore, Yang et al. [84] designed a wireless ventilation control system to monitor various air pollutants beside the CO_2 concentration in 13 different rooms. All in all, five air components are measured (CO_2, total volatile organic compound (VOC), particulate matter, total bacteria, total fungi). The analysis of the concentrations of the observed components suggests that the CO_2 concentration is an adequate indicator for the overall indoor air quality. Consequently, a wireless network containing CO_2 sensors was created. The multiple sensors are connected to ZigBee communication modules, which transmit the data to a centralized computation unit. The computation unit analyses the current concentrations and regulates the ventilation.

Another approach of recent scientific works is the monitoring of VOC concentrations with small distributed sensors. Peng et al. [54] presented a system to monitor the VOC concentration of multiple buildings within a campus. They used a

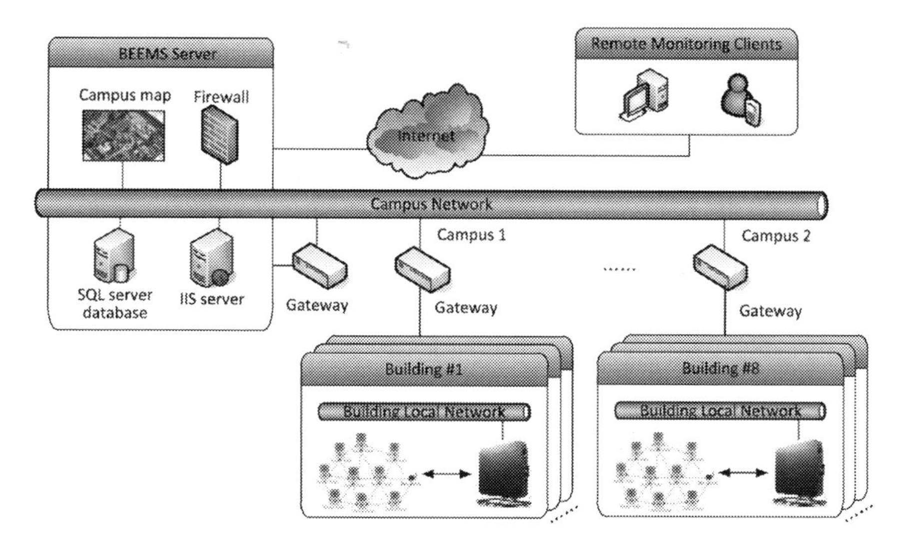

Fig. 5 Architecture of a large scale distributed sensor network for ventilation control [54]

server-client architecture to provide the possibility to monitor and control the indoor air quality from a centralized computation unit. The developed architecture is shown in Fig. 5.

In summary, most scientific works about distributed sensor networks for active ventilation control are focused on the measurement of the CO_2 concentration. An advantage of this approach are the cost-efficient and well-engineered sensors. Hence, the development of a large scale ventilation system based on CO_2 measurement is affordable and sufficiently tested.

In order to control the ventilation system of a whole building a large-scale building automation network may be an adequate approach to observe and control the environment concerning the air quality. The pollution concentration of every particular room can be used to adapt the indoor air quality towards the requirements.

3.2.2 Active Heating Systems

Common heating control applications for thermal comfort are based on the analysis of the indoor temperature and humidity. In order to monitor the thermal comfort with increased accuracy, Torresani et al. [72] designed a distributed wireless sensor network which measures the air flow speed and radiant temperature in addition to temperature and humidity. First results suggest that the system is able to determine the thermal comfort more accurately.

Furthermore, the ability to predict the temperature and the thermal comfort to the purpose of anticipatory control is another issue of recent scientific work. Robol

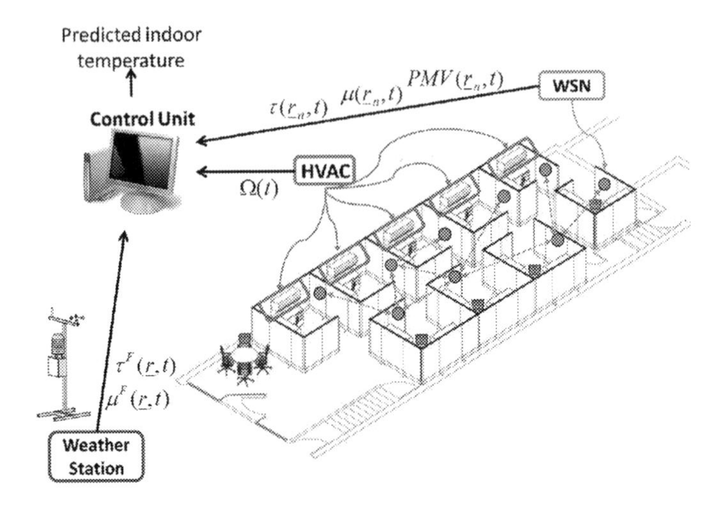

Fig. 6 Architecture of a predictive wireless sensor network for heating control [59]

et al. [59] combine the weather forecast, the predicted mean vote (PMV), and the heating system itself. The system contains 19 wireless sensors, which communicate via ZigBee protocol, a weather station to forecast the thermal influence of the outdoor environment and several radiators. An overview of the system's architecture is shown in Fig. 6. The computation of the multidimensional data is done with a support vector regression algorithm to identify relations between input and output parameter.

Apart from the control of the general temperature, the compensation of temperature differences within the building environment is another issue for heating systems [90]. Differing temperatures inside a building environment can lead to areas with undesired temperature, which have a negative effect on the thermal sensation. An intelligent heating network can measure the temperature at various locations within the building environment to avoid these differences. With the information about occurring differences an intelligent heating system is able to regulate the distributed heating spots to compensate differing temperature areas. Therefore, a computational fluid dynamics model was created to determine the influence of the particular radiators towards the different zones. Such a system requires a heating network with a huge amount of network nodes to cover large areas.

Moreover, Guillemin and Morel [33] combined the control of radiators with an automatic shading system. The shading has a significant effect on the thermal sensation and influences the thermal condition. Hence, these approaches show the requirement of large-scale distributed networks to control every factor which influences the thermal sensation and inhabitant's state of health.

3.2.3 Active Lighting Systems

Active lighting control aims to provide enough light to satisfy the inhabitant's preferences. The fulfillment of lighting preferences directly affects the mood of the inhabitant, which in turn affects well-being and health [78]. The inhabitant's preferences are set prior to the activation of the system. To be aware of uncertainties and to observe the light distribution, distributed photosensitive sensors are used. Wen and Agogino [82] followed this approach and developed a wireless network. The system consists of wireless light sources and wireless sensors to measure the illuminance at different locations. In summary, this approach is able to secure the preferred illuminance within the whole environment even if disruptive outside influences occur.

Based on these findings novel control algorithms were developed to influence the inhabitant's health with adequate lighting. In this context, a lighting network with dynamic light sources was constructed in healthcare facilities to test the effect of the adjusted lighting [1]. The results of the tests showed a general appreciation for the dynamic lighting system. Positive health effects were not observed because of too low illuminance levels during the test phase. This and previous studies proved that the illuminance level is a major factor for lighting control in order to achieve environments with positive health effect [39, 64, 76].

3.3 Adaptive Healthcare Applications

The following examples represent the proceedings in the development of adaptive healthcare applications separated in ventilation systems, heating systems and lighting systems.

3.3.1 Adaptive Ventilation Systems

The ventilation control is able to influence the inhabitant significantly. Hodgson and Murphy [37] summarize several studies, which suggest the effect of different ventilation configurations specifically on patients with respiratory impairments.

A ventilation system which specifically involves inhabitants with respiratory diseases is presented by Fong and Fong [27]. Their system combines a body area network for health monitoring with a building automation network for the measurement of indoor air quality. Moreover, the system is connected with a server for medical observation for abnormality detection. In detail, heart and respiratory rates are used to estimate the inhabitant's state of health and the VOC concentration is monitored to determine the indoor air quality.

Melikov [48] pointed out that a decentralized ventilation system could be an energy efficient solution to supply the inhabitant with an individualized amount of fresh air. The idea behind this approach is that the ventilation is controlled based on the inhabitant's location. Therefore, locations where the inhabitant spends the most time, like work places or seats, have to be equipped with unobtrusive fans and exhausts. In conjunction with an identification system, the directed ventilation is able to adapt the local air change rate individually for every inhabitant. Directed ventilation systems may therefore consist of large networks of fans and exhausts, localization sensors, and identification sensors. Specifically for the implementation of a directed ventilation system in use-cases like office blocks or hospitals, the amount of connected devices is huge, which comes with an increase in computation and communication complexity.

Similarly, Taheri et al. [70] developed a directed ventilation system. Beside these directed fans, the network consists of sensors for the measurement of air temperature, humidity and CO_2 concentration. The results of a short-term study concerning the perceived indoor air quality of the system show minor improvements.

3.3.2 Adaptive Heating Systems

An example for an adaptive heating system is designed by Dovjak et al. [20]. The system's objective is to establish differing heating zones within a hospital room to satisfy the thermal requirements of different patients. In particular burn patients are addressed by the presented system because of their special requirements towards the thermal conditions. Therefore, the scientists created special heating panels to individually regulate the area beyond the panels. To compare the configuration for burn patients and nurses or visitors the particular PMV values are calculated. The thermal condition, which effects the burn patient positively, is rated with a poor PMV value. Hence, environmental conditions with positive health effect are not linked to the thermal sensation in special situations.

Moreover, Feldmeier and Paradiso [25] used a wearable device within a wireless sensor and actuator network to adapt the temperature based on the inhabitant's activity and presence. The wearable device is furthermore an input possibility to rate the thermal condition as hot, neutral and cold. A study with 20 subjects was performed and the comfort achieved by the new control method was rated as enhanced in comparison with the usual system.

One recent field of research is the prediction of the inhabitant's thermal sensation. The inhabitant's perception of the indoor temperature indicates the effect of the current temperature on comfort and health of the inhabitant. Hence, the estimation of the thermal sensation can be used to regulate the temperature according to the inhabitant's requirements. To predict the thermal sensation, various input parameters, like solar radiation and temperature, are analyzed [26]. Multiple complex algorithms, like neural networks or fuzzy controller, are usable in order to execute the analysis [3]. Heating control and air conditioning applications use the predicted thermal sensation to quickly react on environmental changes with the purpose to secure the inhabitant's comfort and health.

Ferreira et al. [26] arranged a large-scale wireless building automation network within a university campus to implement a predictive control algorithm for thermal

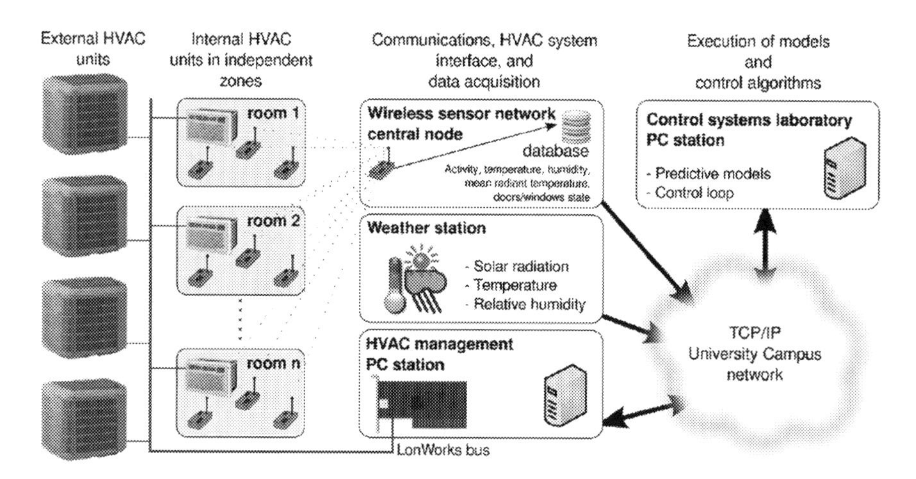

Fig. 7 Architecture of a system for predictive heating control [26]

comfort. Four rooms were equipped with wireless sensors for temperature, air humidity, the state of windows and doors and activity via a passive infra-red sensor. These sensors transmit the acquired data to a centralized computation unit. This central node is connected with the sensor devices via TCP/IP network. Moreover, each room contains its own ventilation and heating unit. Hence, the environmental factors are regulated separately for each room. A PC station manages these separate units and communicates via a LonWorks communication bus. The whole architecture is shown in Fig. 7.

This architecture is used to predict the thermal sensation by the application of an artificial neural network. An advantage of artificial neural networks is that complex non-obvious relations can be identified by the algorithm. But the fact that the algorithm works like a "black-box" and the results cannot be reconstructed is a disadvantage. Furthermore, a major challenge during the design of artificial neural networks for the prediction of thermal sensation is to find the balance between accuracy and execution time. It is of importance to have short execution times to establish a system which is applicable in practice.

3.3.3 Adaptive Lighting Systems

Pan et al. [52] developed a wireless sensor network for adaptive lighting control. The scientists combined photosensitive sensors with wearable devices and two kinds of light sources. The photosensitive sensors' purpose is the measurement of the current light intensity. The wearable device is used for the activity detection and localization of the inhabitant. The information about the inhabitant's location, his set preferences and the current lighting intensity are the base for the regulation of the particular lighting sources.

In a following step, the building automation network for adaptive lighting control was extended by an intelligent lamp which adjusts its position based on the inhabitant's requirements [87]. In order to observe and control the lighting of a whole building, multiple photosensitive sensors and sensors for inhabitant localization are necessary. Hence, for far-reaching adaptive lighting systems adequate architectures and communication methods have to be applied.

The objective of adaptive lighting systems is the adaption of the light based on the requirements of the inhabitant. Therefore, Grigore et al. [32] developed a system, which uses psycho-physical information for lighting control. They used the electro-dermal activity and the electrocardiogram. Hence, the heart rate and the skin conductance are the chosen features to adapt the lighting control. During the tests with two elderly subjects the scientists adapted the light intensity and color temperature to research the effect on the psycho-physical information. Their results show that it is possible to detect the state of relaxation or activation via the measurement of skin conductance and heart rate. The scientists identified the skin conductance response as the most useful parameter for activity estimation. This approach suggests the possibilities of adaptive lighting systems to influence the inhabitant based on the current condition.

4 Opportunities and Limitations

The presented scientific works give a meaningful overview of recent efforts spent on health related building automation networks and control. Although the inhabitant and his preferences are included in the majority of cases, the potential of building automation networks towards healthcare is not yet fully utilized.

The combination of activity recognition and control algorithms for adaptive building automation networks is not widespread. Moreover, varying physical and mental health conditions and thereby different requirements regarding the indoor environment are not in the focus of recent scientific work.

However, the inhabitant's preferences are an important part of several approaches for environmental control. Fanger [24] used findings from psychophysical measurements to develop a method for air supply control years ago. Moreover, the perception of thermal comfort is included in international guidelines, in terms of the PMV [17]. The calculation of the PMV results in an estimation of the amount of persons probably dissatisfied by the current environmental factors. These human-centered approaches are used by several building automation networks for the regulation of the environmental factors [26, 42, 44, 70].

Nevertheless, the approaches are limited because special requirements are not concerned. It has been shown that the perception of life quality is directly influenced by diseases like chronic obstructive pulmonary disease (COPD) [66]. Furthermore, it is suggested that the self-reported health status from COPD patients is related to the perceived indoor air quality, rather than to the measured pollutant concentrations [55]. However, current building automation networks for ventilation control do not involve those circumstances.

Similar to the indoor air quality, the perception of the thermal environment differs for example between healthy people and people with physical paralysis [53]. Accordingly, also building automation networks for heating applications mostly do not involve special requirements of the inhabitant.

Hence, there are various opportunities to develop approaches for the design of more adaptive and individual building automation networks. Beside medical effects of environmental factors, the perception and its influence on the well-being and health of the inhabitant should be considered. Therefore, psychophysical experiments are useful to fill the knowledge gap concerning the special requirements on environmental factors from people with impairments. The resulting design concept for adaptive health related building automation networks is shown in Fig. 8. Initial point of the design concept is the inhabitant and the research on the influence of occurring physical or mental impairments on the perception and medical sensitivity towards the environmental factors. The results from this research are afterwards used to provide the building automation network with the inhabitant's requirements. These requirements are integrated into the control process of the building environment. The control process analyses the current condition of the environmental factors through the data retrieved from an adequate distributed sensor network.

Consequently, the differences between the requirements of the inhabitant's perception and medical condition and the current building environment are compensated through actuator networks. This process leads to an adapted building environment with adequate environmental factors based on the current condition of the inhabitant. Finally, the adjusted environmental factors influence the well-being and health of the inhabitant positively and potentially avoid the worsening of

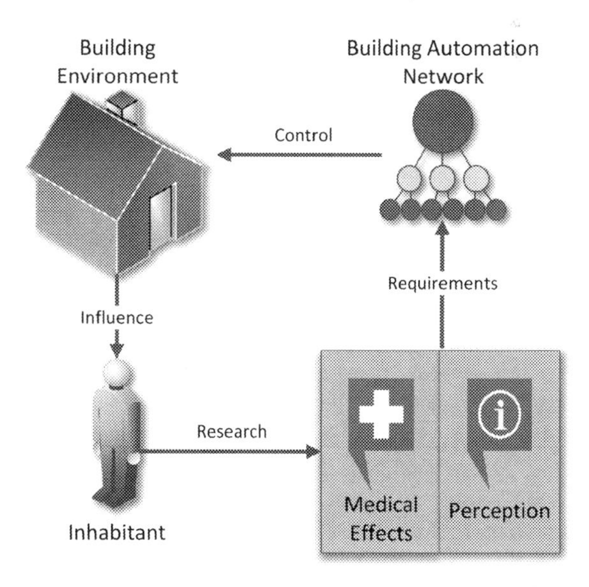

Fig. 8 Concept for the design of more adaptive and health related building automation networks

present diseases. In summary, building automation networks potentially provide the opportunity to establish far-reaching and all-encompassing healthcare applications.

Furthermore, the proceedings in communication and computation technologies established an ideal basis for the monitoring of all relevant environmental factors within a large-scale building automation network [3, 4, 10]. There exist multiple examples for the design of large-scale sensor networks and big data handling. In this context, machine learning models and computational intelligence are promising methods.

Moreover, several approaches were developed to design a gateway connecting the building automation system with medical support and relatives. Building automation networks profit from the use of well tested communication standards, which provide the possibility to involve multiple devices without complications. These improvements open up new possibilities to more holistic applications for healthcare in the building environment.

In this context, creating a connection between the home environments of the neighborhood is an opportunity to build up a widespread network for healthcare. The approach to connect the neighborhood buildings within a network is recently followed by several scientific works addressing the energy efficiency [22, 47, 89]. The achieved proceedings and developed technologies can be adjusted to create a network which fulfills all requirements of a networked healthcare neighborhood. The advantage of a smart and connected neighborhood is that possibly needed aid is always nearby. Moreover, in particular elderly inhabitants often suffer from decreasing social activities. A connected neighborhood has the ability to build a bridge to nearby neighbors and therefore to support social activities.

In addition, the connection of further systems, like medical devices or wearables, with building automation networks is an opportunity to design enhanced healthcare applications. Consequently, interfaces using robust and fast communication methods have to be used to establish a connection. In particular, clothes and watches, which are proposed for fitness activities, are recently upgraded with sensors for the monitoring of heart rate or skin conductance. Additionally, these devices often contain gyroscopes for activity detection. Because of the design and the underlying objective as sportswear and fitness watches, these products are not characterized as medical product. Thus, the acceptance of healthcare applications containing smart clothes or watches is potentially great. Beside the inconspicuousness, no help of experts is required for positioning issues or similar problems. The wearable devices are an opportunity to develop novel approaches in building automation control. The sensor data is useful to react on physical activity or to monitor the inhabitant's health. In this context, Dittmar et al. [18] developed smart clothes and a glove to monitor various physiological parameters. The devices are used for the research into the physical reaction during different situations. Amongst others, the effect of varying environmental factors towards the physical parameters is a current research topic of the scientists.

In summary, there is a large potential to create more adaptive building automation networks based on the recent proceedings in communication and computation methods. Specifically, an individualization of the regulation of the environmental factors will lead to positive health effects.

5 Recommendations

During the design of building automation networks the compliance with communication standards is an important aspect. The building automation networks are significantly easier to extend if they use open and established communication protocols. Hence, in the case that additional nodes within the network are required, sensors or actuators can be easily integrated. The practice to apply established communication protocols simplifies the integration of other systems like wearables, medical devices and car systems. The networking between the building automation system and additional systems may lead to more complex and all-encompassing applications addressing health related issues. An overview about the different wireless machine-to-machine communication standards is given by Zhang et al. [89]. The different standards are ordered in subnetworks with varying application purposes. The ZigBee protocol is thereby dedicated to the building automation networks, which is consistent with the examples described above.

Another challenge for large-scale building automation networks is the handling of the huge amount of data, which are received from the multiple nodes. The interpretation of the data requires intelligent algorithms to control the building automation network based on the sensor data. Different already applied algorithms are described by Dounis and Caraiscos [19]. In order to create an efficient building automation network a computation method has to be chosen which is adequate concerning the particular network components, the environment and the desired application.

A complex challenge for the designers of building automation systems is to be aware of all environmental factors and their dependencies. As mentioned before, the perception of the environmental condition is influenced by several different factors at the same time. In order to fulfill the requirements of the inhabitant as many as possible factors should be considered in the control process.

Another aspect with relevance for the design of building automation networks is the fact that scientific research reveals more and more knowledge about the effect of environmental factors towards the inhabitant's perception and health. Consequently, there should be a novel tendency towards the development of more adaptive building automation networks. In this context, the proceedings in the field of psychophysics and medical research should be included during the design of future building automation applications. Such applications presuppose the monitoring of the mental and physical health and current activity of the inhabitant. Furthermore, existing standards concerning environmental conditions have to be respected but should be enhanced with the gained knowledge from research.

The regulation of the environmental factors via building automation networks to create an adapted environment with positive health effects is potentially able to reduce health related costs for the society.

These environments make a contribution to the decrease of occurring disease symptoms and effect the avoidance of disease worsening positively. Positive long-term health improvements may lead to a shortening of absence periods caused by illness, which results in a relief of costs for health insurance funds.

The development of building automation applications with the focus on health and comfort does not contradict energy issues automatically. In particular presence-based systems are in many cases used for healthcare issues and have the potential to consider the energy efficiency, because the systems conserve energy within unoccupied areas. Accordingly, the top priority should not be assigned to energy efficiency but rather to health related effects.

References

1. Aarts, M.P., Aries, M.B., Straathof, J., van Hoof, J.: Dynamic lighting systems in psychogeriatric care facilities in the netherlands: a quantitative and qualitative analysis of stakeholders responses and applied technology. Indoor and Built Environment p. 1420326X14532387 (2014)
2. Aguirre, E., Led, S., Lopez-Iturri, P., Azpilicueta, L., Serrano, L., Falcone, F.: Implementation of context aware e-health environments based on social sensor networks. Sensors 16(3), 310 (2016)
3. Ahmad, M.W., Mourshed, M., Yuce, B., Rezgui, Y.: Computational intelligence techniques for hvac systems: A review. In: Building Simulation, vol. 9, pp. 359–398. Springer (2016)
4. Alemdar, H., Ersoy, C.: Wireless sensor networks for healthcare: A survey. Computer Networks 54(15), 2688–2710 (2010)
5. Arcelus, A., Jones, M.H., Goubran, R., Knoefel, F.: Integration of smart home technologies in a health monitoring system for the elderly. In: Advanced Information Networking and Applications Workshops, 2007, AINAW'07. 21st International Conference on, vol. 2, pp. 820–825. IEEE (2007)
6. Barroso, A., Den Brinker, B.: Boosting circadian rhythms with lighting: A model driven approach. Lighting Research and Technology p. 1477153512453667 (2012)
7. Bentayeb, M., Norback, D., Bednarek, M., Bernard, A., Cai, G., Cerrai, S., Eleftheriou, K.K., Gratziou, C., Holst, G.J., Lavaud, F., et al.: Indoor air quality, ventilation and respiratory health in elderly residents living in nursing homes in europe. European Respiratory Journal pp. ERJ–00,824 (2015)
8. Berglund, B., Brunekreef, B., Knöppe, H., Lindvall, T., Maroni, M., Mølhave, L., Skov, P.: Effects of indoor air pollution on human health. Indoor Air 2(1), 2–25 (1992)
9. Bose, S., Hansel, N., Tonorezos, E., Williams, D., Bilderback, A., Breysse, P., Diette, G., McCormack, M.C.: Indoor particulate matter associated with systemic inflammation in copd. Journal of Environmental Protection 6(5), 566 (2015)
10. Chen, M., Wan, J., González, S., Liao, X., Leung, V.C.: A survey of recent developments in home m2m networks. IEEE Communications Surveys & Tutorials 16(1), 98–114 (2014)
11. Cook, D.J., Krishnan, N.C., Rashidi, P.: Activity discovery and activity recognition: A new partnership. IEEE transactions on cybernetics 43(3), 820–828 (2013)

12. Corno, F., Sanaullah, M.: Design-time formal verification for smart environments: An exploratory perspective. In: Journal of Ambient Intelligence and Humanized Computing, vol. 5, pp. 581–599. Springer (2014). DOI 10.1007/s12652-013-0209-4
13. Corno, F., Sanaullah, M.: Modeling and formal verification of smart environments. Security and Communication Networks 7(10), 1582–1598 (2014). DOI 10.1002/sec.794. URL http://dx.doi.org/10.1002/sec.794
14. D. Groth, T. Skandier: Network + Study Guide: Exam N10-003: Fourth Edition. Sybex Inc., Alameda, CA (2006)
15. DIN EN 13779: Lüftung von Nichtwohngebäuden–allgemeine Grundlagen und Anforderungen an Lüftungs-und Klimaanlagen. Berlin: Beuth (2005)
16. DIN EN ISO 16484-2:2016-08: Building automation and control systems (bacs) – part 2: Hardware (iso/dis 16484-2:2016)
17. DIN ISO EN 7730: Ergonomie der thermischen Umgebungsanalyse, Bestimmung und Interpretation der thermischen Behaglichkeit durch Berechnung des PMV-und des PPD-Indexes und Kriterien der lokalen thermischen Behaglichkeit. German version of EN ISO 7730: 2006-05 7730 (2005)
18. Dittmar, A., Meffre, R., De Oliveira, F., Gehin, C., Delhomme, G.: Wearable medical devices using textile and flexible technologies for ambulatory monitoring. In: 2005 IEEE Engineering in Medicine and Biology 27th Annual Conference, pp. 7161–7164. IEEE (2005)
19. Dounis, A.I., Caraiscos, C.: Advanced control systems engineering for energy and comfort management in a building environmental review. Renewable and Sustainable Energy Reviews 13(6), 1246–1261 (2009)
20. Dovjak, M., Shukuya, M., Krainer, A.: Individualisation of personal space in hospital environment. International Journal of Exergy 14(2), 125–155 (2014)
21. Eisenhauer, M., Rosengren, P., Antolin, P.: Hydra: A development platform for integrating wireless devices and sensors into ambient intelligence systems. In: The Internet of Things, pp. 367–373. Springer (2010)
22. Fadlullah, Z.M., Fouda, M.M., Kato, N., Takeuchi, A., Iwasaki, N., Nozaki, Y.: Toward intelligent machine-to-machine communications in smart grid. IEEE Communications Magazine 49(4), 60–65 (2011)
23. Fang, L., Wyon, D., Clausen, G., Fanger, P.O.: Impact of indoor air temperature and humidity in an office on perceived air quality, sbs symptoms and performance. Indoor Air 14(s7), 74–81 (2004)
24. Fanger, P.O.: Introduction of the olf and the decipol units to quantify air pollution perceived by humans indoors and outdoors. Energy and buildings 12(1), 1–6 (1988)
25. Feldmeier, M., Paradiso, J.A.: Personalized hvac control system. In: Internet of Things (IOT), 2010, pp. 1–8. IEEE (2010)
26. Ferreira, P., Ruano, A., Silva, S., Conceicao, E.: Neural networks based predictive control for thermal comfort and energy savings in public buildings. Energy and Buildings 55, 238–251 (2012)
27. Fong, A., Fong, B.: Home telemedicine system for chronic respiratory disease surveillance an automated solution for disease control and management to combat the health impact of indoor air pollution. In: Industrial Electronics and Applications (ICIEA), 2012 7th IEEE Conference on, pp. 472–476. IEEE (2012)
28. Gadzheva, M.: Legal issues in wireless building automation: an eu perspective. International Journal of Law and Information Technology 16(2), 159–175 (2008)
29. Gagge, A., Stolwijk, J., Saltin, B.: Comfort and thermal sensations and associated physiological responses during exercise at various ambient temperatures. Environmental Research 2(3), 209–229 (1969)
30. Gao, S., Hoogendoorn, M.: Using Evolutionary Algorithms to Personalize Controllers in Ambient Intelligence, pp. 1–11. Springer International Publishing, Cham (2015)

31. Gasparrini, A., Armstrong, B.: Time series analysis on the health effects of temperature: advancements and limitations. Environmental research 110(6), 633–638 (2010)
32. Grigore, O., Gavat, I., Cotescu, M., Grigore, C.: Stochastic algorithms for adaptive lighting control using psychophysiological features. International Journal of Biology and Biomedical Engineering 2, 9–18 (2008)
33. Guillemin, A., Morel, N.: An innovative lighting controller integrated in a self-adaptive building control system. Energy and buildings 33(5), 477–487 (2001)
34. Guillet, S., Bouchard, B., Bouzouane, A.: Safe and automatic addition of fault tolerance for smart homes dedicated to people with disabilities. In: Ravulakollu, Khan, Abraham (ed.) Trends in Ambient Intelligent Systems, Studies in Computational Intelligence, vol. 633, pp. 87–116. Springer, Berlin, Heidelberg (2016). DOI 10.1007/978-3-319-30184-6_4
35. Jaakkola, H., Thalheim, B.: Architecture-driven modelling methodologies. Frontiers in Artificial Intelligence and Applications (225), 97–116 (2010). DOI 10.3233/978-1-60750-689-8-97
36. Hansel, N.N., McCormack, M.C., Belli, A.J., Matsui, E.C., Peng, R.D., Aloe, C., Paulin, L., Williams, D.L., Diette, G.B., Breysse, P.N.: In-home air pollution is linked to respiratory morbidity in former smokers with chronic obstructive pulmonary disease. American journal of respiratory and critical care medicine 187(10), 1085–1090 (2013)
37. Hodgson, L.E., Murphy, P.B.: Update on clinical trials in home mechanical ventilation. Journal of thoracic disease 8(2), 255 (2016)
38. Huisman, E., Morales, E., van Hoof, J., Kort, H.: Healing environment: A review of the impact of physical environmental factors on users. Building and environment 58, 70–80 (2012). DOI 10.1016/j.buildenv.2012.06.016
39. Ichimori, A., Tsukasaki, K., Koyama, E.: Measuring illuminance and investigating methods for its quantification among elderly people living at home in japan to study the relationship between illuminance and physical and mental health. Geriatrics & gerontology international 13(3), 798–806 (2013)
40. Kephart, J.O., Chess, D.M.: The vision of autonomic computing. Computer 36(1), 41–50 (2003). DOI 10.1109/MC.2003.1160055
41. Khajenasiri, I., Virgone, J., Gielen, G.: A presence-based control strategy solution for hvac systems. In: Consumer Electronics (ICCE), 2015 IEEE International Conference on, pp. 620–622. IEEE (2015)
42. Kolokotsa, D., Tsiavos, D., Stavrakakis, G., Kalaitzakis, K., Antonidakis, E.: Advanced fuzzy logic controllers design and evaluation for buildings occupants thermal–visual comfort and indoor air quality satisfaction. Energy and buildings 33(6), 531–543 (2001)
43. Krishnan, N.C., Cook, D.J.: Activity recognition on streaming sensor data. Pervasive and mobile computing 10, 138–154 (2014)
44. Kumar, A., Hancke, G.P.: An energy-efficient smart comfort sensing system based on the ieee 1451 standard for green buildings. IEEE Sensors Journal 14(12), 4245–4252 (2014)
45. Liu, W., Lian, Z., Liu, Y.: Heart rate variability at different thermal comfort levels. European journal of applied physiology 103(3), 361–366 (2008)
46. Lloyd, E., McCormack, C., McKeever, M., Syme, M.: The effect of improving the thermal quality of cold housing on blood pressure and general health: a research note. Journal of epidemiology and community health 62(9), 793–797 (2008)
47. López, G., Moura, P., Moreno, J.I., De Almeida, A.: Enersip: M2M-based platform to enable energy efficiency within energy-positive neighbourhoods. In: Computer Communications Workshops (INFOCOM WKSHPS), 2011 IEEE Conference on, pp. 217–222. IEEE (2011)
48. Melikov, A.K.: Advanced air distribution: improving health and comfort while reducing energy use. Indoor air 26(1), 112–124 (2016)
49. Mendes, T.D., Godina, R., Rodrigues, E.M., Matias, J.C., Catalao, J.P.: Smart home communication technologies and applications: Wireless protocol assessment for home area network resources. Energies 8(7), 7279–7311 (2015)

50. Merz, Hansemann, Hübner: Building Automation: Communication systems with EIB/KNX, LON und BACnet. Signals and Communication Technology. Springer, Berlin, Heidelberg (2009). DOI 10.1007/978-3-540-88829-1
51. Moreno, M., Santa, J., Zamora, M.A., Skarmeta, A.F.: A holistic iot-based management platform for smart environments. In: Communications (ICC), 2014 IEEE International Conference on, pp. 3823–3828. IEEE (2014)
52. Pan, M.S., Yeh, L.W., Chen, Y.A., Lin, Y.H., Tseng, Y.C.: A wsn-based intelligent light control system considering user activities and profiles. IEEE Sensors Journal 8(10), 1710–1721 (2008)
53. Parsons, K.C.: The effects of gender, acclimation state, the opportunity to adjust clothing and physical disability on requirements for thermal comfort. Energy and Buildings 34(6), 593–599 (2002)
54. Peng, C., Qian, K., Wang, C.: Design and application of a voc-monitoring system based on a zigbee wireless sensor network. IEEE Sensors Journal 15(4), 2255–2268 (2015)
55. Piro, F.N., Madsen, C., Næss, Ø., Nafstad, P., Claussen, B.: A comparison of self reported air pollution problems and gis-modeled levels of air pollution in people with and without chronic diseases. Environmental Health 7(1), 1 (2008)
56. Rahmani, A.M., Thanigaivelan, N.K., Gia, T.N., Granados, J., Negash, B., Liljeberg, P., Tenhunen, H.: Smart e-health gateway: Bringing intelligence to internet-of-things based ubiquitous healthcare systems. In: Consumer Communications and Networking Conference (CCNC), 2015 12th Annual IEEE, pp. 826–834. IEEE (2015)
57. Ransing, R.S., Rajput, M.: Smart home for elderly care, based on wireless sensor network. In: Nascent Technologies in the Engineering Field (ICNTE), 2015 International Conference on, pp. 1–5. IEEE (2015)
58. Raynal, M.: A look at basics of distributed computing. In: 2016 IEEE 36th International Conference on Distributed Computing Systems (ICDCS), pp. 1–11 (2016). DOI 10.1109/ICDCS.2016.109
59. Robol, F., Viani, F., Giarola, E., Massa, A.: Wireless sensors for distributed monitoring of energy-efficient smart buildings. In: Microwave Symposium (MMS), 2015 IEEE 15th Mediterranean, pp. 1–4. IEEE (2015)
60. Rosenthal, N.E., Sack, D.A., Carpenter, C.J., Parry, B.L., Mendelson, W.B., Wehr, T.A.: Antidepressant effects of light in seasonal affective disorder. Am J Psychiatry 142(2), 163–170 (1985)
61. Sánchez-Pi, N., Mangina, E., Carbó, J., Molina, J.M.: Multi-agent System (MAS) Applications in Ambient Intelligence (AmI) Environments, pp. 493–500. Springer, Berlin, Heidelberg (2010)
62. Shikder, S., Mourshed, M., Price, A.: Therapeutic lighting design for the elderly: a review. Perspectives in public health 132(6), 282–291 (2012)
63. Skubic, M., Guevara, R.D., Rantz, M.: Automated health alerts using in-home sensor data for embedded health assessment. IEEE journal of translational engineering in health and medicine 3, 1–11 (2015)
64. Smolders, K.C., De Kort, Y.A., Cluitmans, P.: A higher illuminance induces alertness even during office hours: Findings on subjective measures, task performance and heart rate measures. Physiology & Behavior 107(1), 7–16 (2012)
65. Sprint, G., Cook, D., Fritz, R., Schmitter-Edgecombe, M.: Detecting health and behavior change by analyzing smart home sensor data. In: 2016 IEEE International Conference on Smart Computing (SMARTCOMP), pp. 1–3. IEEE (2016)
66. Stahl, E., Lindberg, A., Jansson, S.A., Rönmark, E., Svensson, K., Andersson, F., Löfdahl, C. G., Lundbäck, B.: Health-related quality of life is related to copd disease severity. Health and quality of life outcomes 3(1), 1 (2005)
67. Sundell, J., Levin, H., Nazaroff, W.W., Cain, W.S., Fisk, W.J., Grimsrud, D.T., Gyntelberg, F., Li, Y., Persily, A., Pickering, A., et al.: Ventilation rates and health: multidisciplinary review of the scientific literature. Indoor air 21(3), 191–204 (2011)

68. Surie, D., Laguionie, O., Pederson, T.: Wireless sensor networking of everyday objects in a smart home environment. In: Intelligent Sensors, Sensor Networks and Information Processing, 2008. ISSNIP 2008. International Conference on, pp. 189–194. IEEE (2008)
69. Suryadevara, N.K., Mukhopadhyay, S.C.: Wireless sensor network based home monitoring system for wellness determination of elderly. Sensors Journal, IEEE 12(6), 1965–1972 (2012)
70. Taheri, M., Schuss, M., Fail, A., Mahdavi, A.: A performance assessment of an office space with displacement, personal, and natural ventilation systems. In: Building Simulation, vol. 9, pp. 89–100. Springer (2016)
71. Tapia, D.I., Alonso, R.S., García, Ó., Corchado, J.M., Bajo, J.: Wireless sensor networks, real-time locating systems and multi-agent systems: The perfect team. In: FUSION, vol. 2013, pp. 2177–2184 (2013)
72. Torresani, W., Battisti, N., Maglione, A., Brunelli, D., Macii, D.: A multi-sensor wireless solution for indoor thermal comfort monitoring. In: Environmental Energy and Structural Monitoring Systems (EESMS), 2013 IEEE Workshop on, pp. 1–6. IEEE (2013)
73. Tunca, C., Alemdar, H., Ertan, H., Incel, O.D., Ersoy, C.: Multimodal wireless sensor network-based ambient assisted living in real homes with multiple residents. Sensors 14(6), 9692–9719 (2014)
74. Valera, A.C., Tan, H.P., Bai, L.: Improving the sensitivity of unobtrusive inactivity detection in sensor-enabled homes for the elderly. In: 2016 IEEE International Conference on Pervasive Computing and Communication Workshops (PerCom Workshops), pp. 1–6. IEEE (2016)
75. Valiente-Rocha, P.A., Lozano-Tello, A.: Ontology and SWRL-Based Learning Model for Home Automation Controlling, pp. 79–86. Springer, Berlin, Heidelberg (2010)
76. Van Hoof, J., Schoutens, A., Aarts, M.: High colour temperature lighting for institutionalised older people with dementia. Building and Environment 44(9), 1959–1969 (2009)
77. VDI 3814:2009-11: Building automation and control systems (bacs)
78. Veitch, J., Newsham, G., Boyce, P., Jones, C.: Lighting appraisal, well-being and performance in open-plan offices: A linked mechanisms approach. Lighting Research and Technology 40(2), 133–151 (2008)
79. Wan, J., Li, D., Zou, C., Zhou, K.: M2M communications for smart city: an event-based architecture. In: Computer and Information Technology (CIT), 2012 IEEE 12th International Conference on, pp. 895–900. IEEE (2012)
80. Wan, J., OGrady, M.J., OHare, G.M.: Dynamic sensor event segmentation for real-time activity recognition in a smart home context. Personal and Ubiquitous Computing 19(2), 287–301 (2015)
81. Wargocki, P., Sundell, J., Bischof, W., Brundrett, G., Fanger, P.O., Gyntelberg, F., Hanssen, S., Harrison, P., Pickering, A., Seppänen, O., et al.: Ventilation and health in non-industrial indoor environments: report from a European multidisciplinary scientific consensus meeting (euroven). Indoor Air 12(2), 113–128 (2002)
82. Wen, Y.J., Agogino, A.M.: Wireless networked lighting systems for optimizing energy savings and user satisfaction. In: Wireless Hive Networks Conference, 2008. WHNC 2008. IEEE, pp. 1–7. IEEE (2008)
83. World Health Organization and others: WHO guidelines for indoor air quality: selected pollutants. WHO (2010)
84. Yang, C.T., Liao, C.J., Liu, J.C., Den, W., Chou, Y.C., Tsai, J.J.: Construction and application of an intelligent air quality monitoring system for healthcare environment. Journal of medical systems 38(2), 1–10 (2014)
85. Yao, Y., Lian, Z., Liu, W., Jiang, C., Liu, Y., Lu, H.: Heart rate variation and electroencephalograph–the potential physiological factors for thermal comfort study. Indoor air 19(2), 93–101 (2009)
86. Ye, J., Stevenson, G., Dobson, S.: Kcar: A knowledge-driven approach for concurrent activity recognition. Pervasive and Mobile Computing 19, 47–70 (2015)
87. Yeh, L.W., Lu, C.Y., Kou, C.W., Tseng, Y.C., Yi, C.W.: Autonomous light control by wireless sensor and actuator networks. IEEE Sensors Journal 10(6), 1029–1041 (2010)

88. Zentralverband Elektrotechnik- und Elektronikindustrie e.V.: Handbuch Geb¨audesystemtechnik: Grundlagen, 4 edn. Europäischer Installations Bus. ZVEI (1997)
89. Zhang, Y., Yu, R., Xie, S., Yao, W., Xiao, Y., Guizani, M.: Home m2m networks: architectures, standards, and qos improvement. IEEE Communications Magazine 49(4), 44–52 (2011)
90. Zhou, P., Huang, G., Zhang, L., Tsang, K.F.: Wireless sensor network based monitoring system for a large-scale indoor space: data process and supply air allocation optimization. Energy and Buildings 103, 365–374 (2015)

Part II
Data Quality and Large-Scale Machine Learning Models for Smart Healthcare

Electronic Health Records: Benefits and Challenges for Data Quality

Abdul Kader Saiod, Darelle van Greunen and Alida Veldsman

Abstract Data quality (DQ) issues in Electronic Health Records (EHRs) are a noticeable trend to improve the introduction of an adaptive framework for interoperability and standards to large-scale health Database Management Systems (DBMS). In addition, EHR technology provides portfolio management systems that allow Health Care Organisations (HCOs) to deliver higher quality of care to their patients than possible with paper-based records. The EHRs are in high demand for HCOs to run their daily services as increasing numbers of huge datasets occur every day. An efficient EHRs system reduces data redundancy as well as system application failures and increases the possibility to draw all necessary reports. Improving DQ to achieve benefits through EHRs is neither low-cost nor easy. However, different HCOs have several standards and different major systems, which have emerged as critical issues and practical challenges. One of the main challenges in EHRs is the inherent difficulty to coherently manage incompatible and sometimes inconsistent data structures from diverse heterogeneous sources. As a result, the interventions to overcome these barriers and challenges, including the provision of EHRs as it pertains to DQ will combine features to search, extract, filter, clean and integrate data to ensure that users can coherently create new consistent data sets.

Keywords Electronic Health Records (EHRs) · Data Quality (DQ) · Health Care Organisations (HCOs) · Database Management Systems (DBMS) · Kilometres (km) · Information and Communication Technologies (ICT) · Health Information Technology (HIT) · Quality Assessment Tools (QAT)

A.K. Saiod (✉) · D. van Greunen · A. Veldsman
Nelson Mandela Metropolitan University (NMMU), Port Elizabeth, South Africa
e-mail: saiodkader@gmail.com
URL: http://www.nmmu.ac.za/DarelleVanGreunen

D. van Greunen
e-mail: Darelle.vanGreunen@nmmu.ac.za

A. Veldsman
e-mail: Alida.Veldsman@nmmu.ac.za

© Springer International Publishing AG 2017

S.U. Khan et al. (eds.), *Handbook of Large-Scale Distributed Computing in Smart Healthcare*, Scalable Computing and Communications,
DOI 10.1007/978-3-319-58280-1_6

1 Introduction

Electronic Health Records (EHRs) refer to implemented structured digital manifestations of real-time, patient-centred health records [1]. EHRs are considered as one of health care's innovation heuristic items and are widely adopted over HCOs and are becoming an important mechanism to perform their daily services [32, 40]. The secure EHR systems provide information available instantly and accurately to the authorized users, so user can coherently create new consistence of data sets [28, 61]. In general, the EHRs is the problem of combining health data that reside at different sources and providing accurate, comprehensive up-to-date patient history [26, 58]. Improvements in the data quality have brought about efficiency, scalability and safety in the implementation of a large scale healthcare DBMS [30]. Health data can therefore be composed, managed by authorised user and consulted by authorised providers from across multiple HCOs nation or global wide and can be shared across them. The EHRs include an enormous range of patient data set, including patient details, history, references, medication, immunisation, allergies, radiology report including images, laboratory data and test reports, admission and discharge details, personal statistics like Body Mass Index (BMI), blood pressure, sugar level etc. These datasets are electronically stored in database as narrative (free text) or encrypted data. The EHR databases are structured to store accurately and securely health information over the time. It can reduce data replication risk as all access points are retrieving data from the main data server and as well as reduces lots of paper work. The principle of data replication is to share information between multiple resources. The replication reduces fault tolerance, increase high accessibility and reliability. Many distributed database systems are using replication to avoid single access point failure and high traffic. It can be possible to dynamically improve load-spreading and load-balancing performance by providing replication [63]. Replication supports restoring replicated databases to the same server and database from which the backup was created [4]. Backup is one of the important processes of database server routine maintenance plans that, to copying and archiving data to an external device. So, backup data can be used to restore the original information after any data loss event. Now a day, electronic data is searchable even from heterogeneous sources and possible to combine them into a single data set. EHRs are even more effective when analysing long term patient medical history [22]. Due to EHRs data being tractable and easy to identify patient preventive visits or screening information, monitor the overall progress, effectively than the paper-based record in HCOs. EHRs improve patient care, increase patient participation, improve care coordination, improve diagnostics and patient outcomes, practice efficiencies for cost savings and allow more case studies for research purposes. Despite the many advantages and functionalities of EHR systems, there are still a considerable number of disadvantages associated with this technology [7]. One of the key concerns is the quality of the data, which includes inconsistency, privacy protection, record synchronisation, lack of standardised terminology, system architecture indexing, deficient standardised terminologies.

The productivity may drop temporally with associated EHRs adaptation as workflows have changed. Several long-standing consequences are emerging from the critical issue of EHRs adaptation [3]. Therefore, it is of utmost importance to advise healthcare organisations to choose the right EHR systems and provide proper setup to establish the complete system to become successful users of EHR systems [42]. Healthcare organizations that are using tangible, augmented EHR systems in their facilities can make better decisions based on the comprehensive information available to them. Improving in healthcare distribution systems are becoming the most consequential technology for medical innovation of all the times. EHR systems exhibit promising potential, which will play the crucial role in HCOs to ensure providing in excellent patient care service, quality management, accurate information, perfect diagnosis, patient information safety, disease management and investigation as advance innovation deftness [56]. In particular, the chapter focuses on large scale DBMS, the data quality introduction of smart interfaces and perfect data mapping in traditional EHR systems as well as mobile and cloud computing. This implies that integrated adoptive EHRs can show inconsistencies, because the data structure and standard from different HCOs are different.

2 Electronic Health Records Background

In our daily lives, data inconsistency may cause with uncertain incidents, if unstructured data composed in the data collection process [35]. An example a web healthcare domain page based on largely composed with free text data. Another example, medical data collections process methods are paper-based and/or archive information.

Information may collect by the data retrieval system and index them by non-text data, so that user can access and find data using special keywords to obtain accurate data sets [41].

Using the non-text data to indexing large text, may lead the data structure design in EHR systems of the other efficient way for accessing and searching information as there are a vast amount of non-text data available [60].

The four latest methods to detect and reduce data inconsistency are:

1. Rough set theory [20];
2. Logic analysis of inconsistent data method [13];
3. Corresponding relational variables of functional dependencies [8];
4. Fuzzy multi-attribute theory [2].

Fuzzy multi-attribute method has ideal performance of the inconsistence data and it can obtain the highest average level of correct information than other solutions [19]. A method for reducing data inconsistency has to be combined with a method for data integration to coherently solve the data inconsistency and the data integration problems simultaneously. The domain ontology may effectively

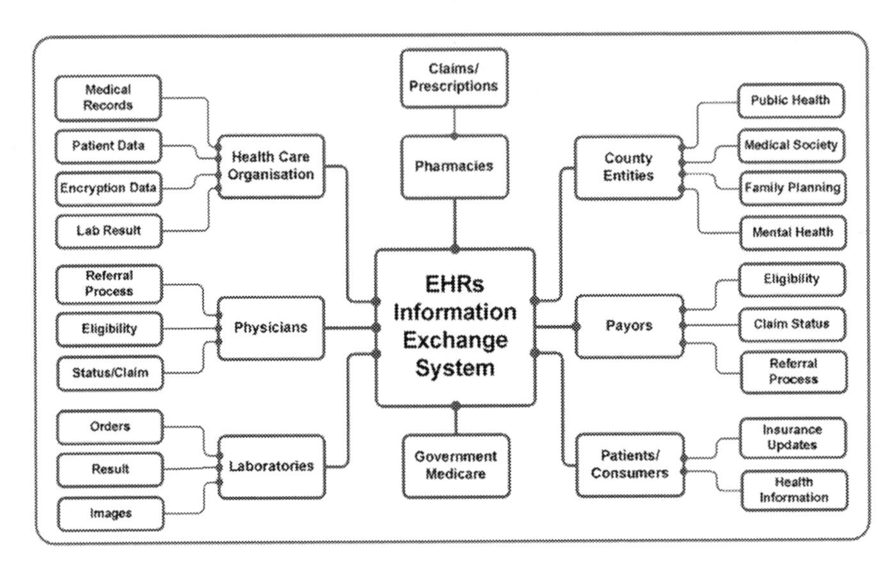

Fig. 1 EHRs information exchange systems architecture

combine data from diverse heterogeneous sources for data integration. The existing ontology data integration methods are, however, not sufficient to implement fuzzy-ontology [24]. The EHRs information exchange systems architecture is shown in Fig. 1.

The benefits of EHRs are numerous when compared to the physician's time and finances, the health benefits for patients and the impact on the environment. The sparse health data may have multi dimensions and it is practically challenging to investigate and analyse for a different reasons such as the heterogeneous features of the system, encompassing quantitative data as well as the categorical information. By the result the random systematic error effect badly and reduces the data quality. Most data integration methods are sufficiently robust to random systematic error for large data sets of input and process. This is commonly identical to bring them on a same scale when using pre-processing principal component analysis and data simplification algorithm [47]. The EHRs systems framework is shown in Fig. 2.

Data quality issues might include patient incorrect unique identification number. Other examples, misplace name, incorrect gender, incorrect date of birth, numeric diagnosis code written in text or saved wrong radiology image, incorrect inserting standard code, such as the National Drug Catalog (NDC) for drugs and derailing bulk analysis (e.g. ICD10 code: International Classification of Diseases Tenth Revision or CPT code: Current Procedural Terminology). Data quality refers to the concepts with immensely large-scale multi dimensional in DBMS, which include not only data search, validation, extract and verification, but also the appropriateness of use to take us even further beyond the traditional concerns with the accuracy of data. The EHR systems design, data structure, aggregation algorithm, simplification methodology and reporting mechanisms highly reflect on data quality.

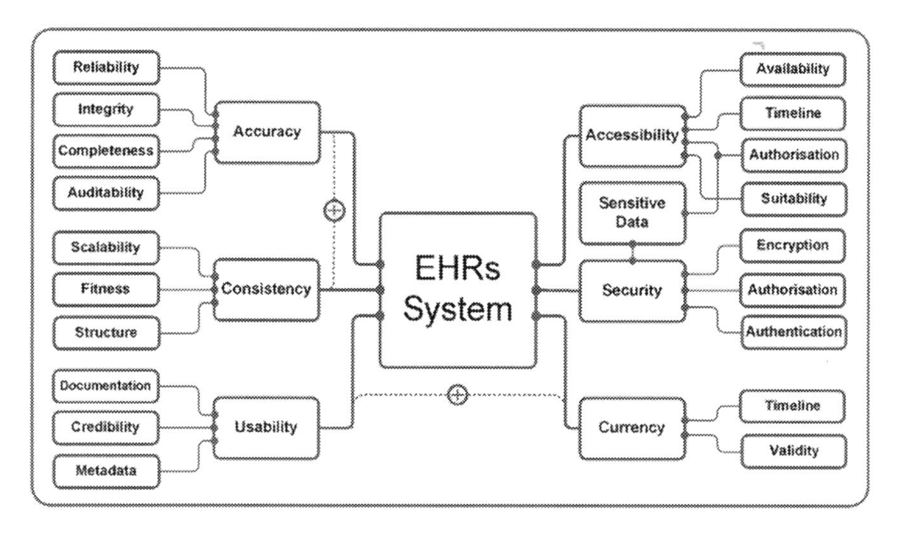

Fig. 2 EHRs systems framework

3 Different Network Architecture and Cloud Computing

In co-operating distributed health information systems and networks, the EHR Systems provided as a lifelong patient record advance towards core applications [6]. Several researchers have shown that only the arbitrary access to patient health information are proximal motive of accurate decision in health care during decision-making and the effective communication between patient care team members [14]. The number of hospitals and clinics are increasing every day, as well as increasing the health information. Health information has digitalised and archived their health record with the universal use of computer and information technology network. There are vast types of wired and wireless network layout, consisting of the type of device including hardware, software, connectivity protocols and communication mode of transmission. It also includes knowledge about the types of networks grouped according to types such as LAN, MAN and WAN. Such as cloud computing, that refers as fast computation and its capability to store large storage space. Now a day cloud computing is a convenient, on-demand network. It is also configurable computing resources to a share group network such as, application, service, server and archive. With the minimal managerial effort cloud computing can be rapidly provided and released the higher productivity. The EHR system can be integrated into cloud computing. Basically, smaller hospital and clinic has limited resources. Cloud computing is to facilitate for those smaller HCO with adequate electronic medical record storage space to provide the exchange and sharing of electronic medical records [12]. Cloud computing has high impact on parallel distributed grid computing systems. The flexibility for the further development of these techniques is recommendable. It is very effective location

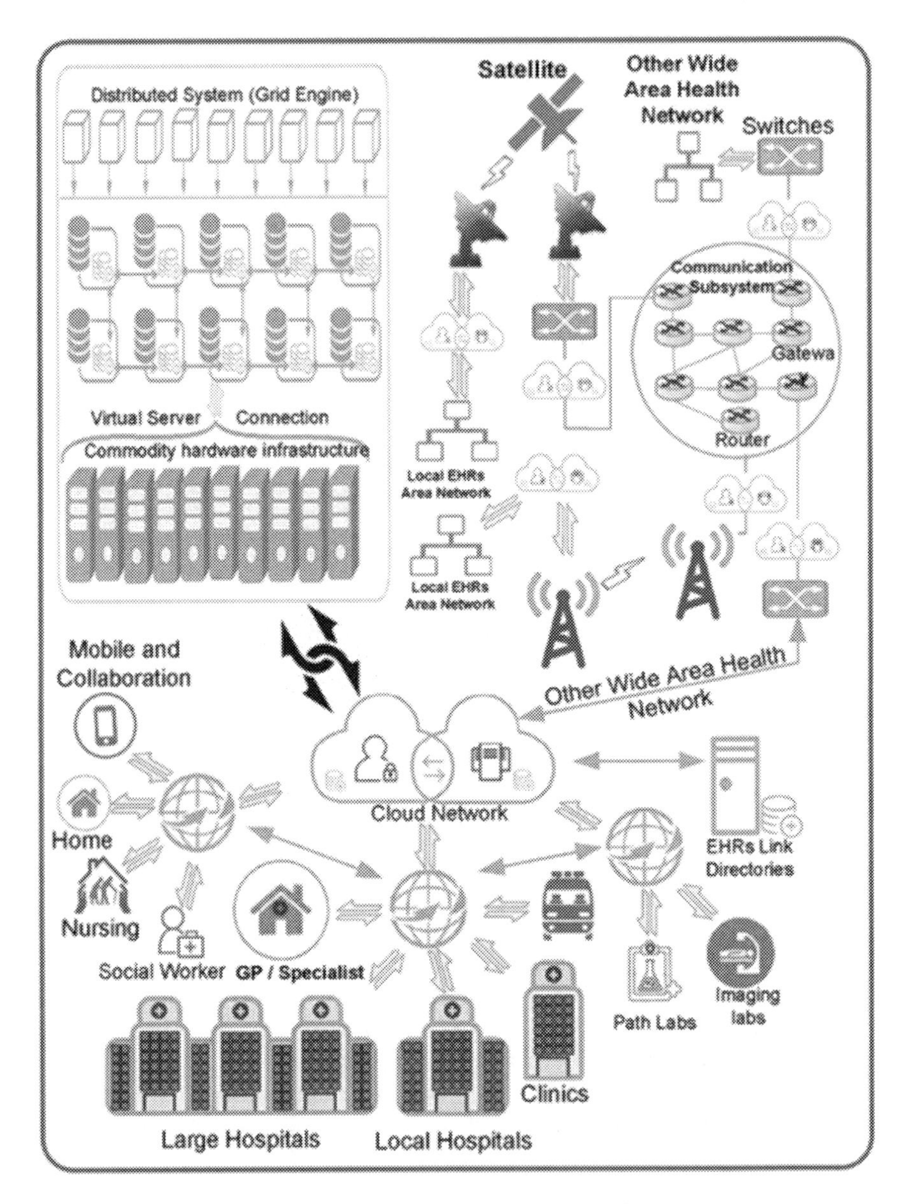

Fig. 3 Large-scale cross platform EHRs system architecture overview

independent technology as well as to enhance the user experiences over the Internet. Now a day, it can provide services for various application scenarios. More and more applications are migrated onto the cloud platform [25].

Mobile Pervasive Healthcare (MPH) service is another innovative technology in EHR system that can provide a wide range of location independent service.

Providing great benefits to both patients and medical personnel of MPH service includes monitoring, telemedicine, location independent medical services, emergency management and response, and pervasive access to healthcare information [39]. There are three specific goals in mobile healthcare systems:

1. The availability location independent of EHRs applications;
2. The location independent health information;
3. The anytime and the invisibility of computing.

There are two categories of EHRs systems: (i) Cloud based technology; (ii) Client server based technology;

Computer with internet connection in order to access via the web, the online data can be stored externally. The cloud computing application allows users on-demand access and provide by third party organisation using the internet. Large-scale cross-platform EHRs system architecture overview is shown in Fig. 3.

There are six benefits of cloud-based systems namely: security, privacy, cost effectiveness, accessibility, reduced IT requirements and it grows with you [29]. The significant risks of each HCO will face when transitioning to cloud-based hosting. The main disadvantage of cloud computing is all data, security, availability, maintenance and control sits to a third party so HCOs have absolutely no control of it. Trusting to the third party service provider is one of the important factors for cloud computing and it takes on a whole different meaning [51]. Despite all the barriers, it's important to remember that cloud health computing paradigms are still under development, but with a lot of chances of being a revolution in a lot of fields. In the near future there will be more services on offer and the development will be greater.

4 The Barriers and Threats of Electronic Health Records

The overarching barriers to EHRs framework are to tackle the indigent quality of data to provide a single, centralised and homogeneous interface for users to efficiently integrate data from diverse heterogeneous sources. Data quality issues may arise when capturing raw data into EHR systems. The data flow process has several factors that influence the quality of information obtained from such datasets at a later stage. The purpose of the data collection processes are data quality management functions include the data flow process application as well as data accumulate, warehousing process systems used to archive data and analyse the process of translating data into meaningful information. The data quality may seriously affect of patient care and even could lead to the death of the patient. This is the key challenges of eradicating treatment errors in the health service process. As patient safety is the key issue in health care service, using effective EHR systems integration and implementation can improve the data quality to reduce medical error. The main consideration for health data includes data accuracy and accessibility, as well as data comprehensiveness, currency, consistency, granularity, precision, relevancy definition, and timeliness. Data quality will empower the tendency of EHRs systems, this emphasises the magnificence of implementing a design-oriented definition. The dimensions of the existing EHRs framework are basically based on historical reviews, understanding intuitive and comparative experiment.

The EHRs structures of an orientation usually vary from framework to framework. For example, the actual use of the data depends on the definition of data quality. It therefore data quality also depends on the application type and what may be deliberated in one application as good quality, but may not good for another. Data quality has emerged as a crucial issue in many application domains. The objective of data quality becomes even more important in the case of patients who need to be identified and notified about important changes in drug therapy or in the case of merging systems of different and similar organisations. The consolidation of information from diverse sources to provide a unified view of an organisation's data assets is technically challenging. The difficulty involves how to practically combine data from disparate, incompatible, inconsistent and typically heterogeneous sources. The other difficult objective in EHRs systems is that data has a structure, which is usually complex and cannot be treated as a simple string of bytes. Often data inconsistency occurs because the data structures may depend on other structures, therefore on a distributed system such data management is very difficult. Another significant aspect of a health data integration system is data mapping. The system must able to materialise data that are mapped from diverse source. Optimally using routinely collected data increases poor quality data, which automatic mechanism would raise the need of the semantic interoperability as well as quality data measurement [34]. Quality improvement and error reduction are two of the justifications for healthcare information technologies. Despite their concerns, HCOs are generally very interested in adopting and implementing EHR systems. A major concern of success of implementing is the large gap between planning for the introduction of EHR systems and medical maintenance system in hospitals. The primary purpose of the successful EHR systems implementation depends on these application systems and maintains the application significantly to achieve the benefit desired and expected. The real barriers causing this gap may not be the availability of technology to the HCOs, as information systems are actually becoming available almost everywhere, but the deficiency in providing proper support before, during and after implementation of the EHR system. The financial constrains are another important matter of the migration from the paper-based health record to an EHR system. Generally there are two principle barriers and challenges in the method of prosperous EHR system integration, namely:

1. Human barriers (e.g. professional and beliefs);
2. Financial barriers (e.g. available money or funding opportunities).

The human factors become even more important as the benefits are only anticipated after the successful integration and implementation of the EHRs systems. The information security is the most important for the quality health care service. It improves the potential of EHRs as well as accuracy, accessibility, productivity, efficiency and to reducing the costs of healthcare and medical errors. Most HCO administrators are aware that it is time consuming to migrate from paper base record system to an EHR system. It is also important to change the provider behaviors and health care practitioner with regard to electronic healthcare systems, but time is also needed. Few things also need to be addressed regarding to successful implementation of an EHR system, such as attitudes, impressions and beliefs. The most important factor is essential to understand the reasons for and the purpose of the implementation of EHR systems in the whole subject [46]. Research and statistics showed EHRs estimated potential savings as well as the costs of the widespread adoption of EHRs systems. Important health and safety benefits were modelled and concluded that effective EHR system implementation and networking, could improve healthcare efficiency and safety. It also showed that Health Information Technology (HIT) could enhance the prevention and management of chronic diseases, which could eventually double the savings, while increasing health and other social benefits. The feasibility of introducing an EHR system to improve data quality is the meaningful association between the heterogeneous data source and the integration into HCOs to improve healthcare service. The integrity constraints are specified in the global scheme of data mapping, which can be used to promote EHRs data quality as well. The uncertainties are the other important integration aspect in EHRs that should be minimised to improve data quality. The most important barriers and constraints to high quality datasets in order to promote must solved the integration of EHR systems and electronic health record, to achieve maximum benefit of the healthcare services. Finally, it is noted that the query answer in the context of data exchange, contributes to data quality.

5 Literature Review

Existing literature shows that several techniques and major EHRs systems currently exist to deal with data quality issues, which historically have faced DBMS. After a profoundly analysis of various cutting-edge commercial accomplishment existing on the software market and an intensive review of literature, it appears there are still some limitations to practical tools for EHRs systems. Physically access of diverse information sources of robust support is provided, but only if these are standard database structure tables. At the moment, there are no automatic mechanisms to solve existing integration problem [43]. Peer-to-Peer (P2P) topology is used when system-individual participants contact a localised server to search other data and to contact other participants directly, to exchange information or share resources. However, Gribble et al. [23] stated that generic P2P systems often do not take care of the semantics of the data exchanged. This is a serious drawback, especially considering that when the network grows, it becomes hard to predict the location and the quality of the data provided by the system. Tania et al. [57] propose a mediated query service, which is a system that is used for configuring mediation systems for building and maintaining multi-dimensional multimedia data warehouses. Considerable disadvantages are, however, involved in moving data from multiple, often highly disparate data sources, into a single data warehouse. This translates into long implementation time, high cost, lack of flexibility, outdated information and limited capabilities.

A subsequent representation by Gilson et al. [21] for data integration was proposed using middleware architecture. The middleware can encompass dynamic scheduling, performance management and transport services for distributing scientific visualisation tasks in a grid environment. Middleware, however, has a high development cost, the implementation thereof is time and resource consuming, few satisfying standards exist, its tools are not good enough and often threatens real-time performance of a system and middleware products are not very mature. Load-balancing issues, limited scalability, low levels of fault tolerance and limited programmer access area, for example, are some of the main disadvantages of middleware.

Combining Aggregation Operators (AO) and fuzzy Description Logics (DL), Vojtáš [59] presents a fuzzy DL with general AOs. The expressiveness of the logic is, however, very limited. An additional evaluation of this strategy was also done for data and multimedia sources using an ontology-based data integration system. A Mediator Environment for Multiple Information Sources (MOMIS) data integration system was proposed using a single ontology approach to overcome this limitation. The system combines the MOMIS framework with the STASIS framework. MAFRA [38] is an ontology mapping framework for distributed ontology, which supports an interactive, incremental and dynamic ontology mapping process in the semantic web context. Using ontology integration, the conflicts in the result can be solved by satisfying the consistence criterion. An approximation technique has been identified as a potential way to reduce the complexity of reasoning over ontology's in expressive languages such as OWL 1 DL and OWL 2 DL [49]. A vast amount of research concerning EHR mechanisms has been carried out over the last few years. Fuzzy-ontology is moving forward to express fuzzy properties, membership functions and linguistic hedges [11]. The fuzzy-ontology definitions that are found in the literature are quite naturally influenced by fuzzy set theory, fuzzy logic and existing ontology languages. Shaker et al. [55] performed an exercise using fuzzy-ontology integration to solve the problem of equivalently matching concepts to avoid pairs of mismatching concepts and conflicts regarding multiple entities to reduce data inconsistency. Another related work was performed by Sanchez et al. [52], which considers fuzzy-ontology with general quantifiers that could be used for some type of quantifier-guided aggregation.

Cristiane et al. [15] used a DISFOQuE system to analyse the fuzzy-ontology to perform semantic query expansions. This is an ontology-based data integration system for data and multimedia sources, which is essentially performed manually by the integration designer. A few studies handle fuzziness and give support for uncertainty in their conceptual models for multimedia materials. The studies by Aygün et al. [5] and Özgür [45] try to handle this uncertainty by supporting fuzzy attributes. Different types of databases exist, but the type most commonly used in healthcare is the Online Transaction Processing (OTP) database. For the most part, healthcare databases are used as the foundation for running the many transactional system databases, which structures accommodate the creation of a wide range of transactional applications such as EHRs lab systems, financial systems, patient satisfaction systems, patient identification, data tracking, administration, billing and payment processing and research. The EHRs database servers are to replace the old paper-base documents, files, folders and filing cabinets. Data is therefore now more convenient and current. It's obvious that the benefits of EHRs are equal to the benefits of the applications that run on them. Significant advances in automation and standardisation of business and clinical processes can be attributed to these applications and databases. With EHR databases, data can also be stored externally and backed up in a secure place to prevent data loss. Because front-end software can provide tip text and enforce data integrity, the back-end data can therefore become more standardised and accurate. Lastly, because the data is electronic, it allows for quicker processing of typical transactions such as lab results and payment claims. One of the biggest benefits of all these databases is the amount of data healthcare organisations have been able to capture. They now have huge data stores that can be used to inform better and more cost-effective care. EHRs focus on strategies for combining data residing at different heterogeneous sources and providing the users with a unified view of the data. A vast amount of work has been developed in the EHRs area and some interesting results have shown the effectiveness of this approach. It has, however, not been extensively evaluated with regard to ease of data access to dynamic her systems and their widely implementation over HCOs. The aim is to avoid the theoretic pitfalls of monolithic ontologies, facilitate interoperability between different and independent ontologies and provide flexible EHRs capabilities. In addition, not all the existing EHRs integration techniques are sufficient, as many healthcare organizations are still capturing their data in spreadsheets and often mismatch information and formats, which cause incorrect report generation and reduce the quality of the data. There is thus a need to develop or use an efficient EHRs system, using a template screen, which is efficiently mapped to the online transaction-processing database. ***An important objective of EHRs systems is the way it needs to be adapted to address the data quality issue to achieve all possible benefits and address, all problems described above***.

6 Electronic Health Records Data Structure

Most HCOs data are highly structured and heavily depend on claims data, but absence the prosperous scope provided by health data. Furthermore, leverage health data basically depend on vendor-delivered implementation, communication, such as a Continuity of Care Documents (CCDs) is the few analytics applications. They also stick limitations via both design and integration that make them insufficient for populating health and productivity analytics, until CCDs offer a consolidated and expedient way to implement electronic health data. Methods for data capturing in EHR systems include direct capturing, capturing on the screen template, scanning hand written documents or importing transcribed data from other information systems in different data exchange formats, such as JSON, XML, CSV, TXT, REBOL, Gellish, RDF, Atom, YAML and other data exchange technologies. Each one of these methods has strengths and weaknesses that may have an impact on data quality. Only the quality of the data can ensure that healthcare providers have confidence in EHRs systems to deliver the best service possible. To capture, store as well as develop and implement structured health data to avoid data quality gap must use the integrated analysis program. In order to effectively solve the challenge of data quality gaps, there is a need to discuss further relevant points. Valid data capturing techniques require that when a clinical encounter takes place and provider and/or automated systems insert information into an EHR system, it is for example, captured accurately into the EHR of a patient. Valid data structures need to be used both in the way in which data is captured as well as storage of the data in an appropriate format and location. If an integer is captured in a VARCHAR field, its feasibility for reporting, analysis and quality will be reduced, even if it is captured in a structured field. If the template or screen structure is not properly mapped or configured in the database, the value may still be stored in an incongruous location. The analysis or reporting purposes for this information is extracted from the server and made instant and available to authorised user. There is no needing include extracting all pertinent information when it is back end database connection. How data will extract or how data will select from the query table, are the key factors in how the exchange of create the data set in how the exchange tackle impacts on the application quality of the outgoing data quality. It is of importance to identify the point at which data quality gaps are introduced. This will in turn lead to focused initiatives to eliminate such gaps.

Data security is a key concern in healthcare interoperability whether paper-based or electronic health records. According to the human rights, every individual can keep personal data confidential and not being disclosed for surveillance or interference from another organisation or even to the government. All confidential information should be protected and encrypted while data that is shared as a result of the clinical relationship [50]. Patient data can only be released when the patient gave his/her consent or when stipulated by law. Information may disclose information sharing only if the patient is unable to do so because of age or mental incapacity, data sharing decision should be made by the legal representative or legal guardian of the patient. The information is considered confidential and must be protected when a result the query result of clinical cooperation. The identity of the patient cannot be ascertained when information is populated, for instance, the number of patients with HIV in a government hospital, does not fall in this denomination [50].

7 Electronic Health Records Data Synchronisation

The gradual harmonisation of the data overtime, so called data synchronisation is the procedure of establishing consistency between information from a diverse source to the destination data server and vice versa. Considering large-scale computing, dataflow between multi-user clinicians and one central server, definitely entails a multi-way synchronisation model. Since, the server must send a client the data previously created by other clients. The patient is not conscious of the entire data structure as it is the server data structure algorithm to figure out the modifications so called he rights management rules. In many cases, data should be available in more than one directory server using three different techniques for achieving this. This includes a directory replication protocol, direct synchronisation between a pair of directory servers and indirect synchronisation between two or more servers. Replication has the best operational characteristics but the lowest functionality, which can differ between the various techniques. The majority of replication techniques entail indirect synchronisation, which has the highest functionality and the poorest operational characteristics, while direct synchronisation is intermediate. There are numerous reasons why data in one directory server needs to be made available in another directory server. These include availability, load sharing, locality, reaching data on other servers, data access restrictions as well as data mapping. Figure 4 depicts the two-way data synchronisation workflow model:

Generally synchronisation between a client and a server follows five steps:

1. The data administrator rules prepares the data for a “go/no-go” response when the authorised user initialises the request;

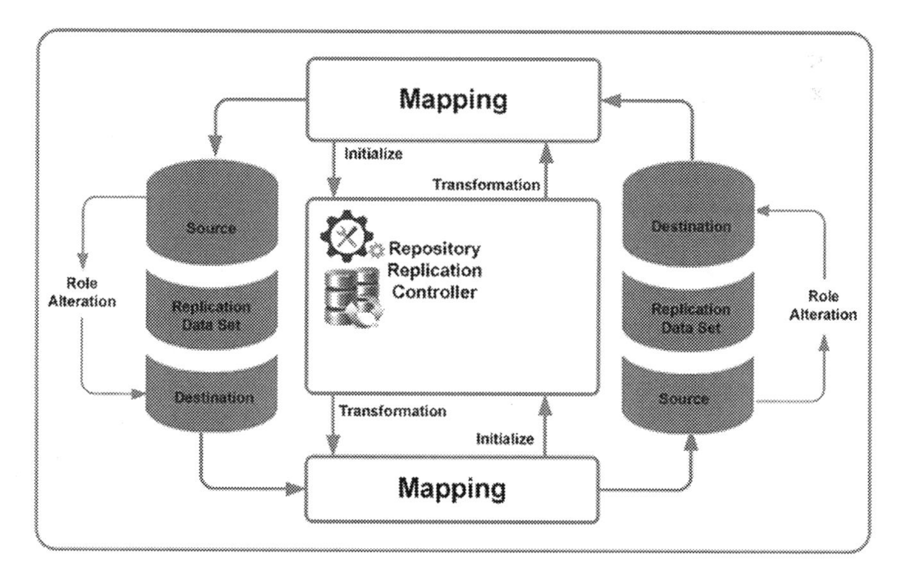

Fig. 4 Two way data synchronisation workflow

2. The server algorithm rules checks the user authentication to accomplish whether synchronisation is required and finally checks for all possible conflicts;
3. The authorised user submit the data trees;
4. Before to nodes and stores data the server assigns new IDs to trees;
5. The server uniquely identify the data in the network to these collective IDs and the collective database.

It should be noted that only the authorised user allows viewing the sent to the client according to the accurate management rules. Finally, before replacing the local IDs with collective ones and storing the new trees to the server, the authorised user updates it's to local database [17]. The overall practice shows that EHRs and the ability to exchange health information electronically can help HCOs to provide higher quality and safer care for patients, while creating tangible enhancements for healthcare. EHR systems thus enable healthcare providers to not only improve the care management plan for their patients, but to also provide improved healthcare through accurate, up-to-date and complete information sets about patients. This enables quick access to patient records for an improved and coordinated care plan. This is achieved by securely sharing electronic information with patients and other clinicians that in turn helps providers to diagnose more effectively and thus reduce the medical errors. It contributes to the provision of safer care, improved patient and provider interaction and communication. Add to this healthcare convenience, more reliable prescribing, promotion of legible and complete documentation supported by accurate, streamlined coding and billing. Other improvements include enhancing privacy and security of patient data, helping providers improve productivity and work-life balance, enabling providers to improve efficiency and meet their business goals, reducing costs through decreased paperwork, improved safety, reduced duplication of testing and improved healthcare services. Figure 5 depicts a typical model of the data synchronisation architecture of a healthcare risk manager's organisation:

It therefore became necessary, to implement adaptive, interoperable EHR systems to improve the quality of data, which addresses the current EHRs challenges. As a result, the proposed solution will focus on a novel approach based on different methods and existing systems, to reduce the challenges of EHRs and data quality. EHRs technology will be applied to not only perform the function of receiving and displaying information, but to automatically and accurately extract information from diverse heterogeneous data sources that use makes use of healthcare services. For data to equivalently match two concepts across different data sources and automatically resolve any inconsistency arising from multiple data entities is the challenge of EHRs. The important expected contribution of this study will be to realise a method to improve on EHRs data quality from heterogeneous and inconsistent data sources. The key outcome of EHRs will be to discover a new merged concept by finding consensus among conflicting data entries.

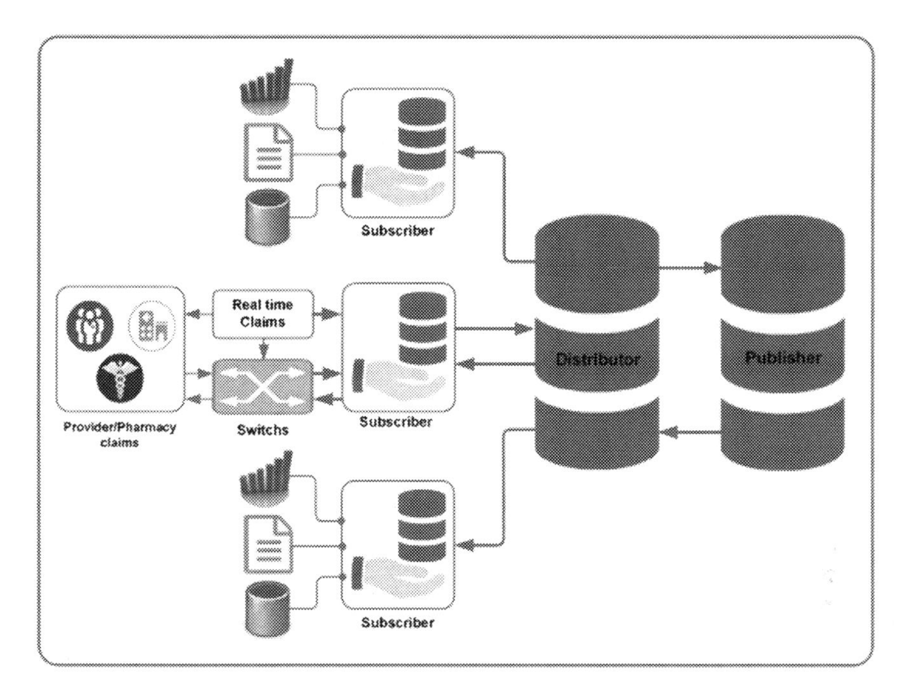

Fig. 5 A healthcare risk manager's organisation data synchronisation architecture

8 Electronic Health Records Data Collection

Data collection is defined as the on-going, systematic assembling and measuring of information, analysis and illustration of health data necessary for integration, implementing, designing, and evaluating public health prevention programmes, which then enables one to answer relevant questions and evaluate outcomes [62]. The HCOs collect data to observe health to handle subsidies and services as well as inform bankroll and resource allocation, identify and appraise healthcare services, inform the development of health policies and interventions, assist clinical decisions about patient care and meet legislative requirements. Surveillance is undertaken to inform disease prevention and control measures, identify health emergencies as an early warning system, guide health policies and strategies and measure the impact of specified health interventions. Few people are, for example, dying from infectious diseases, but for instance, due to changing patterns of physical activity and expenditure of drug, tobacco, alcohol and food more people are suffering from chronic diseases. The survey process is conducted to maximise accuracy and participation to generate statistics. Using a different data collection algorithm, these statistics are generated from diverse sources, including household surveys, routine reporting by health services, public registration and censuses and disease observation systems. HCOs involve a different civil data set and private data collection systems, including clinical surveys, administrative enrolments, billing records and medical records used by various entities, including hospitals, physicians and healthcare plans. The possibility of each to facilitate data on patients or enrolees data on race, ethnicity and language are also collected to some extent by all of these entities suggesting [16]. Data breaches in healthcare come in a variety of forms such as different healthcare capturing and storing methods as well as technology used such as excel, access, SQL and Oracle. Manual data collection from ward-based sources captured only 376 (69%) of the 542 in-patient episodes, captured by the hospital's administrative electronic patient management programme. Administrative data from the electronic patient management programme had the highest levels of agreement with in-patient medical record reviews for both length of stay (93.4%) data and discharge destination (91%) data [53]. Currently, fragmentation of dataflow occurs because of silos of data collection. In HCOs data are often collected by clinical assistants, clinical nurses, clinicians and practice staff.

Compare the completeness of data capturing and level of agreement between three data collection methods is prospective observational studies:

1. Manual data collection from ward-based sources or paper based: Paper & Pencil, Surveys, Chart abstraction and Weekly return card;
2. Administrative data from an electronic patient management program: Dedicated electronic data collection systems, EHRs-based, Images and Audio and video recording (qualitative research);
3. Inpatient medical record review for hospital length of stay and discharge destination.

With specific diseases in clinical and genomic research, the objective of EHRs is to generate large cohorts of patients. The electronic phenotype selection algorithms are to find such cohorts a rate-limiting step is the development.

This study evaluated the portability of a published phenotype algorithm to identify Rheumatoid Arthritis (RA) patients from electronic health records at three different institutions, using three different EHR systems. EHR systems are seen by many as an ideal mechanism for measuring the quality of healthcare and monitoring ongoing provider performance. It is anticipated that the availability of EHRs-extracted data will allow quality assessment without the expensive and time-consuming process of medical record abstraction. A review of the data requirements for the indicators in the Quality Assessment Tools (QAT) system, suggests that only a third of the indicators would be readily accessible from EHRs data. Other factors such as the complexity of the required data elements, provider documentation habits and the EHRs variability make the task of quality assurance more difficult than expected. Accurately identifying eligible cases for quality assessment and validly scoring, those cases with EHRs extracted data will pose significant challenges, but could potentially lower costs and therefore expand the use of quality assessment. Improving the data collection process across the healthcare system is one of the key challenges to improve data quality.

9 Improving Data Collection Processes

Overreaching opportunities abound for increased quantities of EHRs, for improved quality of data and for new data elements that were once considered too burdensome or expensive to capture. This wealth of EHRs can be used to validate or calibrate health demand models, for inpatient care information systems analysis and for modelling mobile source emissions across a healthcare network. These data collection and processing advancements are however, costly and should be implemented with caution. The focus of healthcare is on data accuracy issues pertaining to the mechanism chosen for data collection and data processing, using EHRs technology. Vast amounts of technology spreads exist throughout the transportation field, which are automating numerous manual data collection processes. These advances generally reduce labour costs and manual capturing errors. Automation of survey data collection allows EHR systems to collect new data streams without increasing respondent burdens. When data are combined from diverse heterogeneous sources, the data that are syntactically identical (same format, same units) can show important inconsistencies, as data elements that supposedly represent the same concept, actually represent different concepts at each site. The term semantic variability expresses the data variability caused by differences in the meaning of data elements. Differences in data collection, abstraction and extraction methods, or measurement protocols can result in semantic variability. Figure 6 depicts the dataflow control system in large-scale DBMS.

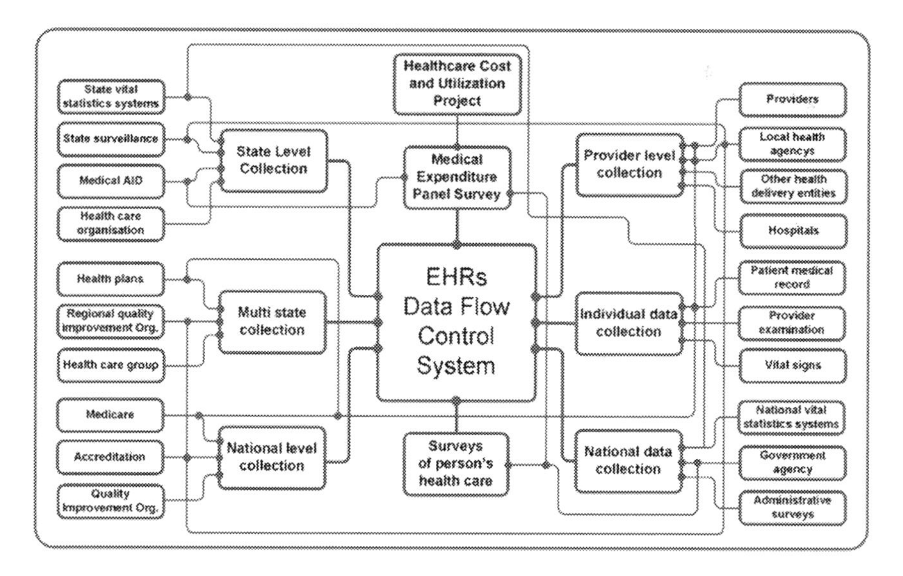

Fig. 6 The data flow control system in large scale DBMS

Failure to distinguish between fasting and random blood glucose, finger-stick or venipuncture sampling or serum or plasma measurements would, for example, result in glucose values that do not represent the same concept. Semantic variability is difficult to detect using single-site data alone, because data semantics tend to be consistent within an institution. Only when the data are combined from multiple heterogeneous sources can such semantic differences be detected. The above discussion regarding the challenges faced by various healthcare professionals and healthcare institutions, highlights the importance of accurate data capturing and data quality in order to overcome HIT constraints and minimise respondent and organisational resistance. Integration of data systems has the potential to streamline collection processes, so that data can be reported on easily and that an individual would not need to self-identify race, ethnicity, and language requirements during every health encounter. Integrating the various data systems, enhancing legacy HIT systems, implementing staff training, and educating patients and communities about the reasons for, and importance of collecting these data, can help improve data collection processes. Not all data systems capture the method through which the data were collected, and some systems do not allow for data overrides. The interoperability of data systems may, for example, prohibit a provider from updating a patient's data, which were provided by the patient's healthcare plan. Self-reported data should therefore trump indirect, estimated data or data from an unknown source. Ways of facilitating this process logistically warrant further investigation. Data overriding should be used with caution, as overriding high-quality data with poor-quality data reduces the value for analytic processes.

Currently, one specific data collection effort under evaluation for automation is the patient update survey, which traditionally has been administered to obtain a comprehensive up-to-date patient history. The fundamental concern associated with the need to change medical practice tendencies and the way of interacting with patients, created barriers to EHRs implementation and use. The adaptation to EHR systems were also considered a major threat to practitioner professionalism, because of the corresponding requirements for providers to adhere to the requirements of the EHRs, including electronic documentation and compliance with standardisation guidelines. Even though current data collection methods are subject to numerous errors, the survey data collected are used to forecast regional health data such as demographics, hospital admissions and discharge notes, medical history of patients, improvement notes, outpatient clinical health notes, medication prescription records, medication and allergies, immunisation statuses, radiology reports and images, laboratory data and test reports, essential symptom, personal statistics like BMI, blood pressure, age and weight information etc. In addition, the availability of EHRs databases makes the automated processing of such data feasible. With the application of these technologies, however, care and caution should be applied when using and interpreting the datasets obtained from the data collection method used.

10 Data Quality Issues in Electronic Health Records

Quality data, appropriate for use, comprise of characteristics that include completeness, uniqueness, consistency, accuracy, validity, correctness and accurate timelines. The quality of data can be analysed from multiple dimensions. One such dimension is a measurable data quality property that represents some aspect of the data accuracy and consistency that can be used to guide the process of understanding quality [44]. Though EHRs data quality is often only considered within the narrow scope of data verification and validation, it should also concern equally critical aspects of assuring that EHRs data is appropriate for a specific use. Alternatively, the quality of data is comprehended as in high demand, according from this denomination, as the volume of data increases and the question of internal consensus within data become significant, regardless of its appropriateness for use for any particular external purpose. Even when discussing the similar set of data used for the same intention, confluence's prospect on data quality can often be in uniqueness. Some information quality problems may arise from when the raw data is collected until it becomes useful information. The majority of EHRs data is captured by a large number of individuals from heterogeneous sources and data exchange accessed these days to index text object use data rescue systems devised. Due to unit measurement without different definitions and may be captured in the EHR system. It will absolutely impossible or may not comparatively and assessment to interpret what is being reported by other clinician when validated psychometric scales to assess patient status are not used. The objective deficiency that these problems, classify idiosyncratic data quality features.

The data inconsistencies can be identified directly, which can lead to inaccuracies and bias, as the data is collected geographically and over time and might be adjusted differences over to account for unequal measures over time [9]. The main concern of EHRs is the feasibility of introducing EHR systems in HCOs to improve the data quality in order to achieve all possible benefits pertaining to healthcare services. To effectively address this concern, the following issues need to be taken in account:

1. What are the most meaningful associations among heterogeneous health data sources that can be explored to improve EHRs data quality?
2. What kinds of integrity constraints are specified in the global scheme of data mapping that can be explored to improve EHRs data quality?
3. What are the uncertainties in data integration that when minimised, results in an improved EHRs data quality?

Schaal et al. [54] motivate the adoption of accessible data based on its definition of data that comprises of clarity and consistency. The intimidation posed during data storage and transmission, EHRs are seen as a hopeful accomplishment to problems in EHR managements and despite them. One of the key barriers is to optimally use routinely collected data, as the increasingly poor quality remains in the data. This raises the need for automating the mechanisms used to measure data quality and semantic interoperability. This framework is a result of filtering the existing data quality dimensions in many research sources and checking its suitability to the nature of e-health systems. In many research sources and verifying its praiseworthiness to the behaviour of e-health systems, this skeleton is a outcome of percolation the subsist data quality dimensions.

11 Methodology

The main contribution of EHR systems consists of mathematical modelling of a heuristic methodology based on a combination of the perfect matching and similarity measurement for distributed concepts unanimity techniques for inconsistency and conflict resolution performance to improve data quality. Creating a consensus between perfect matching and similarity measurement can be resolved unite of data inconsistency, mismatches and conflict ontology entity regarding diverse data sources. Data quality, consistency, reliability, validity, accuracy, completeness and timeliness are the eventual significant list of EHR systems. Matching is a process of finding alignment between sets of correspondences with a semantic verification output of the matching process. This merging is a process of creating a new set of possibly overlapping data. However, the aim of the main task is to determine best illustrate object to find semantically fundamental equivalent motive in EHR systems. This provides a strong theoretical and practical framework to work with heterogeneous, complex, conflicting and automatic consensus methods for EHRs. A concept detection method could be semantically more meaningful, if multimedia data integration process is a subset of the annotation process for trustable automatic data mapping, such as image, sound or video indexing by special code. This means that each and every EHRs amalgamated data associate to a distinguishable adumbration characteristic. So, conflict may happen on EHRs data integration, if a diverse amalgamated data associate to the same apprehension in the diverse EHR system. Discovering the interrelation in EHR systems is a significant phenomenon among entities manifested in diverse EHRs values. The similarity measurement often discovered that those conflicting entities are approximately identical among EHRs entities. Specially, with a chronic health circumstance, the EHRs statistic predicts individual development and effectuation, since EHRs adoption better meets the needs of the growing modern community. Currently, there are five principles that contribute to data quality. These principles are listed as:

1. Formal Concept Analysis;
2. Conceptual Clustering;
3. Generation;
4. The Grid-File for Multi-attribute Search;
5. Semantic Representation Conversion.

This will be done to ease data access, extract information, search mechanisms, synchronises and establish semantic connections, filter data and provide different levels of security, provide data inconsistency solutions, resolve equivalently matching or conflicting information in multiple entities, resolve queries and achieve data compression and automatic EHRs integration simultaneously. Conflicts based on the occurrence of the same names or the same structures for different concepts, were solved by using the concept of Potentially Common Parts (PCP) propagation. Other aforementioned conflicts such as associated value conflicts and conflicts on a concept level, were also resolved using consensus methods. Specific criteria can be attributed to the representation. The criteria comprise of:

Comparability consists and specify designate of the analytical data quality, in observing the variation in performance critical measures to the Triad as the Triad emphasises collaborative data sets. Various analytical methods show that there are three different types of divers can be identified in collaborative data sets. These variations are individual-level variations (for example age, sex, co-morbidities), provider level variations and random/residual variations. It is obvious that challenges in data availability and comparability issues are numerous national and international comparisons.

Completeness is defined as the extent to which all data elements are integrated. One of the most important aspect for integration result that the completeness is the guarantee of appearance of all ingredients when integrating. Each data element should be captured in an EHR system, so that a provider could create a data set for a patient's characteristics. Either, it will not possible for a provider to create an accurate diagnosis for a patient characteristic. Incomplete data can't provide accurate diagnosis even when the corresponding information supplied by EHR systems. The data will remain incomplete, until providers are not completed with the approximate group value associating to semantic categories. Finally, the inconsistencies of the patient diagnosis with appropriate values, with the inconsistency of any value in these appropriate values are the intention acceptability of total designation for the EHRs completeness.

Consistency is defined as the absence of any inconsistencies in the EHRs result and been solved all appearing conflicts among elements when integrated. When stream data appended dependent interpretative variables from diverse heterogeneous sources, often integrate data refers to the similar subject, but apprehend different inconsistence information. The time (T) dimensional observation data could be large and are asymptotically valid for certain time. The data could be repeat approximately same value over the time such a situation is called a conflict.

Identification is defined as structure similarity among entity source and the EHRs result. The EHRs domain apprehensions often contain entities that have interrelated among the property value. This defines that each EHRs entity accompanied to certain concepts. If identical characteristic associating to the identical apprehension in various ontologies, the conflict in the EHRs are also associated with different associated EHRs value, it also manifested as conflict.

Timeliness is defined as associate between the registration and diagnosis entity and the determination time to the observation diagnosis of the occurrence statistical report. The EHRs statistics reports improve provider observation of patient outcome. Overall statistic indicated that the use of EHR systems could sustain improves productivity of health care service, such as timeliness statistic report or invoices etc.

12 The Similarity Measurement

The importance of EHRs data integration is to find the correlation among entities manifested in diverse EHRs. The similarity measure technology may discover those conflicting entities are approximately identical among EHRs entities. With the tremendous growth in the adoption of EHRs, heterogeneous sources of patient health information are becoming available. It is practically challenging to discover significant similarity entity and how to measure and leverage providers inputs. It is a very important aspect to identify accurate subsidiary uses of EHRs data to achieve the goal [31]. Figure 7 shows the workflow and architecture of the similarity detection service as follows:

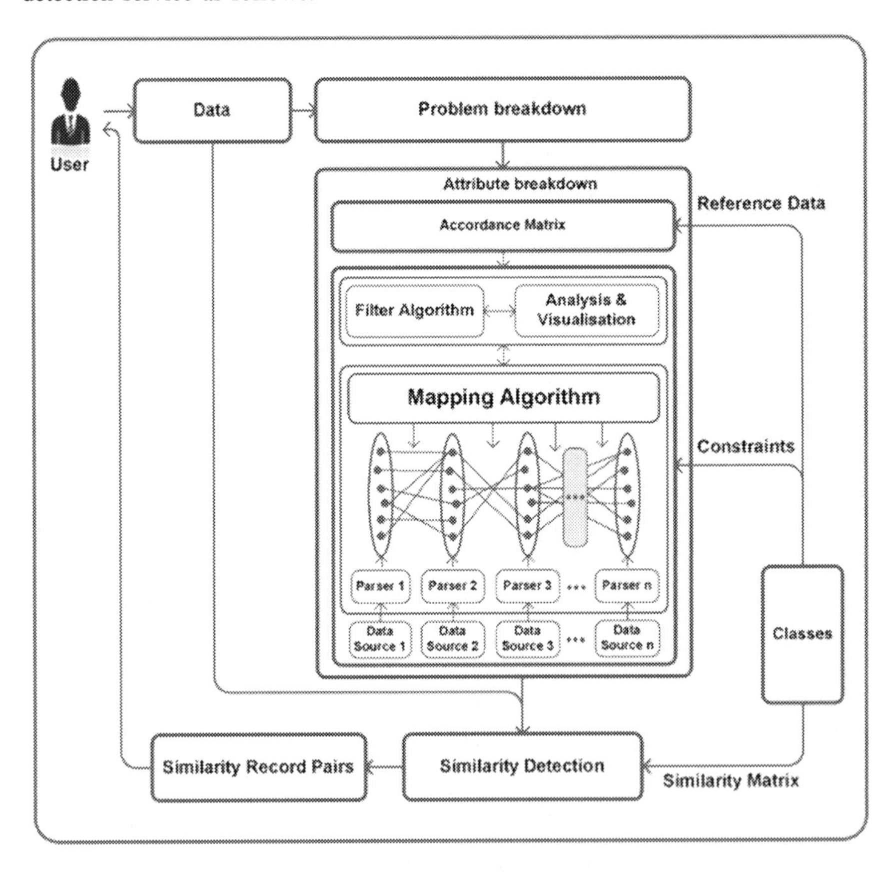

Fig. 7 Workflow and architecture of the similarity detection service

The objective of similarity becomes even more important, when measuring the similarity among equivalent patient entity based on their EHRs data. There are three effective similarity measurement types are appropriate in many applications, such as:

1. Case-based retrieval of similar;
2. Treat similarity between the batch similarity;
3. Cohort comparison and comparative effectiveness.

According to the aforementioned EHRs integration, the similarity measurement technology assorted in four different groups:

Instance-Based Similarity: The similarity between concepts is determined by common instances, as well as comparing new problem instances with instances and stores in memory, instead of performing explicit generalisation. Instance-based ontology mapping is a promising solution to a class of ontology alignment problems. The similarities between concepts define as ordinary instance and matching new entity issues and store them, but not executing the exact generation. The common entity is the key value of similarity among two concepts. The promising solution is instance-based ontology mapping for a class of ontology classification. Measuring among similarity and annotated entity sets crucially depends on it. A set of abstractions evolved from significant entities do not maintain by Instance-based algorithms. If it has the large storage capability, then this approach reaches the nearest neighbour algorithm. The classification accuracy significantly reduced the large storage requirements, but its performance degrades rapidly.

The instance-based similarity equation is:

$$Similarity(x, y) = -\sqrt{\sum_{a=1,n} (x_a - y_a)^2} \tag{1}$$

where, x and y are instances in an n-dimensional instance space [18].

1. ***Lexical-Based Similarity***: The similarity between two concepts is based on the analysis of the linguistic interpretation of associated names. An example, let's find a most similar words for word W, to combine an estimate. Weight the evidence provided by word W' by a function of its similarity to W. Combining information among similar words is a similarity measuring function between words. Which word pairs require a similarity-based measurement is determined by a scheme method. If word W_1' is "alike" to word W_1, then W_1' can participating entity about the probability of invisible word pairs involving W_1 [27]. The Lexical-Based Similarity methods for language modelling of combining evidence evaluated as:

$$P_{sim}(W_2|W_1) = \sum_{w_1' \in S(w_1)} \frac{W(w_1, w_1')}{N(w_1)} P\left(w_2|w_1'\right) \tag{2}$$

$$N(w_1) = \sum_{w_1' \in S(w_1)} W(w_1, w_1') \tag{3}$$

$S(W_1)$—The set of words most similar to W_1;
$W(W_1, W_1')$—Similar function.

2. ***Scheme-Based Similarity***: The similarity among amalgamated characteristic is the analysis of similarity among two intentions. There are two types of structure based similarity:

    1. The internal structure-based similarity;
    2. The external structure-based similarity.

It can be the alteration of $P_{sim}(W_2|W_1)$ in the back of Eq. (2), such as interpolating with the unigram probability $P(w_2)$:

$$P_r(w_2|w_1) = \gamma P(w_2) + (1 - \gamma) P_{SIM}(w_2|w_1) \tag{4}$$

The linear combination illustrate in yielding between the similarity estimate and the back-off estimate:
if $\gamma = 1$, Then possibly to make γ depended on w_1.
So, the similarity allotment for achievement could vary between words [33].

3. ***Taxonomy-Based Similarity***: The structural relationship breakdown is the base of similarity among two concepts in Taxonomy-Based Similarity. It considers the relations as links connecting concepts. If two concepts are already matched, their neighbours (concepts are collected along with the links from the already matched concepts) may also be somehow similar.

Let's consider two gene products W_1 and W_2, and being represented by collections of terms $W_1 = T_{11}, \ldots, T_{1i}, \ldots, T_{1n}$ and $W_2 = T_{21}, \ldots, T_{2i}, \ldots, T_{2n}$.
Based on the two sets, the goal is to define a natural similarity between
The main goal is to determine a natural similarity, based on two sets among W_1 and W_2, denoted as $S(W_1, W_2)$ [48]. Considerable two principle approaches are:

1. ***First approach***: *The similarity is computed pair-wise, say $S_{ij}(T_{1i}, T_{2j})$ and then the aggregation is performed using, for example, the average as*:

$$S_a(W_1, W_2) = \frac{\sum_{i=1}^{n} \sum_{j=1}^{m} S_{ij}}{mn} \tag{5}$$

It is an interesting factor, when the objects T_{1i}, T_{2j}, belong to a given ontology.
Here, the pair wise similarity can be determined as in [37] using shortest paths and information theoretic constructs. The problem rise, only if the average is used with this approach.
Even when the two sets are very similar, $S_a(W_1, W_2)$ may not be 1.
When W_1 and W_2 have only one common entity, then the similarity is 1 and it will ignore the other. Then real trouble is to choose the maximum.

13 The Perfect Matching

Every apex of the nodes is incident and to exactly one edge of the matching is an assignment of nodes, called perfect matching. The concept of perfect matching is n/2 edge, it means that perfect matching only possible on nodes with the even vertices number only. Complete matching or 1-factor is the other name of perfect matching. Here, the dynamic Hungarian algorithm is presented, appropriate to optimally solve the assignment task in condition with changing edge costs, time and as well as improving the healthcare service. The combinatorial optimisation algorithm of Hungarian method is to solve the assignment issues in polynomial time and which expected later primal-dual methods. The assignment problem is widely-studied and exists in many application domains, known as the maximum weighted bipartite matching problem [10]. The Hungarian algorithm undertakes the existence of a bipartite graph, G = (H, P; E) that have illustrated in Fig. 8, where E is the set of edges and H and P are the sets of nodes in each baffler of the diagram.

Let us call a function $y\colon (H \cup P) \to R\, a\, potential\, if, y(i) + y(j) \leq c(i,j) for\, each\, i \in H, j \in P$. The potential value of y is $\sum_{v \in H \cup P}^{n} \mathrm{y(v)}$.

The time of each perfect matching is the latest value of each potential.

The perfect matching of tight edges discover by the Hungarian method: an edge ij is called tight for a potential y, if $y(i) + y(j) = c(i,j)$. Let us denote the subgraph of the tight edges by G_y. The time of a perfect matching in G_y (if there is one) equals the value of y.

Suppose, there are four hospitals (same group hospital) in a big city to which a model is assigned tasks on a one-to-one basis. The time of assigning a given resource to a given task is also known. Figure 8 shows a bipartite graph of Hungarian algorithm as follows:

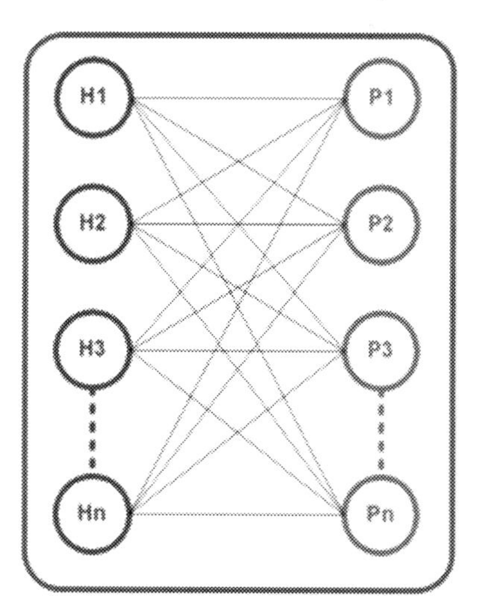

Fig. 8 Bipartite graph of the Hungarian algorithm

An optimal assignment needs to be found, which minimises the total time to better service. The central hospital call centre receives emergency phone calls and decides from which hospital to send the ambulance and to which hospital the minimum distance is between the hospitals (H) and the patient call location (P). A decision-making model is designed using the Hungarian algorithm to calculate how the ambulance should respond to the patient for emergency services to minimise the total time, as time is the biggest factor which can save the life of patients. The distance in kilometres (km) between the hospital H (ambulance location) and the patient call location P are given below:

P \ H	H1	H2	H3	H4
P1	110	95	95	100
P2	55	105	75	85
P3	145	115	110	125
P4	165	130	115	135

Step 1*: *Subtract row minima: This step is to determine the lowest element. Then in that row, subtract it from each element. In row 1 subtract 95, in row 2 subtract 55, in row 3 subtract 110, and in row 4 subtract 65 as the lowest element.

$$\begin{bmatrix} 110 & 95 & 95 & 100 \\ 55 & 105 & 75 & 85 \\ 145 & 115 & 110 & 125 \\ 65 & 130 & 115 & 135 \end{bmatrix} \sim \begin{bmatrix} 15 & 0 & 0 & 5 \\ 0 & 50 & 20 & 30 \\ 35 & 5 & 0 & 15 \\ 0 & 65 & 50 & 70 \end{bmatrix}$$

Step 2*: *Subtract column minima: In this step similarly as step 1 for each column let's determine the lowest element then, subtract it from each element in that same column. In column 1 subtract 0, in column 2 subtract 0, in column 3 subtract 0 and in column 4 subtract 10.

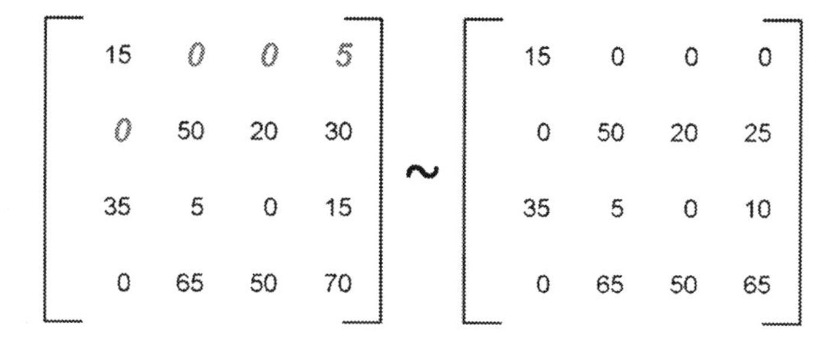

Step 3: ***Cover all zeros with a minimum number of lines***: This step is to cover all zeros in the resulting matrix. Minimum number of horizontal and vertical lines should be use to cover all zeros. An optimal assignment exists between the zeros, if *n* lines are required. The algorithm stops.

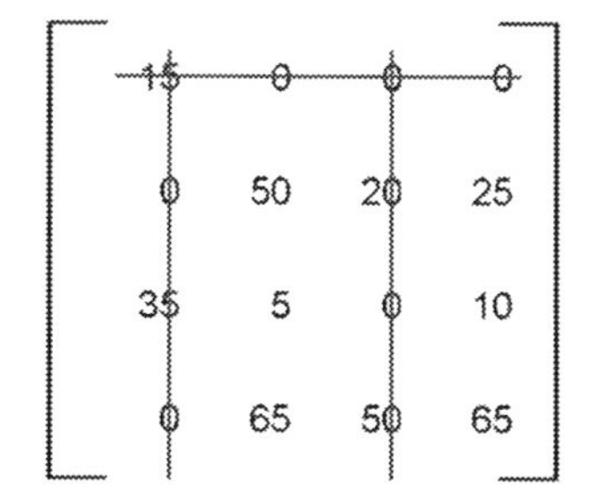

The step 4 will continue, as it required less than *n*th lines.
Step 4: ***Create additional zeros***: This step is to determine the smallest element (call it k) in step 3. This smallest element didn't cover by a line. All uncovered elements must subtract by k, here is the smallest element. Then if the element covered twice then add k to all elements. We have to proceed to Step 5, as we have the minimal number of lines is less than 4.
Step 5: This step is to determine the smallest entry (5) that is not covered by any line. So, in each uncovered row subtract 5.

$$\begin{bmatrix} 15 & 0 & 0 & 0 \\ 0 & 50 & 20 & 25 \\ 35 & 5 & 0 & 10 \\ 0 & 65 & 50 & 65 \end{bmatrix} \sim \begin{bmatrix} 15 & 0 & 0 & 0 \\ -5 & 45 & 15 & 20 \\ 30 & 0 & -5 & 5 \\ -5 & 60 & 45 & 60 \end{bmatrix}$$

Now add 5 to each covered column.

$$\begin{bmatrix} 15 & 0 & 0 & 0 \\ -5 & 45 & 15 & 20 \\ 30 & 0 & -5 & 5 \\ -5 & 60 & 45 & 60 \end{bmatrix} \sim \begin{bmatrix} 20 & 0 & 5 & 0 \\ 0 & 45 & 20 & 20 \\ 35 & 0 & 0 & 5 \\ 0 & 60 & 50 & 60 \end{bmatrix}$$

And now let's, return to the ***Step 3***.

Step 3: Again cover all the zeros in the resulting matrix. Minimum number of horisontal and vertical lines should be use to cover all zeros.

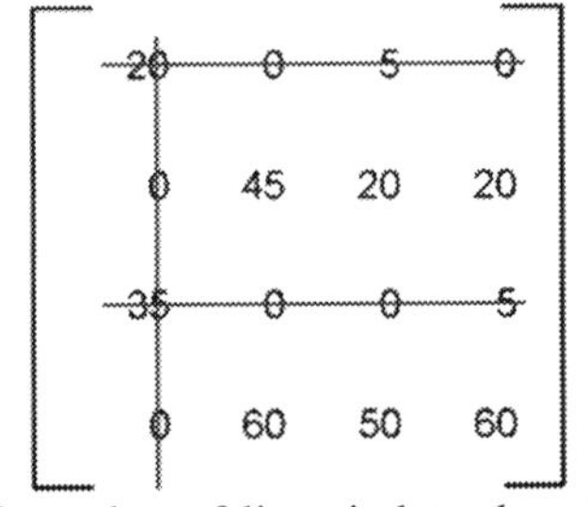

Step 4: Since the minimal number of lines is less than 4, return to Step 5.
Step 5: Note that 20 is the smallest entry not covered by a line. Subtract 20 from each uncovered row.

$$\begin{bmatrix} 20 & 0 & 5 & 0 \\ 0 & 45 & 20 & 20 \\ 35 & 0 & 0 & 5 \\ 0 & 60 & 50 & 60 \end{bmatrix} \sim \begin{bmatrix} 20 & 0 & 5 & 0 \\ -20 & 25 & 0 & 0 \\ 35 & 0 & 0 & 5 \\ -20 & 40 & 30 & 40 \end{bmatrix}$$

Then add 20 to each covered column.

$$\begin{bmatrix} 20 & 0 & 5 & 0 \\ -20 & 25 & 0 & 0 \\ 35 & 0 & 0 & 5 \\ -20 & 40 & 30 & 40 \end{bmatrix} \sim \begin{bmatrix} 40 & 0 & 5 & 0 \\ 0 & 25 & 0 & 0 \\ 55 & 0 & 0 & 5 \\ 0 & 40 & 30 & 40 \end{bmatrix}$$

Now return to ***Step 3***.

Step 3: Cover all the zeros in the matrix with the minimum number of horizontal or vertical lines.

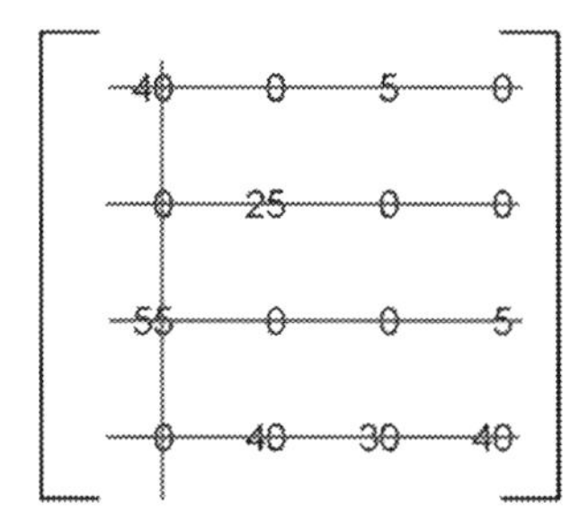

Step 4: Again determine the smallest element of lines is 4. This smallest element didn't cover by a line. The calculation is finished as an optimal assignment of zeros is possible.

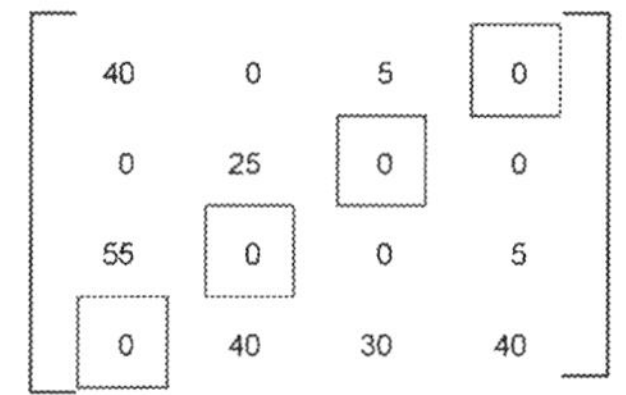

We have found the zero as the total cost for this assignment. So, it must be an optimal assignment.

Now, let's return to the original time matrix of the same assignment.

$$\begin{bmatrix} 110 & 95 & 95 & \boxed{100} \\ 55 & 105 & \boxed{75} & 85 \\ 145 & \boxed{115} & 110 & 125 \\ \boxed{65} & 130 & 115 & 135 \end{bmatrix}$$

So the hospital should send ambulance H4 to Site P1, ambulance H3 to Site P2, ambulance H2 to Site P3, and ambulance H1 to Site P4.

14 Analysis of Results

Information and Communication Technologies (ICT) in healthcare organisations can be used in a beneficial way to address the key benefits and challenges faced by EHR systems, and policy makers increasingly recognise this potential. ICT enabled solutions support the provision of effective, efficient and good quality services, when implemented on a larger scale DBMS.

Healthcare policy makers and strategists inevitably will have to find some way in which to deliver more and more complex services to meet the increasing demand and expectations for promotion and maintenance of health, treatment and care. It is a significantly essential component to confirm that expected benefits must actualize by healthcare professionals to ensure EHRs adoption. There is associating the specific impact of isolating and organisational factors in designating EHRs adoption called a knowledge base gap. Therefore need to be assessed on the adoption of EHRs in healthcare settings, the unique contributions of isolating and organisational factors, as well as the possible interrelations between these factors.

All experimental measured units such as time, distance and motion are a continuous variable and calculated in standard deviations and units in standard time formats. Time is estimated using a count of the incidences of an activity within a certain time period and reported as proportions. To facilitate comparisons across studies, taking in account the different sampling units, such as ambulance encounter versus ambulance total emergency service time, a relative time difference was calculated. The relative time difference was determined for each, considering the time it took to document using a computer, minus the time it took to document on paper, divided by the time it took to document on paper, producing a negative value if the EHRs was time efficient. 95% Confidence intervals were calculated for differences in means and proportions to assess the significance of reported differences, when there was insufficient information to compute 95% confidence intervals. The weighted averages were calculated for both types of sampling unit ambulance encounter and emergency service time, to accumulate for the changeability across our test studies. The following formulas have used to calculate the weighted averages [36]:

$$WA = \frac{\sum_{i=1}^{n}[SW(i)*RTD(i)]}{\sum_{i=1}^{n}SW(i)} \tag{6}$$

In which,

$$(SW) = \left(n_{group1} + n_{group2}\right) \quad (7)$$

$$(RTD) = \frac{(documentation\ time_{group2} - documentation\ time_{group1})}{documentation\ time_{group1}} \quad (8)$$

where *WA—Weighted Average, SW—Sampling Weight, RTD—Relative Time Difference.*

The overall research identified that to achieve the benefits, depends on successful EHRs system implementation and use. Only data quality can provide confidence about the EHRs data to providers so that the benefits of using EHRs, such as best service, data accessibility, quality and safety measurement, improvement and reporting can be seen.

15 Conclusions

The main contribution of this chapter is the improvement of a novel framework for an effective method for electronic health records to achieve its maximum benefits and reduce data quality challenges in healthcare organisations to the minimum. A consensus method was also applied to solve the matching conflicts in EHRs integration. In practice, a dynamic Hungarian algorithm-matching tool was implemented by combining PCP and consensus techniques. The EHRs consist of the following essential steps to achieve the goal: the formal concept analysis the conceptual clustering, the ontology generation, the Grid-File for multi-attribute search and the semantic representation conversion. EHR technology became even more essential for modern healthcare services as increasing the communication network (Internet) and ICT technologies. The aim of EHR systems are not only to improve the healthcare service and wellbeing, it is indispensable demand to design a novel framework for EHRs services to reach beyond independent towards sustainability of our modern society and adaptation. Introducing EHRs systems in healthcare service can, however, offer vast benefits to HCOs and society. The social and ethical acceptance is an important factor for the EHR systems adoption, such as services relies to trust between patients and providers have towards. In this chapter, we discussed the possible benefits and challenges of data quality by introducing efficient EHRs systems in HCOs.

The dynamic Hungarian algorithm shows how a decision-making system for the assignment problems with emergency services saves time and reduces service costs and the results showed that both accuracy and completeness have a large impact on the approach effectiveness. In real-time scenarios, the goal of the method algorithm is to efficiently integrate health data and repair inconsistence data instantly and accurately, when changes in the edge time and costs appear. The overall scenario and challenges discussed above shows data quality in EHRs systems, which demonstrate the method to be effective with regard to accurate performance of the provider's service. This method presents the result of the principle theoretical characteristics that are considered to tackle any thereafter theoretical and practical problems for both qualitative and quantitative methodologies of implementing EHRs. The EHRs system will not have any limits and the system can be modified efficiently to benefit scalability.

References

1. Abdel, N. H. Z., Mohammed, E. and Seham, A. E. (2015), Electronic Health Records: Applications, Techniques and Challenges; International Journal of Computer Applications (0975 – 8887) Volume 119 – No. 14, June 2015
2. Abdolhadi, N., Mohammad, M. S., Abbas, A. B. (2012). Landfill site selection by decision-making tools based on fuzzy multi-attribute decision-making method. DOI 10.2007/s12665-011-1137-2
3. Andrea, H. and Barbara, P. (2005), Software Quality by Misuse Analysis, Case study in section 6 was removed because it is confidential
4. Andrew, D. B., Scott, M. A., Scott, B. and Brandon, J. R. (2015). Data replication tracing; Publication number: US8935612 B2
5. Aygün, R. S. and Yazici, A. (2004). Modeling and Management of Fuzzy Information in Multimedia Database Applications. Multimedia Tools Appl. vol. 24, pp. 29–56
6. Bernd, B. (2006). Advanced and secure architectural EHR approaches, International Journal of Medical Informatics (2006) 75, 185—190
7. Brent A. Metfessel (2014) Financial Management Strategies for Hospitals and Healthcare Organizations; ISBN-13: 978-1466558731
8. Bernhard, T. (2013). Dependencies in Relational Databases, December 1, ISBN: 9783663120186
9. Bruce, BK., Tom, B., Lucy, S., Andrew, L., Masica, M., Nilay, S., Neil, S. (2013). Fleming. Challenges in Using Electronic Health Record Data. CER. ISSN: 0025-7079/13/5108-0S80
10. Burkard, R. E. and Ela, E. (1999). Handbook of Combinatorial Optimization. pp. 75–149
11. Carlos, B., Roberto, Y., Fernando, B., Sergio, I., Jorge, B., Eduardo, M., Raquel, T., Ángel, LG. (2015). Emerging Semantic-Based Applications; DOI: 10.1007/978-3-319-16658-2_4
12. Charalampos, D., Thomas, P., and Ilias M. (2010). Mobile Healthcare Information Management utilizing Cloud Computing and Android OS. 978-1-4244-4124-2/10/$25.00 ©2010 IEEE
13. Cheng, H. (2014). Analysis of panel data, Third Edition, ISBN: 978-1-107-65763-2
14. Chery, R., Mary, DW. and Suzanne, AB. (2012). Patient-Centered Care and Outcomes: A Systematic Review of the Literature. DOI: 10.1177/1077558712465774
15. Christian, B., Sabine, H. S., Silke R. (2010). Data Bases, the Base for Data Mining, Data Mining in Crystallography, Volume 134. pp 135–167, DOI: 10.1007/430_2009_5
16. Citro, C. F., Martin, M. E. and Straf, M. L. (2009). Principles and Practices for a Federal Statistical Agency: Fourth Edition. ISBN: 978-0-309-12175-0, DOI: 10.17226/12564
17. Consuela, H., Dominique, S., Philippe, A., Marie, C. J., and Patrice, D. (2005). Author information, AMIA AnnuSymp Proc.: 296–300. PMCID: PMC156070
18. David, W. A.(1992). Tolerating noisy, irrelevant and novel attributes in instance-based learning algorithms. Journal—International Journal of Man-Machine Studies—Special issue: symbolic problem solving in noisy and novel task environments archive, Volume 36 Issue 2, Feb.1992, Academic Press Ltd. London, UK, UK, DOI: 10.1016/0020-7373(92)90018-G
19. Evangelos, T. (2013). Multi-criteria Decision Making Methods: A Comparative Study. ISBN: 9781475731576
20. Ewa, O. (2013), Incomplete Information: Rough Set Analysis. ISBN: 9783790818888

21. Gilson, A., Giraldi, Fabio, P., Bruno, S., Vinicius, F., and Dutra, M. L. (2005). Data Integration Middleware System for Scientific Visualization., RJ, ZIP 25651-070, Brazil
22. Gombert, B. G. and Rochester, (2015). Systems and Methods for Attaching Electronic Versions of Paper Documents to Associated Patient Records in Electronic Health Records; United States Patent Application 20150339441 Kind Code: A1
23. Gribble, S., Halevy, A., Ives, Z., Rodrig, M. and Suciu, D. (2001). What can databases do for peer-to-peer? In Proceedings of the Fourth International Workshop on the Web and Databases, WebDB
24. Hai, B. T., Trong, H. D. and Ngoc, T. N. (2013). *A Hybrid Method for Fuzzy Ontology Integration*. An International Journal, 44, pp. 133–154
25. Hsu. J. T., Hsieh, S. H., Cheng, P.H., Chen, S. J. and Lai, F. P. (2011) "Ubiquitous mobile personal health system based on cloud computing," in Proc. IEEE Region 10 Conf. TENCON, Bali, Indonesia, Nov. 2011, pp. 1387–1390
26. Ibrahim, AFS. (2016). New Secure Solutions for Privacy and Access Control in Health Information Exchange; http://dx.doi.org/10.13023/ETD.2016.307
27. Ido, D. and Lillian, L. (1997). Fernando Pereira. Similarity-based methods for word sense disambiguation. DOI: 10.3115/979617.979625
28. Illhoi, Y., Patricia, A., Miroslav, M., Keila, PH., Rajitha, G., Jia-Fu, C. and Lei, H. (2012). Data Mining in Healthcare and Biomedicine: A Survey of the Literature, DOI: 10.1007/s10916-011-9710-5
29. Jasmine, P. (2013). 6 Advantages of Using a Cloud-Based EHR System for Physician Practices, http://hitconsultant.net/2013/11/19/6-advantages-of-using-a-cloud-based-ehr-system-for-physician-practices/ (Accessed 12 November 2016)
30. Jens, M., Stefan, O., Daniel, F., Christoph, H., Janina, K. and Wolfgang, H. (2012). Efficient data management in a large-scale epidemiology research project, Computer Methods and Programs in Biomedicine; http://dx.doi.org/10.1016/j.cmpb.2010.12.016
31. Jimeng, S., Fei, W. and Jianying, H. (2016) Shahram Edabollahi Supervised Patient Similarity Measure of Heterogeneous Patient Records, IBM TJ Watson Research Center, http://www.kdd.org/exploration_files/V14-01-03-Sun.pdf (Accessed 23 August 2016)
32. Jinyuan, S., Yuguang, F. and Xiaoyan, Z. (2010). Privacy and emergency response in e-healthcare leveraging wireless body sensor networks; DOI: 10.1109/MWC.2010.5416352
33. Karov, Y. and Edelman, S. (1996). Learning similarity-based word sense disambiguation from sparse data. pp. 42–55. Somerset, New Jersey: Association for Computational Linguistics
34. Liaw, S.T. (2012). Towards an ontology for data quality in integrated chronic disease management: A realist review of the literature. International journal of medical informatics, pp. 1–15
35. Leonardo, C. B., Jéssica, O. de S., Fábio, R. J., Caio, S. C., Márcio, R. de C., Vânia, P. de A., N. and Regina, B. de A. (2015). Methodology for Data and Information Quality Assessment in the Context of Emergency Situational Awareness, DOI: 10.1007/s10209-016-0473-0
36. Lise, P., Jennifer, P, Robyn, T., and Yuko, K. (2005). The Impact of Electronic Health Records on Time Efficiency of Physicians and Nurses: A Systematic Review, doi:10.1197/jamia.M1700
37. Lord, P.W., Stevens, R.D., Brass, A. and Goble, C. A. (2003). Semantic similarity measure as a tool for exploring the gene ontology, pp. 601–612. 2003
38. Maedche, A., Motik, B., Silva, N. and Volz, R. (2002). Mafra - a mapping framework for distributed ontologies. DOI: 10.1007/3-540-45810-7_23, Print ISBN: 978-3-540-44268-4, Online ISBN: 978-3-540-45810-4
39. Maglogiannis, I., Doukas, C., Kormentzas, G. and Pliakas, T. (2009). Wavelet-Based Compression With ROI Coding Support for Mobile Access to DICOM Images Over Heterogeneous Radio Networks, vol. 13, no. 4, pp. 458–466, July 2009
40. Matthew, G. C., Russel, K., Marisa, R. and Richard, S. (2016). Utility of Daily Mobile Tablet Use for Residents on an Otolaryngology Head & Neck Surgery Inpatient Service; DOI: 10.1007/s10916-015-0419-8

41. Moon, F., Juan, M., Campos, I. and Luis, M. (2016). Personalizing xml information retrieval; ISBN: 9788491250548
42. Nir, M. and Taleah, H. (2011). Risk Management and Healthcare Policy. Department of Health Care, Organisation and Policy, USA; DOI: 10.2147/RMHP.S12985
43. Nirase, F. A., Azreen, A., Shyamala, D., Masrah, A. and Azmi, M. (2016). An integrated method of associative classification and neuro-fuzzy approach for effective mammographic classification. DOI: 10.1007/s00521-016-2290-z
44. Nuno, L., Seyma, N. S. and Jorge, B. (2015). A Survey on Data Quality: Classifying Poor Data. Conference Paper. DOI: 10.1109/PRDC.2015.41
45. Özgür, N. B. (2007). An Intelligent Fuzzy Object Oriented Database Framework for Video Database Applications. Computer Engineering Department, METU, Ankara, Turkey
46. Pagliari, C., Donnan, P., Morrison, J., Ricketts, I., Gregor, P. and Sullivan, F. (2005). Adoption and perception of electronic clinical communications in Scotland. 13 (2), 97–104
47. Peter, B. Jensen1, L. J. and Søren B. (2012). Mining electronic health records: towards better research applications and clinical care. DOI:10.1038/nrg3208
48. Raychaduri, S. and Altman, R.B. (2003). A literature-based method for assessing the functional coherence of a gene group, Bioitt Jonnafics, 19(3), pp. 396–401
49. Reb, Y., Pan, J. Z., and Zhao, Y. (2010). Soundness Preserving Approximation for TBox Reasoning. In the Proc. of the 25th AAAI Conference (AAAI2010)
50. Rinehart, T. L. A., Harman, L. B. (2006). Ethical Challenges in the Management of Health Information. Jones and Bartlett. Privacy and confidentiality; p. 54. Chapter 3
51. Rodney, L., MD (2012). Cloud Computing in the Health Care Setting: Advantages and Disadvantages. ISSN 1559-4939
52. Sanchez, E. and Yamanoi, T. (2006). Fuzzy Ontologies for the Semantic Web. 7th International Conference on Flexible Query Answering Systems (FQAS 2006), Milan, Italy. pp. 7–10
53. Sarkies, M. N., Bowles, K. A., Skinner, E. H., Mitchell, D., Haas, R., Ho, M., Salter, K., May, K., Markham, D., O'Brien, L., Plumb, S. and Haines, T. P. (2015). Data Collection Methods in Health Services Research, Hospital Length of Stay and Discharge Destination. DOI:10.4338/ACI-2014-10-RA-0097
54. Schaal, M., Smyth, B., Mueller, R. M. and MacLean R. (2012). Information Quality Dimensions for the Social Web, in Proceedings of the International Conference on Management of Emergent Digital EcoSystems, ser. MEDES '12. New York, NY, USA: ACM, pp. 53–58
55. Shaker, E. S., Mohammed, E. and Riad A.M. (2015). A fuzzy-ontology-oriented case-based reasoning framework for semantic diabetes diagnosis. Volume 65, Issue 3, Pages 179–208, DOI: http://dx.doi.org/10.1016/j.artmed.2015.08.003
56. Sumit Chakraborty (2014). Healthcare System Innovization through Digital Transformation. Reference: HSIDT/ V1.0/ CR 15082014
57. Tania, C., Genoveva, V., Jose, L. and Zechinelli, M. (2004). Building Multimedia Data Warehouses from Distributed Data. e-Gnosis [online], Vol. 2, Art. 10
58. Terence, H. L. (2015). Regression Analysis of Cloud Computing Adoption for U.S. Hospitals; http://scholarworks.waldenu.edu/dissertations (Accessed 31 Oct 2016)
59. Vojtáš, P. (2006). A fuzzy EL Description Logic with crisp roles and fuzzy aggregation for web consulting. Knowledge-Based Systems (IPMU 2006)
60. Wang, C., Zhang, J. and Qin, L. (2016). Design & Research of Legal Affairs Information Service Platform Based on UIMA and Semantics. ISSN: 2233-7857 IJFGCN
61. Weng, C. C., Hao, H., Carolina, O. L. U. and Yong, C. (2013). Benefits and Challenges of Electronic Health Record System on Stakeholders: A Qualitative Study of Outpatient Physicians, DOI: 10.1007/s10916-013-9960-5
62. WHO: http://www.who.int/violence_injury_prevention/surveillance/en/ (Accessed 24 July 2016)
63. Yeturu, A., Michael, P. and Naeem, A. (2016). Methods, devices and systems enabling a secure and authorized induction of a node into a group of nodes in a distributed computing environment; Publication number US9264516 B2

Large Scale Medical Data Mining for Accurate Diagnosis: A Blueprint

Md. Sarwar Kamal, Nilanjan Dey and Amira S. Ashour

Abstract Medical care and machine learning are associated together in the current era. For example, machine learning (ML) techniques support the medical diagnosis process/decision making on large scale of diseases. Advanced data mining techniques in diseases information processing context become essential. The present study covered several aspects of large scale knowledge mining for medical and diseases investigation. A genome-wide association study was reported including the interactions and relationships for the Alzheimer disease (AD). In addition, bioinformatics pipeline techniques were implied for matching genetic variations. Moreover, a novel ML approaches to construct a framework for large scale gene-gene interactions were addressed. Particle swam optimization (PSO) based cancer cytology is another discussed pivotal field. An assembly ML Random forest algorithm was mentioned as it was carried out to classify the features that are responsible for Bacterial vaginosis (BV) in vagina microbiome. Karhunen-Loeve transformation assures features finding from various level of ChIP-seq genome dataset. In the current work, some significant comparisons were conducted based on several ML techniques used for diagnosis medical datasets.

Keywords Medical data mining • Machine learning • Particle swarm optimization • Alzheimer disease • Cancer • Bacterial vaginosis • Karhunen-Loeve transformation • Random–forest algorithm

Md.Sarwar Kamal
Computer Science and Engineering, East West University Bangladesh, Dhaka, Bangladesh
e-mail: sarwar.saubdcoxbazar@gmail.com

N. Dey (✉)
Department of Information Technology, Techno India College of Technology, Kolkata, India
e-mail: neelanjan.dey@gmail.com

A.S. Ashour
Faculty of Engineering, Department of Electronics and Electrical Communications Engineering, Tanta University, Tanta, Egypt
e-mail: amirasashour@yahoo.com

© Springer International Publishing AG 2017

S.U. Khan et al. (eds.), *Handbook of Large-Scale Distributed Computing in Smart Healthcare*, Scalable Computing and Communications,
DOI 10.1007/978-3-319-58280-1_7

1 Introduction

Biological processing is considered the imperative part of the world computing. Thus, biological research has a great impact in data arrangement, analysis and measurement due to its robust mechanical and automated techniques. Mining techniques are significant for retrieving meaningful information from the biological data. It is a dynamic and systematic demonstration. However, more powerful methods, algorithms, software and integrated tools are required for the biological processing. Machine learning is one of the key methods for handling biological datasets and very large DNA (Deoxyribonucleic acid) sequences [1–4]. Computers and other digital systems assist large biological data processing, thus the discovery and development of new systems is essential with the rapid growth of large biological dataset. New research and computations are generating huge volume of datasets in each and every moment. Moreover traditional approaches are unable to manage very large biological data with accurate and fast computations. Consequently, biological mining techniques which are hybrid mechanisms with computer science, physics, chemistry, biology, mathematics, statistics, genetic engineering, molecular biology and biochemistry; become indispensable. Furthermore, sets of evolutionary computing algorithms can govern the large biological dataset processing [5–10]. These techniques achieve faster biological data processing with accuracy and perfections. Moreover, cloud computing, data sciences and bioinformatics are examples for popular new fields for assisting biological data processing. Furthermore, due to the massive amount of the biological information, big data in biological processing become a common phenomenon in current industry and laboratories. Organizing and arranging information from these big dataset is a challenging issue as well as a key factor in knowledge mining. Statistical and mathematical illustrations are supportive for retrieving meaningful and hidden information. Data mining techniques are equally important for information exaction [11–15].

In the age of wireless communications and faster digitization, very large bio centric information have been growing in exponential manner due to the rising of faster processing on microarray datasets. Moreover, DNA sequencing, RNA (Ribonucleic acid) synthesis, protein-protein interactions are also some prime factors that increase the datasets volume. Big data analysis techniques support these datasets to obtain meaningful information from the human and animal dataset. The growth of the data volume in the recent era is significantly huge compared to few years back. Recent growth is so rapid, which is almost twenty times more than three years back collections as reported in Fig. 1. The primary assessments are done for 12 years as 2000–2015.

In Fig. 1, the X-axis and Y-axis illustrated the years, and the datasets outcome for each year; respectively. All the four lines are merged due to the similarities among the datasets collections. There are very less changes from 2009 to 2015,

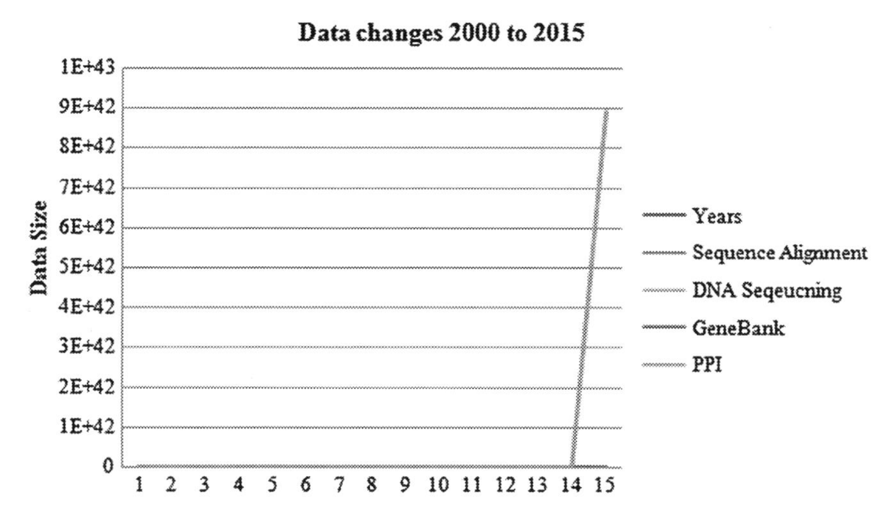

Fig. 1 Various datasets growth from 2000 to 2012 [16]

but there are sudden changes from 2011 to 2015. Currently, these changes are automated and reached the apex points without return [17–29]. One of the pivotal reasons behind the large biological datasets is the diversity of human, animal and plant life. Despite the variations, the biological details interrelated with the universal sets of living organs.

The main contribution of the current work is to highlight the machine learning role in the large scale medical data mining. Innovative data mining techniques in diseases information processing was addressed due to the excessive data generation in the medical experiments and very big scopes in human centric diseases. In addition, consecutive tissue networks have been discussed to identify the AD existence in the tissue. The PSO role to assess the infected parts of cells was addressed. The current work included also extensive discussion related to the statistical epitasis networks for checking gene-gene interactions for obesity. Furthermore, the concept and applications of big data in health informatics was included.

The chapter is organized as follows. Background study is demonstrated at Sect. 2 with delineating the AD related associations including the gray matter functionalities of this disease as well as introducing cancer based computational analysis. Big data and its impacts on health informatics are narrated in Sect. 3. In Sect. 4, the machine learning techniques based supervised learning analysis is addressed. Web semantics is demonstrated in Sect. 5, while the HIV-1 computational classifications, as well as the findings of obesity under gene-gene interaction, Microbial communities, and Bacterial Vaginosis, are addressed in Sect. 6. Finally, the conclusion is given in Sect. 7.

2 Background

General mining can be groped in several ways; however most popular mining processes can be categorized as predictive -or descriptive-data mining as reported in Table 1. Image processing, signal processing, business data processing, DNA sequencing or protein interactions are easily manageable using one of these techniques. Predictive data mining techniques are used frequently to get faster and accurate data. Most of the predictive techniques are based on statistical processing as well as mathematical analysis. There are lots of mathematical models and techniques that are under predictive models. Irrespective of areas and subjects, predictive data mining approaches are imperative to obtain exact information from lots of datasets. Moreover, simulations and other computing are also easily adjustable by predictive mining. It enables ML approaches to learn and train datasets based on the historical data demonstrations and computing. These analysis and synthesis bridge biological mining from present to upcoming future.

There are set of predictive approaches which are frequently used in the digital era, such as the neural networks, principal component analysis, independent component analysis, particle swarm intelligence, self-organization map, regressions, support vector machine (SVM), classification and regression tree (CART), decision tree (DT), deep neural networks (DNN), discriminate analysis (DA), Bayesian Network (BN), Boosting (BT) and Random Forest (RF). In addition, several experiments have been crowned using various methods of bioinformatics related to identification of gene factors behind enormous devastating diseases. Nonetheless, all the previous works transpire only a low segment of gene-gene

Table 1 Sources of data mining

Predictive biological analysis	Descriptive biological analysis
The primary goal is to separate the large dataset into small groups	This process generates set of rules for controlling whole dataset
Set of statistical analysis support to get the exact meaning of the desired items	There are set of descriptive analysis that indirectly used the predictive mining algorithms. As for example Smith waterman and Needleman Wanch algorithms were applied to find the sequences under predictive environments
All features associated in the training datasets are equally important for all data levels	Group of training data clustering is used to handle the large volume of biological datasets. Popular clustering processes are frequently using to get the meaningful ideas
Training and testing features determine the overall outcomes of the experiments	Features are collected in a group rather being individual
In each experiment, there must get some outcomes. If outcomes have probabilities greater than 70% it is said to be acceptable	Experimental outcomes are determined by group results. Sometimes single results are not measured due to the excessive volumes of datasets exist in a group

interaction or difference due to DNA sequence switch, which is liable for rapidly increasing rate of demolishing disease like Alzheimer's. The AD is one kind of neurological disturbance, which occurs due to damages of brain cells. Though Alzheimer's diseases start lightly, it widens rapidly causing short time memory loss and cognitional degeneration. Long term process of this disease leads to dementia, which is responsible for enormous damage of human brain's usual activities [30]. Various algorithms belong to bioinformatics can be applied to identify the principal genetic codes behind some crucial diseases like Alzheimer. Various studies regarding AD have been illustrated that almost 70% damage is associated with genetics for this diseases [31–33]. Even one of the significant gene APOE (Apo lipoprotein E), which is the principal cholesterol server to human brain is engaged with the genes accused of spreading AD.

Basically, developed NetWAS which is one of the ML based algorithms is considered to recognize the symphony among the associated genes. Furthermore, the Network Interface Miner for Mutagenic Interactions (NIMMI) combines protein-protein interaction data and GWAS data for better and reliable performance [34]. So, a new ML approach for tissue-specific internal reaction to override the previous findings from the method GWAS was implemented. Specific tissue features that may play prime role for determining the root cause for every devastating disease, such as the AD and can overcome various critical challenges were reported in [35]. Thus, the source code and overall findings of this work can simplify the way to develop approaches of various methods for best outcome and better efficiency.

Several studies were conducted related to the genetics computing for grey matter density in Alzheimer's disease, where the AD has no exact known cure [36–38]. In [37], a full concentration on bioinformatics approach to the genetic analysis of grey matter density to result in deceased outset of the AD was provided. Various kinds of ML were carried out by assembling them together for better execution than previous works. Full concentration on gene factors movement and internal reaction behind them along with functional genomics data for entrancing biological relationship was specified. Considering all the undiscovered facts, this study is based on genome wide association study (GWAS) and applied on the datasets which belong to the AD Neuroimaging Initiative (ADNI) using grey matter density methods implemented process. A new method was implemented to cope with polymorphisms and their regression to make an obstacle for rapidly growing AD. Functional magnetic resonance imaging (fMRI) methods on approximately 818 peoples as well as 733 genetic data categories for experiment were applied. After that both fMRI and GWAS has been embedded successfully to enhance the possibility of bringing to pass voxel-wise genome-wide association studies (vGWAS) for managing better opportunity to generate various mapping based problems. In the first stage, the Quantitative Multifactor Dimensionality Reduction (QMDR) process was engaged to classify the total number of genes along with SNPs, which can overcome the requirement of the first stage till execution. Basically, the QMDR helps to detect non-linear SNP–SNP interactions [39]. In the second phase, bioinformatics approach was applied on genes enrolled in the first phase to diminish the number of genes factors as in [40]. Furthermore, gene factor evolution using microarray proves the complication of breast cancer disease. A lot of methods have been proposed by various researchers and scientists to identify the main culprit factors behind this devastating disease.

The most liable genes for this heinous disease are BRCA1 and BRCA2 [41]. Various recent studies represent several microarray resolution to get a better way to identify the sub graphs for the cure of breast cancer [42]. From the perspective of clinical science, one of the heterogeneous diseases is breast cancers which obstacle for improving the diagnosis of tumors classifications clinically [43]. Currently, multi-gene lists and single sample predictor models provide better performance to reduce the multidimensional complexity level of this disease. The incapability of some established model to deal with high dimensional data limits the opportunity of gaining desired result, however various new studies contributing a great role to compete with this mysterious disease. A new iterative powerful strategy for computably biased subtypes and enhancing class prediction while using METABRIC dataset were performed.

Typically, the traditional methods help largely for clinical decision making creating various discoveries. The PAM50 methods are used for assigning the molecular subtypes based on various gene expressions. Other various methods are also correlated to clinical diagnosis [44, 45]. All the methods work on low dimensional datasets as well as individual sets of data.

From bioinformatics, the ensemble learning with various algorithms results in a great extent. Actually the main advantage of ensemble learning is it can easily comprehend decreased over fitting as well as improvise performance of classification. There's a lots of ensemble approaches among which select-bagging and select-boosting are the main approaches to work efficiently and in a faster way. Although, the iterative approach was used alone or along with CM1 score then the outcome was quite disappointed, whereas the iterative approach with combination of an ensemble learning mechanism provides faster and efficient performance than others [46]. Besides, practically this work's improvised methods titled iterative method with CM1 score and ensemble learning approach represents a great effectively for foretelling more accurate and exact sample subtypes in the METABRIC breast cancer dataset.

Generally, several cancer diseases are identified by the human cell which is primarily affected [47–49]. Meanwhile, next-generation sequencing and microarrays already have disclosed enormous number of genomic features like DNA copy number alterations (CNA), mRNA expression (EXPR), microRNA expression (MIRNA), and DNA somatic mutations (MUT). Therefore, lots of exploration for a particular type of this genomic data produces various types of prediction biomarkers in cancer. Various predictive biomarkers have mentioned for research basis on various number of biological components simply, such as genomic, proteomic, metabolomics, pathological, imaging and psychological features. Thus, the genomic biological features have been used in a great extent although here National Cancer Institute and the National Human Genome Research Institute plays the main role [49].

In [49], a Cox proportional hazard model was proposed for feature selection algorithm. In addition, the constraint PSO process was also interpreted based on biological behavior. Completing various iterations using bootstrap beta coefficients have been detected going through the log-likelihood (NFS and CPSO) or a penalized maximum likelihood function. The used CPSO was basically associated with biological behavior of flock. Therefore, these particles belong to the swarm of particles representing the positions and velocity. This CPSO randomly set the positions vectors and velocity together. The velocities and positions are updated automatically updated analyzing their performance and types of elements. The authors have used 4 types of datasets which are online based associated with almost 100 types of elements including EXPR, MIRNA, CNA, and MUT in the TCGA assortment while accession. The CPSO was used to evaluate basis components of the sophisticated dataset using its ability to produce various user defined elements that is used as the basic survival model.

The network feature selection model is also used to detect protein-protein interaction network for evaluation of feature selection. Therefore, it is also used for producing poly-cancer biomarkers. This NFS established best performance, while the datasets were more complicated and sophisticated to deal with. It evaluated any kinds of data and represented the desired result [50] and also successfully explored the complicated data with noticeable success rate. This algorithm performed the best efficient process of finding the basic features for detecting cancer disease. Using similar algorithms all the models were evaluated and were compared using the concordance index (c-index) for obtaining the better performance.

This work differentiated the predictive level of various features genomic for characterize genomic related data. The integration process of enormous genomic datasets produced higher class models of datasets which are more powerful than that from single survival data simply like mRNA. From the source of genomic data, the mRNA gene reproduced stronger highly preserved models for integration of cancer genes data sets.

From the preceding studies, it is clear that the collected data from various scientific experiments or movements are massive which require efficient data management, analyze, providing, manipulating to reach in a goal [51]. Thus, big data analytics become essential to handle such huge data amount.

3 Big Data Computing

Big data computing is an overgrowing technique for mining multidimensional data from scientific discovery along with various large-scale structures [52]. Big data analysis system is designed in such a way that it can identify any meaningful data from a vast crowd of data. Big data technologies are currently gaining the opportunities in medical science, bioinformatics, health informatics, computer science, management system and lots of fields. Various recent articles have been reported statistical information for the big data computing benefits in several applications such as mobile devices, tablet computers, internet of things, and cloud computing [53, 54]. The most significant fields are scientific exploration, health care, governance, financial and business management analysis, web analytics, internet of things along with mobile health informatics, and bioinformatics. Compared to big data computing, service-oriented technologies, such as cloud computing is also capable of storing data, analyzing and manipulating large size of data but sometimes it becomes challenging working with cloud computing, that time big data computing is must. The overall architecture of big data was demonstrated in Fig. 2.

Figure 2 illustrated the big data computing along with closer innovation or discussion on architecture, technologies, tools, mobile technologies, health technologies and many more paradigms working behind big data computing. Typically, big data technologies have been used widely medical science and health-care informatics research. A huge numbers of data sets have been gathered and generated using various bioinformatics approach for the sake of research in the fields of medical science [56, 57]. In order to compete with this increasing amount of dataset, algorithms of informatics science to explore the hidden discoveries from them were performed. In spite of all this there's a lots of obstacle with big data among which store, search, analysis, processing, sharing, viewing, discovering knowledge from those data though exploring knowledge from these type of big data has become burning question for the scientists and researchers of last decades [58].

Traditionally, there are various types of sources for genomics and proteomics information. Each and every source has its own styles, mythology though most of source use ontology like genome ontology. Precision medicine asserts the entire requirement needed to acquire the best clinical outcome. Therefore, precision of medical data refers to analyze, to interpret and to integrate the increasing number of unequal sources [59]. The benefits of machine learning, supervised learning, and data mining were used to replace the current traditional use of various algorithms. Informatics approaches for analyzing, integrating, and detaching the medicine legibility for better performance of current medical science were introduced in [59].

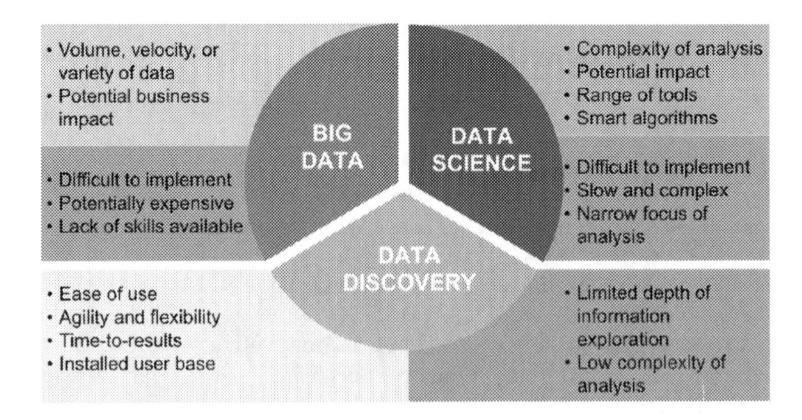

Fig. 2 Overview architecture of big data computing [55]

The authors differentiated between the traditional strategies and next generation informatics approaches to evaluate data of medical science for making a pathway to cope with any kind of diseases and explore new drugs analyzing the output produced using various modern informatics approaches.

Consequently, for going towards the goal of precise, medicine and healthcare in the current systems require bioinformatics approaches along with developed accurate storing capability for information regarding genomic data. Additionally, more emphasizes are compulsory to characterize genetic factors for accurate assessment for developing the health outcomes [60]. Health informatics is associated with health care technologies to develop more reliable health care system. Its basic elements are basically engaged with information science, computer science, social science, behavioral science, management science, and others [61]. Actually, health informatics is involved with the resources, devices, storages, backups with other computers, clinical guidelines, and information/communication system [62, 63]. For gaining knowledge from this vast amount of data, health informatics will require a potential limitless process to cope with this kind of data. The most challenging consequence working with vast data is investigating this data in a reliable manner. The main use of health informatics is to develop various bioinformatics process to illustrate vast medical data in an easy way. In addition, the health informatics cooperates with the population data which is executed in a particular subfield [64]. A big velocity for big data is happen when new update of current population's health care system is providing to data center in a great speed by means of health sensor or mobile devices [65].

The basis goal of health informatics is to provide answer of any patient's frequently asked question regarding health issue in a constant possible time via mobile devices, internet services, and tablet computers. Furthermore, mobile health monitors refers the use of improved modern technologies like mobile device, computers for monitoring health issue and providing alarm for risky situations [66]. Presently, the mobile health has risen as sub-segment of eHealth, use of information technologies like mobile phones, tablets, communications technologies, and patients monitoring [67]. It monitors the symptoms, signs of various diseases via mobile phone technologies [68, 69]. Sometimes this issue becomes challenging to tackle the big data problems. The spreading of mobile health technologies spectrum is shown in Fig. 3 [70].

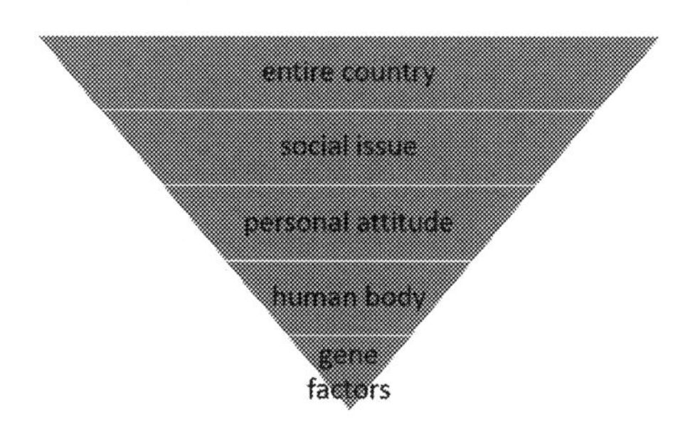

Fig. 3 The overall mobile health technologies process [70]

Such biomedical big data is considered the most challenging task for the active researchers and it indicates investigating, analyzing, storing data, visualizing in lower dimension of higher data. It generally extracts desired value from data [71, 72]. Therefore, big data requires a set of new techniques with new forms of integration to form better performance [73]. Recently, parallel computing which was proposed by Google has created a wide vision of working with big data. Cloud computing is also an approach of dealing with biological big data because of its ability to develop system ability, and to speed up the system. Cloud computing also diminishes system requirements. Biomedical research indicates analyzing the biological data in molecular or macromolecular stages. Next generation sequencing technologies and big data techniques in bioinformatics assist to access into biomedical research data sets. The Hadoop and MapReduce technologies are playing a great role recent years for dealing with the vast amount of data. Big data has great significant efforts in clinical informatics. Clinical informatics refers to health care technologies in medical science along with all kinds of health related issues. Overall there's a lot of use of big data in various fields like clinical science, biomedical research, and imaging informatics. By the sake of various ML algorithms, all the liable gene factors or symptoms as well as risk factors can be determined. Clinical and practically observed data actually helps to accomplish precautionary steps for type 2 diabetes [74–82].

4 A Supervised Learning Process to Validate Online Disease Reports

All the bioinformatics algorithms that determine the main risk gene factors or gene variations behind each and every disease of medical science must require a large number of data to manipulate. For this situation, the pathogen distribution model is widely used for its high predictive ability of any factors. It also demonstrates largely to create diseases maps depending on each disease's variation and liable gene factors. Production of data for these methods comes from online health based data system such as Genbank. One of the major problem of online data base is all the data may not be valid and there is no such method for validation of dynamically providing online based data. Depending on environmental and socio-economic condition the occurrence possibility of each disease in a particular position is defined by the location of disease occurrence.

4.1 Targeted Learning in Healthcare Research

From the beginning of availability of big data electronic health care technologies and claims data sets are arising in a great extent for answering the drug safety measures all over the world. The ever-growing rate of these current technologies towards investigational data sets such as genomic information, laboratory results, and radiologic images [83]. These big data sets in health care technologies are increasing day by day and the questions are widening. Compared to this trend the new approaches are not improved enough to get rid of this trend. The old parametric modeling approaches are inadequate for analyzing the coefficients of the big data source. Therefore, the illustration of these coefficients is largely depends on various covariant. All the traditional approaches feel obstacle for the higher dimensionality of big data. They can't convert this higher dimension to its lower one [84]. Realizing this context, big data problems can be solved using a new approach namely targeted learning (TL).

Targeted learning (TL) is a current approach for dealing with big data problems which is implemented using semi parametric approach along with supervised machine learning mechanisms. This approach targets on higher dimensional data and helps previewing lower dimension of higher dimensional data. The specific focus of targeted learning algorithms is to minimize the bias of any targeted parameter and make it simple to reach in a discovery point. Basically the targeted learning (TL) algorithm is the combination of two bioinformatics approaches which are Super learning (SL) and targeted minimum loss- based estimation (TMLE). Actually, the TMLE is applied on data which is analyzed by Super learning (SL) before. First, the big clinical data is manufactured by SL, after that TMLE is used. Because of this combination the targeted learning (TL) approach outputs sound findings analyzing big health data. Nowadays, the TL is basically applied in a wide range of spheres like genomics, precision medicine, health policy, and drug safety. Therefore, this paper illustrated the significant contribution because of the combination of two bioinformatics approach named Super learning (SL) and targeted minimum loss- based estimation (TMLE).

4.2 *Lumping Versus Splitting for Mining in Precision Medicine*

In recent years, the rise of data severe biology, advancement in molecular biology and technological biology along with the way the health care is delivered to the patient of current world paves the biologists working on these new diseases to find a particular cure using precision medicine models [85]. Medical science is utilizing the advantage of modern improvised data mining methodologies in various aspects of detection of liable DNA codes or gene factors for better outcome of devastating diseases which are invented recently. It is one of the most challenges for medical science finding prevention or cure from such kinds of recent invented diseases. Consequently, thousands of people die because of not finding the exact gene factors or DNA codes working behind the disease. With the renovation of bioinformatics, a new movement has been seen in medical science because of getting the related genes factor corresponding to each and every disease [86]. Therefore, nowhere the data mining is needed for precision medicine. The capability of representing each and every disease's risk for treatment purpose is one of the correlating factors for precision medicine. This achieved a great measure from the last era for ongoing technology improvement. A lot of current powerful approaches rely on unilabiate and linear evaluations that can be easily avoid the structure of complicated criterion [87, 88]. One of the successful example for the precision medicine model is to drug development involving the drug Crizotinib, a vanquisher for the MET and ALK kinases which started the practical improvement with a widen number of population in a great extent.

Several studies tried to prove that using accurate types of data mining and making working portion for each disease will be fruitful for the scientists and researchers determining subtype graphs in low cost along with less time consumption. With the determination of subtypes for various diseases, a great opportunity can be found to keep compete with the increasing rate and approaches of development of diseases along with accurate liable factors of that particular disease and also if this happens then it will be start of a new era from the perspective of medical science. Using enough specific small groups and perfect small types of data can improve the precision medicine models. Thus, the biological data mining process has a great effect in biological large data to play a sensitive role in finding responsible culprit accurately. It also can be used for many clinical and practical contexts to ensure better treatment for the patients and also for exploring reason behind recent invented diseases along with devastating diseases like diabetes or cancer.

5 Mining Drug-Drug Interactions on Semantic Web Technology

Drug-drug attraction has the most priority for showing its tremendous effect on patients [89–93]. A sufficient knowledge should be mandatory for prescribing or taking the medicine for both the clinical association and patients. The new improved process regarding investigation of various diseases risk factor for patients should be broadening to decline the death rate for such diseases. In order to improve genetic tests for finding the suspicion of various diseases, DDI-induced ADEs is required to diminish the risk of prescribing harmful medication [93]. Providing information investigating the DDIs data is full of challenge for medical science. However, using improved informatics approach can easily easy to beat the challenge.

A vast number of new drugs have been invented using various bioinformatics still processing. One of the main significant discoveries is taxon related drugs. Paclitaxel and docetaxel are considered the best performance giving anticancer taxon related drugs though they have lots of bad side effects [94]. In clinical statistics, singular machinery to protest cancer gene for diminishing growth rate makes the Texans related drugs differ from the other related drugs. Besides it is considered most hopeful treatment of cancer disease over worldwide [95, 96].

6 Machine Learning Based Health Problems Manipulation

The HIV (human immunodeficiency virus) is one of the deadly disease from the last three or four decades. The prevention process for the HIV can be improved either scanning the responsible mutants or scanning the resistive capabilities of resistive drugs [97]. Several expert groups have been working on both genotypic and phenotypic consequence of genes for HIV although genotypic is faster and cheaper than phenotypic. In [98], protease and reverse transcriptase cross-resistance information for improved drug resistance prediction by means of multi-label classification were introduced. Therefore, 2 protease sequence and 715 reverse transcriptase sequences along with specific genotypic and phenotypic data have been manipulated using various ML techniques including binary relevance classifiers, classifier chains, and ensembles of classifier chains. Multi-level classification models along with cross-counteraction intelligence were applied to portend the two of the best resistive drug classes used for antiretroviral therapy for the disease HIV-1. The two basic drugs are named as protease inhibitors (PIs) and non-nucleoside reverse transcriptase inhibitors (NNRTIs). Completing overall process the authors have successfully achieve a stage that is quite predicted to be accurate compared to other investigation till today.

Another health problem that obstacle the individuals is the obesity. Recently, obesity becomes a common problem for almost everyone both in developed and developing countries as well [99, 100]. Recent studies have proven the necessity of epistasis or gene-gene interactions for explaining the harmful factor of overweight and obesity. Various network-based models play a great role to explain the basis reason. It is also challenging for the researchers to analyze the data pairwise. The network based algorithms play a great tribute as it has the ability continuing pairwise operation. A network based approach was implemented in [100] which is called statistical epistasis network (SEN) to classify the SNP-SNP interaction in every gene associated with obesity or overweight. The interactions which exceed a specific terminate point build the SEN network. This study represented a traditional properties for identification of genetic interaction from genome based arrays and also invention of various nodes of biological substances to diminish the obesity problem specifying the accurate gene responsible for overweight or obesity problems.

Bacterial vaginosis which is known as vagina microbiomes consists of various types of biological bacteria although all of them a few are quite dangerous for human body [101]. In [102], a relationship between bacterial viagnosis and a microbial community was extracted. For microbial community, the subsets of every community are justified with various bioinformatics algorithms. For classification and identification of relationship between bacterial vaginosis and microbial communities the logistic regression (LR) and random forests (RF) have been used. The authors successfully represented the relationships between BV and MC by adding some features to machine learning methods of bioinformatics. The ML achieved great accuracy to determine similar patterns; therefore it can be used to detect the similar patterns of bacterial vaginosis and microbial community.

From the preceding survey, it is established that big data mining has a significant role in clinical medicine for prediction of disease development, guidance of rational use of drugs, medical management, and evidence-based medicine as well as disease risk assessment, and clinical decision support. Big data is generated everywhere during monitoring, and medical healthcare and imaging processes as well as from social media applications [102–114]. Machine learning proved its efficiency in predicting and classifying several disease, however big data mining techniques including Dempster–Shafer theory, rough set theory [115], fuzzy theory, artificial neural network [116], cloud theory, inductive learning theory, genetic algorithm, decision tree, Bayesian network, pattern recognition, statistical analysis, and high-performance computing can be studied in future work.

7 Conclusion

Health informatics ensures faster and accurate medical data and symptoms processing. There are several analysis that support information mining from large volume of raw data. Drug design, big data analyses, diabetes factors predictions, cancer gene analyses, machine learning based scoring system, semantic web synthesis, Epigenetic internal functionalities, type-1 HIV intersections, computational obesity simulations and Microbial Communities and Bacterial picture are some areas that are sketched. Each and every area is the key filed that control the better life of human being. Adverse Event Report System (AERS) can be applied to assess the drugs-drugs interactions that help for perfect drug design simulation. For recent adverse disease, the HIV (human immunodeficiency virus) datasets are also verified by binary relevance classier, which dynamically categorized the infected data.

Computational mining and simulations help to get new dimensions in these sectors. Accurate measurements are vital for better health. Now-a-days, robots are frequently used to complete the critical operations of the human body. Moreover, lots of devices are employed to control the exact amount of chemicals during drug design, disease identifications, pathological interactions for HIV monitoring and organic chemical reactions. Subsequently, large data mining approaches for scientific measurement are essential for ever.

References

1. Aenenhaus Arthur, Philippe Cathy, Guillemot Vincent, Cao A. Kim, and Frouin Vincent. 2014. *Variable selection for generalized canonical correlation analysis.* Biostatistics. 15(3): 569–83.
2. Alon, 2003. *Biological networks: the tinkerer as an engineer.* Science, 301:1866–1867.
3. Al-Shahrour Fatema, Minguez Pabel, Vaquerizas M. Jaun, and Dopazo Jaoquin. 2005. *BABELOMICS: a suite of web tools for functional annotation and analysis of groups of genes in high-throughput experiments.* Nucleic Acids Res. 33(Web Server issue): W460–4.
4. Alexander Stojadinovic, Anton Bilchik, and Smith David. 2013. *Clinical decision support and individualized prediction of survival in colon cancer: Bayesian belief network model.* Ann Surgery Oncology 20(1):161–74.
5. Ahn Yoel, Bagrow P. James, and Lehmann Sune. 2011. *Link communities reveal multiscale complexity in networks.* Nature 20, 466:761–764.
6. Ashburner Michael, Ball A. Catherine, Blake A. Judith, Botstein David, Butler Heather, and Eppig T. Midori. 2000. *Gene ontology: tool for the unification of biology.* The Gene Ontology Consortium. Natural. Genetics. 25, 25–29.
7. Batagelj Valadimir, and Mrvar Andrej. 1998. *Pajek—Program for Large Network Analysis.* Connections, 21:47–57.
8. Banks A. Charles, Kong E. Stephen, and Washburn P. Michael. 2012. *Affinity purification of protein complexes for analysis by multidimensional protein identification technology.* Protein Expression and Purification, 86:2, 105–119.
9. Bader D. Gray and Hogue W. Christopher. 2003. *An automated method for finding molecular complexes in large protein interaction networks.* BMC bioinformatics, 4:1.
10. Bader D. Gray, and Hogu W. Crishtopher. 2003. CWV: *An automatedmethod for findingmolecular complexes in large protein interaction networks.* BMC Bioinformatics, 4:2.
11. Breitkreutz Bobby, Stark Chris, and Tyers Mike. 2003. *Osprey: a network visualization-system.* Genome Biology, 4(3):R22.
12. Crippen Gordan, Havel F. Timothy. 1988. *Distance Geometry and Molecular* Conformation. New York: Wiley.
13. Cao A. Kim, Rossouw Debra, Robert-Granié Chiristele, and Besse Philippe. 2008. *A sparse PLS for variable selection when integrating omicsdata. Stat Application of Genetic* Molecular Biology, 7(1):35.
14. Cao A. Kim, Martin G. Pascal, Robert-Granié Christele, and Besse Phillippe. 2009. *Sparse canonical methods for biological data integration: application to a cross-platform study.* BMC Bioinformatics.10:34.
15. Chung Dongjun, Chun Hyonho and KelesSunduz. *Sparse Partial Least Squares (SPLS) Regression and Classification.*
16. Zou Dong, Ma Lina, Yu Jun, and Zhang Zhang, 2015. *Biological Databases for Human Research.* Genomics Proteomics Bioinformatics, 13,55–63.
17. Chuang Han, Lee Eunjun, Liu Yu, and Ideker Trey. 2007. *Network-based classification of breast cancer metastasis.* Molecular System Biology, 3:140.
18. Chintapalli R. Venkateswara, Wang Jing, and Dow A. Julian. 2007. *Using FlyAtlas to identify better. Drosophila melanogaster models of human disease.* Natural Genetic. 39:7, 15–20.
19. Chatr-Aryamontri Andrew, Breitkreutz J. Bobby, and Heinicke Sven. 2013. *The BioGRID interaction database: 2013 update.* Nucleic Acids Research, 41:1, D816–D823.
20. Chen S. Ming, Han Jaiwei, and Yu S. Philip. 1996. *Data mining: An overview from a database perspective.* IEEE Trans. Knowledge and Data Engineering, 8:866–883.
21. Chopra Pankaj, Kang Jaewoo, Yang Jiang, and Lee M. Goo. 2008. *Microarray data mining using landmark gene-guided clustering.* BMC Bioinformatics, 9:92.

22. Costa G. Ivan, Krause Roland, Opitz Lennart, and Schliep Alexnder. 2007. *Semi-supervised learning for the identification of syn-expressed genes from fused microarray and in situ image data*. BMC Bioinformatics, 8:10, S3.
23. Croft David, Mundo F. Antonio, Haw Robin, Milacic Marija, Weiser Joel, and Wu Guanming. 2014. *The Reactome pathway knowledgebase*. Nucleic Acids Res. 42:D472–7.
24. Cserháti Tibor, Kósa Agnes, and Balogh Sandor. 1998. *Comparison of partial least-square method and canonical correlation analysis in a quantitative structure-retention relationship study*. Journal of Biochemistry Biophysics Methods. 36(2–3):131–141.
25. D'andrade Roy. 1978. *U-Statistic Hierarchical Clustering*. Psychometrika. 4:58–67.
26. Dahlquist D. Kam. 2004. *Using GenMAPP and MAPPFinder to view microarray data on biological pathways and identify global trends in the data*. Bioinformatics, Chap. 7, Unit 75.
27. Fern X. Zhang Fern and Brodley E. Carla. 2003. *Solving cluster ensemble problems by bipartite graph partitioning*. In Proceedings of the 21st International Conference on Machine Learning: 2003; Banff, Alberta. New York, NY: ACM Press; 182–189.
28. Fruchterman M. Thomas, Reingold M. Edward. 1991. *Graph Drawing by Force-Directed Placement*. Software. Practice and Experience, 21:1129–1164.
29. Frey J. Brendan, and Dueck Delbert. 2007. *Clustering by passing messages between data points*. Science, 315(5814):972–976.
30. Corder, E.H., A.M. Saunders, W.J. Strittmatter, D.E. Schmechel, P.C. Gaskell, GWet Small, A.D. Roses, J.L. Haines, and Margaret A. Pericak-Vance. "Gene dose of apolipoprotein E type 4 allele and the risk of Alzheimer's disease in late onset families." *Science* 261, no. 5123 (1993):921–923.
31. Goate A, Chartier-Harlin MC, Mullan M, Brown J, Crawford F, Fidani L, Giuffra L, Haynes A, Irving N, James L, Mant R. *Segregation of a missense mutation in the amyloid precursor protein gene with familial Alzheimer's disease*. Nature. 1991 Feb 21; 349(6311): 704–6.
32. Lambert JC, Ibrahim-Verbaas CA, Harold D, Naj AC, Sims R, Bellenguez C, et al. Meta-analysis of 74,046 individuals identifies 11 new susceptibility loci for Alzheimer's disease. Nat Genet. 2013; 45(12):1452–8.
33. Younghee Lee, Haiquan Li, Jianrong Li, Ellen Rebman, Ikbel Achour, Kelly E Regan, Eric R Gamazon, James L Chen, Xinan Holly Yang, Nancy J Cox, and Yves A Lussier, Network models of genome-wide association studies uncover the topological centrality of protein interactions in complex diseases, J Am Med Inform Assoc. 2013 Jul; 20(4): pp. 619–629. Published online 2013 Jan 25. doi:10.1136/amiajnl-2012-001519.
34. N. Akula, A. Baranova, D. Seto, Jeffrey, M.A. Nalls, A. Singleton, L. Ferrucci, T. Tanaka, S. Bandinelli, Y.S. Cho, Y.J. Kim, Jong-Young Lee, Bok-Ghee Han, J. McMahon, A Network-Based Approach to Prioritize Results from Genome-Wide Association Studies, Published: September 6, 2011.
35. Goate A, Chartier-Harlin MC, Mullan M, Brown J, Crawford F, Fidani L, Giuffra L, Haynes A, Irving N, James L, Mant R. Segregation of a missense mutation in the amyloid precursor protein gene with familial Alzheimer's disease. *Nature*. 1991 Feb 21; 349(6311): 704–6.
36. Rogaev EI, Sherrington R, Rogaeva EA, Levesque G, Ikeda M, Liang Y, Chi H, Lin C, Holman K, Tsuda T, Mar L. Familial Alzheimer's disease in kindreds with missense mutations in a gene on chromosome 1 related to the Alzheimer's disease type 3 gene. *Nature*. 1995 Aug 31; 376(6543):775–8.
37. Bertram L, McQueen MB, Mullin K, Blacker D, Tanzi RE: Systematic meta-analyses of Alzheimer disease genetic association studies: the AlzGene database. Nat Genet 2007, 39:17–23.
38. Mullan M, Crawford F, Axelman K, Houlden H, Lilius L, Winblad B, Lannfelt L. A pathogenic mutation for probable Alzheimer's disease in the APP gene at the N–terminus of β–amyloid. Nature genetics. 1992 Aug 1; 1(5):345–7.
39. Ritchie MD, Hahn LW, Roodi N, Bailey LR, Dupont WD, Parl FF, Moore JH, Multifactor-dimensionality reduction reveals high-order interactions among

estrogen-metabolism genes in sporadic breast cancer, Am J Hum Genet. 2001 Jul; 69 (1): pp. 138–47. Epub 2001 Jun 11.
40. Kononen J, Bubendorf L, Kallionimeni A, Bärlund M, Schraml P, Leighton S, Torhorst J, Mihatsch MJ, Sauter G, Kallionimeni OP. Tissue microarrays for high-throughput molecular profiling of tumor specimens. *Nature medicine. 1998 Jul 1; 4(7):844–7.*
41. Perou CM, Sørlie T, Eisen MB, van de Rijn M, Jeffrey SS, Rees CA, et al. Molecular portraits of human breast tumours. Nature. 2000; 406(6797):747–52. doi:10.1038/35021093.
42. Parker JS, Mullins M, Cheang MC, Leung S, Voduc D, Vickery T, et al. Supervised risk predictor of breast cancer based on intrinsic subtypes. J ClinOncol. 2009; 27(8):1160–1167. doi:10.1200/JCO.2008.18.1370.
43. Wang Y, Klijn JG, Zhang Y, Sieuwerts AM, Look MP, Yang F, et al. Gene-expression profiles to predict distant metastasis of lymph-node-negative primary breast cancer. The Lancet. 2005; 365(9460):671–9. doi:10.1016/S0140-6736(05)17947-1.
44. Curtis C, Shah SP, Chin SF, Turashvili G, Rueda OM, Dunning MJ, et al. The genomic and transcriptomic architecture of 2,000 breast tumours reveals novel subgroups. Nature. 2012; 486(7403):346–52. doi:10.1038/nature10983.
45. David J. Dittman, Taghi M. Khoshgoftaar, Amri Napolitano, Selecting the Appropriate Ensemble Learning Approach for Balanced Bioinformatics Data, Proceedings of the Twenty-Eighth International Florida Artificial Intelligence Research Society Conference, pp. 329–334.
46. K. Gao, T. Khoshgoftaar, R. Wald, Combining Feature Selection and Ensemble Learning for Software Quality Estimation, Proceedings of the Twenty-Seventh International Florida Artificial Intelligence Research Society Conference, pp. 47–52.
47. Heim S, Mitelman F. Cancer cytogenetics: chromosomal and molecular genetic aberrations of tumor cells. John Wiley & Sons; 2015 Aug 17.
48. Folkman J. Angiogenesis in cancer, vascular, rheumatoid and other disease. Nature medicine. 1995 Jan 1; 1(1):27–30.
49. Hudson TJ, Anderson W, Artez A, Barker AD, Bell C, Bernabé RR, et al. International network of cancer genome projects. Nature. 2010; 464(7291):993–8. doi:10.1038/nature08987.
50. Qian Wang, Jiaxing Zhang, Sen Song, Zheng Zhang, Attentional Neural Network: Feature Selection Using Cognitive Feedback, arXiv:1411.5140v1[cs.CV] 19 Nov 2014.
51. Dean J, Ghemawat S. MapReduce: simplified data processing on large cluster. Communications of the ACM 2008; 51(1): 107–113.
52. IDC, The digital universe in 2020: big data, bigger digital shadows, and biggest growth in the Far East, www.emc.com/leadership/digital-universe/index.htm [last accessed 20 November 2014].
53. Chen C.L.P, Zhang C.Y. Data-intensive applications, challenges, techniques and technologies: a survey on big data, Inform. Sci, doi:10.1016/j.ins.2014.01.015.
54. Chen M, Mao S, Liu Y. Big data survey. Mobile Networks and Applications 2014; 19(2): 171–209.
55. Chen M, Mao S, Liu Y. Big data: a survey. Mobile Networks and Applications. 2014 Apr 1; 19(2):171–209.
56. Jake Luo, Min Wu, Deepika Gopukumar and Yiqing Zhao, Big Data Application in Biomedical Research and Health Care: A Literature Review, libertas academia, freedom to research, published on 19 Jan 2016. doi:10.4137/BII.S31559.
57. Dr. Xin Deng, Dr. Donghui Wu, Big Data Analytic Technology for Bioinformatics and Health Informatics, Call for Papers: Special Session at 2015 IEEE Symposium on Computational Intelligence in healthcare and e-health (IEEE CICARE 2015).
58. Emdad Khan, Addressing Bioinformatics Big Data Problems using Natural Language Processing: Help Advancing Scientific Discovery and Biomedical Research, Modern Computer Applications in Science and Education, pp. 221–228.
59. Cambridge Healthtech Institute's Eighth Annual, Integrated Informatics Driving Translational Research & Precision Medicine, March 7–9, 2016, Moscone North Convention

Center, San Francisco, CA, Part of the 23rd International Molecular Medicine Tri-Conference.
60. Tonia C. Carter and Max M. He, Challenges of Identifying Clinically Actionable Genetic Variants for Precision Medicine, Journal of Healthcare Engineering Volume 2016 (2016), Article ID 3617572.
61. Coiera E. Guide to health informatics. CRC press; 2015 Mar 6.
62. O'donoghue, John; Herbert, John (2012). "Data management within mHealth environments: Patient sensors, mobile devices, and databases". Journal of Data and Information Quality (JDIQ). 4 (1):5.
63. Mettler T, Raptis DA (2012). "What constitutes the field of health information systems? Fostering a systematic framework and research agenda". Health Informatics Journal. 18 (2): 147–56. doi:10.1177/1460458212452496. PMID 22733682.
64. Chen J, Qian F, Yan W, Shen B (2013) Translational biomedical informatics in the cloud: present and future. BioMed Res Int 2013, 8.
65. Brown-Liburd H, Issa H, Lombardi D. Behavioral implications of Big Data's impact on audit judgment and decision making and future research directions. Accounting Horizons. 2015 Jun; 29(2):451–68.
66. Adibi, Sasan, ed. (February 19, 2015). Mobile Health: A Technology Road Map. Springer. ISBN 978-3-319-12817-7.
67. Sohn H, Farrar CR, Hemez FM, Shunk DD, Stinemates DW, Nadler BR, Czarnecki JJ. A review of structural health monitoring literature: 1996–2001. Los Alamos National Laboratory, USA. 2003.
68. Frank J, Di Ruggiero E, Mowat D, Medlar B. Developing knowledge translation capacity in public health. Canadian Journal of Public Health. 2007 Jul; 98(4).
69. Schatz B, Marsh C, Patrick K, et al. Research challenges in measuring data for population health to enable predictive modeling for improving healthcare. ACM SIGHIT Rec. 2012; 2:36–41.
70. Jiang Y, Liao Q, Cheng Q, et al. Designing and evaluating a clustering system for organizing and integrating patient drug outcomes in personal health messages. AMIA Annu Symp Proc. 2012; 2012: 417–426.
71. Becker T, Curry E, Jentzsch A, Palmetshofer W. New Horizons for a Data-Driven Economy: Roadmaps and Action Plans for Technology, Businesses, Policy, and Society. In New Horizons for a Data-Driven Economy 2016 (pp. 277–291). Springer International Publishing.
72. Magoulas, Roger; Lorica, Ben (February 2009). "Introduction to Big Data". Release 2.0. Sebastopol CA: O'Reilly Media (11).
73. Snijders, C.; Matzat, U.; Reips, U.-D. (2012). "'Big Data': Big gaps of knowledge in the field of Internet". International Journal of Internet Science. 7: 1–5.
74. Wild S, Roglic G, Green A, et al. Global prevalence of diabetes estimates for the year 2000 and projections for 2030. Diabetes Care 2004; 27:1047–1053.
75. Centers for Disease Control and Prevention. Estimates of diabetes and its burden in the United States. National Diabetes Statistics Report. Atlanta, GA: US Department of Health and Human Services. 2014.
76. Lindstro M. J, Louheranta A, Mannelin M, et al. The Finnish Diabetes Pre-vention Study (DPS): Lifestyle intervention and 3-year results on diet and physical activity. Diabetes Care 2003; 26:3230–3236. 20.
77. Li G, Zhang P, Wang J, et al. The long-term effect of lifestyle interventions to prevent diabetes in the China Da Qing Diabetes Prevention Study: A 20-year follow-up study. Lancet 2008; 371:1783–1789. 21.
78. Ramachandran A, Snehalatha C, Mary S, et al. The Indian Diabetes Pre-vention Programme shows that lifestyle modification and metformin prevent type 2 diabetes in Asian Indian subjects with impaired glucose tolerance (IDPP-1). Diabetologia 2006; 49:289–297.
79. Kahn HS, Cheng YJ, Thompson TJ, et al. Two risk-scoring systems for predicting incident diabetes mellitus in US adults age 45 to 64 years. Ann Intern Med 2009; 150:741–751. 24.

80. Stern MP, Williams K, Haffner SM. Identification of persons at high risk for type 2 diabetes mellitus: Do we need the oral glucose tolerance test? Ann Intern Med 2002; 136:575–581. 25.
81. Chen L, Magliano DJ, Balkau B, et al. AUSDRISK: An Australian Type 2 Diabetes Risk Assessment Tool based on demographic, lifestyle and simple anthropometric measures. Med J Aust 2010; 192:197–202. 26.
82. Lindstro M J, Tuomilehto J. The diabetes risk score: A practical tool to predict type 2 diabetes risk. Diabetes Care 2003; 26:725–731.
83. Groves P, Kayyali B, Knott D, et al. The 'big data' revolution in healthcare. Boston: McKinsey Quarterly. 2013.
84. Bellman RE. The theory of dynamic programming. Rand Corporation technical report, 1957.
85. van Regenmortel MH, Fauquet CM, Bishop DH, Carstens EB, Estes MK, Lemon SM, Maniloff J, Mayo MA, McGeoch DJ, Pringle CR, Wickner RB. Virus taxonomy: classification and nomenclature of viruses. Seventh report of the International Committee on Taxonomy of Viruses. Academic Press; 2000.
86. National Institutes of Health. Precision medicine initiative cohort program, 2015.
87. National Institutes of Health. Precision Medicine Initiative Cohort Program. 2016.
88. Francis S. Collins, M.D., Ph.D., and Harold Varmus, M.D, A New Initiative on Precision Medicine, the new England journals of medicine, N England J Med 2015; 372:793–795 February 26, 2015 doi:10.1056/NEJMp1500523.
89. Seripa D, Panza F, Daragjati J, Paroni G, Pilotto A. Measuring pharmacogenetics in special groups: geriatrics. Expert opinion on drug metabolism & toxicology. 2015 Jul 3; 11(7): 1073–88.
90. Siobhan Dumbreck, Angela Flynn, Moray Nairn, Martin Wilson, Shaun Treweek, Stewart W Mercer, Phil Alderson, Alex Thompson, Katherine Payne, Guthrie, Drug-disease and drug-drug interactions: systematic examination of recommendations in 12 UK national clinical guidelines, *BMJ* 2015; 350.
91. Caterina Palleria, Antonello Di Paolo, Chiara Giofrè, Chiara Caglioti, Giacomo Leuzzi, Antonio Siniscalchi, Giovambattista De Sarro, and Luca Gallelli, Pharmacokinetic drug-drug interaction and their implication in clinical management, journal of research in medical science, J Res Med Sci. 2013 Jul; 18(7): 601–610.
92. Becker ML, Kallewaard M, Caspers PW, Visser LE, Leufkens HG, Stricker BH. Hospitalisations and emergency department visits due to drug-drug interactions: a literature review. Pharmacoepidemiol Drug Saf. 2007; 16(6):641–51.
93. Daly AK. Pharmacogenomics of adverse drug reactions. Genome med. 2013; 5(1):5.
94. Verma RP, Hansch C, QSAR modeling of taxane analogues against colon cancer, Eur J Med Chem. 2010 Apr; 45(4):1470–7. doi:10.1016/j.ejmech.2009.12.054. Epub 2010 Jan 13.
95. Fauzee NJS, Dong Z, Wang YI. Taxanes: promising anti-cancer drugs. Asian Pac J Cancer Prev. 2011; 12:837–51.
96. Song L, Chen QH, She XE, Chen XG, Wang FP. Conversional synthesis and cytotoxic evaluation of novel taxoid analogs. J Asian Nat Prod Res. 2011; 13(9):787–98.
97. Niko Beerenwinke, Martin Däumer, Mark Oette, Klaus Korn, Daniel Hoffmann, Rolf Kaiser, Thomas Lengauer, Joachim Selbig, and Hauke Walter, Geno2pheno: estimating phenotypic drug resistance from HIV-1 genotypes, Nucleic Acids Res. 2003 Jul 1; 31(13):3850–3855. PMCID: PMC168981.
98. Soo-Yon Rhee, Jonathan Taylor, Gauhar Wadhera, Asa Ben-Hur, Douglas L. Brutlag, Robert W. Shafer, Genotypic predictors of human immunodeficiency virus type 1 drug resistance, vol. 103 no. 46, Soo-Yon Rhee, 17355–17360.
99. Kelly T, Yang W, Chen C-S, Reynolds K, He J. Global burden of obesity in 2005 and projections to 2030. Int J Obes (Lond). 2008; 32:1431–7.
100. Ogden CL, Carroll MD, Kit BK, Flegal KM. Prevalence of childhood and adult obesity in the United States, 2011- 2012. JAMA. 2014; 311:806–14.

101. Ravel J, Gajer P, Abdo Z, Schneider GM, Koenig SS, McCulle SL, et al. Vaginal microbiome of reproductive-age women. Proc Natl Acad Sci. 2011; 108(Supplement 1):4680–687.
102. Kamal S, Ripon SH, Dey N, Ashour AS, Santhi V. A MapReduce approach to diminish imbalance parameters for big deoxyribonucleic acid dataset. Computer methods and programs in biomedicine. 2016 Jul 31; 131:191–206.
103. Kamal S, Dey N, Nimmy SF, Ripon SH, Ali NY, Ashour AS, Karaa WB, Nguyen GN, Shi F. Evolutionary framework for coding area selection from cancer data. Neural Computing and Applications.:1–23.
104. Acharjee S, Dey N, Samanta S, Das D, Roy R, Chakraborty S, Chaudhuri SS. Electrocardiograph Signal Compression Using Ant Weight Lifting Algorithm for Tele-Monitoring. Journal of Medical Imaging and Health Informatics. 2016 Feb 1; 6(1): 244–51.
105. Dey N, Das P, Chaudhuri SS, Das A. Feature analysis for the blind-watermarked electroencephalogram signal in wireless telemonitoring using Alattar's method. In Proceedings of the Fifth International Conference on Security of Information and Networks 2012 Oct 25 (pp. 87–94).
106. Cinque M, Coronato A, Testa A. Dependable services for mobile health monitoring systems. International Journal of Ambient Computing and Intelligence (IJACI). 2012 Jan 1; 4(1):1–5.
107. Van Hoof J, Wouters EJ, Marston HR, Vanrumste B, Overdiep RA. Ambient assisted living and care in The Netherlands: the voice of the user. Pervasive and Ubiquitous Technology Innovations for Ambient Intelligence Environments. 2012 Sep 30:205.
108. Odella F. Technology Studies and the Sociological Debate on Monitoring of Social Interactions. International Journal of Ambient Computing and Intelligence (IJACI). 2016 Jan 1; 7(1):1–26.
109. Tapia DI, Corchado JM. An ambient intelligence based multi-agent system for Alzheimer health care. International Journal of Ambient Computing and Intelligence (IJACI). 2009 Jan 1; 1(1):15–26.
110. Favela J, Tentori M, Segura D, Berzunza G. Adaptive awareness of hospital patient information through multiple sentient displays. International Journal of Ambient Computing and Intelligence (IJACI). 2009 Jan 1; 1(1):27–38.
111. Baumgarten M, Mulvenna M, Rooney N, Reid J. Keyword-Based Sentiment Mining using Twitter. International Journal of Ambient Computing and Intelligence. 2013; 5(2):56–69.
112. Odella F. Technology Studies and the Sociological Debate on Monitoring of Social Interactions. International Journal of Ambient Computing and Intelligence (IJACI). 2016 Jan 1; 7(1):1–26.
113. Araki T, Ikeda N, Dey N, Chakraborty S, Saba L, Kumar D, Godia EC, Jiang X, Gupta A, Radeva P, Laird JR. A comparative approach of four different image registration techniques for quantitative assessment of coronary artery calcium lesions using intravascular ultrasound. Computer methods and programs in biomedicine. 2015 Feb 28; 118(2):158–72.
114. Araki T, Ikeda N, Dey N, Acharjee S, Molinari F, Saba L, Godia EC, Nicolaides A, Suri JS. Shape-based approach for coronary calcium lesion volume measurement on intravascular ultrasound imaging and its association with carotid intima-media thickness. Journal of Ultrasound in Medicine. 2015 Mar 1; 34(3):469–82.
115. Roy P, Goswami S, Chakraborty S, Azar AT, Dey N. Image segmentation using rough set theory: a review. International Journal of Rough Sets and Data Analysis (IJRSDA). 2014 Jul 1; 1(2):62–74.
116. Dey N, Ashour AS, Chakraborty S, Samanta S, Sifaki-Pistolla D, Ashour AS, Le DN, Nguyen GN. Healthy and Unhealthy Rat Hippocampus Cells Classification: A Neural Based Automated System for Alzheimer Disease Classification. Journal of Advanced Microscopy Research. 2016 Jun 1; 11(1):1–0.

Machine Learning Models for Multidimensional Clinical Data

Christina Orphanidou and David Wong

Abstract Healthcare monitoring systems in the hospital and at home generate large quantities of rich-phenotype data from a wide array of sources. Typical sources include clinical observations, continuous waveforms, lab results, medical images and text notes. The key clinical challenge is to interpret these in a way that helps to improve the standard of patient care. However, the size and complexity of the data sets, which are often multidimensional and dynamically changing, means that interpretation is extremely difficult, even for expert clinicians. One important set of approaches to this challenge is Machine Learning Systems. These are systems that analyse and interpret data in a way that automatically recognizes underlying patterns and trends. These patterns are useful for predicting future clinical events such as hospital re-admission, and for determining rules within clinical decision support tools. In this chapter we will provide a review of machine learning models currently used for event prediction and decision support in healthcare monitoring. In particular, we highlight how these approaches deal with multi-dimensional data. We then discuss some of the practical problems in implementing Machine Learning Systems. These include: missing or corrupted data, incorporation of heterogeneous and multimodal data, and generalization across patient populations and clinical settings. Finally, we discuss promising future research directions, including the most recent developments in Deep Learning.

C. Orphanidou (✉)
Department of Electrical and Computer Engineering, University of Cyprus, Nicosia, Cyprus
e-mail: orphanid@ucy.ac.cy

D. Wong
Leeds Institute of Health Sciences, University of Leeds, Leeds, UK
e-mail: d.c.wong@leeds.ac.uk

© Springer International Publishing AG 2017

S.U. Khan et al. (eds.), *Handbook of Large-Scale Distributed Computing in Smart Healthcare*, Scalable Computing and Communications,
DOI 10.1007/978-3-319-58280-1_8

1 Introduction

Advances in the development of smart sensors and intelligent communication systems combined with the proliferation of smart devices and access to cheaper and more effective power and storage mechanisms have led to an explosion in healthcare data in the past few years. In 2012 healthcare data worldwide amounted to approximately 500 petabytes and by 2020 the amount is projected to be 25,000 petabytes [1]. The large quantities of data, generated in hospital and at home, present the opportunity to develop data-driven approaches for delivering best practice and improving patient outcomes. The key clinical challenge is to interpret the available data in order to provide better and faster decision-making and thus improve the standard of patient care and, consequently, patient health outcomes. Data-driven systems being developed aim to provide disease diagnosis, offer online patient tracking, identify physiological deterioration, provide risk assessments, as well as predict the occurrence of severe abnormalities such that suitable interventions can be put in place in a timely manner.

One important set of approaches to this challenge is Machine Learning Systems. These are computer algorithms that analyse and interpret data in a way that automatically recognizes underlying patterns and trends. Compared to more traditional statistics-based approaches where prior information about the process to be modelled is required, machine learning favours a black box approach: the relationship between different variables does not need to be fully understood. For instance in disease diagnosis systems, the underlying labelling processes are not particularly important; the system just needs to learn how to replicate them. While this black-box approach does not provide any knowledge into the way the different parameters are associated with outcomes, it is particularly suitable for healthcare monitoring applications where the available information to be processed is very complex. Variables to be combined are often present in a plethora of different formats, such as lab-results, clinical observations, imaging scans, continuous waveforms and more, and the associations between the different variables are not always clearly understood. The human expert, the gold standard of clinical decision-making gains clinical acumen in large part through experience. The basic principle of Machine Learning is not far-off: for a computer to be taught how to perform a task we need to provide it with enough examples of how it should be done. As more information is added to the system, the "experience" grows and the decision-making is improved.

The potential of machine learning clinical applications is enormous. In complex medical cases, the inclusion of aggregate data may reveal new information that is not seen by the individual. Machine learning systems additionally offer the possibility of dynamic, online monitoring at home and the hospital and are particularly useful in situations where real-world constraints may restrict the number of clinical staff attending to the patients. Moreover, the ability of machine learning models to analyse massive amounts of constantly refreshed, diverse information in real-time, via Big Data/Deep Learning approaches, offers the potential of quick and effective decision-making at a decreased cost. Additionally, machine learning can provide input which is similar to that of a truly independent expert since it circumvents the confirmation bias of the clinical expert [2]. However, the size and complexity of the data sets, which are often multidimensional and dynamically changing, means that interpretation is extremely difficult, even for expert clinicians. Prediction accuracy depends on the amount of data available to build the system's "experience". Additionally, because the researcher is searching for patterns without knowing what may emerge, findings need to be validated using stringent methods, in order to ensure that they are not occurring by chance.

In this chapter we will introduce the principles of machine learning and review models currently used for event prediction and decision support in healthcare monitoring. In particular, we highlight how these approaches deal with multi-dimensional and heterogeneous data. We then discuss some of the practical problems in implementing Machine Learning Systems. These include: how to process missing or corrupted data and how to process heterogeneous and multi-modal data. Finally, we discuss promising future research directions, including the most recent developments in Deep Learning.

2 Machine Learning Models

Machine learning models are computer programs that can "learn" important features of a data set (the *training* set) such that the user can make predictions about other data which were not part of the training set (the *test* set). Applications arising from these models include classifiers which can separate datasets into two or more classes based on characteristics measured in each data set [3] or regression models which can estimate continuous variables. In the context of clinical applications, classifiers have been proposed for disease diagnosis (computer-aided diagnosis-CAD), event prediction, forecasting of patient outcomes, even to predict hospital mortality. Regression models, on the other hand, have been proposed for estimating risk scores and for estimating disease stage and predicting clinical progression.

A machine learning model considers a large set of N D-dimensional *feature vectors* $\{X_1, \ldots, X_N\}$, $X \in R^D$, called the *training* set which is used in order to tune the parameters of an adaptive model. In order to build a machine learning model, for each one of the feature vectors, we need to have a corresponding *target* value $\{Y_1, \ldots, Y_N\}, Y \in R^K$. When building a binary classifier, $Y \in \{0, 1\}$ (the *label)*, while in the case of building a regression model, Y takes a continuous value from a usually predefined range. The goal of building a machine learning model is to build a rule which can predict Y given X, using only the data at hand. Such a rule is a function $h: X \rightarrow Y$ which is essentially the *machine*. The exact form of the function $h(X)$ is determined during the *training* phase (sometimes also referred to as the *learning* phase), using the training data: this type of learning is called *supervised*. Once the model is trained, it can then be used to determine Y for new values of X, not used in the training set, i.e., the *test* set. The ability to predict Y correctly from new values of X is known as *generalization* and it is a central goal in machine learning and pattern recognition [4].

It is also possible to build a machine learning model based only on the input vectors X, without any corresponding target values. These type of *unsupervised* learning approaches aim to discover groups of similar attributes within the dataset (*clustering*), to determine the distribution of data within the input space (*density estimation*) or to reduce the dimensionality of the input space for the purpose of *visualization* [4].

The steps involved in building a machine learning algorithm are:

- Choosing the analysis model
- Choosing the attributes of the data set that will comprise the features of the system
- Training the model
- Validating the model on the test data

In the following sections we will review current approaches for addressing every step of the process and discuss considerations related to clinical applications.

2.1 Model Selection

The first applications of machine learning in biomedicine were based on Artificial Neural Networks (ANN) and the promise of building systems modelled after the structure and functioning of the brain [5]. The systems showed a lot of promise and led to many applications in biomedical image and signal analysis. However, the complexity and lack of understanding about how the different components of the systems are connected made it difficult to interpret the outputs in a clinical context. Further effort was then made to create linear models for pattern recognition in biomedicine, which have the advantage of being easier to analyse and interpret in a meaningful way and are also computationally efficient. An example of a linear model, which has been used extensively in biomedical applications, is Support Vector Machines (SVM). An attractive property of this approach is the fact that while it uses a linear process for separating high-dimensional feature data, it allows the input data to be modelled non-linearly in order to obtain the high-dimensional feature space [6]. It is often the case, however, that clinical data contain high amounts of noise (for example physiological signals obtained via wearable sensors). To address this uncertainty in the data and at the same time to incorporate prior knowledge into the decision-making process, methods based on Bayesian inference have been introduced and have made significant impact in the detection and assessment of disease in biomedicine [5]. In the next sections we will describe the methodologies employed in ANNs, SVMs and Bayesian Networks and discuss the respective advantages and disadvantages of each technique when applied to the analysis of multidimensional clinical data.

2.1.1 Artificial Neural Networks

Artificial Neural Networks (ANNs) are mathematical models which attempt to simulate the structure and functionality of the brain. The building blocks of such networks are mathematical functions which are interconnected using some basic rules. The parameters of each building block are learnt during the process of training. ANNs have shown great potential in approximating arbitrary functions, however, in some practical applications it was found that the brain-like structure could sometimes impose entirely unnecessary constraints [4]. *Feed-forward neural networks*, e.g., the multilayer perceptron, have shown to be of greatest practical value and have been widely applied to biomedical clinical data analysis. Figure 1 shows a general structure of a feed-forward neural network. In a feed-forward neural network the route from the multidimensional input space to the multidimensional output space involves a series of functional transformations via the so-called *hidden layers*. The first step is to construct M linear combinations of the input variables $x_1, x_2, \ldots, x_D$ in the form

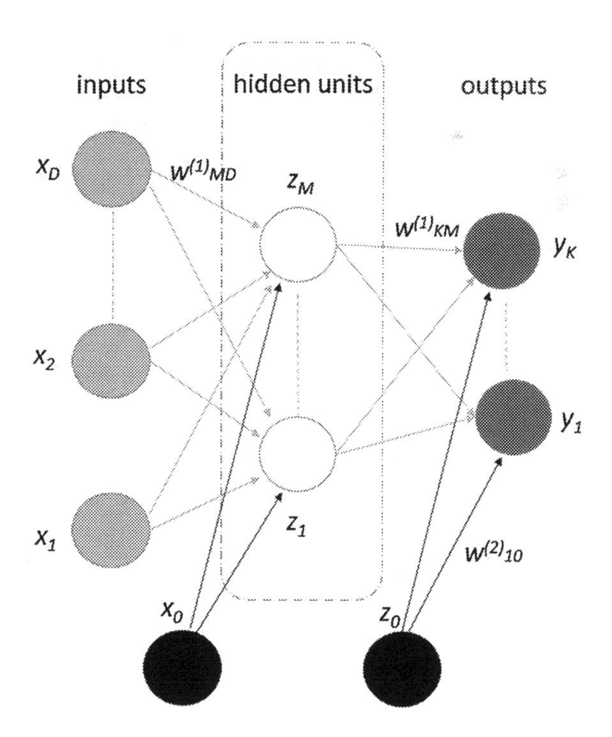

Fig. 1 Feed-forward neural network (adapted from [4])

$$a_j = \sum_{i=1}^{D} w_{ij}^{(1)} x_i + w_{j0}^{(1)} \tag{1}$$

where $j = 1, \ldots, M$ and M is the number of hidden units and the superscript (1) indicates which layer the parameters $w_{ij}^{(1)}$ (the *weights*) and $w_{j0}^{(1)}$ (the *biases*-nodes allowing for any fixed offset on the data) originate from [4]. The outputs a_j, known as activations are then transformed using nonlinear activation functions $h(\cdot)$ to give

$$z_j = h(a_j) \tag{2}$$

which are the *hidden units* of the network. The same procedure is then repeated in order to produce the output unit activations:

$$a_k = \sum_{j=1}^{D} w_{kj}^{(2)} z_j + w_{k0}^{(2)} \tag{3}$$

where $k = 1, \ldots, K$ and K is the number of outputs. The output unit activations are then transformed using another activation function to give the outputs, y_k.

$$y_k = l(a_k) \tag{4}$$

The choice of activation functions in all layers of the network is usually determined by the type of application and data characteristics. Sigmoidal functions are often used (logistic sigmoid or the *tanh* function), especially for binary classification problems [4].

2.1.2 Support Vector Machines

In its most common formulation, the Support Vector Machines approach considers N-dimensional input patterns x_i and output labels y_i. The input and output data are trained in order to estimate a function $f: R^N \rightarrow \{\pm 1\}$ such that $f(x) = y$ for new input/output examples (x, y). Both training and new data are assumed to have been generated from the same underlying probability distribution $P(x, y)$ [6]. The SVM classifier is based on the class of hyperplanes

$$(w \cdot x) + b = 0, w \in R^N, b \in R, \tag{5}$$

where the decision function is given by

$$f(x) = sign((w \cdot x) + b) \tag{6}$$

The optimal hyper-plane can be uniquely determined by solving a constrained optimization problem whose solution **w** has an expansion $w = \sum_i v_i x_i$ in terms of data of the training set which lie on maximal margin of separation between the two classes (the support vectors). Since Eqs. (4) and (5) depend only on dot products between patterns, the training data can be mapped nonlinearly to a higher-dimensional feature space F, via a map Φ such that the optimal separating hyper-plane can now be constructed in F. This is achieved by substituting $\Phi(x_i)$ for each x_i and applying simple *kernels* k, such that

$$k(x, x_i) := ((\Phi(x) \cdot \Phi(x_i)) \tag{7}$$

The decision boundary then becomes

$$f(x) = sign\left(\sum_{i=1}^{l} v_i \cdot k(x, x_i) + b\right), \tag{8}$$

where the parameters v_i are computed as the solution of a quadratic programming problem.

In essence, in input space the separating hyper-plane corresponds to a nonlinear decision function whose form depends on the type of kernel used [6] (see Fig. 2). Depending on the application at hand, different kernels may be used. Commonly used kernels include the radial basis function (RBF) given by

$$k(x, y) = \exp(-\|x - y\|^2)/2\sigma^2, \tag{9}$$

where σ is a scaling factor [6] and the polynomial given by

$$k(x, y) = (x \cdot y)^{\mathrm{d}}, \tag{10}$$

where d is the order of the polynomial.

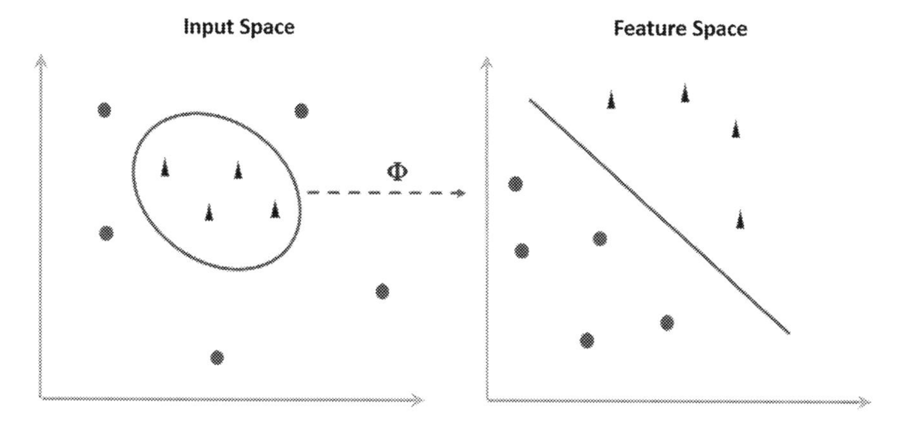

Fig. 2 The kernel trick in Support Vector Machines formulation (adapted from [6])

2.1.3 Bayesian Networks

Clinical datasets are often noisy and incomplete, making the building of machine learning models challenge. A way of dealing with noisy observations is to consider measured variables as latent states from which noisy observations are made [7]. Because many patient aspects are not directly measurable, state-space approaches have been extensively considered for obtaining reliable estimates of physiological states under uncertain conditions. Kalman Filters (KFs), are a good choice for dealing with noisy data since they treat measurements as noisy observations of an underlying state and update the state only if high confidence in the current state is high, conditioned on the previous observation [7]. Noisy observations are then naturally rejected and not taken into account in the calculation of the state. Bayesian approaches are also able to meet these challenges by incorporating uncertainty into the decision-making process. In the recent years, Bayesian methods have experienced a huge popularity for the development of biomedical applications and have shown promising performance in modelling a range of problems relevant to biological learning [5]. In classification problems, for instance, Bayesian approaches consider class conditional distributions, $P(D/C)$, (where D is the data and C is the class) which can be trained for each different class. The conditional probability of each class given data D can then be calculated using Baye's rule to obtain

$$P(C/D) = \frac{P(D/C)P(C)}{P(D)} \tag{11}$$

Classification of novel examples can then be performed by computing the likelihood over each model.

Bayesian networks are graphical models where each node represents a random variable and each link represents the dependencies between the linked variables. Along with the graphical structure of the network, a joint probability distribution *Pr* is learnt using the training data; for each random variable V_i represented by a node, a set of conditional probability distributions is determined connecting it to all the nodes it follows (sometimes referred to as the *parent* nodes and symbolized by $\pi(\cdot)$), $\Pr(V_i/\pi(V_i))$. The conditional probability distributions between each variable and node then define a unique joint probability distribution over the graph's structure as [8]:

$$\Pr(V_1, \ldots, V_n) = \prod_{i=1}^{n} \Pr(V_i/\pi(V_i)) \tag{12}$$

A restriction in the graphical models defined is that there can be no directed cycles, i.e., that the structure of the graph does not permit for a path which starts and ends at the same node, for this reason such graphs are also called *acyclic graphs* [4].

An advantage of Bayesian Networks compared to other approaches such as SVMs and ANNs is that they allow for interpretation of the interactions between different variables which makes them easier to combine with findings from clinicians.

2.2 Feature Extraction and Selection

The number and choice of features is critical to the success of a machine learning model. Using too many features relative to the "true" dimensionality of the process to be modelled may result in *overfitting*, a result of the classifier learning the training data instead of the intrinsic trends of the data [3]. Using a large number of features also requires a large training dataset in order to reliably estimate the relationships between the multidimensional variables, a phenomenon known as *the curse of dimensionality*. While there is no widely accepted rule for the ratio of features to "events", as a rule of thumb, at least ten events are needed per feature to achieve a reasonable predictive performance [9]. The choice of features is another crucial issue. Depending on the application of the machine learning model, the features selected are usually picked such that they have some bearing on the associated physiological process. These features would be the ones a clinician would review in order to assess the physical state of the patient. For example when building a system which may predict exacerbations in patients with Traumatic Brain Injury (TBI), intracranial pressure (ICP) should be included since it is the most important identifier of an exacerbation. For people with chronic cardiorespiratory problems elevations in heart rate (HR) and respiration rate (RR) and a drop in oxygen saturation (% SpO_2) are the most important precursors of an exacerbation. As a result HR, RR and % SpO_2 are obvious choices for features to be used in a predictive model for such exacerbations. It is often the case, however, that more abstract characteristics are used as features for a machine learning model. Examples are frequency characteristics of the ECG signal, such as the amount of entropy in different frequency bands, used for the diagnosis of Atrial Fibrillation (AF) [10] or statistical texture features extracted from medical images in order to identify malignant tumours [11]. While these abstract characteristics cannot be directly linked with assessments a clinician would make for making a decision, they often reveal strong links with medically relevant information.

2.3 Training, Testing and Evaluation Metrics

The data required for training and testing machine learning models are most often collected via clinical trials. The protocols of these clinical trials need to reflect the requirements of the algorithm to be designed. Collected data naturally need to correspond to the variables defined in the model. Enough data need to be collected, guided by the dimension of the feature space, so that the relationships between the different variables can be reliably derived. Target values need to be carefully defined. For example, when designing systems to identify "events", such as physiological exacerbations, the training data need to be chosen as to contain enough clearly marked occurrences of such events. This is often a challenge when building systems for diagnosing rare events and diseases.

In classification problems, human labelling, the "gold standard" of clinical diagnosis, is usually done by clinicians. Human labelling, however, suffers from inconsistencies, known as intra- and inter-rater variability. To alleviate this, often, multiple raters are used and only data with consistent labels across raters are used for building the classifiers.

Performance evaluation of machine learning algorithms is usually assessed based on predictive accuracy compared to the "gold standard". Sensitivity, Specificity, and Accuracy are the metrics most often used and in many cases a trade-off between true positive and true negative rate needs to be defined since the "cost" of each different type of error varies depending on the application. Sensitivity, given by TP/(TP + FN) where TP are true positives and FN are false negatives, measures the proportion of "positives" that have been correctly identified as such. Specificity, given by TN/(TN + FP) where TN are true negatives and FP are false positives, measures the proportion of "negatives" that have been correctly identified as such. Accuracy corresponds to overall proportion of correct classifications. Receiver Operating Characteristic (ROC) curves serve as a graphical representation of the trade-offs between the Sensitivities and Specificities of each model specification. While accuracy could be used as a metric for evaluating the performance of the system, the "cost" of a false positive (i.e., a signal identified as acceptable which is actually unacceptable) may be higher in practice than that of a false negative (i.e., an acceptable signal identified as unacceptable). The former would result in a false measurement whereas the latter would result in the rejection of signal which could actually have been used. In such situations, decision functions may be defined where the relative cost of each error is weighted or thresholds may be set in the minimum acceptable value of each metric, such that the best model for every application may be chosen.

Cross-Validation

Cross-validation is a method often used in order to evaluate machine learning models which allows all data points to be used in both the training and testing phases of the model evaluation procedure. In K-fold cross-validation all available data are firstly divided randomly into K different equally sized groups. At each iteration, one group is treated as the test set and the remaining K − 1 groups are used as the training set. A model is then trained K times, each time using one of the training sets and the associated test set and the overall accuracy is measured as the average of the accuracy measures of over the K iterations [4] (Fig. 3).

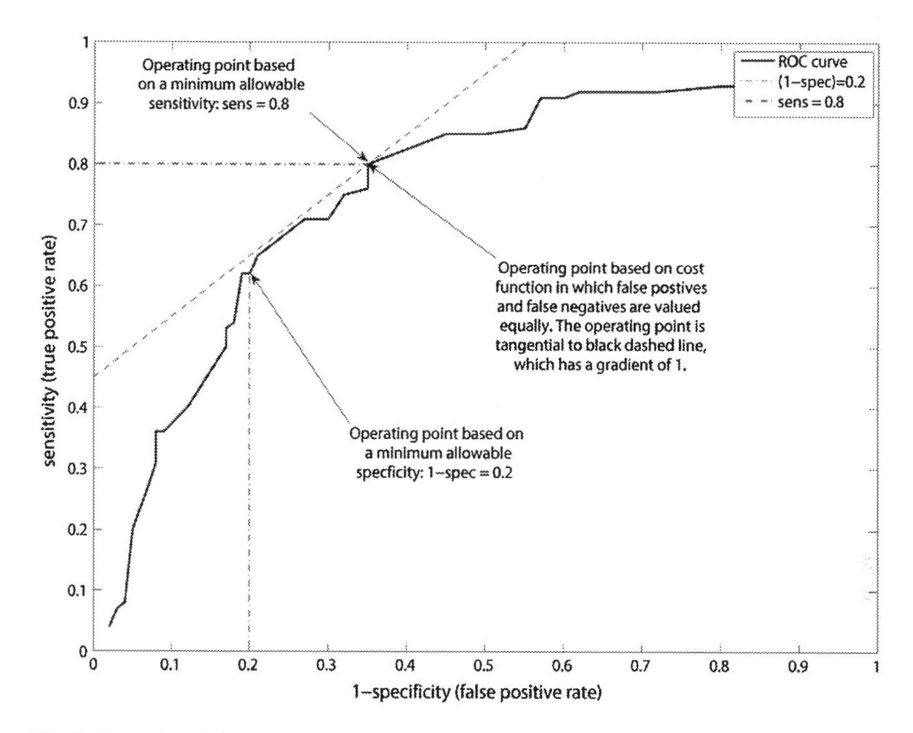

Fig. 3 Example ROC curve indicating operating point selection based on different criteria

3 Challenges Related to Clinical Applications

For real-life clinical problems, analysis of data is not straightforward, and cannot simply be reduced to the application of standard machine learning algorithms. Whilst data quality and analysis issues are not unique to healthcare, the acquisition of data from human patients brings additional challenges that do not occur in other fields. Two prominent challenges are the analysis of datasets with missing or corrupted data, and the analysis of heterogeneous and high-dimensional data.

3.1 Corrupted and Missing Data

Corrupted data occurs when a recorded measurement does not accurately reflect the true state of the object or person being measured. Missing data occurs when there is no recorded measurement at a given point in time. If left unrecognised, analysis that does not take into account missing or corrupted data may to lead to inaccurate decision-making. In the worst cases, this could mean patients being assigned the

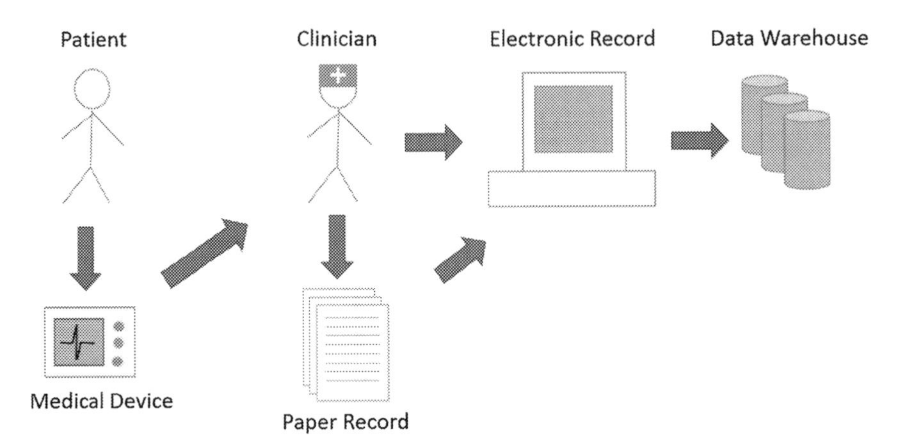

Fig. 4 Data flow during the collection of health data from patients. Multiple stages of data transfer are usually necessary before the final data items are stored securely within a data warehouse

wrong course of treatment. In the UK healthcare system alone, data of poor quality has previously been linked to unnecessarily cancelled operations, and undetected outbreaks in C. difficile infections [12].

To understand why health data are often of poor quality, it is helpful to first consider the steps typically involved during data collection. In general, the clinical data from patients involves multiple stages (Fig. 4), each allowing possibility of data corruption. Two of these stages are now discussed in greater detail.

Patient-Medical Device: In many common scenarios, the first opportunity for data corruption occurs when patient measurements are recorded using medical equipment. Incorrect use of medical equipment has been associated with erroneous measurements in a wide variety of clinical situations. For instance, Boba et al. [13] found that many breast core needle biopsies produced false-negative results due to sampling from an inappropriate site.

Vital sign monitoring is particularly prone to error caused by patient-device interaction. In the case of pulse oximeters, that measure the level of oxygen in the blood (SpO_2), corrupted data are often due to poor attachment of the device to the finger [14]. The relative motion between finger and device leads to physiologically implausible measurements known as motion artefact. Motion artefacts are a common problem for other physiological measurements including heart rate (via ECG) and activity detection (via accelerometers) [15, 16].

The problem of poor device attachment is becoming increasingly important as attempts are made at medium and long-term ambulatory monitoring outside of the hospital environment to reduce pressure on emergency services [17]. In these cases, the state-of-the-art is to apply an adhesive patch to the patient's sternum. Each patch contains a set of integrated sensors that can monitor multiple vital signs concurrently [18, 19]. The patients monitored tend to be more physically active than those monitored in-hospital which leads to greater levels of motion artefact. These artefacts are compounded by the practical problem of deterioration of patch adhesion over time.

Even if reliable device attachment can be guaranteed, the accuracy of the medical devices themselves may vary. In many cases, medical instrumentation is subject to regulations that guarantee tolerance (that is, variation from the true value). For instance, the US Food and Drug Administration mandates that all pulse oximeters for medical use have a maximum root mean squared error of <3% over the normal operating range [20]. However, multiple reviews of pulse oximeters have shown much greater variability when tested on healthy individuals [21].

Finally, we note that in some instances, there are multiple clinically-accepted methods for measuring the same data item. This can lead to instances in which variability is due to the measurement method, rather than the patient's true state. Core body temperature may be measure using either oral mercury, oral electronic, or tympanic electronic thermometers [22]. Blood pressure is traditionally measured using a mercury sphygmamometer. During measurement, an inflatable cuff temporarily cuts off blood flow to the arm. As the cuff is deflated, characteristic 'Korotkoff' sounds are used to identify the peak (systolic) and trough (diastolic) of the blood pressure waveform [23]. Modern semi-automatic blood pressure monitors take a different approach. The monitors measure the amplitudes of oscillations in the blood pressure cuff caused by the expansion of the arteries as blood is being forced through. These measurements are then converted into systolic and diastolic blood pressures derived empirically [24]. Pavlik et al. tested semi-automatic against manual methods, showing that the semi-automatic method produced consistently higher blood pressure readings [25]. Similar studies showing discrepancies between the two methods have since been reported for hypertensive patients and home-monitoring devices [26, 27].

Clinical Expert—Paper/Electronic Record: Having successfully taken a patient's measurements, the next step is for the clinician to interpret and validate the measurement. Error in clinical interpretation can occur through misreading information. For example, the oversight of a decimal point has led to high profile medication errors [28]. In response, national agencies have specific recommendations for numbers, including the avoidance of trailing zeros (to differentiate 1.0 and 10, for example) [29]. Clinical interpretation may also involve combining raw information into aggregate scores. For instance, the overall level of patient severity may be assessed through the use of Early Warning Scores (EWS). These scores assign an integer value to vital sign measurements; the sum of these values forms an EWS that is used to inform level of in-hospital care. These relatively simple calculations have repeatedly been shown to be erroneous approximately 20% of the time [30, 31].

The final clinically-validated data are transcribed to an official clinical record, which may be paper-based or electronic. The process of data transcription is prone to further error. For instance, Callen et al. [32] describe, for an Australian metropolitan hospital, how both handwritten and electronic systems contained clinically significant medication transcription errors in discharge summaries (handwritten: 12.1% and electronic: 13.3% for 13,000+ medications). The authors suggest numerous potential factors that may contribute to the level of error, including heavy workload and distractions from the current task. Further causes of transcription error include unintuitive design and lack of training [33, 34].

3.1.1 Reducing Corrupt Data

The previous section showed the multiple steps required to collect health data, and how each step is prone to data corruption. In instances when data collection is on-going, it is highly desirable to optimise these steps to maximise the reliability of the data for retrospective analysis.

One way to reduce patient-medical device errors is to improve the sensors within the device. Whilst integrated adhesive patches represent the current clinically viable method for recording vital signs, novel techniques are being developed that may reduce the problem of motion artefact. Batchelor et al. tackle motion artefact by using alternative methods of affixation [35]. Their prototype transfer tattoo electrodes provide a strong attachment to the skin and higher durability than traditional electrodes whilst producing similar data reliability (as evidenced through signal-to-noise ratios). Tarassenko et al. [36], as well as multiple others [37, 38], take another approach. Rather than ensuring the best possible contact, they attempt to measure vital signs with no patient contact, using video images. Results using the contactless techniques are comparable to traditional monitoring methods for patients at rest, with a mean absolute difference of approximately 3 beats/min for heart rate measurements.

Another way to reduce data corruption is to eliminate the amount of interpretation and transcription of clinical measurements. For vital sign data, incorrect calculations of EWS has been virtually eliminated with the help of electronic data entry at the bedside [39]. These so-called e-Obs systems allow users to type data; the system then automatically calculates the EWS and may provide care recommendations [40, 41]. This idea has been extended by medical device manufacturers, who have created integrated vital signs monitors that automatically send the EWS score and vital signs directly to the hospital's Electronic Patient Record [42].

Automated systems that reduce transcription have become increasingly commonplace in modern healthcare. The rise of Computer Physician Order Entry (CPOE) systems to standardise and automate the ordering of medication has been associated with reductions in nursing transcription errors [43]. Another electronic systems designed to reduce transcription error is the Bloodtrack system for blood transfusions [44]. Bloodtrack electronically allocates compatible red blood cell units by using barcode scanners to identify both the patient and blood packet. The introduction of the system has been associated with improvements in safety checks during blood sample collection, in addition to reduction in time to deliver blood [45, 46].

A final way to increase data quality is to identify corrupt data in real-time and encourage human intervention. In the simplest cases, this means preventing a user from entering implausible data. For instance, in the case of CPOE systems, drug-drug interactions data can be used to prevent prescription of potentially dangerous drug combinations [47].

A more sophisticated example is the Phillips Intellivue vital sign monitor. These devices measure multiple types of vital signs continuously and are used to monitor patients at risk of rapid deterioration. These devices generate audible alarms that indicate when the monitor data are unreliable and the vital signs sensors need to be reattached. The technical details for determining periods of unreliable data (typically via Signal Quality Indices) are explained in Sect. 3.1.2.

Whilst the adoption of processes that reduce corrupt and missing data is helpful for a wide range of healthcare related tasks, such as medical research and hospital management, there are multiple other competing aims within real clinical practice. Most importantly, standards of patient care should not be compromised. Bonnici et al. [48] highlight this in the context of wireless sensors, implying that patient choice and comfort is of paramount importance for successful implementation of remote monitoring systems.

Financial cost also needs to be considered. There is a trade-off between using the best (and most costly) equipment, and the level of improvement in staff efficiency and data quality that can be achieved [49]. For some in-hospital electronic solutions, improvements in data quality have been offset by significant increases in time to complete clinical tasks [50].

3.1.2 Identifying Corrupt Data

In reality, data corruption cannot be eliminated completely during the measurement and documentation process. Methods are therefore required to process and analyse low quality data. The first step of this process is to correctly identify the corrupt portions of the data set. In particular, it is important to accurately distinguish between an unusual, but true, measurement that may have clinical significance and abnormal data due to artefact. One common way to identify artefactual data is through Signal Quality Indices (SQIs). A SQI is a measure of confidence in the reliability of a data point. Typically, the development of an SQI begins by selecting relevant attributes, or features, that should be present in high quality data. Three popular types of features are:

Range Checking compares the data to physiologically plausible ranges. Any measurement outside the range is considered to be low quality. Tat et al. [51] implement range checking to evaluate the quality of an ECG signal. Part of their SQI involves converting the raw signal to a heart rate. Heart rates outside of the range 30–210 are considered bad quality.

Inference based on simultaneously recorded data—relies on the fact that measurements are often not independent. For instance, there is strong correlation between continuous blood pressure signal and ECG. Johnson et al. [52] make use of this by developing a SQI for heart rate, in which a high data reliability is estimated when the two signals peak at similar times.

Comparison to previous values compares the current data to previously measured values. If the difference between the current and previous values is deemed to be improbable, the measurement is considered to be invalid. Clifton et al. showed one implementation of this approach for tympanic thermometers. By using Bayesian changepoint detection, natural variation in temperature was distinguished from an unexpected step-change in temperature due to calibration error [53].

If the original waveform data are available, more complex features may be used. These may include morphological features (that is, recognition of typical shapes of data), and frequency features generated after the raw signal has been converted into its frequency components using a Fourier transform. For instance, Orphanidou et al. show, for ECG signals, how differences in morphology may be measured using an average cross-correlation between a template and unknown data [54]. A review from [55] indicated that this approach was particularly specific for ECG signal quality in comparison to alternative features.

SQI may be derived from one or more of these features. If multiple features are used, they must be combined in some way to produce a single result. The synthesis of multiple features is often completed using machine learning methods, like the example covered in case study 2 [56].

Setting the threshold between good and bad data quality is itself a challenging problem. In the previous example, the threshold was determined via clinical experts who were asked to label the training data. In many cases however, acceptable signal quality is often task dependent. For instance, in the case of PPG, respiratory rate is often detected using the small amplitude, low-frequency part of the signal—a high threshold on data quality is required. In contrast, heart rate can be computed from portions of the signal that typically have greater amplitude and less prone to random noise. Practically, this means that signal quality indices are highly specific to the clinical setting, a finding supported by Nizami's review of 80 artefact detection methods used in critical care medicine [57].

3.1.3 Processing Corrupt and Missing Data

After the identification of corrupt data, there are, broadly, two possible options: to use the corrupted data, or to discard the data.

Using corrupt data

Correction of corrupted data is possible when the mechanism by which the data were corrupted is known. For instance, in the case of an ECG signal, the observed signal is often subject to baseline wander caused by respiration, motion, or gradual changes in the ECG electrodes (Fig. 5). The baseline wander artefact is known to primarily affect low frequencies, so a high pass filter can be used to eliminate the spurious part of the signal [58].

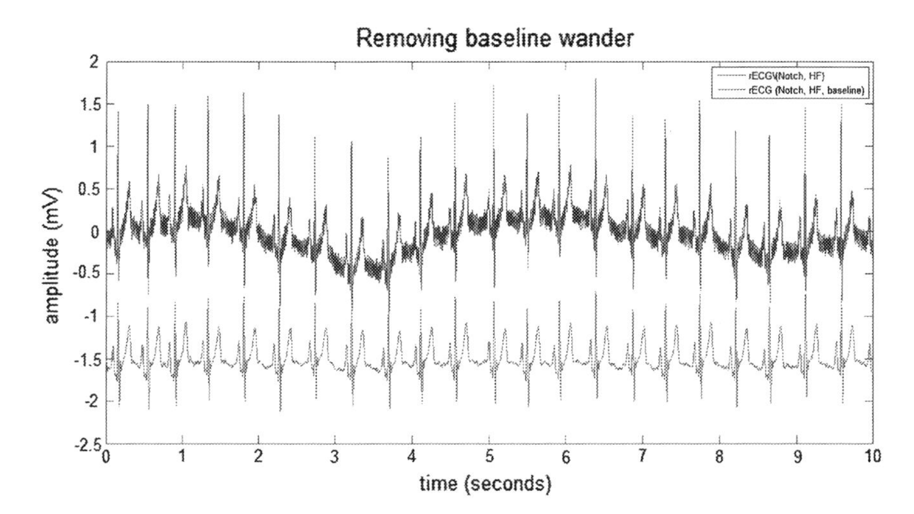

Fig. 5 Baseline wander in an ECG signal. The original signal (in *blue*) has a low frequency variation associated with respiration rate. By applying a high-pass filter (in *red*) the baseline wander can be removed to allow easier signal processing [59]

In the majority of cases, it is not possible to correct artefacts. However, even then, artefact may be non-random and can be used to infer additional useful information. For instance, in the case of EEG signals that measure brain activity, artefactual changes in the signal may be caused by muscle movement as the eyes blink. In many applications, the blink artefact is a nuisance, and there have been many attempts to identify and remove eye-blink artefacts [60, 61]. However, for certain applications, knowledge about blinking may be useful. For instance, the clinical standard for determining level of consciousness is partly determined by whether a patient's eyes are open [62]. If one were to attempt to ascertain consciousness level using EEG (as has been attempted by [63, 64]), the eye-blink artefact may contain useful information.

Even if artefactual data does not present useful information for the task at hand, a curated and annotated set of known artefacts can be used as exemplars to improve future artefact detection. Lawhern et al. use this approach for EEG signal classification to identify jaw and eye motion artefacts. Sections of EEG signal were first parameterised in an autoregressive model. The model parameters were then were successfully classified using Support Vector Machines, such that real signal was distinguished from multiple types of EEG artefact [65].

When data cannot be reasonably corrected, they are often removed from analysis. The way that missing data are handled is of paramount importance; it is easy to inadvertently introduce bias that leads to spurious results. One example of this is an early version of the cardiovascular risk score, QRISK [66]. QRISK (and its successor, QRISK2 [67]) outputs, for a patient, a percentage risk of cardiovascular disease within the next ten years. The output is based on an extensive range of variables including family history, smoking status and age. When data are missing, it attempts to estimate the missing values. However, the effect of this has led to unexpected outcomes, including an implausible null association between cholesterol level and cardiovascular risk [68]. Problems with imputation in QRISK have since been corrected and the algorithm revalidated [69].

Missing data can be categorised in three ways. Data Missing Completely At Random (MCAR) means that data points are missing at random, AND the missing value is independent of any other values in the data set. Data Missing At Random (MAR) means that data points are missing at random, but that the missing data can be partially explained by other variables in the data set. Data Missing Not At Random (MNAR) means that data points are not missing at random, such that the probability of the data being missing is associated with its value. In practice, it is often difficult to distinguish between these three categories, as the missing values are not known. However, knowledge of these missing data mechanisms is useful for recognising potential bias introduced by techniques for analysing incomplete data sets.

Listwise Deletion

The simplest technique for analysing incomplete data sets is to remove records with missing data, known as listwise deletion. This process ensures that only completed sets of data are used to construct models. Listwise deletion is typically appropriate when only a small percentage of data are missing (e.g. 1%) [70]. Listwise deletion has two significant drawbacks. First, the remaining data set will be biased, with reduced variability in the missing variable, if data are not MCAR. Second, valid information is unnecessarily discarded when there are multiple variables for each data record.

Data Imputation

Rather than removing missing records, one can attempt to replace the missing data elements with values estimated from the observed data, a process known as data imputation. A simple method for imputation, *mean imputation*, is to replace the missing data with the mean of the all other observations of that variable. This approach has been adopted within clinical software for detection of physiological deterioration from continuous vital signs [71]. In this case, the speed and simplicity of mean imputation was a useful practical method that allowed assessments of deterioration to be conducted in real-time. Mean imputation should be applied with caution, as the variance of the complete data set after imputation will lower than the true value. To avoid this problem, we may instead randomly sample from the distribution rather than selecting the mean, a process known as *stochastic imputation*. Unbiased sampling from an arbitrary distribution can be achieved using Gibbs sampling, or other Monte Carlo Markov Chain approaches [72].

If data are MAR (not MCAR), the underlying relationship between the observed and missing data can be used to provide a more precise imputation. One such method is *regression mean imputation*. Under this scheme, complete data records are used to regress (typically linear regression) the variable with missing data onto all other variables. The resulting equation is then used to impute the missing data points. Like simple mean regression, this deterministic approach (the unknown value is completely determined by the observed variables) artificially reduces data variability.

The regression approach can be extended to non-continuous variables. For example, logistic regression can be used for categorical variables [73]. In the case of censored data where values outside of a given range are unknown (for instance, due to limited time for study follow-up, or when the dynamic range of a sensor is too small) the Tobit model for truncated regression provides a non-biased estimate [74].

Another simple method for imputation, used in particular for time series data, is 'last value carried forward' also known as 'sample-and-hold'. Under this scheme, missing data are replaced with the last known value. Compared to the mean imputation approaches, sample-and-hold makes the additional assumption that subsequent observations are likely to be more similar than observations taken at random times.

The primary limitation of each of these methods is that the inherent uncertainty of missing data are discarded. More complex approaches, including multiple imputation, maximum-likelihood, and Gaussian process regression, circumvent this by using probability distributions to model the missing data.

Multiple imputation uses stochastic imputation to create multiple possible versions of the missing data record. All versions of the data set are analysed separately, and the outputs are averaged to get an overall result. Standard errors on the output parameters are calculated using Rubin's rules [75]. Rubin's rules take into account the variance of the missing data variable (determined as the variance within the completed records) and the variance of the multiple imputations. The reliability of multiple imputation estimates depends on the number of imputations used. Whilst initial research suggested a small number (3–5) imputations, Graham et al. showed that this was insufficient for estimating variance accurately [76]. Instead, they suggest using at least 20 imputations, a number that may increase depending on the overall percentage of missing data [77]. A more detailed tutorial on multiple imputation can be found in [78].

One popular implementation of multiple imputation when more than one variable has missing data is Multiple Implementation by Chained Equations [79]. Under this scheme, all missing data are initialised using mean imputation. Multiple imputation is then used to provide a more accurate estimate for each variable in turn. This process is repeated several times until convergence criteria are met.

An alternative approach is Maximum-Likelihood (ML) estimation. A full description is provided in [80] and is summarised briefly here. ML methods model all of the measured data as a joint probability distribution function, f. The distribution function is parameterised by a set of free parameters, θ. For the simple case in which each variable is normally distributed, the joint pdf is a multivariate Gaussian that is fully defined by the mean and covariance.

If each data record, x_i, is independent, then the probability of attaining a given set of n observed data is provided by the likelihood function:

$$L = \prod_{i=1}^{n} f(x_i|\theta) \quad (13)$$

In the case when some of the data records contain missing elements, the probability can be described by marginalising f over the missing variables so that the likelihood of single data record, in which the set of M variables are missing, is:

$$\int_M f(x_i|\theta) \quad (14)$$

ML attempts to find the most likely model instance by maximising the likelihood through adjustment of θ. In some instances, the maximum likelihood may be calculated analytically. However, in practice, the likelihood function may be highly non-linear and a closed form solution is not possible. In these cases, the likelihood function is maximised iteratively using methods such as the Expectation-Maximisation algorithm. Because the parameter set, θ, fully describes the variables and the correlations between them, the parameters can then be converted to regression equation parameters if specific instances of imputation are required.

Gaussian process regression extends these principled approaches by taking into consideration temporal relationships. In Gaussian process regression, n data points from a time series are modelled as a single sample from an n-dimensional Gaussian distribution (Fig. 6), defined by a covariance matrix. Any missing data are then simply represented by the conditional distribution: *P(missing data | observed data)*, which is also Gaussian.

The elements of the covariance matrix are determined via a covariance function that describes the expected change of the time series through time. In the simplest cases, the covariance functions simply describe how local measurements are highly correlated, and that correlation decreases as data samples become further apart in time. Alternatively, the covariance function can be based on domain-specific knowledge. For instance, Stegle et al. use a covariance function that takes into account periodic circadian rhythm for inferring missing heart rate [81].

Roberts provides a more comprehensive introduction to Gaussian process regression [82]. If multiple time series data are captured simultaneously, correlations between variables can also be modelled. Two similar approaches that model both temporal and inter-variable correlations using Gaussian processes are multi-task GPs and dependent GPs [83, 84].

Wong et al. show how Gaussian process regression in conjunction with other machine learning methods were used to generate alerts for abnormal vital sign data [85]. Likely distributions of the missing data were first imputed. The distributions were inputs to a model that generated alerts based on the vital sign abnormality, and the level of certainty in the data.

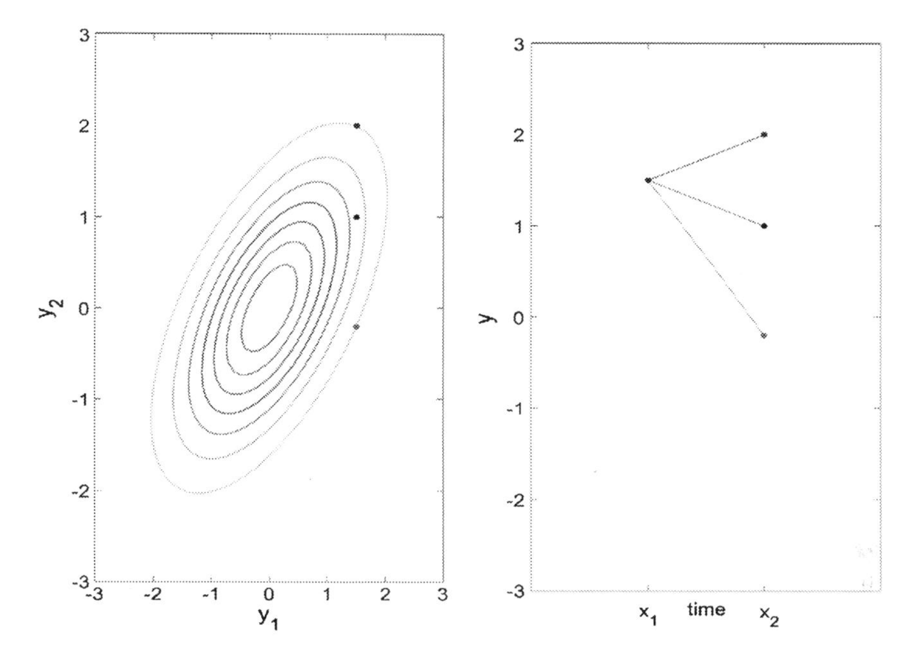

Fig. 6 Simple example of a Gaussian process for two time points. The *left figure* shows the joint probabilities of all possible pairs of points as a bivariate Gaussian distribution. The *right figure* shows the time series plots for the three points on the distribution highlighted in *blue*, *black* and *red*

In summary, analysis of missing data remains a complex problem. The optimal choice of data imputation technique depends on the specific problem, and should consider practical problems such as speed of implementation in addition to accuracy of the imputed data. Simple imputation may be used for some cases, but care should be taken to ensure that biases are identified. The fundamental limitation of such approaches is that a single value is used to represent the missing data point—thereby losing information about the uncertainty or 'missingness'. By contrast, stochastic approaches such as multiple imputation, maximum likelihood and Gaussian process regression attempt to model missing data as distributions. Whilst these are more principled methods, they require more complex and time-consuming calculations.

3.2 *Integrating Heterogeneous Data Sources*

Typical care for a patient in a modern health service involves multiple types of data collected from a disparate range of sources. Data analytics that combines multiple sources of data, a process known as data fusion, is useful for two main reasons.

First, the multiple data sources may provide *complementary* information that provides a more complete description of the problem. Secondly, the multiple sources may measure the same event, providing redundant information. Whilst the data itself may not provide any new information, the independent sources can be used to corroborate a given measurement and may be useful for assessing data corruption via Signal Quality Indices.

In practice, the process of integrating data sources is fraught with difficulty. We now address three issues in data analysis with multiple sources and address how they are commonly dealt with in practice.

3.2.1 Dimensionality and Feature Selection

Combining multiple data sources into a super-set used for analysis increases both the volume and variety of data items. As the number of variables increases, the amount of data required to derive meaningful results increases exponentially—a phenomenon commonly referred to as the Curse of Dimensionality. Figure 7 demonstrates this phenomenon for categorical data. In the example, three data points are represented by red squares. For two variables (a 2D data space), this represents coverage of 3/9 possible states. The addition of a third variable (a 3D data space) means that the same number of data points represents a much smaller proportion of the possible states, 3/27.

One solution to the Curse of Dimensionality is to determine an *optimal* subset of variables, a process known as *feature selection*. If done correctly, only unimportant variables are discarded. Multiple methods for feature selection have been proposed in the literature, and Saeys et al. provide a detailed discussion of a wide range of feature selection techniques [86].

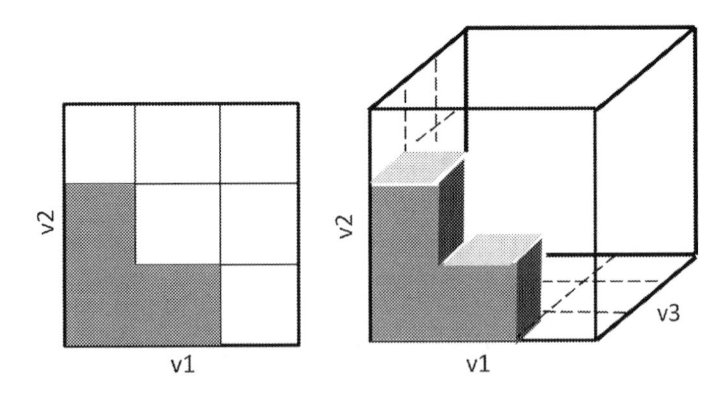

Fig. 7 An example of the Curse of Dimensionality. **a** Variables v1 and v2 can take three possible values each. The three data points (in *red*) provide examples in 3/9 (33%) of possible combinations. **b** The addition of a new variable, v3, reduces the coverage to 3/27(11%) of possible combinations

The most conceptually simple of feature selection techniques is **Univariate Feature Selection** and is appropriate when the target variable is known (i.e. supervised learning). In this method, each variable is taken in turn to see how it correlates with the target variable. Variables that have poor correlation are discarded. One drawback of this approach is that data redundancy is not considered.

Another intuitive way of selecting features is **Backward feature elimination/ Forward feature construction**. In backward feature elimination, all variables are initially included in a model that tries to explain the target variable. After this, one input is removed from the initial set of n, and the model is re-run. There are n possible variables to remove, leading to n different model results. The model that best describes the target variable is kept, and the associated input variable is discarded. This process is repeated until a pre-determined criterion is met. Forward feature construction uses the same iterative approach, but instead begins with only one input variable, and adds the most useful variable at each iteration.

One model that lends itself well to feature elimination and construction methods is random forests, an extension of the decision tree algorithm [87]. In the case of feature elimination, a random forest model is first applied to all input variables. The variable that is least informative is the first to be removed. The level of information is determined through a scoring function. The function may include information about how many times a feature appears in the individual decision trees, and the classification accuracy of each tree. Specific examples of scoring function are described in [88].

Unlike the univariate feature selection, both feature elimination and construction naturally deal with redundant information. If once an input variable is included, a similar input will only be incorporated if it provides significant additional information. Both approaches are also 'greedy' algorithms. This means that they select the best available choice on each iteration. Such approaches only guarantee an optimal solution under specific conditions [89].

The methods described so far find a subset of the original input variables. However, in some cases, input variables may themselves be based on some smaller set of unmeasured, latent variables. The process of recasting the initial input variables into the smaller set of latent variables is known as dimensionality reduction. Each new variable will be a function of the initial inputs, and may have no inherent meaning itself. Mathematically, dimensionality reduction can be considered a transformation of the initial data space into a feature space that can be used to describe most of the variance within the data set. Because these techniques solely rely on properties of the input data, they can be applied without reference to an output target variable.

One common dimensionality reduction techniques is Principal Component Analysis [90]. PCA transforms data sets described by N-input variables to a data set described by M features. The M features are linear combinations of the input variables. They are derived by projecting the dataset onto the eigenvectors corresponding to the M largest eigenvalues. Figure 8 demonstrates PCA for a simple case in which $N = M = 2$. The PCA output results in a linear rotation of the data so

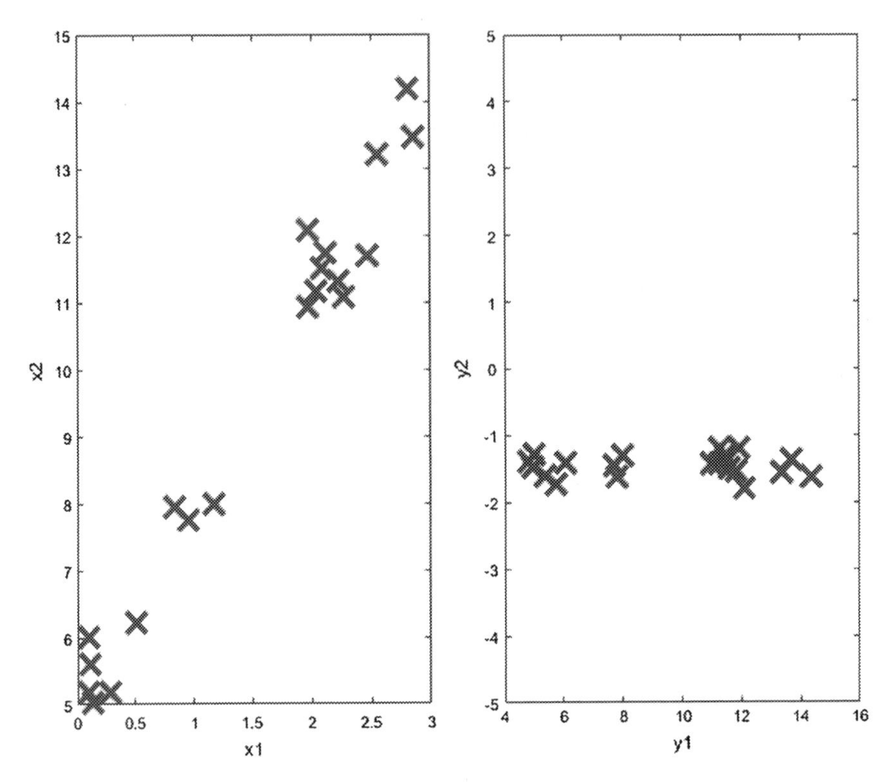

Fig. 8 Demonstration of principle component analysis with two features. Initially, the data are fully described in terms of x1 and x2. PCA linearly transforms the data along the directions with greatest variance. In this case [y1 y2] = [a b; c d] [x1 x2]. After the transformation, data are primarily a function of y1, and y2 can be ignored with minimal loss of information

that the data align with the principal axes y1 and y2. The y2 axis has a smaller range than the untransformed data, so may be disregarded (such that the data are described only in terms of y1) with minimal loss of information.

Sammon maps [91] are another dimensionality reduction technique that attempts to maintain the Euclidean distance between points in the initial feature space, and a reduced-feature output space. In this case, the axes of the output space represent non-linear combinations of the original features. The method considers all distances between data points so that a data set with n records requires $n!$ computations—intractable for large values of n. For such data sets, approximations may be derived using a sparse set of comparisons [92] or by explicitly learning the transform function [93]. Due to its reliance on Euclidean distance, Sammon maps are not easily applicable to data sets that contain categorical or binary features.

3.2.2 Data Fusion of Heterogeneous Data

The combination of multiple sources and types of data to provide a single, more informative, variable is known as data fusion. Many of the key data fusion concepts were developed within robotics and have since been adapted to healthcare data. A detailed discussion of data fusion can be found in [94]. Here, we describe two specific data fusion approaches, their engineering application, and their subsequent use for healthcare problems.

Kalman filters have found wide-spread application in many different data fusion problems using clinical data [94]. The Kalman filter (KF) is a recursive linear estimator which calculates estimates for a continuous valued state that evolves over time on the basis of existing observations of the state [94]. The underlying assumptions are Bayesian (explained in Sect. 2.1.3) where estimations of parameters are made based on conditional probabilities. In the case of the KF the condition parameters are the probabilistic observations of the values of the variable in time. The evolution of the parameter of interest $x(t)$ is, thus, described using an explicit statistical model. Another statistical model is also used to describe the way that the observations, $z(t)$, are related to $x(t)$. The gains of the KF are then chosen such that the resulting estimate of the parameter of interest $\hat{x}(t)$ minimises mean-squared error and is thus the conditional mean, $\hat{x}(t) = E[x(t)/Z^t]$. This means that the estimated value is calculated as an average and not as a most likely value as in other probabilistic approaches. Because of the explicit description of process and observations, and the consistent use of statistical measures of uncertainty, the Kalman Filter framework makes it possible to incorporate different sensor models into the basic form of the algorithm. Additionally, at each point in time, it is possible to evaluate the role each sensor plays in the performance of the system, making it an ideal approach for data fusion.

Example successful applications can be found in [95] and in [96]. In the former, a KF framework was employed in order to fuse heart rate (HR) estimates extracted from different signals based on individual Signal Quality metrics for each signal. In the latter, an extension of the basic KF framework was used, the Factorial Switching Kalman Filter (FSKF) which applies a third set of variables, in addition to the *observations* and *states* of the classic KF framework, called the *factors*. The FSKF in this case, was used in order to estimate the true values of vital signs in the Neonatal Intensive Care (NICU) at times where the measurements were obscured by artefact. The *factors* incorporated into the system in this case were related to possible system failures causing artefact, such as probe dropouts, incubator open, etc. These factors had a range of possible settings and at each given point, the existing setting was taken into account in the estimation model.

One other approach to data fusion is novelty detection. Novelty detection methods are used when we wish to classify normal and abnormal data records, but only have very few abnormal training examples. In this case, the challenge is often to accurately differentiate between extreme, but normal data, and truly abnormal data. When a single source of information is used, differentiation is sometimes impossible. For instance, for heart rate data, a low value can either indicate good health, or underlying problems with the heart's electrical activity. In these cases, integrating data from multiple different sensors allows for more accurate classification. Multi-sensor data fusion is an approach that has been applied to traditional engineering applications such as jet engine monitoring [97], and adapted for use with healthcare data. One specific data fusion algorithm for vital sign monitoring is described in greater detail in Sect. 4.1.

Whilst these multi-sensor data fusion approaches are useful in specific healthcare settings, they do not address one of the unique aspects for healthcare data analysis: the rich variety of data acquired. Health data sets often contain variables of multiple data types—a property known as heterogeneity. A data type defines the set of values that a data item may take; common data types include text, binary, categorical, ordinal and continuous (or floating point). Whilst some data fusion and machine learning methods may be adapted (e.g. see [98]), most are unable to deal with multiple data types simultaneously.

One promising approach for fusing heterogeneous data is Multiple Kernel Learning (MKL). In traditional kernel learning methods, such as SVMs (see Sect. 2.1.2), a kernel function outputs a measure of similarity, given a pair of data inputs. The kernel function is typically chosen a priori, based on known properties of the data. MKL methods differ by learning and using the optimum linear sum of a family of kernel functions:

$$K = \sum_i b_i k_i \tag{15}$$

Due to the property of kernel functions, K is also a kernel function, so standard techniques can then be applied (for example, [99]). If each individual kernel is tailored for use with particular data types, the kernel, K, provides a blend that allows us to process fuse multiple data types optimally.

MKL has been successfully applied to heterogeneous data in the healthcare setting. One example, from Ye et al. [100] showed how MRI image data could be fused with patient demographics and genomic results to help diagnose Alzheimer's disease more effectively than by using any one data type.

3.2.3 Technical and Sociological Issues

The use of multiple data sources brings many practical obstacles that are exacerbated in the healthcare space. Currently, clinical data are collected by multiple devices, belonging to multiple organisations. The data are stored in separate databases, a phenomenon referred to as data compartmentalisation. The barriers to successful data sharing are manifold.

First, the linkage of databases poses ethical and legal concerns. Many countries have legislation that governs the use of personal health information [101]. In the UK, this means that personal data can only be used under specific circumstances.

Individual databases may be released more generally if the data set is anonymised so that individuals cannot be identified. One prominent example of anonymised health care data is MIMIC-II, which provides access to over 30,000 de-identified hospital patient records. If data are not de-identified properly, there remains a risk that individuals can be identified by piecing together information from complementary data sources. For instance, Gymrek et al. [102] showed how de-identified genomic data could be traced to individuals by linkage with genealogy databases.

Secondly, there are non-trivial technical challenges in linking databases. Many of these, including minimising levels of data redundancy, are addressed through the academic discipline of data integration theory (See [103] for further information). Practically, successful data integration requires well-defined standards to ensure that database fields can be interpreted unambiguously, and that the field contents are harmonious. One such standard, SNOMED-CT, provides a comprehensive collection of codes for medical terms that could to help structure database items [104]. Unfortunately, the use of multiple competing standards has hindered data integration. Most notably, until recently, the majority of UK healthcare IT systems used an alternative dictionary, Read codes [105].

Finally, database linkage may require cooperation between competitive system manufacturers. In some cases, the data providers may simply disagree with the intended use of the data [106]. More typically, there may be willingness to share data sets, but details such as ownership of the data or the rights of any generated intellectual property [107] means that data sharing agreements are often complex.

3.2.4 Large-Scale and Distributed Computing Methods

The large volume of clinical data available for processing, the variety of data types and structures, as well as the velocity required in the production and processing of clinical data have led to the development of novel and robust technologies for extracting useful information and for enabling more broad-based healthcare solutions [108]. Large-scale and distributed computing methods provide solutions for the retrieval and reliable storage of clinical data, as well as data security, sharing, and analysis. Distributed processing systems such as the Apache Hadoop [109] have been proposed as solutions for the storage of electronic health records (EHRs) [110] and the storage of physiological signals [111]. The enabling of reliable and rapid computations in such infrastructures, provides the potential for building novel machine learning algorithms. Similar systems, intended for the storing and querying of large amounts of physiological data (e.g., EEG), as well as their visualization, have also been proposed using Hadoop-based data processing modules, and have shown reductions in computational time [112, 113]. *Home-Diagnosis* [114], a cloud-based framework employing a Lucene-based distributed search cluster has been proposed to deal with issues of privacy protection, to ensure highly concurrent and scalable medical record retrieval and to facilitate data analysis in a self-caring setting. The issue of privacy and data protection is a particularly important one with respect to distributed computing systems since a data breach may occur when multiple nodes conspire. To address this issue secure computing methods have recently been proposed ensuring confidentiality of the data used by each different party even in that case that all of the other parties conspire to crack the data [115]. In terms of data analysis, a predictive modelling platform for healthcare analytic research (PARAMO) has been proposed recently [116], which employs parallel computing in a cluster environment supporting the pipeline of necessary tasks (cohort construction, feature selection and construction, cross-validation and classification), such that predictive models can be built based on electronic health records (EHRs). In addition to predictive accuracy, such systems hold promise for use for the analysis of multidimensional and heterogeneous clinical data since they facilitate the use of Big Data analytics for sorting out "messy" clinical data, identifying causalities and associations amongst large amounts of data and improving health care quality, in general.

4 Case Studies

4.1 *Application of Machine Learning for the Prediction of Patient Deterioration in an Emergency Department*

Studies have shown that patients experiencing adverse events in hospitals (such as cardiac arrest or admission to the ICU) present with abnormal vital signs before the event, with many of those, presenting abnormalities up to 24 h in advance [117]. Because the current standard of recording vital sign observations is paper-based and observations are taken intermittently outside of the ICU, these abnormalities are often missed, especially in busy clinical environments. Additionally, current alerting strategies rely on single parameters or in the calculation of Early Warning Scores (EWS) based on a rule-based pre-set thresholds. The first case study we review concerns the automation of the process of calculating the health status of the patient via a data-driven, rather than rule-based, machine learning model. Firstly, we will present the approach and then discuss its application in an emergency department.

4.1.1 System Overview

The system, initially presented in [71], tracks patient health status in real time by fusing the patient's vital signs collected by monitors in a general hospital ward. The parameters used are heart rate, respiration rate, blood pressure, arterial oxygen saturation (SaO_2) and skin temperature. Vital signs were measured every 5 s except for blood pressure which was measured every 30 min using an inflatable cuff placed over the medial artery. The proposed system does not extract any rules connecting these five parameters to patient deterioration, it simply *learns* a model of normality directly from the available data. The system produces a single index of the patient's health status, Patient Status Index (PSI), by fusing the five vital signs. This PSI is calculated via a *probabilistic model of normality* in five dimensions, which was previously *learnt* from the data taken from a representative sample of high-risk adult patients. The PSI is calculated continuously and whenever the vital signs fall outside the learnt envelope of normality, an alert is generated [71]. The aim behind the development of such a system is for generating alerts (early warning system) in real-time, triggering the intervention of a Medical Emergency Team (MET). Such systems can be integrated with existing patient monitors or a central station on the relevant ward to such of a large number of patients can be monitored at the same time, without increasing the burden of the clinical staff.

4.1.2 Training Data and Pre-processing

The training data set included 3500 h of vital sign data collected from 150 general-ward patients at the John Radcliffe Hospital, Oxford (average length of stay of 24 h per patient), who were classified as "high-risk" based on a set of assessments proposed by the attending clinicians. The feature vector was defined as $x = \{x_1, \ldots, x_5\}$, the vector of the five vital signs. Because the units and dynamic ranges of each parameter are different (i.e. an increase of 0.5 °C in temperature is more significant than an increase of 0.5 mmHg in blood pressure or 0.5 beats per minute (bpm) in heart rate), the vital signs were normalized before forming the feature vector **x**. Observation of the data revealed that all except for arterial oxygen saturation (SaO_2) followed a near-Gaussian distribution (SaO_2 was one-sided as it cannot exceed 100%) so pre-processing included a standard zero-mean, unit variance normalization. To deal with the noise in the data caused by patient movement, data were short-term median filtered. Median filtering was also used in order to deal with missing parameter streams that occurred. Additionally, if no valid measurement of a parameter was acquired for 1 min, the value from a historic median filtered was used, derived from the most recent 5 min of valid data (blood pressure was excluded from this rule since it was only recorded every 30 min). If the gap in a measurement persisted for 30 min (possibly because of a disconnected probe), then the mean of the training set was used instead, thus replacing the missing values by the 'most normal' value in the parameter vector x.

4.1.3 Model Overview

The model of normality was defined as the unconditional probability density function, $\hat{p}(x)$, and was estimated using the training data using a combination of k-means clustering and Parzen windows. Initially, the k-means clustering algorithm is used in order to select 500 cluster centers from the thousands of normalized feature vectors in the training set. Each center x_j (also called a prototype pattern) then forms a kernel in the Parzen windows estimator of the pdf given by:

$$\hat{p}(x) = \frac{1}{N(2\pi)^{d/2}\sigma^d} \sum_{j=1}^{N} \exp\left(\frac{-\left\|x - x_j\right\|^2}{2\sigma^2}\right), \tag{16}$$

where each spherical kernel has the same global width σ and d is equal to 5. This probability is then used in order to calculate the PSI such that it quantifies deviations from “normality”. The aim is that alert will be generated when the PSI exceeds a pre-determined threshold. The PSI is then calculated by:

$$PSI = log_e\left[\frac{1}{\hat{p}(x)}\right] \tag{17}$$

A PSI of 3.0, corresponding to a probability value of 0.05 was chosen for the alerting threshold and an alert was generated when the PSI was above this threshold of 3.0 for 4 out of 5 min.

4.1.4 Testing of the PSI in the Emergency Department

The system described was validated on several different clinical trials. Here, we present its validation on the emergency department (ED) of a medium-sized teaching hospital [118]. In this particular study, the aim was to investigate whether employment of the PSI, as calculated using the learnt model, would be able to detect patient deterioration and generate an alert earlier than the standard practice of manually recording vital sign and Track and Trigger (T&T) data (also known as Early Warning Scores). Data were collected from adults entering the resuscitation room, ‘majors’ and observation ward of the ED. For calculating the PSI, continuous vital sign data (RR, heart rate, blood pressure and SpO_2) were acquired from the bedside monitors and saved to a server. Observation charts were also collected retrospectively. The “gold standard” of patient deterioration was captured by recording escalations of care. This was done by two clinicians who retrospectively and independently reviewed the clinical notes to identify escalations. In the case of disagreement, a third clinician reconciled the discrepancies.

4.1.5 Results

Out of the 400 patients for whom continuous vital signs were collected and PSI scores were calculated, 35 had an escalation after arriving at the ED. 15 of them had no PSI score at the time around the escalation either because of equipment failure, unavailability for monitoring at the time of escalation, or because their escalation was deemed to have been due to ongoing conditions rather than a new deterioration occurring at the ED. Of the remaining 20 patients who experienced deterioration while in the ED, 15 were detected by the PSI. PSI greatly outperformed T&T and there were many cases where the PSI would predict deterioration before the traditional paper-based T&T.

4.1.6 Conclusions

This study highlighted the potential of machine-learning data fusion approaches for predicting events in patients. Because such scores can be calculated continuously deterioration can be detected earlier compared to systems relying on documented intermittent observations. Additionally, small deviations in one or more parameters can be recognised promptly whereas in current practice an alert would be generated when a parameter shows a big deviation from normality. This study also showcased some of the problems in using automatic machine-learning based systems using clinical data, in that data are very often incomplete or absent altogether due to practical problems (power failure, server failure, movement of patients or monitors or removal of leads from the patient). Machine learning approaches need to have the flexibility to allow for this kind of failures if they are to be incorporated systematically into clinical practise.

4.2 Application of Machine Learning for Assessing the Clinical Acceptability of Electrocardiograms

The explosion of m-health applications both in the developing and developed world has the potential to deliver information and decision support to people that would not otherwise have had access to medical treatment, it is important that stringent quality controls are put into place such that the measurements that reach the untrained recipient are reliable and that noisy measurements are not used. The second case study we will review concerns the creation of a system which is intended to provide real-time feedback on the diagnostic quality of the Electrocardiogram (ECG). The purpose of such a system is to be able to prompt an inexperienced user for example, to adjust recording conditions (e.g. sensor placement) until the quality is sufficient that a reliable medical diagnosis can be made, primarily of arrhythmias [56]. The study was developed as part of the PhysioNet/Computing in Cardiology challenge 2011, which further required that the algorithm should be efficient enough such that it may run in near real-time on a mobile phone device.

4.2.1 Training Data and Annotating

Data to support development and evaluation of challenge entries were collected by the Sana Project and provided freely via PhysioNet. The dataset includes 1500 10 s recordings of standard 12-lead ECGs, which were sampled at 500 Hz for a minimum of 10 s by nurses, technicians and volunteers with varying degrees of experience. 1000 recordings were available as training data and 500 recordings as test data. Each ECG recording was annotated by a minimum of 3 and a maximum of 18 annotators who assigned a rating to the sample related to its quality. The final label of each sample was determined by the average rating and some pre-set thresholds, such that recordings were divided into three classes: acceptable (70%), unacceptable (30%) and indeterminate (<1%). Because of the discrepancy in the number of records from the acceptable and unacceptable classes, bootstrapping was employed in order to increase the samples in the "unacceptable" class by using additive real noise to clean data taken from other ECG databases. In the resulting database, 20,000 10s ECG samples were used for training and 10,000 for testing, both sets of which were balanced for "acceptable" and "unacceptable" recordings [56].

4.2.2 Model Overview

Initially, each ECG channel was down-sampled to 125 Hz using an anti-aliasing filter. QRS detection was then performed using two different open-source QRS detectors. Next, seven quality indices were extracted for each one of the 12 leads, resulting in 84 features per recording. Those 7 indices were the percentage of beats detected on each channel which were detected in all channels, the percentage of beats detected by both QRS detectors, the relative power in the QRS complex, the third and fourth moments of the distribution, the percentage of the signal that was a flat line and the relative power in the baseline of the signal. All features which were not given by percentages were normalized by subtracting the median such that all features were in the range of [0 1]. The features were then used to train a classifier using two different models: a Support Vector Machine (SVM) and a standard feed-forward Multi-Layer Perceptron Neural Network (MLPNN). Classifiers were tested using all 12 leads simultaneously, i.e. using 84 features and using a single lead only, i.e., using only 7 features. Additionally, different combinations of the seven features were tested in order to find the best.

4.2.3 Results

For the single-lead case, the best overall results were obtained for the SVM with a classification accuracy of 96.5% on the test data and corresponding Sensitivity and Specificity of 97.2% and 95.8%, respectively, using only four out of the seven features. For the 12-lead case, the best results were given using five out of the seven features, using the SVM with an accuracy of 95.9% and Sensitivity and Specificity of 96.0% and 95.8%, respectively.

4.2.4 Conclusions

The proposed system achieved training accuracies of 98% and test set accuracies up to 97% which indicate that extremely accurate classification of noisy ECGs is possible. Important improvements were noted when the training sets were balanced using artificial data. Lastly, by examining the incorrectly classified data, it was found that in most cases the labels were 'borderline' and could be relabelled either way, thus indicating that test accuracy could be considered to approach 100%.

5 Concluding Remarks and Future Directions

In this chapter, we provided an overview to the current processes and techniques used to analyse heterogeneous and high dimensional healthcare data. We addressed some of the technical challenges and highlighted the real-world issues that are unique to healthcare.

As health data analysis continues to develop as a research field, one may expect to see new analysis methods tailored towards big health data. Currently, we have seen a trend towards the redevelopment of adaptation of traditional machine learning approaches for use with large data sets. IBM Watson's success in natural language processing follows on from a wealth of previous research. Similarly, Google's Deepmind extends artificial neural network methods via the field of deep learning. These new approaches have already shown great promise in other fields. Most notably, in early 2016, the AlphaGo program used deep learning (in combination with other methods) to defeat the world-class Lee Sedol at the game of Go—a scenario thought improbable 10 years ago. Both IBM and Google have since expressed interest in healthcare data. Whilst output from both parties has been limited at the time of writing, there is precedent for using deep learning methods on medical images [119, 120].

As machine learning methods are applied to increasingly large data sets, we expect the associated challenges to also increase. In particular, the current trend is towards using data collected within routine clinical care—potentially providing data sets many orders of magnitude larger than from research studies. As these routinely-collected datasets are not carefully curated, resulting data are very likely to be of lower quality, such that corrupt and missing entries are more common. The combination of larger datasets and poorer data quality means that automated methods of reliably and accurately processing missing data will be increasingly necessary.

The use of routine data also offer new opportunities to link multiple sources of data. Whilst we have touched on the benefits of data fusion, future research is likely to bring together data from surprisingly disparate sources. For instance, recent research is starting to link consumer research data from supermarket loyalty cards with health data. The increasing number of data features means that robust methods must be found to ensure that the underlying features are not lost amongst the plethora of variables. The complexities and disparities need to be carefully considered by the research community, so that the potential of machine learning applications in clinical data may be reached. Once many of these issues are resolved, machine learning has the potential to deliver a step-change in the manner in which the monitoring of patients and diagnosis of disease is performed for a sustainable future of healthcare management.

References

1. Roski J, Bo-Linn GW, Andrews TA. Creating value in health care through big data: opportunities and policy implications. Health Affairs. 2014 Jul 1;33(7):1115–22.
2. Krumholz HM. Big data and new knowledge in medicine: the thinking, training, and tools needed for a learning health system. Health Affairs. 2014 Jul 1;33(7):1163–70.
3. Foster KR, Koprowski R, Skufca JD. Machine learning, medical diagnosis, and biomedical engineering research-commentary. Biomedical engineering online. 2014 Jul 5;13(1):1.
4. Bishop CM. Pattern recognition and Machine Learning. Springer-New York 2006.
5. Sajda P. Machine learning for detection and diagnosis of disease. Annu. Rev. Biomed. Eng. 2006 Aug 15;8:537–65.
6. Hearst MA, Dumais ST, Osman E, Platt J, Scholkopf B. Support vector machines. IEEE Intelligent Systems and their Applications. 1998 Jul;13(4):18–28.
7. Johnson AE, Ghassemi MM, Nemati S, Niehaus KE, Clifton DA, Clifford GD. Machine learning and decision support in critical care. Proceedings of the IEEE. 2016 Feb;104(2): 444–66.
8. Lucas PJ, van der Gaag LC, Abu-Hanna A. Bayesian networks in biomedicine and health-care. Artificial intelligence in medicine. 2004 Mar 1;30(3):201–14.
9. Peduzzi P, Concato J, Kemper E, Holford TR, Feinstein AR. A simulation study of the number of events per variable in logistic regression analysis. Journal of clinical epidemiology. 1996 Dec 31;49(12):1373–9.
10. Asgari S, Mehrnia A, Moussavi M. Automatic detection of atrial fibrillation using stationary wavelet transform and support vector machine. Computers in biology and medicine. 2015 May 1;60:132–42.
11. Oliver A, Freixenet J, Marti R, Pont J, Pérez E, Denton ER, Zwiggelaar R. A novel breast tissue density classification methodology. IEEE Transactions on Information Technology in Biomedicine. 2008 Jan;12(1):55–65.
12. Healthcare Commission. Report of the healthcare Commision's visit to Maidstone and Tunbridge Wells NHS Trust on 12 and 13 December 2007. Retrieved 20-Jul-2016 url: http://webarchive.nationalarchives.gov.uk/20060502043818/http://healthcarecommission.org.uk/_db/_documents/Maidstone_and_Tunbridge_Wells_follow_up_visit_report_-_Dec_07.pdf.
13. Boba M, Kołtun U, Bobek-Billewicz B, Chmielik E, Eksner B, Olejnik T. False-negative results of breast core needle biopsies–retrospective analysis of 988 biopsies. Polish Journal of Radiology. 2011 Jan;76(1):25.

14. Clarke GW, Chan AD, Adler A. Effects of motion artifact on the blood oxygen saturation estimate in pulse oximetry. In Medical Measurements and Applications (MeMeA), 2014 IEEE International Symposium on 2014 Jun 11 (pp. 1–4). IEEE.
15. Hamilton PS, Curley MG, Aimi RM, Sae-Hau C. Comparison of methods for adaptive removal of motion artifact. In Computers in Cardiology 2000 2000 (pp. 383–386). IEEE.
16. Yang CC, Hsu YL. A review of accelerometry-based wearable motion detectors for physical activity monitoring. Sensors. 2010 Aug 20;10(8):7772–88.
17. Celler BG, Sparks RS. Home Telemonitoring of Vital Signs—Technical Challenges and Future Directions. IEEE journal of biomedical and health informatics. 2015 Jan;19(1):82–91.
18. Hernandez-Silveira M, Ahmed K, Ang SS, Zandari F, Mehta T, Weir R, Burdett A, Toumazou C, Brett SJ. Assessment of the feasibility of an ultra-low power, wireless digital patch for the continuous ambulatory monitoring of vital signs. BMJ open. 2015 May 1;5(5): e006606.
19. Steinhubl SR, Feye D, Levine AC, Conkright C, Wegerich SW, Conkright G. Validation of a portable, deployable system for continuous vital sign monitoring using a multiparametric wearable sensor and personalised analytics in an Ebola treatment centre. BMJ Global Health. 2016 Jul 1;1(1):e000070.
20. SO80601-2-61:2011: Medical electronical equipment — Particular requirements for basic safety and essential performance of pulse oximeter equipment. International Organization for Standardization, Geneva, Switzerland.
21. Milner QJ, Mathews GR. An assessment of the accuracy of pulse oximeters. Anaesthesia. 2012 Apr 1;67(4):396–401.
22. Modell JG, Katholi CR, Kumaramangalam SM, Hudson EC, Graham D. Unreliability of the infrared tympanic thermometer in clinical practice: a comparative study with oral mercury and oral electronic thermometers. Southern medical journal. 1998 Jul;91(7):649–54.
23. Beevers G, Lip GY, O'Brien E. Blood pressure measurement: Part II–conventional sphygmomanometry: Technique of auscultatory blood pressure measurement. British Medical Journal. 2001 Apr 28;322(7293):1043.
24. Baker PD, Westenskow DR, Kück K. Theoretical analysis of non-invasive oscillometric maximum amplitude algorithm for estimating mean blood pressure. Medical and biological engineering and computing. 1997 May 1;35(3):271–8.
25. Pavlik VN, Hyman DJ, Toronjo C. Comparison of Automated and Mercury Column Blood Pressure Measurements in Health Care Settings. Journal of clinical hypertension (Greenwich, Conn.). 2000 Mar;2(2):81–6.
26. Wong WC, Shiu IK, Hwong TM, Dickinson JA. Reliability of automated blood pressure devices used by hypertensive patients. Journal of the Royal Society of Medicine. 2005 Mar 1;98(3):111–3.
27. Akpolat T, Dilek M, Aydogdu T, Adibelli Z, Erdem DG, Erdem E. Home sphygmomanometers: validation versus accuracy. Blood pressure monitoring. 2009 Feb 1;14(1): 26–31.
28. Thimbleby H. Improving safety in medical devices and systems. In Healthcare Informatics (ICHI), 2013 IEEE International Conference on 2013 Sep 9 (pp. 1–13). IEEE.
29. Thimbleby H. Ignorance of interaction programming is killing people. interactions. 2008 Sep 1;15(5):52–7.
30. Wilson SJ, Wong D, Clifton D, Fleming S, Way R, Pullinger R, Tarassenko L. Track and trigger in an emergency department: an observational evaluation study. Emergency Medicine Journal. 2012 Mar 22:emermed-2011.
31. Prytherch DR, Smith GB, Schmidt P, Featherstone PI, Stewart K, Knight D, Higgins B. Calculating early warning scores—a classroom comparison of pen and paper and hand-held computer methods. Resuscitation. 2006 Aug 31;70(2):173–8.
32. Callen J, McIntosh J, Li J. Accuracy of medication documentation in hospital discharge summaries: A retrospective analysis of medication transcription errors in manual and electronic discharge summaries. International journal of medical informatics. 2010 Jan 31; 79(1):58–64.

33. Wallace DR, Kuhn DR. Failure modes in medical device software: an analysis of 15 years of recall data. International Journal of Reliability, Quality and Safety Engineering. 2001 Dec;8 (04):351–71.
34. Obradovich JH, Woods DD. Special section: Users as designers: How people cope with poor HCI design in computer-based medical devices. Human Factors: The Journal of the Human Factors and Ergonomics Society. 1996 Dec 1;38(4):574–92.
35. Batchelor JC, Casson AJ. Inkjet printed ECG electrodes for long term biosignal monitoring in personalized and ubiquitous healthcare. In 2015 37th Annual International Conference of the IEEE Engineering in Medicine and Biology Society (EMBC) 2015 Aug 25 (pp. 4013–4016). IEEE.
36. Tarassenko L, Villarroel M, Guazzi A, Jorge J, Clifton DA, Pugh C. Non-contact video-based vital sign monitoring using ambient light and auto-regressive models. Physiological measurement. 2014 Mar 28;35(5):807.
37. Takano C, Ohta Y. Heart rate measurement based on a time-lapse image. Medical engineering & physics. 2007 Oct 31;29(8):853–7.
38. Verkruysse W, Svaasand LO, Nelson JS. Remote plethysmographic imaging using ambient light. Optics express. 2008 Dec 22;16(26):21434–45.
39. Pullinger R, Wilson S, Way R, Santos M, Wong D, Clifton D, Birks J, Tarassenko L. Implementing an electronic observation and early warning score chart in the emergency department: a feasibility study. European journal of emergency medicine: official journal of the European Society for Emergency Medicine. 2016 Feb 17.
40. Wong D, Bonnici T, Knight J, Morgan L, Coombes P, Watkinson P. SEND: a system for electronic notification and documentation of vital sign observations. BMC medical informatics and decision making. 2015 Aug 13;15(1):1.
41. Smith GB, Prytherch DR, Schmidt P, Featherstone PI, Knight D, Clements G, Mohammed MA. Hospital-wide physiological surveillance–a new approach to the early identification and management of the sick patient. Resuscitation. 2006 Oct 31;71(1):19–28.
42. Meccariello M, Perkins P, Quigley LG, Rock A, Qiu J. Vital Time Savings: Evaluating the Use of an Automated Vital Signs Documentation System on a Medical/Surgical Unit. J Healthc Inf Manag 2010 24(4):46–51.
43. Mekhjian HS, Kumar RR, Kuehn L, Bentley TD, Teater P, Thomas A, Payne B, Ahmad A. Immediate benefits realized following implementation of physician order entry at an academic medical center. Journal of the American Medical Informatics Association. 2002 Sep 1;9(5):529–39.
44. Murphy MF, Fraser E, Miles D, Noel S, Staves J, Cripps B, Kay J. How do we monitor hospital transfusion practice using an end to end electronic transfusion management system?. Transfusion. 2012 Dec 1;52(12):2502–12.
45. Davies A, Staves J, Kay J, Casbard A, Murphy MF. End-to-end electronic control of the hospital transfusion process to increase the safety of blood transfusion: strengths and weaknesses. Transfusion. 2006 Mar 1;46(3):352–64.
46. Staves J, Davies A, Kay J, Pearson O, Johnson T, Murphy MF. Electronic remote blood issue: a combination of remote blood issue with a system for end-to-end electronic control of transfusion to provide a "total solution" for a safe and timely hospital blood transfusion service. Transfusion. 2008 Mar 1;48(3):415–24.
47. Resetar E, Reichley RM, Noirot LA, Dunagan WC, Bailey TC. Customizing a commercial rule base for detecting drug-drug interactions. In AMIA 2005.
48. Bonnici T, Orphanidou C, Vallance D, Darrell A, Tarassenko L. Testing of wearable monitors in a real-world hospital environment: What lessons can be learnt?. In 2012 Ninth International Conference on Wearable and Implantable Body Sensor Networks 2012 May 9 (pp. 79–84). IEEE.
49. Wahlster P, Goetghebeur M, Kriza C, Niederländer C, Kolominsky-Rabas P. Balancing costs and benefits at different stages of medical innovation: a systematic review of Multi-criteria decision analysis (MCDA). BMC health services research. 2015 Jul 9;15(1):1.

50. Yeung MS, Lapinsky SE, Granton JT, Doran DM, Cafazzo JA. Examining nursing vital signs documentation workflow: barriers and opportunities in general internal medicine units. Journal of clinical nursing. 2012 Apr 1;21(7–8):975–82.
51. Tat TH, Xiang C, Thiam LE. Physionet challenge 2011: improving the quality of electrocardiography data collected using real time QRS-complex and T-wave detection. In2011 Computing in Cardiology 2011 Sep 18 (pp. 441–444). IEEE.
52. Johnson AE, Behar J, Andreotti F, Clifford GD, Oster J. Multimodal heart beat detection using signal quality indices. Physiological measurement. 2015 Jul 28;36(8):1665.
53. Clifton DA, Wong D, Clifton L, Wilson S, Way R, Pullinger R, Tarassenko L. A large-scale clinical validation of an integrated monitoring system in the emergency department. IEEE journal of biomedical and health informatics. 2013 Jul;17(4):835–42.
54. Orphanidou C., Bonnici T., Charlton P. Vallance D., Darrell A. and Tarassenko L., Signal Quality Indices for the Electrocardiogram and Photoplethysmogram: Derivation and Applications in Wireless Monitoring, in IEEE Journal of Biomedical and Health Informatics, 19(3), pp. 832–838, 2015.
55. Daluwatte C, Johannesen L, Galeotti L, Vicente J, Strauss DG, Scully CG. Assessing ECG signal quality indices to discriminate ECGs with artefacts from pathologically different arrhythmic ECGs. Physiological Measurement. 2016 Jul 25;37(8):1370.
56. Clifford GD, Behar J, Li Q, Rezek I. Signal quality indices and data fusion for determining clinical acceptability of electrocardiograms. Physiological measurement. 2012 Aug 17;33(9): 1419.
57. Nizami S, Green JR, McGregor C. Implementation of artifact detection in critical care: A methodological review. IEEE reviews in biomedical engineering. 2013;6:127–42.
58. Kaur M, Singh B. Comparison of different approaches for removal of baseline wander from ecg signal. In Proceedings of the International Conference & Workshop on Emerging Trends in Technology 2011 Feb 25 (pp. 1290–1294). ACM.
59. ECG baseline wander. Reproduced with permission from http://joachimbehar.comuv.com/ECG_tuto_1.php.
60. Hoffmann S, Falkenstein M. The correction of eye blink artefacts in the EEG: a comparison of two prominent methods. PLoS One. 2008 Aug 20;3(8):e3004.
61. Li Y, Ma Z, Lu W, Li Y. Automatic removal of the eye blink artifact from EEG using an ICA-based template matching approach. Physiological measurement. 2006 Mar 14;27(4): 425.
62. Teasdale G, Jennett B. Assessment of coma and impaired consciousness: a practical scale. The Lancet. 1974 Jul 13;304(7872):81–4.
63. Paul DB, Rao GU. Correlation of Bispectral Index with Glasgow Coma Score in mild and moderate head injuries. Journal of clinical monitoring and computing. 2006 Dec 1;20(6): 399–404.
64. Beridze M, Khaburzania M, Shakarishvili R, Kazaishvili D. Dominated EEG patterns and their prognostic value in coma caused by traumatic brain injury. Georgian Med News. 2010 Sep;186:28–33.
65. Lawhern V, Hairston WD, McDowell K, Westerfield M, Robbins K. Detection and classification of subject-generated artifacts in EEG signals using autoregressive models. Journal of neuroscience methods. 2012 Jul 15;208(2):181–9.
66. Hippisley-Cox J, Coupland C, Vinogradova Y, Robson J, May M, Brindle P. Derivation and validation of QRISK, a new cardiovascular disease risk score for the United Kingdom: prospective open cohort study. Bmj. 2007 Jul 19;335(7611):136.
67. Hippisley-Cox J, Coupland C, Vinogradova Y, Robson J, Minhas R, Sheikh A, Brindle P. Predicting cardiovascular risk in England and Wales: prospective derivation and validation of QRISK2. Bmj. 2008 Jun 26;336(7659):1475–82.
68. Sterne JA, White IR, Carlin JB, Spratt M, Royston P, Kenward MG, Wood AM, Carpenter JR. Multiple imputation for missing data in epidemiological and clinical research: potential and pitfalls. Bmj. 2009 Jun 29;338:b2393.

69. Collins GS, Altman DG. An independent and external validation of QRISK2 cardiovascular disease risk score: a prospective open cohort study. Bmj. 2010 May 13;340:c2442.
70. Allison PD. Missing data: Quantitative applications in the social sciences. British Journal of Mathematical and Statistical Psychology. 2002;55(1):193–6.
71. Tarassenko L, Hann A, Young D. Integrated monitoring and analysis for early warning of patient deterioration. British journal of anaesthesia. 2006 Jul 1;97(1):64–8.
72. Gilks WR, Wild P. Adaptive rejection sampling for Gibbs sampling. Applied Statistics. 1992 Jan 1:337–48.
73. Kirkwood BR. Essentials of medical statistics. Blackwell Scientific Publications; 1988.
74. Tobin J. Estimation of relationships for limited dependent variables. Econometrica: journal of the Econometric Society. 1958 Jan 1:24–36.
75. Rubin DB. Multiple imputation for nonresponse in surveys. John Wiley & Sons; 2004 Jun 9.
76. Graham JW, Olchowski AE, Gilreath TD. How many imputations are really needed? Some practical clarifications of multiple imputation theory. Prevention Science. 2007 Sep 1;8(3): 206–13.
77. Bodner TE. What improves with increased missing data imputations?. Structural Equation Modeling. 2008 Oct 22;15(4):651–75.
78. Schafer JL. Multiple imputation: a primer. Statistical methods in medical research. 1999 Feb 1;8(1):3–15.
79. Azur MJ, Stuart EA, Frangakis C, Leaf PJ. Multiple imputation by chained equations: what is it and how does it work?. International journal of methods in psychiatric research. 2011 Mar 1;20(1):40–9.
80. Allison PD. Handling missing data by maximum likelihood. In SAS global forum 2012 Apr 22 (Vol. 23).
81. Stegle O, Fallert SV, MacKay DJ, Brage S. Gaussian process robust regression for noisy heart rate data. IEEE Transactions on Biomedical Engineering. 2008 Sep;55(9):2143–51.
82. Roberts S, Osborne M, Ebden M, Reece S, Gibson N, Aigrain S. Gaussian processes for time-series modelling. Phil. Trans. R. Soc. A. 2013 Feb 13;371(1984):20110550.
83. Dürichen R, Pimentel MA, Clifton L, Schweikard A, Clifton DA. Multitask Gaussian processes for multivariate physiological time-series analysis. IEEE Transactions on Biomedical Engineering. 2015 Jan;62(1):314–22.
84. Boyle, P. and Frean, M., 2004. Dependent gaussian processes. In *Advances in neural information processing systems* (pp. 217–224).
85. Wong D, Clifton DA, Tarassenko L. Probabilistic detection of vital sign abnormality with Gaussian process regression. In Bioinformatics & Bioengineering (BIBE), 2012 IEEE 12th International Conference on 2012 Nov 11 (pp. 187–192). IEEE.
86. Saeys Y, Inza I, Larrañaga P. A review of feature selection techniques in bioinformatics. bioinformatics. 2007 Oct 1;23(19):2507–17.
87. Breiman L. Random forests. Machine learning. 2001 Oct 1;45(1):5–32.
88. Breiman L, Friedman J, Stone CJ, Olshen RA. Classification and regression trees. CRC press; 1984.
89. Edmonds J. Matroids and the greedy algorithm. Mathematical programming. 1971 Dec 1; 1(1):127–36.
90. Joliffe IT, Morgan BJ. Principal component analysis and exploratory factor analysis. Statistical methods in medical research. 1992 Mar 1;1(1):69–95.
91. Sammon JW. A nonlinear mapping for data structure analysis. IEEE Transactions on computers. 1969 May 1;18(5):401–9.
92. Wong D, Strachan I, Tarassenko L. Visualisation of high-dimensional data for very large data sets. In Workshop Mach. Learn. Healthcare Appl., Helsinki, Finland 2008.
93. Lowe D, Tipping ME. Neuroscale: novel topographic feature extraction using RBF networks. Advances in Neural Information Processing Systems. 1997:543–9.
94. Durrant-Whyte H, Henderson TC. Multisensor data fusion. In Springer Handbook of Robotics 2008 (pp. 585–610). Springer Berlin Heidelberg.

95. Li Q. and Clifford G. D., Signal quality and data fusion for false alarm reduction in the intensive care unit, Journal of Electrocardiology, 45(6):596–603, Nov 2012.
96. Williams C, Quinn J, McIntosh N. Factorial switching Kalman filters for condition monitoring in neonatal intensive care.
97. Clifton DA, Bannister PR, Tarassenko L. A framework for novelty detection in jet engine vibration data. In Key engineering materials 2007 (Vol. 347, pp. 305–310). Trans Tech Publications.
98. Ma M, Gonet R, Yu R, Anagnostopoulos GC. Metric representations of data via the Kernel-based Sammon Mapping. In The 2010 International Joint Conference on Neural Networks (IJCNN) 2010 Jul 18 (pp. 1–7). IEEE.
99. Hu M, Chen Y, Kwok JT. Building sparse multiple-kernel SVM classifiers. IEEE Transactions on Neural Networks. 2009 May;20(5):827–39.
100. Ye J, Chen K, Wu T, Li J, Zhao Z, Patel R, Bae M, Janardan R, Liu H, Alexander G, Reiman E. Heterogeneous data fusion for alzheimer's disease study. In Proceedings of the 14th ACM SIGKDD international conference on Knowledge discovery and data mining 2008 Aug 24 (pp. 1025–1033). ACM.
101. Blumenthal D. Launching hitech. New England Journal of Medicine. 2010 Feb 4;362 (5):382–5.
102. Gymrek M, McGuire AL, Golan D, Halperin E, Erlich Y. Identifying personal genomes by surname inference. Science. 2013 Jan 18;339(6117):321–4.
103. Lenzerini M. Data integration: A theoretical perspective. InProceedings of the twenty-first ACM SIGMOD-SIGACT-SIGART symposium on Principles of database systems 2002 Jun 3 (pp. 233–246). ACM.
104. Donnelly K. SNOMED-CT: The advanced terminology and coding system for eHealth. Studies in health technology and informatics. 2006 Jan;121:279.
105. O'Neil M, Payne C, Read J. Read Codes Version 3: a user led terminology. Methods of information in medicine. 1995 Mar;34(1–2):187–92.
106. Lopez AD. Sharing data for public health: where is the vision?. Bulletin of the World Health Organization. 2010 Jun;88(6):467.
107. van Panhuis WG, Paul P, Emerson C, Grefenstette J, Wilder R, Herbst AJ, Heymann D, Burke DS. A systematic review of barriers to data sharing in public health. BMC Public Health. 2014 Nov 5;14(1):1.
108. Luo, Jake et al. "Big Data Application in Biomedical Research and Health Care: A Literature Review." Biomedical Informatics Insights 8 (2016): 1–10. *PMC*. Web. 8 Nov. 2016.
109. White T. Hadoop: The Definite Guide. Sebastopol, CA:O'Reilly Media, Inc.;2012.
110. Jin Y, Deyu T, Yi Z. A distributed storage model for EHR based on HBase. In: 2011 International Conference on Information Management, Innovation Management and Industrial Engineering (ICIII), Shenzhen, China; IEEE. 2011:369–72.
111. Dutta H, Kamil A, Pooleery M, et al. Distributed storage of large-scale multidimensional electroencephalogram data using Hadoop and HBase. In: Fiore S, Aloisio G, eds. Grid and Cloud Database Management. Berlin: Springer; 2011:331–47.
112. Sahoo SS, Jayapandian C, Garg G, et al. Heart beats in the cloud: distributed analysis of electrophysiological 'Big Data' using cloud computing for epilepsy clinical research. J Am Med Inform Assoc. 2014;21(2):263–71.
113. Jayapandian CP, Chen C-H, Bozorgi A, et al. Cloudwave: distributed processing of "Big Data" from electrophysiological recordings for epilepsy clinical research using Hadoop. In: AMIA Annual Symposium Proceedings, Washington, DC; AMIA. 2013:691.
114. Lin W, Dou W, Zhou Z, et al. A cloud-based framework for home-diagnosis service over big medical data. J Syst Software. 2015;102:192–206.
115. Kimura E., Hamada K., Kikuchi R., Chida K., Okamoto K., Manabe S., Kuroda T., Matsumura Y., Takeda T. and Mihara N., Evaluation of Secure Computation in a Distributed Healthcare Setting, in A. Hoerbst et al. (Eds.), Volume 228: Exploring Complexity in Health: An Interdisciplinary Systems Approach, Studies in Health Technology and Informatics, pp. 152–156, 2016.

116. Ng K, Ghoting A, Steinhubl SR, et al. PARAMO: a PARAllel predictive MOdeling platform for healthcare analytic research using electronic health records. J Biomed Inform. 2014;48:160–70.
117. Goldhill DR, White SA, Sumner A. Physiological values and procedures in the 24 h before ICU admission from the ward. Anaesthesia. 1999 Jun 1;54(6):529–34.
118. Wilson SJ, Wong D, Pullinger RM, Way R, Clifton DA, Tarassenko L. Analysis of a data-fusion system for continuous vital sign monitoring in an emergency department. European Journal of Emergency Medicine. 2016 Feb 1;23(1):28–32.
119. Cireşan DC, Giusti A, Gambardella LM, Schmidhuber J. Mitosis detection in breast cancer histology images with deep neural networks. In International Conference on Medical Image Computing and Computer-assisted Intervention 2013 Sep 22 (pp. 411–418). Springer Berlin Heidelberg.
120. Havaei M, Davy A, Warde-Farley D, Biard A, Courville A, Bengio Y, Pal C, Jodoin PM, Larochelle H. Brain tumor segmentation with deep neural networks. Medical Image Analysis. 2016 May 19.

Data Quality in Mobile Sensing Datasets for Pervasive Healthcare

Netzahualcóyotl Hernández, Luis A. Castro, Jesús Favela, Layla Michán and Bert Arnrich

Abstract Mobile sensing is becoming a popular approach for inferring patterns of activity and behavior to determine how they affect health and wellbeing. This data-driven approach has the potential to become a major tool in the field of epidemiology, aimed at determining the causes of disease in populations, as well as motivating behavior change. These sensing technologies are generating large datasets that demand significant processing and data management resources. Studies in mobile sensing for healthcare have motivated the creation of large, complex datasets with information opportunistically gathered from distributed sensors in mobile devices. In this chapter, we discuss some of the architectural challenges regarding data gathering in this distributed data-intensive environment such as the healthcare industry, as well as issues regarding the organization and sharing of the large amounts of data collected. Some of these issues include the heterogeneity of the devices, diversity of sensors used, and the need for data provenance when integrating datasets from diverse studies. We highlight that assessing data quality is of paramount importance for conducting longitudinal studies and building on historical knowledge as new data become available.

N. Hernández (✉) · J. Favela · L. Michán
Department of Computer Science, CICESE, Ensenada, Mexico
e-mail: netzahdzc@cicese.mx; netzahdzc@gmail.com

J. Favela
e-mail: favela@cicese.mx

L.A. Castro
Department of Computing and Design, Sonora Institute of Technology, Ciudad Obregon, Mexico
e-mail: luis.castro@acm.org

L. Michán
Facultad de Ciencias, UNAM, Mexico City, Mexico
e-mail: laylamichan@ciencias.unam.mx

B. Arnrich
Department of Computer Engineering, Boğaziçi University, Istanbul, Turkey
e-mail: bert.arnrich@boun.edu.tr

© Springer International Publishing AG 2017

S.U. Khan et al. (eds.), *Handbook of Large-Scale Distributed Computing in Smart Healthcare*, Scalable Computing and Communications,
DOI 10.1007/978-3-319-58280-1_9

Finally, we identify future research topics in the growing field of mobile sensing and its application to healthcare and wellbeing. We discuss aspects of data curation, data quality, and data provenance, and we provide suggestions on how these challenges could be addressed in the near future.

Keywords Mobile sensing • Healthcare • Standards • Data curation • Data harmonization

1 Introduction

Mobile and wearable technologies incorporate advanced computing, communication, and sensing capabilities that enable collecting data related to their users and their surroundings. The augmented capabilities of these devices and their ubiquity, have contributed to an emerging field known as mobile sensing. This area aims at collecting and analyzing data from several devices scattered around a particular geographical area worn or carried by users, particularly outside the clinic. This emerging area is of particular interest for researchers in healthcare as it provides an unusual lens for better understanding human behavior associated to disease outbreaks, disease onsets, medical care, and health status, as it is often the case in epidemiology. Clinical sensors, although clearly useful for pervasive healthcare, are not the main focus of this chapter. We rather focus on emerging technologies such as smartphones and wearable devices that are to be used in naturalistic conditions by individuals, meaning that they are used in contexts upon which researchers have no control, and they tend to be challenging for collecting data that can be useful. Besides, the ubiquity of these devices makes it possible to collect massive amounts of behavioral data from large populations.

This emerging area, known as mobile sensing uses a data-driven paradigm of scientific discovery through data, since the body of knowledge generated deeply associates to data captured by mobile devices. Preserving and sharing datasets are paramount to the growth and maturity of the field. Thus, the amount of data gathered through mobile sensing imposes important demands on the communication, storage, and processing infrastructure.

The involvement of a large number of volunteers in participatory sensing campaigns[1] is an important component of data-driven science. In other fields, this is referred to as citizen science or crowd-sourced science, which is scientific research

[1]A sensing campaign is a data collection campaign following a research protocol. A sensing campaign can involve tens or thousands of participants carrying one or more mobile devices, which opportunistically collect data from the user or her surroundings, or ask the user to carry out certain task (e.g., take a picture when feeling sad or answer a question).

conducted, in whole or in part, by amateur or nonprofessional scientists. At times, this turns out to be fundamental for science, as the amount of unstructured data to be analyzed can be overwhelming for scientists and current infrastructure for supporting analysis. Gathering data from a diverse population is particularly important for healthcare applications, notably to uncover how behavior influences healthcare.

In mobile sensing for pervasive healthcare, one of the main concerns is generating reliable datasets that can be used to push forward the boundaries of the area, which necessarily involves providing structure to the data. While current efforts have yielded promising results, our vision is that scientists could tap into a distributed repository of healthcare datasets. These datasets are to be curated and integrated to facilitate conducting new research in healthcare such as generalizing previous findings when comparing with new data from a different population and creating longitudinal studies controlling for the conditions in which data were gathered over long periods of time. These types of endeavors are paramount for research in fields such as epidemiology. Efforts to create repositories of datasets are not new in the computer science discipline. The machine learning community has made available numerous repositories, including some in pervasive healthcare, aimed at detecting daily life activities [1]. Examples of these repositories include the UCI Machine Learning Repository [2] and Keel [3]. These datasets however are not consolidated or homogenized. They are meant to be used independently to test new learning algorithms or to be used by students as a learning tool.

Closer to our aim are efforts such as Registry of Research data Repositories (re3data) [4], Dryad [5] with data from papers, DataOne [6], a repository on Earth and environmental data, and a repository of datasets for ecological modeling and forecasting [7]. Within the domain of healthcare, the Observational Health Data Sciences and Informatics (OHDSI) is an open-source initiative hosted at the Columbia University with the purpose of standardizing observational data and analytics of healthcare data [8]. This is achieved through a common data model and a series of tools. OHDSI however uses patient registries rather than data obtained from mobile sensors.

The Open mHealth [9] initiative recognizes the importance of mobile sensing data for healthcare research and is developing mechanisms to standardize data and integrate data streams to encourage the development of new pervasive healthcare apps. It also offers an Application Program Interface (API) to access data from a repository and to conduct data analytics. While the effort to standardize data from different sensors is encouraging, the platform is meant for applications for the end user, rather than as a research platform. MD2K [10] is a Center for Excellence for Mobile Sensor Data-to-Knowledge funded by the National Institutes of Health (NIH) in the United States with the purpose of facilitating gathering, analyzing and interpreting health data generated by mobile and wearable sensors. The current effort is focused on two application domains with a long-term vision of acting as a repository of mobile data using Open mHealth standards.

Of particular interest here is the Precision Medicine Initiative, initiated in 2015 in the US,[2] and aimed at creating a cohort of one million participants that will contribute biological and genetic data, and of particular interest to this chapter, behavioral and lifestyle information gathered from mobile sensors.

This chapter elaborates on some of the issues in large-scale studies involving off-the-clinic mobile sensors, and challenges to carry out mobile phone sensing campaigns for pervasive healthcare. As mentioned, we focus our discussion on mobile/wearable sensors producing heterogeneous data from multiple contexts. These varying contexts wherein data are collected come with unprecedented challenges for pervasive healthcare such as quality assurance or architectural aspects related to data processing demands imposed on the infrastructure. Lastly, this chapter presents a mobile sensing platform and a multi-site sensing campaign, which is a way to illustrate how the aforementioned challenges and issues could be addressed.

2 Mobile Sensing Opportunities for Healthcare Research

Human activities are complex and dynamic. Activities at different levels of granularity can be performed concurrently and they might be interwoven. Hence, the development of activity-aware applications requires appropriate representations of computational activities that are relevant to the services provided by systems.

One of the trends that have promoted activity recognition research is the significant increase in available data due to the incorporation of sensors such as GPS, accelerometers and microphones, in mobile phones. The ubiquity of these devices also makes them ideal platforms for the deployment of pervasive healthcare solutions. Relevant examples to healthcare include the use of accelerometer data to reliably determine if a person is standing, walking or running, and to estimate energy expenditure. The automatic estimation of these activities is relevant for wellness applications that measure periods of moderate or intense activity.

In this context, mobile devices can be used to infer and manage patient-related information, perform medical diagnostics, and provide nutrition-related information and wellness recommendations. For instance, unobtrusively monitoring gait speed along a period of time over a route, could provide early evidence of fatigue; where accelerometer and location data can be used to assess the perception of physical fatigue (commonly associated to fragility) on elderly population [11]. Wearable devices have also been used to infer periods of anxiety among caregivers of people with dementia [12].

The capacity and ubiquity of smartphones have catalyzed the biosensing mobile phone and wearable market. For instance, public and private initiatives participation have started to growth vertically and horizontally in sectors aimed at sensing and

[2]https://www.nih.gov/research-training/allofus-research-program.

inferring: movement [13], heart rate [14], sleep [15], temperature [16], respiration [17], oxygen consumption [18], skin [19], attention [20], food ingestion [21], blood levels [22], among others. The common vision consists on collecting data to test pharmacogenomics, provide new pharmacology ideas for non-therapeutic treatments, proactively identify disease risk on populations, and explore the feasibility of case studies with patients for better understanding how mobile technology could improve health outcomes, individually or collectively.

3 Architectures and Data Issues in Large-Scale and Distributed Sensing Environments

Mobile sensing for healthcare faces a number of challenges related to data gathering and sharing, some of which are similar to those found in other areas, while differing in other aspects. First, healthcare research involving mobile devices, if they are to have a profound impact on daily life, are to be carried out in a large scale, involving a number of mobile devices distributed across large regions such as a country or across borders. Several diseases studied by epidemiology are known to be caused not only by genetic or biological factors but also by environmental and behavioral ones. Thus the need to understand the interplay among the various factors that have an effect on disease onset, development, and care affecting diverse populations.

3.1 Software Architecture Issues

Gathering and processing large amounts of mobile sensing data imposes important demands on the hardware and software infrastructure. A mobile sensing platform is generally composed of the following elements: sensors, computing devices, networks, and storage. Each node might combine these elements in different ways. For instance, a smartphone has sensing capabilities, processing power, but somewhat limited network and storage capabilities; while servers usually possess no sensing capabilities, but rate very high in processing power, communication network, and storage.

As show in Fig. 1, a common mobile sensing architecture follows a tree-like structure, involving mobiles devices with sensing capabilities at the leaves. One of the factors influencing latency is how distributed computing power is within the layers of the architecture. For instance, most mobile sensing studies reported in the literature typically perform little processing in the leaves. However, in some scenarios, and mainly due to privacy and latency, it is desirable to perform some computing at the lower levels (leaves). However, depending on the configuration of the architecture chosen, the latency derived from the amounts of data to be transferred over the network can vary significantly, as show in Table 1.

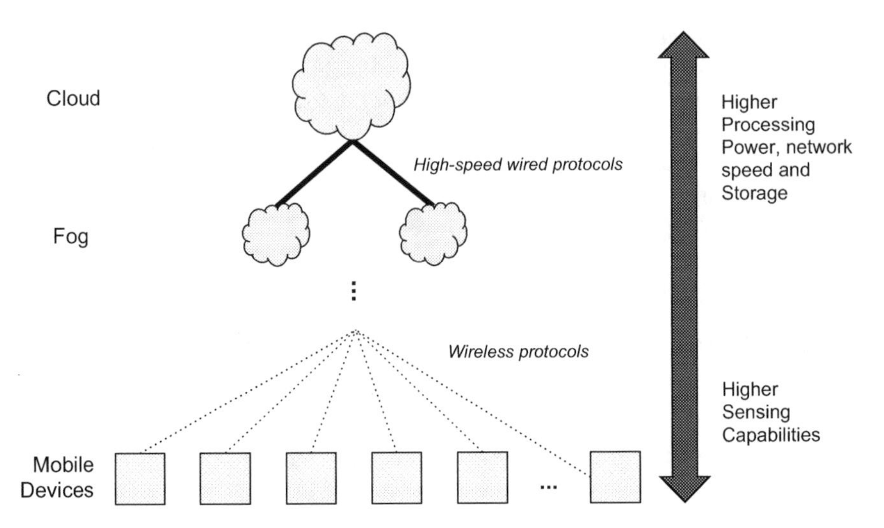

Fig. 1 Hierarchical view of a mobile sensing architecture

Table 1 Cost-benefit relationship for the three levels from the cloud computing perspective

Scenario	Amount of data	Latency	Cost	Complexity
Full cloud-based computing	Large	High	Low	Low
Fog computing	Middle	Middle	Middle	Mid
Fully distributed computing	Small	Low	High	High

3.2 *Data Issues*

In Table 2, we present some of the data issues currently faced by the research community in mobile sensing in order to achieve the goal of having a data infrastructure from which to continuously construct new knowledge and validate previous findings. This is particularly important in healthcare research involving mobile or wearable devices in large-scale and distributed environments, as the issues are to be increasingly present.

3.2.1 Heterogeneity in Data Gathering

While mobile phones have become the most popular means for gathering mobile data, there are important differences in the manner in which information is collected. The sensors available in each device might have different accuracies or the data might be sampled at different frequencies due to the restrictions of each sensing campaign. For instance, to avoid battery depletion, it might be decided to record location information once every 5 min, or due to privacy, to record it only Monday to Friday from 09 to 14 h. As mobile devices evolve and new and more powerful

Table 2 Data management and collection issues for mobile sensing at large

Category	Issue	Responsible
Research	Heterogeneity in data gathering	Researchers
	Data annotation	Researchers
	Data pre-processing	Researchers
	Limited data sharing	Researchers
Legal	Privacy	Participants/researchers
	Ethics	Researchers
Engineering	Heterogeneity in sensor data	Hardware vendors
	Dispersion	Researchers/stakeholders

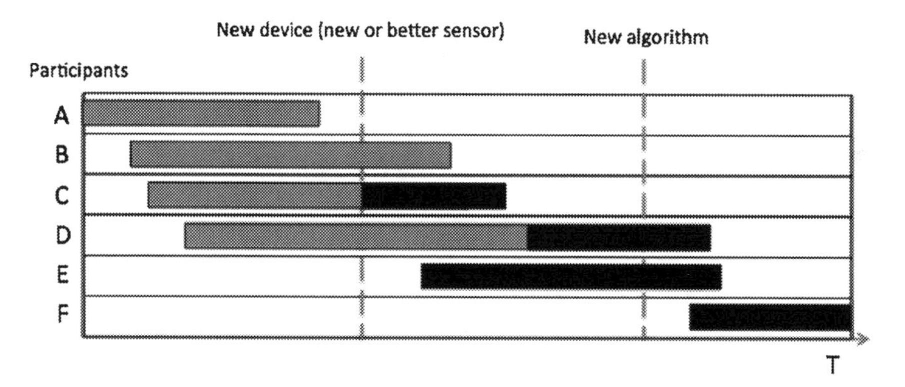

Fig. 2 Example of data retrieved at different periods and under different conditions (mobile sensing device and/or algorithm). The change in color in each *horizontal bar* represents when the user adopted a new sensing device. The *blue dashed lines* represent that a significant event during the study, such as the introduction of a new device or inference algorithm (color figure online)

sensing and storage capacity becomes available, we might face the issue of how to compare recordings from the same individual who over the years has used different recording devices (i.e., from fitness trackers, to a smartphone, a smart-watch or intelligent clothing). One relatively straightforward alternative is to turn to the lowest common denominator but this has the inconvenience of losing the advantage provided by richer data. Another option is to interpolate data in datasets with sparser information and consider the uncertainty raised by using this approach during data analysis.

A dataset for a longitudinal analysis might include individuals who join the study at different times and with different devices. Consider a span of the study that involves a change in technology, for instance, the incorporation of an altimeter in a mobile device. The new sensor can be used to estimate the number of stairs a person walks each day. Furthermore, sometime after the new sensor is available, a new algorithm is proposed that uses the accelerometer and altimeter to better estimate the number of calories burned each day. As illustrated in Fig. 2, participant A joins the study from the beginning and leaves the study before the device with the new sensor is available. Participant B is still in the study when the new device is introduced, but it never adopts it. The new algorithm for calculating calories burned cannot be used with the data from these two participants. In contrast, participant C adopts the new device as it is introduced. Metadata needs to be used to indicate that the data collected from this person differs given the device used. In addition, when the new algorithm is made available, caloric expenditure during the period the person had the new device can be re-calculated, but cannot be directly compared to the initial phase when an older device was used. Participant E enters the study with the new device and, as the new algorithm is introduced, her calories expended can be estimated more accurately, and the ones previously recorded re-calculated. Finally, participant F joins the study with the new device and after the new algorithm was introduced, and thus the estimation of the calories the participant burned are estimated using the same device/algorithm. This example highlights the need for metadata to better understand the conditions in which the data were gathered and calculated; what is generally referred as data provenance. The researcher might for instance decide to use calories estimated with the original algorithm, since it can be used with all the data in the dataset.

Data harmonization between heterogeneous studies involves defining common data and agreeing on a data scheme to which different datasets can be transformed.

3.2.2 Data Annotation

Due to the naturalistic conditions in which mobile sensing studies are conducted, annotating data and establishing ground truth can require significant effort. Mobile sensing studies often rely on user participation to annotate the data, which might compromise their reliability. In addition, the annotation might be incomplete if the user is not always able or willing to provide the data.

3.2.3 Data Pre-processing

Some sensors such as microphones, accelerometers, or cameras have the potential to generate considerable amounts of data. For instance, one minute of uncompressed audio at 44 kHz requires approximately 5 MB of storage capacity. If continuous audio is recorded from several subjects for days or weeks it quickly becomes impractical to store all this information. Besides, specific studies might be interested in detecting only some events, for instance, when the individual is involved in a conversation, or detecting that he/she is outdoors. In addition, location or audio data might be processed to preserve the anonymity of the subject. The consent agreement might specify, for instance, that the audio recorded will be processed so that the content of the conversation or the identity of the interlocutors could not be inferred. Thus, it is a common practice to process the data gathered in a manner that some information is lost. If years later, a new study wants to use these findings, it needs to be aware of how the data were processed. As an example, speaker identification in a legacy study might have 93% accuracy, compared to 97% for a new study, with which we want to conduct an integrated analysis. Since the original data from the legacy study are not available, the new algorithms cannot be run on that dataset. The researcher needs to be made aware of these differences, and, if possible, be provided with tools to take them into account during the analysis.

3.2.4 Limited Data Sharing

While several research teams in mobile sensing have made their datasets available to other researches, this is not the norm, and different groups might use different formats and metadata. To a large degree it reflects the novelty of the field, but also the fact that the effort to make the data available (e.g., adding metadata, put in adequate format, anonymize), might not be compensated.

3.2.5 Privacy

Due to their nature, many personal data are considered sensitive. Examples include location, behavior, or personal health records. Other data, on the other hand, can be disclosed without much concern. In the case of personal data, some people may be willing to share them only if authorized individuals can access them or the data is anonymized for analysis. For instance, individuals can be willing to share health records with authorized healthcare professionals, but not with certain government agencies. For this, mechanisms such as proper anonymously data anonymization are paramount, releasing data with certain restrictions (data license for commercial or research use), or providing some sort of private/public keys to access data.

3.2.6 Ethics

Making sure that participants understand the prolonged validity of the data they are contributing is important, as the data could be used in future studies. Consent forms should be handled in such a way that participants are fully aware of the reach of the study in which they participate. A recent example of how remote informed consents are handled is through Apple's Research Kit [23] in which participants sign in through the mobile phone. However, there are certain issues that may arise, such as deriving new behavior information from previously recorded data without the participants' knowledge or consent. For instance, if new research finds that visiting certain places increases the risk of developing certain disease, there may be ethics and privacy issues that, because knowledge was not available at the time of the sensing campaign, bring about the question of whether those data can be used, even if they may benefit the participants.

3.2.7 Heterogeneity in Sensor Data

Due to the great diversity in the market of mobile phones and chipset vendors, sensor data generated by mobile devices can vary greatly. For instance, the wireless Received Signal Strength Indicator (RSSI), which is a measurement of the power presented in a received radio signal, is commonly used to infer indoor location. Depending on the chipset vendor, the RSSI may vary as they use different RSSI_Max value; which might lead to different measures or samples even in the same network. Heterogeneity remains an issue since there are many actors involved, but for the purposes of this area, the peculiarities of the hardware used for creating/collecting the data should be made public.

3.2.8 Dispersion

In some large-scale and distributed computing scenarios, one of the main issues can be dispersion. Having low dispersion is desirable in distributed systems, but can have high costs. In the case of mobile sensing, dispersion can be derived from having multiple sites generating, processing, and curating data. Depending on the circumstances, this can be an issue if there are multiple healthcare organizations either public or private helping to collect, annotate, curate, and store data that plan to be aggregated into a single cloud-based, consolidated dataset. For instance, take the example of Mexico in which there are three main national public healthcare systems insuring 58, 55, and 13 million Mexicans nationwide. Those three systems are often managed through local administrations, which can have access to different types of infrastructures. Under this scenario, aggregating data from those three systems with different infrastructures in terms of storage, processing power, and communication service can be challenging. Leaving aside all private institutions and physicians providing care, as the number of actors involved in collecting, annotating, curating, and storing data increases in number, and presumably criteria, this can become a growing issue of great implications for research in healthcare.

4 The m^k-sense Mobile Sensing Platform

In this section we present the m^k-sense platform; a cloud-based computing architecture which uses mobile phones as sensing elements (leaves). The configuration of the platform illustrates some of practical compromises made in the design of multi-site sensing campaigns.

m^k-sense is an extension of the open source framework Funf [24], developed to collect data through mobile devices. It consists of a bimodal implementation: (1) a client-side application, and (2) a server-side to dynamically create surveys and monitor data completeness. m^k-sense aims to support multiple sensing campaigns

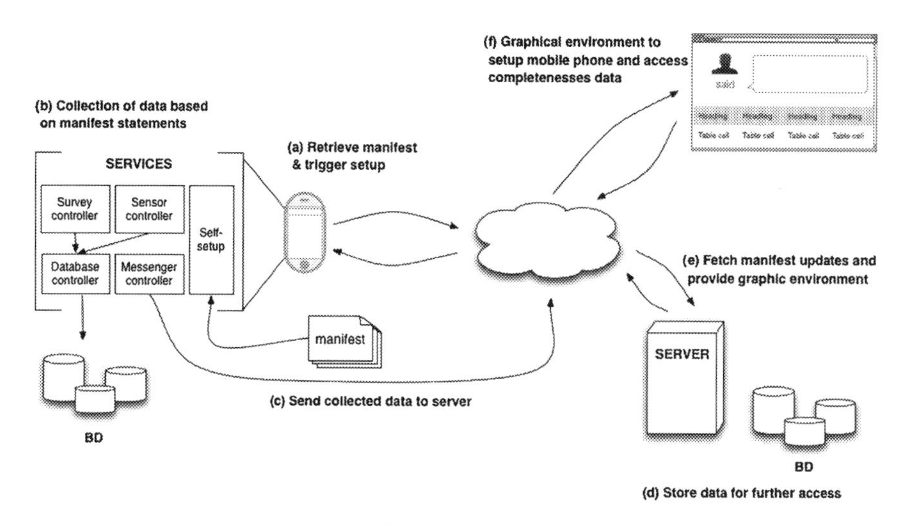

Fig. 3 Data collection architecture in m^k-sense

with minimal configuration effort. Thus, researchers avoid investing resources in developing dedicated software.

m^k-sense has been designed to require minimal technical knowledge from users to effectively operate the platform, it is based on a concept of packing in which researches are allowed to address multiple studies in parallel. m^k-sense is implemented on a three-layer architecture. The presentation-layer provides a graphical environment to create study-packages and monitor data completeness. The data-layer stores data into a relational database. Finally, the business-layer manages resources on the client-side (e.g., questionnaires) before and after they are sent to the server-side, as illustrated in Fig. 3.

Data collection involves two main stages:

1. **Collection of data**. Once the client-side application is installed on a mobile phone and a study package has been selected, m^k-sense retrieves a configuration manifest as a first approximation for auto-setup of the sensing mechanism in the mobile device. The manifest is fetched from the server to automatically setup the device as illustrated in Fig. 3a.

   a. If the manifest specifies that a sequence of surveys should be replied, then they will be scheduled accordingly to be launched on the mobile phone.
   b. Otherwise, the application will start collecting sensor data; based on pre-defined characteristics (e.g., intervals, frequency) specified at the manifest.

2. **Messenger service**. Both sensor and surveys data are temporarily sheltered in the mobile phone. In order to send data to the server-side, m^k-sense enables a messenger service to opportunistically transfer batches of data. The service is performed using a wireless connection as presented on Fig. 1b–d.

A more detailed description of m^k-sense is presented in [25].

4.1 Walkability: A 21-Day Sensing Campaign

Walking is one of the many activities of daily life that have a positive impact on health and wellbeing, environmental pollution, and economic benefits. In addition, studies in Ambien Assisted Living (AAL) have focused on developing intelligent environments that might be suitable for elderly population and people with disabilities to remain active and independent despite their physical limitations [26]. In this context, walking is an activity commonly recommended by physicians to improve wellbeing. This is mainly due to its effectiveness and simplicity, since it does not require specialized equipment or controlled conditions.

Trying to provide a better understanding of walkable areas, several initiatives have advanced mechanisms to define and compute a walkability score [27, 28]. Evaluations might be based on several sources of information. For instance, on user's feedback provided voluntarily, or by retrieving social medial information from sites such as Flickr and Foursquare to automatically identify safe and walkable streets [29].

The 21-day sensing walkability sensing campaign is a study designed to explore a mechanism based on mobile phones' sensors to further analyze how friendly a road/path is for walking. Walkability is in an important concept in urban design that includes aspects such as infrastructure (e.g., sidewalks, street layout), places of interest (e.g., markets, schools, retails, home), among others. In addition, walkable areas might be an incentive to promote activities to benefit health like going out and perform physical activities such as walk, socialize with neighbors and relatives, and so on. Several walkability scores exist as of today, which are mainly based on several aspects such as counting people in a certain area or region (e.g., street).

The study presented in this work was addressed with the voluntary participation of subjects who work or study at universities campuses. Hence, the walkability evaluation focuses on a common area shared by several participants. The sensing campaign was conducted in Mexico, Turkey, and Spain with an overall participation of 65 people, as presented on Table 3.

Table 3 Population characteristics

	Group A	Group B	Group C
No. of participants	29	21	15
City, Country	Ensenada, Mexico	Istanbul, Turkey	Toledo and Castille-La Mancha, Spain
Size of the city	Medium (500k)	Large (14M)	Small (84k) and Large (2M)
Density of population	9/km^2	2600/km^2	362/km^2 and 27/km^2
Gender	15 male; 14 female	17 male; 4 female	4 male; 9 female
Average age (S.D.)	28.48 (5.79)	23.24 (3.62)	28.42 (9.08)

The study's protocol was replicated under strict supervision; same directions and training procedure were provided. As part of the methodology, each participant received a survey under two conditions: automatically triggered by detecting a continued walking interval of 5 min or on-demand requested by the participant.

There were up to two software updates during the study due to technical issues reported by the participants, and software improvements. Participants completed a simple survey at different moments during the study. Based on preliminary data, the Walkability survey was voluntarily completed 3 times per day; approximately. Data were collected throughout a 21-day period with an optional extension of 7 days.

5 Data Management Issues in the Walkability Study

In this section, we aim at illustrating previously discussed issues rather than proposing definitive answers to them. Thus, along this section we discuss how the data management issues raised in Sect. 3 were addressed in the Walkability Study.

5.1 Data Curation Lifecycle Models

As part of the planning of the project, we defined a data lifecycle model to address the Walkability study. The data collection models are ad hoc reference protocols for the design, management, and implementation of data collections. It can be used to help identify additional steps that may be required—or actions not required by certain situations or disciplines—and to ensure that processes and policies are adequately documented, their main objectives are: (1) to provide a graphical, high-level overview of the stages required for the successful curation and preservation of data from initial conceptualization or receipt through the iterative curation cycle, (2) to plan activities within a group, organization, consortium or institution to ensure that all of the necessary steps in the curation lifecycle are covered, there are cycles it may enter at any stage of the process depending on their current needs by forward or, (3) to provide a granular function to be mapped against it to define roles and responsibilities and build a framework of standards and technologies to implement.

There are several data lifecycle models have been proposed, including:

- DataONE data life cycle for of Earth and environmental data [6].
- Data life cycle UCSD [30].
- Digital Life Cycle [31].
- DCC Curation Lifecycle Model [32].

5.2 *Data Management Plan for the Walkability Study*

A Data Management Plan (DMP) is a document that outlines a process from the bid-preparation stage through and after the project is completed. The purpose of DMPs is to keep record of the many aspects of data management (e.g., digital assets management, archiving, digital preservation, content and record diligence) to achieve a data-preservation in the future.

To illustrate our DMT, we adopted a DCC Curation Lifecycle Model; previously mentioned. Hence, we used DMPonline[3] from the Digital Curation Centre to create a Data Management Plan for the Walkability Study. The project planning included the following aspects:

- **Administration details**. The project is presented through a brief description of the study and expected results in the production of scientific data. In addition, detailed information like: grant funder, project name, and research leader, is provided for further contact reference.
- **Data types**. It is elaborated regarding the variety of data-types that are expected to result from the project, including the raw data arising directly from the research, the reduced data derived from it, and published data.
- **Data preservation**. It describes which data will be preserved and how this will be achieved. Software and metadata that will be retained to enable the data to be read and interpreted were described as well as the period of time the data might be shielded.
- **Data sharing**. It specifies and justifies which data might have value to others and should be shared. It takes into account the cost of curation, the potential long-term demand for the data and the feasibility for the data to be reused by others.
- **Resources**. It defines the amount of resources required to preserve the dataset that will result from the Walkability study, as well as the implicit cost and for sharing respective data.

5.3 *Structural, Descriptive, and Administrative Metadata*

Metadata is structured information that describes, explains, locates, or otherwise makes it easier to retrieve, use, or manage an information resource. Metadata is often called data about data or information about information [33]. There are three main categories of metadata: descriptive, structural, and administrative metadata. To illustrate them, we present a set of categories based on the Walkability dataset (e.g., demographic, privacy, questions, sensors, surveys), classified according to the metadata associated to these data as presented in Table 4.

[3]https://dmponline.dcc.ac.uk/.

Table 4 Example of metadata classification for walkability study dataset

Metadata type	Data-section	Metadata
Descriptive; provide information to reach other data	Demographic	participant_id: Unique participant Id
		device_id: Unique participant's device Id
	Questions	question_id: Question unique id
Structural; facilitate navigation to resources	Surveys	question_(38 and 40): Answers for question number 38. This element content includes the physical location and format specifications
	Experimental	event: Unique code for events which require a reply from both the researcher and the participant
Administrative; provide technical data to facilitate further data-processing	Privacy	timestamp_db: Time recorded from database manager when temporarily recording data into participant's device (client-side)
	Questions	question_type: Question type (reference to bellow description section for more details)
	Sensors	timestamp_db: Date recorded from database manager when recording data into participant's device (client-side)
		accuracy: Accuracy of the event
		type: Accelerometer data type
		mAccuracy: Get the estimated accuracy of this location, in meters
		mAltitude: Get the altitude if available
		mBearing: Get the bearing, in degrees
		mProvider: Returns the name of the provider that generated this fix. Null if it has not been set
		mSpeed: Get the speed if it is available, in meters/second over ground. If this location does not have a speed then 0.0 is returned
	Surveys	timestamp_db: Time recorded from database manager when temporary recording data into participant's device (client-side)
		survey_name: Survey name
	Experimental	timestamp_db: Date when the event happened
		type: Purpose of the message: {message, service, question, answer}
		description: Type of the message: {welcome, code, technical, privacy,

(continued)

Table 4 (continued)

Metadata type	Data-section	Metadata
		study, complaint, drop, experience, access2data}
		direction: Flow of interaction event: {researcher => participant, participant => researcher}
		media: Mechanism of how the interaction event happened: {face2face, email, app, phonecall, other [facebook, whatsup, phonetextmessage]}

5.4 *Standards and Protocols*

Defining the data types to be used in the study should include establishing the standards to be used for each data type when available. There are some international standards and protocols for scientific and technical data that were adopted for the Walkability study, to describe data such as gender (ISO/IEC 5218), dates (ISO 8601), countries (ISO 3166-1) and cities (ISO 3166-2), and languages (ISO 639-3:2007).

5.5 *Privacy*

The information collected in the Walkability study was segmented into 5 categories (i.e., level of activity, sites visited, battery consumption, shared photographs, and completed questionnaires). Then users assigned a level of privacy to each item based on the six ordered Blue to Crimson sample data-tags [34], as shown in Table 5.

To address this issue, in the Walkability study we directly requested our participants to answer a set of questions, as illustrated on Table 6.
Data description:

A. What level of privacy would you set to your ACTIVITY LEVEL (obtained from the accelerometer sensor of your phone)?
B. What level of privacy would you set to your VISITED PLACES along the study (obtained from the GPS sensor of your phone)?
C. What level of privacy would you set to you BATTERY LEVEL collected from you phone?
D. What level of privacy would you set to PHOTOGRAPHS shared through questionnaires?
E. What level of privacy would you set to shared QUESTIONNAIRES RESPONSES?

Table 5 Sharing sensitive data with confidence: the data-tags system

BLUE	The information could be made public revealing my identity.
GREEN	The information could be made public while respecting my anonymity.
YELLOW	I believe that this information is sensitive and personal. From what I could authorize it to be shared only in certain cases.
ORANGE	I believe that this information is personal and could put at risk my identity. From what I could authorize to share it under my supervision.
RED	Very sensible. I could allow sharing it in a few exceptions.
CRIMSON	Extremely sensitive. I could allow sharing it under limited occasions.

Table 6 Privacy level from a sample of participants of Mexico, from the walkability study

PARTICIPANT	A	B	C	D	E
51	GREEN	GREEN	GREEN	GREEN	GREEN
57	GREEN	GREEN	GREEN	GREEN	GREEN
59	GREEN	YELLOW	GREEN	GREEN	GREEN
60	YELLOW	RED	GREEN	RED	GREEN
61	GREEN	YELLOW	GREEN	GREEN	GREEN
62	GREEN	ORANGE	GREEN	GREEN	GREEN
67	GREEN	GREEN	GREEN	YELLOW	RED
69	RED	RED	GREEN	CRIMSON	GREEN
70	GREEN	GREEN	BLUE	BLUE	BLUE
82	GREEN	GREEN	GREEN	GREEN	GREEN

5.6 *Data Quality and Quantity*

To accurately assess data quality, we took into account both researchers and participants' perspectives. Hence, we requested each participant to score their participation commitment using a Likert scale of 7 levels. In addition, we asked the researcher responsible for each site to use a similar rating to indicate his assessment of the commitment of the participant to the study.

Another aspect we took into account was missing data. To do so, we used a data monitoring service available at the server-side of m^k-sense platform. In this context, the server collects data and allows researchers to have a glance of the amount of

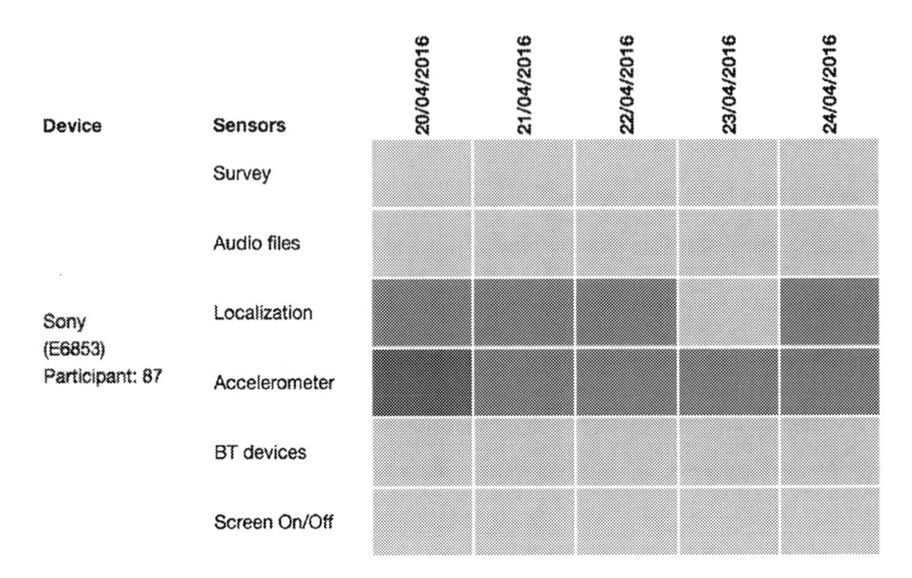

Fig. 4 Data completeness visualization from a study in which only location and acceleration data were collected. Each row corresponds to one feature and each *square* corresponds to one day of data collected. Color-coding indicates the amount of data collected: *light color* indicates little to no data; *dark color* stands for higher amounts of data

data that has been collected to a certain period of time. A graphical interface (a.k.a. a dashboard) is activated once the server begins to receive mobile phone data; Fig. 3e and f, it enables a service to directly communicate with participants by text messages, among others. For instance, Fig. 4 shows a sample of the list of features available on m^k-sense; where a lighter color represents a small amount of data, and a darker one represents a higher amount of data collected. This visualization allows researchers to have a quick glance of the amount of data, effortlessly and opportunistically. For instance, a researcher might have recognized that Participant #87 was lacking location data on April 23rd, 2016. Hence, the researcher might get in touch with the participant to provide respective support.

In addition, we asked participants their thoughts and/or decision to enable/disable the location sensor during the study, as presented on Table 7. We believe this information might further clarify misleading assumptions regarding participants' commitment.

Data description:

A. What do you think the lack of data is due? Be as descriptive as possible
B. Along the study: Did you considered to disable the application (m^k-sense) or GPS location service, so your data were not shared? [Yes, No]

Table 7 Sample of data quality's tags based on participants' perception

Participant	A	B	B (Justification)
51	Technical issues	Yes	Traveling issues
57	Traveling	Yes	Ran out of battery, traveling issues
59	Unclear directions, motivation	Yes	Ran out of battery
60	Availability	Yes	Ran out of battery, traveling issues
61	Traveling	No	Commitment
67	Technical issues	No	No reason provided
62	Technical issues	No	No reason provided
69	Availability	Yes	Ran out of battery
70	Unknown	No	Privacy reasons
82	Traveling	Yes	Traveling issues

Table 8 Adapted quality flag schema

Quality control (QC)	
Data treatment	Evaluation
No QC performed	No QC performed
No problem noted	QC performed; good data
Data is uncertain	QC performed; probably good data
Data were changed as a result of the QC	QC performed; acceptable data
Data were interpolated as a result of the QC	QC performed; probably bad dada
Data suspicious, check manually before use	QC performed; bad data

Table 9 Report of quality control based on the walkability dataset

Collected data	Pre-parse	Post-parse (final dataset)
Sensor-accelerometer	Data were changed as a result of the QC	QC performed; acceptable data
Sensor-location	No problem noted	QC performed; good data

5.7 Data Quality Control

To keep a record of how our dataset was prepared (pre-sharing) and their level of quality, once the study finished, we clustered and evaluated them based on a quality flag schema proposed in the literature [35]. As illustrated in Table 8, we identified two levels of interest: data treatment; in which we tag our data based on a pre-parse perspective, and evaluation; in which we score a post-parse dataset product of any potential data-treatment. To do so, we conducted an inspection in two phases: pre-parse; in which we defined a timestamp value due to inconsistencies found on a number of devices (as discussed in Sect. 2.1 Software architecture issues) and post-parse; as a final step to score out dataset, as showed on Table 9.

As noted, this report of quality control (Table 9) enabled certain strategies linked to data management issues raised in Sect. 3. The Walkability Study presented in this section illustrated how these issues were present at different levels.

6 Conclusions

Mobile sensing is becoming an important component in advancing research by disclosing ubiquitous data, for instance mobile devices are able to collect daily-life data, which could be used to conduct healthcare research in both naturalistic and controlled conditions. There are many challenges to be considered when conducting large study campaigns, such as the heterogeneity of the sensing technology, which implies that devices might use different sets of specifications or a data model to expand the sensing campaign through third parties. The importance lies in the potential enrichment of information that could result from different data analyzes like: longitudinal studies, comparison among different studies, or retrospective legacy-analysis that might have an impact in areas like epidemiology.

The problem with current efforts for standardizing datasets can be summarized in two main issues: on the one hand, current alternatives seem not to be interoperable with others, which restricts the opportunity to intersect datasets. On the other hand, their methodology suggests that data will be standardized from the time of adopting respective schemas; meaning that legacy data collected in the past could be ignored.

In this chapter, we illustrated how the aforementioned issues will be present in sensing campaigns, as many of these issues have not any foreseeable answer in the near future. However, researchers need to be aware of these, and design appropriate data management strategies. Although these issues were observed and discussed using a relatively small, and arguably controlled, sensing campaign, they can be easily exacerbated in large-scale distributed scenarios such as the ones mentioned earlier in this chapter. Clearly, some of the issues and types of studies discussed in this chapter require the aggregated effort of the research community, government, and the industry. Future work of the research community should aim at creating a unified schema of data types and associated metadata for datasets of this kind, if emergent areas such as mobile sensing are to have a profound impact on research and daily life.

References

1. Calatroni, A., Roggen, D., Tröster, G. (2011). Collection and curation of a large reference dataset for activity recognition. In Systems, Man, and Cybernetics (SMC), 2011 IEEE International Conference on (pp. 30–35). IEEE.
2. Lichen, M. (2013). UCI Machine Learning Repository [http://archive.ics.uci.edu/ml]. Irvine, CA: University of California, School of Information and Computer Science.

3. Alcalá, J., Fernández, A., Luengo, J., Derrac, J., García, S., Sánchez, L., and Herrera, F. (2010). Keel data-mining software tool: Data set repository, integration of algorithms and experimental analysis framework. Journal of Multiple-Valued Logic and Soft Computing, 17 (255–287).
4. Rücknagel, J., et al. Metadata Schema for the Description of Research Data Repositories: version 3.0, 29 p, DOI:http://doi.org/10.2312/re3.008.
5. White, Hollie C., et al. "The Dryad data repository: A Singapore framework metadata architecture in a DSpace environment." Universitätsverlag Göttingen (2008): 157.
6. Data Observation Network for Earth (DataONE). Data Citation and Attribution; https://www.dataone.org/citing-dataone (accessed Sep. 2016).
7. Boose, E, A Ellison, L Osterweil, L Clarke, R Podorozhny, J Hadley, A Wise, and D Foster (2007) Ensuring reliable datasets for environmental models and forecasts. Ecological Informatics, 2(3):237–247.
8. Voss, EA., Makadia, R., Matcho, A., Ma, Q., Knoll, C., Scheme, M., DeFalco, FJ., Lonche, A., Zhu, V., Ryan, PB. (2015). Feasibility and utility of applications of the common data model to multiple, disparate observational health databases. Journal of the American Medical Informatics Association. 22(3):553–64.
9. Estrin D, Sim I. Health care delivery. Open mHealth architecture: an engine for health care innovation. Science 2010 Nov 5;330(6005):759–760.
10. Kumar, S., Abowd, G. D., Abraham, W. T., al'Absi, M., Beck, J. G., Chau, D. H., Genevan, D. (2015). Center of excellence for mobile sensor Data-to-Knowledge (MD2K). Journal of the American Medical Informatics Association, 22(6), 1137–1142.
11. Netzahualcóyotl Hernández, and Jesús Favela. Estimating the Perception of Physical Fatigue Among Older Adults Using Mobile Phones. Human Behavior Understanding. Volume 9277 of the series Lecture Notes in Computer Science. 978-3-319-24194-4.
12. Darien Miranda, Jesus Favela, Catalina Ibarra, Netzahualcóyotl Cruz. Naturalistic Enactment to Elicit and Recognize Caregiver State Anxiety. Journal of Medical Systems, 2016.
13. Tactiohealth. Retrieved at November 14th 2016, from http://www.tactiohealth.com/
14. Garmin. Retrieved at November 14th 2016, from http://www.garmin.com/en-US
15. Fitbit. Retrieved at November 14th 2016, from https://www.fitbit.com/mx
16. Owletcare. Retrieved at November 14th 2016, from http://www.owletcare.com/
17. Zephyrhealth. Retrieved at November 14th 2016, from https://zephyrhealth.com/
18. Withings. Retrieved at November 14th 2016, from http://www.withings.com/us/en/
19. Neumitra. Retrieved at November 14th 2016, from https://www.neumitra.com/
20. Jins-meme. Retrieved at November 14th 2016, from https://jins-meme.com/en/
21. Proteus. Retrieved at November 14th 2016, from http://www.proteus.com/
22. Ihealthlabs. Retrieved at November 14th 2016, from https://ihealthlabs.com/
23. ResearchKit framework. Retrieved 22/09/2016, from http://researchkit.org/
24. Aharon, N., Gardner, A., Sumter, C., Peatland, A.: Funf: Open Sensing Framework. http://funf.media.mit.edu (2011).
25. Hernández, N., Arnrich, B., Favela, J., Yavuz, GR., Demiray, B., Fontecha, J., Ersoy, C. mk-sense: An extensible platform to conduct multi-institutional mobile sensing campaigns. Ubiquitous Computing & Ambient Intelligence. Health, AAL, HCI, IoT, Smart Cities, Sensors & Security. UCAmI 2016 (Accepted for publication).
26. Gersch, M., Lindert, R., Hewing, M.: AAL-business models: Different Prospects for the Successful Implementation of Innovative Services in the Primary and Secondary Healthcare Market. In: AALIANCE Conference, Malaga, Spain (2010).
27. Walkonomics. Retrieved at November 14th 2016, from http://walkonomics.com
28. Walkscore. Retrieved at November 14th 2016, from http://walkscore.com
29. Daniele Quercia, Luca Maria Aiello, Rossano Schifanella, and Adam Davies. 2015. The Digital Life of Walkable Streets. In Proceedings of the 24th International Conference on World Wide Web (WWW '15). International World Wide Web Conferences Steering Committee, Republic and Canton of Geneva, Switzerland, 875–884.

30. The Library. Data Management. Retrieved 22/09/2016, from http://libraries.ucsd.edu/services/data-curation/data-management
31. Van den Lynden, V., Corti, L., Willard, M. & Bishop, L. (2009). Managing and Sharing Data: A Best Practice Guide for Researchers. Retrieved 22/09/2016, from http://www.data-archive.ac.uk/media/2894/managingsharing.pdf
32. DCC Curation Lifecycle Model. Retrieved 22/08/2016, from http://www.dcc.ac.uk/resources/curation-lifecycle-model
33. Radebaugh, J. Understanding Metadata. National Information Standards Organization, 2004. 20 pp. ISBN: 978-1-880124-62-8.
34. Sweeney L, Crosas M, Bar-Sinai M. Sharing Sensitive Data with Confidence: The Datatags System. Technology Science. 2015101601. October 16, 2015. http://techscience.org/a/2015101601
35. Reiner Schlitzer. Oceanographic quality flag schemes and mappings between them. Alfred Wegener Institute for Polar and Marine Research. Retrieved 22/09/2016, from http://odv.awi.de/fileadmin/user_upload/odv/misc/ODV4_QualityFlagSets.pdf

Part III
Internet-of-Things, Fog Computing, and m-Health

Internet of Things Based E-health Systems: Ideas, Expectations and Concerns

Mirjana Maksimović and Vladimir Vujović

Abstract Even the interaction between technology and healthcare has a long history, the embracing of e-health is slow because of limited infrastructural arrangements, capacity and political willingness. Internet of Things (IoT) is expected to usher in the biggest and fastest spread of technology in history, therefore together with e-health will completely modify person-to-person, human-to-machine and machine-to-machine (M2M) communications for the benefit of society in general. It is anticipated that the IoT-based e-health solutions will revolutionize the healthcare industry like nothing else before it. The rapid growth of IoT, Cloud computing and Big data, as well as the proliferation and widespread adoption of new technologies and miniature sensing device, have brought forth new opportunities to change the way patients and their healthcare providers manage health conditions, thus improving human health and well-being. The integration of IoT into the healthcare system brings numerous advantages, such as the availability and accessibility, the ability to provide a more "personalized" system, and high-quality cost-effective healthcare delivery. Still, the success of the IoT-based e-health systems will depend on barriers needed to overcome in order to achieve large-scale adoption of e-health applications. A large number of significant technological improvements in both hardware and software components are required to develop consistent, safe, effective, timely, flexible, patient-centered, power-efficient and ubiquitous healthcare systems. However, trust, privacy and security concerns, as well as regulation issues, identification, and semantic interoperability are pivotal in the widespread adoption of IoT and e-health together. Therefore, developing a climate of trust is one of the most important tasks that must be accomplished for successful e-health implementations. This chapter analyzes the ideas and impacts of

M. Maksimović (✉) · V. Vujović
Faculty of Electrical Engineering, University of East Sarajevo,
Vuka Karadzica 30, 71123 East Sarajevo, Bosnia and Herzegovina
e-mail: mirjana@etf.unssa.rs.ba

V. Vujović
e-mail: vladimir_vujovich@yahoo.com

© Springer International Publishing AG 2017

S.U. Khan et al. (eds.), *Handbook of Large-Scale Distributed Computing in Smart Healthcare*, Scalable Computing and Communications,
DOI 10.1007/978-3-319-58280-1_10

IoT on the design of new e-health solutions and identifies the majority of challenges that determine successful IoT-based e-health system adoption.

Keywords Internet of Things · E-health · Expectations · Concerns

1 Introduction

Healthcare, as an essential human right, is in the interest of every human being and can be considered as fundamental for a functioning society. The research of healthcare systems' role and the importance in the quality of life and social welfare in modern society nowadays is broadly performed in order to help produce better decisions on policy design and implementation of healthcare systems at global, national and sub-national scales [6, 116]. Longer and healthier human's life makes the population more productive what implies the important contribution of health to economic well-being.

Healthcare systems and services in a new era in medicine and technology are essential for accomplishing the healthcare needs of individuals and populations. Thus, effective public health systems are designed to take care of the health of target populations which constant growth requires new, more advanced and efficient healthcare solutions [91]. To develop and evaluate innovative approaches for improving the quality of healthcare, innovations in the organization, funding, roles of health professionals as well as the use of technology, are equally important. With the present Information and Communication Technology (ICT) development, healthcare, as well as every aspect of human life today, has been revolutionized. In other words, the impact of technology in healthcare is immense—the rapid advancements in the ICT have changed healthcare systems locally and globally. Hence, a fundamental change over the last decades in both ICT and the medical sector, has switched the traditional view of health, where healthcare delivery has been designed around the provider (located in hospitals or clinics), to a new and multifaceted scenario, where the care goes to the patient, instead of the patient going to the care [38, 75]. The application of ICT to human health is one of the leading research goals for the 7th and 8th Framework Programs of European Union (EU). Beyond the technological factors, it is important to highlight that socioeconomic and political factors have also a significant influence on the evolution of digital healthcare (Fig. 1).

As can be seen in Fig. 1 healthcare is outstandingly affected by technological advancements [61]. Technological breakthroughs change healthcare in all its areas, creating a new vision of healthcare known as e-health. E-health with the help of ICTs creates novel opportunities for information distribution, interaction and joining forces of all participants in healthcare sector (the public, institutions, health professionals and healthcare providers). E-health, despite its social, political, ethical, technological and economic constraints, became a major part of a modern 21st Century society [38]. Development of new technologies, particularly the Internet

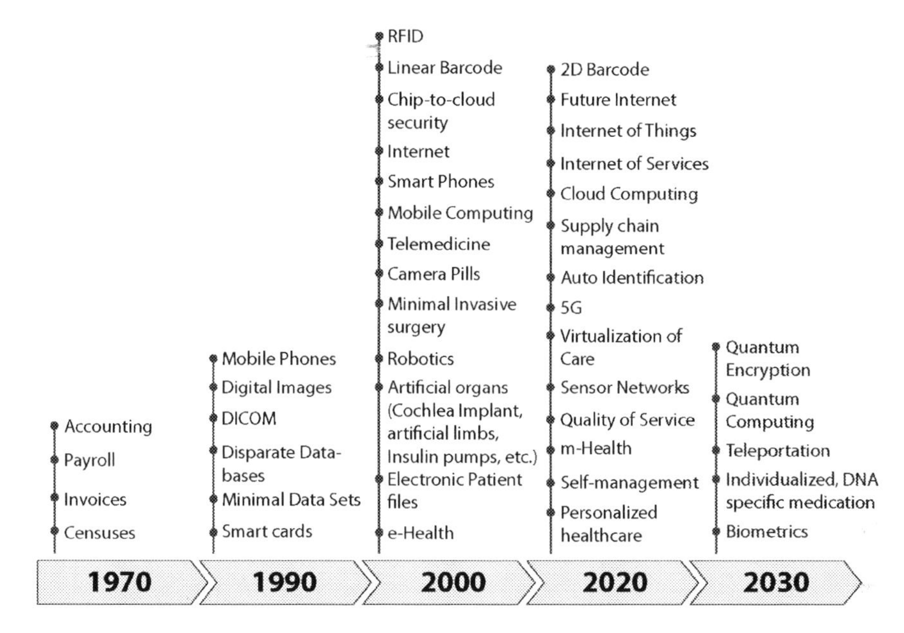

Fig. 1 Digital health evolution [36]

and Wireless Sensor Networks (WSNs) that together make the new unique concept called "Internet of Things" (IoT), has created a new horizon in the healthcare sector. As an emerging paradigm and a cutting edge technology, IoT connects the world via smart objects [56] and holds enormous potential for transforming the healthcare delivery system in the modern healthcare systems of 21st Century. Communications in IoT vision relates to communications among devices and objects, as well as among diverse devices (machine-to-machine (M2M) communications), supporting people daily patterns within a smart environment. These principles provide abilities to human to interact with various types of smart (intelligent) devices, converge and make applications, and commonly participate without outstanding interworking technologies [62]. It is considered that the IoT has greatest potential in the healthcare sector. This can be seen in many current healthcare solutions, which are already applied to enhance the availability and quality of care, and above all to avoid unnecessary healthcare costs and efforts. Using smart IoT devices, remote health monitoring and notification can be done easily, accurately and in a timely manner, what is essential in emergency cases [60, 103]. In theory, emergency admissions could be reduced with the help of proactive IoT-driven e-health systems which should be able to address the problems before they become more serious or irreversible. Relying on these facts, new concepts and technologies like network architectures, services, applications, interoperability, and security and privacy issues represent leading research trends in the IoT-based healthcare. In addition, there is a need for continuous work on legislation, policies, and guidelines in order to successfully implement the IoT principles in the medical field [59].

From an economic point of view, healthcare, as the global largest and fastest growing industry, is one of the areas that are expected to progress notably over years to come. McKinsey Global Institute [80] reveal prognosis and economic feasibility of the IoT-based healthcare. Figure 2 shows that by 2025 the highest percentage of the IoT incomes will go to the healthcare sector and hopefully will lead to fully customized, available, and on-time healthcare services for everyone.

Evidently, technology is increasingly playing a role in almost all healthcare processes, creating e-health services which provide better healthcare accompanied with improved availability, efficiency, responsibility and satisfaction of consumers. However, with the e-health industry growth more questions and challenges are faced in healthcare research. In other words, despite the potential of IoT-based e-health systems and services to improve the quality of healthcare, its wider uptake is hampered by a number of factors, such as the lack of access to capital by healthcare providers, resistance to change on the part of healthcare professionals and patients as well, standardization issues connected with security, privacy and confidentiality concerns, legal barriers and lack of technical skills.

To get as much as possible insights into the IoT role in progressive healthcare, this chapter examines the ideas and current impacts of IoT on the design of new e-health solutions and future directions for incorporating IoT into the clinical practice of medicine. It begins with a recapitulation of the literature, which includes the currently available systems on the market, as well as technological approaches for their implementation. A detailed analysis of the e-health system benefits, together with the objectives which must be fulfilled for their progress and significant improvement, are presented too. Relying on these objectives and modern technologies, a comprehensive analysis of applying the IoT in healthcare has been given. The study also includes the technological and methodological approach for the implementation of IoT-based healthcare systems. Alongside this, the IoT-based e-health system architecture was presented coupled with analysis of numerous recent studies that include the latest trends and challenges for integrating the modern technology in the IoT healthcare system. As a part of the performed research, benefits and expectations are especially highlighted, and challenges, risks and concerns which deal with various factors that have a direct or indirect impact on

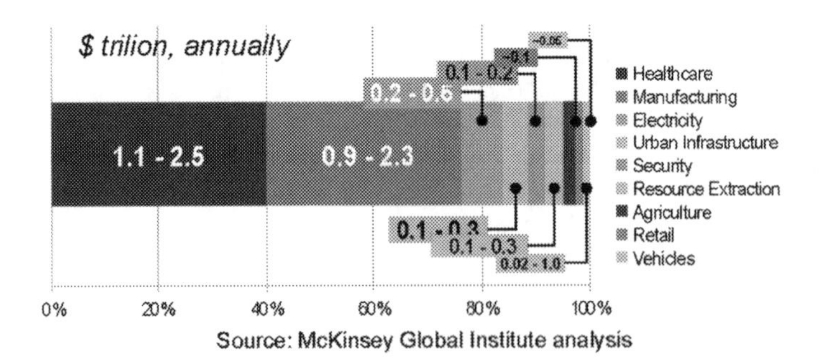

Fig. 2 The IoT leading applications and their economic impact in 2025 [55]

the implementation of IoT in healthcare are discussed as well. The chapter is concluded with summary representation of facts and includes SWOT analysis to evaluate the Strengths, Weaknesses, Opportunities, and Threats of presented concepts which determine successful IoT-based e-health system adoption.

2 E-health

E-health, as one of the results of the Internet expansion and appearance of e-terms during the 1990s, becomes an indispensable term which represents a mean of improving health services access, efficiency and quality by applying ICTs to health. Nowadays, e-health as a way of achieving healthcare reform represents one of the main research goals by many academic institutions, professional bodies and funding organizations. There are various currently used forms of e-health:

- Electronic Health Record (EHR)—an electronic version of a comprehensive report of the patient's overall health that make all information available immediately and in a secure way to authorized users [20],
- Electronic Medical Record (EMR)—a digital report that encompasses all of patient's medical history from one practice [50],
- Personal Health Record (PHR)—a health report where the patient keeps his health-related data in a private, secure, and confidential environment [70],
- Virtual healthcare teams and decision support teams—teams of healthcare professionals who cooperate, exchange information on patients through digital equipment with aim to improve their knowledge and make better decisions [40, 128],
- e-prescribing—a technology framework that allows writing and sending prescription electronically and directly from the healthcare institution to the pharmacy [20],
- e-appointments—an online service that makes scheduling an appointment for any health institution fast and easy, while reducing waiting time [135],
- m-health (mobile health)—a universal term that encompasses health practices enabled by mobile devices and other wireless technology [70, 74],
- Telemedicine—the ICT based remote delivery of healthcare information and services [51, 78, 131, 132],
- Telehealth—the distribution of health-related services and information via ICTs [25],
- Internet-based technologies and services, and more.

These are some of the many digital health technologies that serve to make easier the health-related data aggregation, storage, transfer, retrieval and processing; improve interaction between patients and healthcare providers; monitor various (biological and physiological) parameters, and ensure distant healthcare services [36].

Some of well-known intelligent pervasive healthcare systems, among others, are [86, 94, 125]: *@Home system* (enables remote monitoring of patient's vital parameters); *HEARTFAID* (enables on-time diagnosis and more effective insights in heart diseases within old people); *ALARM-NET* (an Assisted-Living and Residential Monitoring Network for ubiquitous, adaptive healthcare); *CAALYX* (Complete Ambient Assisted Living Experiment based on the usage of wearable lightweight devices that measure vital signs of a patient and automatically alert care provider in an emergency case); *TeleCARE* (enables the development of a configurable common infrastructure useful for the elderly people and the healthcare providers); *CHRONIC* (an integrated IT (Information Technology) environment for the care of chronic patients); *MyHeart* (with the help of smart electronic and textile systems and adequate services offers the means for dealing with cardiovascular diseases); *OLDES* (enables a wider range of services to old people using an innovative low-cost technology); *SAPHIRE* (implements the patient monitoring by using agent technology and intelligent decision support systems); *MobiHEALTH* (facilitates the online, continuous monitoring of vital signs, via GPRS (General Packet Radio Service) and UMTS (Universal Mobile Telecommunications System) technologies); *SAPHE* (allows intelligent, unobtrusive continuous healthcare monitoring via telecare networks with small wireless body sensors and sensors integrated in homes); *DITIS* (an e-health mobile application which supports networked collaboration for home healthcare); *AXARM* (an extensible remote assistance and monitoring tool for neurodegenerative disease telerehabilitation); *VirtualECare* (an intelligent multi-agent system for health monitoring and interacting with elderly people). The list of pervasive healthcare systems grows constantly along with the rapid advancements in ICTs and their widespread adoption can benefit patients, healthcare providers, managers and policy makers as well (Fig. 3) [2].

From a patient's point of view, e-health makes easier access to quality healthcare services through associated networked-monitoring equipment, particularly to

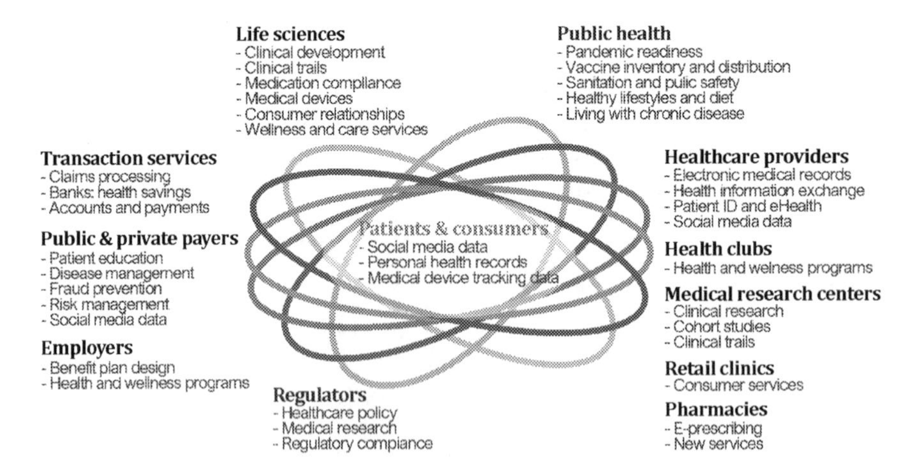

Fig. 3 The role and importance of participants in healthcare sector [2]

people in remote, rural and isolated communities. The old and less "physically" mobile patients, especially benefit from these health services over distance because they require fewer visits to the healthcare professional and institutions and thus they are more capable of living on their own. In the case of a potentially dangerous situation or detected anomalies (when dataset goes beyond the normal range, approaching to potential emergency), the system can generate an alarm [21]. Thus, e-health gives health professionals faster, secure access to all the data they need to care for the patient (Fig. 4). Recent surveys on patients' behavior to digital health (according to Frost & Sullivan) show that about 16% of them use wearable sensors, 24% use mobile applications to track their health and wellness, and 29% use electronic PHR. It is anticipated that this tendency will continue as 47% of patients would consider using wearable devices in the closest future [26]. The benefits of these self-monitoring devices are the removal of the need to run expensive and long tests as well as the realized connection with healthcare expert systems. These systems are essential in providing accurate information for diagnosis, decision-making, reducing medical errors and enabling prompt healthcare [91].

Since relevant health data are available to healthcare providers when required, e-health is seen as an opportunity to make healthcare more efficient by facilitating communication and enhancing patient care offering new services and types of treatments, alongside reduced delays, errors and administrative costs [47]. Multidisciplinary teams of health professionals, through e-health, have faster and secure access to all the information required to treat the patients in an adequate and timely manner. They can exchange health information and arrange health interventions in an effective way, thereby avoiding tasks duplications and cutting costs. Possible errors and complications, especially medication errors and adverse drug reactions, can be deflected through the role of e-prescribing systems. If an order is made for medications to which a patient is known to be allergic or there are potential contra-indications and drug interactions, this system flags alerts. Consequently, the less time is spent to clarifying and rewriting illegible prescriptions, and thus can be better used. However, Li et al. [71] identify and synthesize factors which influence healthcare providers' acceptance of e-health vision: healthcare provider characteristics (experience and knowledge in IT sector, gender, age, race, professional role and experience); medical practice characteristics (practice size and level, single or multi-specialty, location, teaching status, patient age range); voluntariness of use;

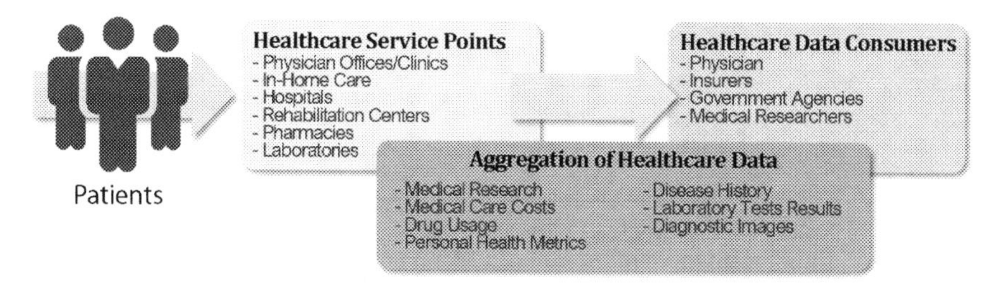

Fig. 4 The massive aggregation of healthcare data in the healthcare ecosystem

performance expectancy (the usefulness and needs, relative advantage, job-fit, payment and financial stimulus); effort expectancy (simplicity of usage and complexity); social influence (the subjective norm, competition, supportive organizational culture for change, and friendship network) and facilitating or inhibiting conditions (legal concerns, patient privacy issues, financial limitations, IT support). Having in mind that healthcare providers are the key enablers of e-health initiatives, their acceptance of e-health systems and applications is essential to reform and revolutionize healthcare.

Easy access, dissemination, use and exchange of accurate and reliable information, enable policy makers to made correct healthcare investment decisions (Fig. 4). In this way, health service interventions are conducted to where they are instantly required. Managers, through access to national health data summaries, can better supervise and evaluate health intervention programs.

Therefore, e-health has many benefits to offer. Organizations and governments worldwide are choosing to implement e-health in order to enhance quality of care as well as the patient experience. The major benefits can be summarized in [65]:

- Technology usage effectively saves time (increased timeliness of treatment and decreased transfer rates) and eases financial pressures.
- Quality of care is enhanced through more informed decision making processes. Diagnoses are on-time and more accurate.
- Online healthcare services are provided for members, employers, providers and brokers. Wireless devices' usage enables real-time treatment, while telemedicine and remote in-home monitoring support senior wellness and preventative care, as well as expert diagnosis and treatment to rural residents. Remote consultations, whether urgent or diagnostic saves lives.
- Delivery of care is more efficient, cost-effective and convenient. Customer experience is more satisfied while staff and doctor satisfaction is also improved.
- ICTs usage can enable health processes to cover more cases without raising staff numbers or related costs. Thus, costs are reduced and administrative efficiency and coordination are improved.
- Revenue cycle management is speeded through electronic payment technology.
- Enhanced access to a patient's health information decreases the incidence of medical errors.

As can be noticed, e-health is rapidly growing and changing and owns the enormous potential to improve the quality and efficiency of healthcare. However, its widespread use is obstructed by a number of barriers, ranging from technical to financing to political issues (Fig. 5) [30].

As technology is rapidly changing, new e-health solutions are constantly progressing to satisfy the needs of current practice. Appropriate technology infrastructure, systems integration, standardization as well as social, ethical, and economic questions, represent the main challenges for ubiquitous e-health adoption and achieving higher quality and more productive healthcare. To achieve healthcare

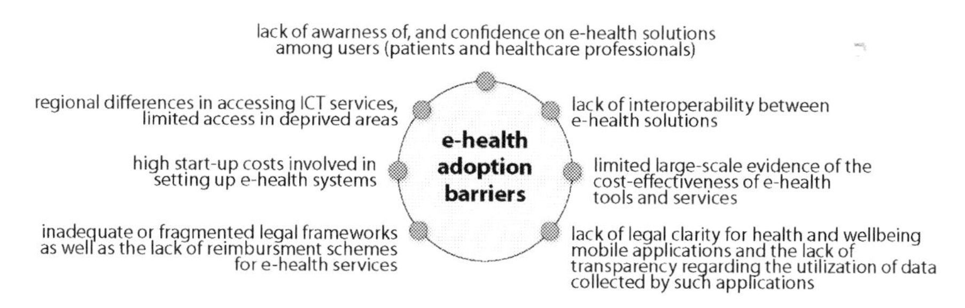

Fig. 5 The major barriers to wider uptake of e-health

improvements, it is recognized that every healthcare system should accomplish next six goals [57], Steinwachs and Hughes (2008):

- *Patient safety*—includes the prevention of errors and adverse effects to patients associated with healthcare. To accomplish this goal, it is necessary to perform certain actions such as correct identification of the patient, enhancing communication, enabling adequate care and reducing the risk of undesired outcomes.
- *Effective care*—is based on scientific evidence (laboratory experiments, clinical research, epidemiological studies…) that treatment will lead to desired health outcomes.
- *Timeliness*—considers that healthcare organization should be organized to provide care to patients in a timely manner. Although occasionally harmless, a misdiagnoses or failure to timely diagnose a medical condition, illness, or injury could lead to worsening of the condition and outcomes to worsen.
- *Efficiency*—is based on identifying and eliminating waste of resources (equipment, energy, supplies and ideas).
- *Patient-centered* healthcare—involves the creation of individualized healthcare services according to the patient's needs, values, and preferences.
- *Equity*—means providing the same quality of care regardless of personal characteristics such as gender, race, education, geographic location, and socioeconomic status.

These six goals represent a guideline for creating a contemporary, Internet-based healthcare system, and in the rest of this chapter a discussion will show their significance.

3 The IoT Based E-health Systems and Services

In the past, sensing in the healthcare was applicable mainly in healthcare institutions, and rarely outside of hospitals. Additionally, sensing unit at an early stage, were simple devices for measuring parameters of interest and creating some form of the output signal (mechanical, electrical, or optical). Nowadays, a development of

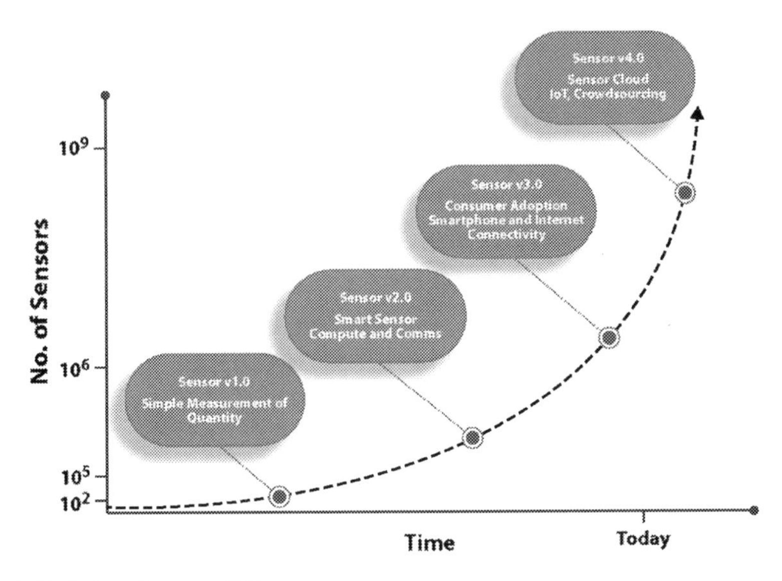

Fig. 6 Evolution of sensors [79]

computing and pervasive communications, connectivity to the Internet and Cloud integration as well as use of mobile smart devices, have added outstandingly to the capabilities of sensor devices, their number and scope (Fig. 6) [79].

Society is currently witnessing ICT influences on the evolution of sensors and their applications which can be almost everywhere: from health and fitness, aging demographics, personalized healthcare, public health, national security, IoT, water and food traceability and production. Consequently, using new concepts and approaches like IoT, Big data and Cloud computing, novel healthcare solutions have a huge potential to easily meet all of six improvements goals.

IoT-powered healthcare systems of 21st Century rely on the fundamental definition of the IoT as a network of intelligent, interconnected devices (which are usually equipped with microcontrollers or microprocessors, memory, wireless transceiver, sensing unit and autonomous power supply) based on existing and evolving interoperable ICTs [56]. To realize the integration of IoT principles in e-health, a variety of sensors (wearables and ingestible devices) gather patient's health-related data; microcontrollers process and wirelessly transmit those data; microprocessors provide user interfaces and displays while healthcare-specific gateways and the Cloud are used to analyze and store the data. The analyzed data are then transmitted wirelessly to medical professionals for further medical analysis, the remote control of certain medical treatments or parameters or real-time feedback [69, 89, 121].

To continuously monitor several vital signs of patients and transmit the data to the server, different health sensors either embedded in some device, like a smartphone, or wearable by users, are utilized. Ideally, the chosen sensors should be invisible, unobtrusive and non-invasive, able to protect user privacy and data confidentiality, to consume low-power and demand minimal computational resources, to be cheap and easy to install and have low-maintenance overhead [130]. For example, various sensors like temperature sensors, voice-sensors (microphone), video sensors, image sensors, IR (infrared) sensors, optical sensors, ultrasonic sensors, piezoelectric sensors, accelerometer, and more, can be used to address the same or different problems (fall detection, child care, disabled care, etc.) [120]. Connecting diverse medical devices (e.g., thermometers, glucometers, smart heart rate monitors, fitness tracking device, blood pressure cuffs, asthma inhalers, etc.) creates a new paradigm commonly referred the "Internet of Medical Things" (IoMT) [108]. To allow synchronization of the real world with its virtual representation and therefore enable enhanced process and decision-making support, these smart objects used for medical purposes should be unique in its context or system (to have an identity), have abilities to gather the information and to interact with environment (sensors and actuators), determine the current position, communicate with other objects, store data (memory) and act autonomously to accomplish a predefined goal [127]. Relying on these principles, according to report by the Atlantic Council [44] a four categories of medical devices led by IoT concepts are identified: consumer-based (e.g., fitness tracking devices), wearable, external devices (e.g., insulin pumps), internally embedded devices (e.g., pacemakers, within the body sensors) and stationary devices (e.g., home-monitoring devices, IV (intravenous) pumps and fetal monitors). These four categories of medical devices may be considered as the foundation of any modern healthcare system nowadays.

With the rapid technological advancements, the new generation of "medical" or "clinical wearables" has more advanced performances in the sense of sensing, capturing and analyzing, making them more clinical useful [76]. Using a new type of networks, various communication technologies like GSM (General System for Mobile communication), RFID (Radio Frequency Identification), GPS (Global Positioning System), Bluetooth, Wi-Fi, ZigBee and NFC (Near Field Communication) for interconnecting wearable health sensors, and transferring sensor data to the central server [100, 120] enables making the human body as a part of the IoT, bringing in such way integration to a completely new level. Following these principles, in the next few years it is expected that the 5G network, with its superfast connectivity, intelligent management, and data capabilities, will provide new possibilities in healthcare, including diagnostics, data analytics, and treatment [126]. More specifically, the IETF (Internet Engineering Task Force) has standardized 6LoWPAN (IPv6 over Low-Power Wireless Personal Area Networks), ROLL (Routing over Low power and Lossy-networks), and CoAP (Constrained Application Protocol) to equip constrained devices used in IoT vision [72].

How to deal and process a large amount of gathered data is one of the biggest challenges in present healthcare systems. The large quantity of data is usually stored in the Cloud where they are reachable worldwide, by a virtually unlimited number of participants, even simultaneously. Private information of a patient, are usually accessible to himself and to the healthcare givers but they are also anonymously available to anyone, so that can be effectively aggregated for research or statistical worldwide analysis [38]. A variety of techniques, such as artificial intelligence, machine learning, intelligent data mining, computer vision, Big data and analytics and more, are used to discover hidden patterns, anomaly detection, perform predictive modeling and to make actionable decisions. In this way, using smart devices equipped with evidence-based algorithms increase the possibility to significantly reduce the number of medical errors. Alongside this, information regarding health should be always accessible to both healthcare provider and patient in the most understandable formats for each [42]. In order to understand the life cycle of the device, researchers propose the usage of six C's: Connection (the path showing how device is connected to the ecosystem); Collection (how data are collected from the sensing element); Correlation (mapping the data to a context and perform correlation to produce relevant and concise data); Calculation (making a decision based on filtered and processed data); Conclusion (taking appropriate actions); and Collaboration (the patient and the healthcare teams' work together). Relying on six C's definition, the architecture for e-health must support diverse devices, applications, and backend systems to enable the free information flow (satisfying the needs of six C's life cycle) in order to make on-time and right decisions [69]. Therefore, gateways, medical servers, and health databases, are crucial in making medical records and bringing health services to authorized stakeholders whenever required [59].

The elements defined above for gathering, storing, transmitting and analyzing data are essential regardless of different technologies and architectures of IoT healthcare solutions that can be found in a review of literature [4, 21, 46, 82, 84, 86, 90, 93, 97, 104, 110, 134]. In addition to technology, that creates the capacity to provide health services, the structure of healthcare also includes the facilities (e.g., hospitals and clinics) and personnel (e.g., physicians and nurses) [109]. Enabling simple and cost-effective collaboration of patients, hospitals and healthcare organizations, via smooth and secure connectivity, is a significant trend [59].

The representative cases of IoT/IoMT include remote monitoring of people health (chronic or long-term conditions); tracking patient medication orders and the location of patients admitted to hospitals; and patients' wearable mobile health devices, which can send data of interest to healthcare providers. In other words, nowadays the Internet and smart mobile devices provide a quite simple interactive environment for all, fulfilling the principles of IoT-based e-health: to enable anyone to access e-health services anytime, anyplace and on any device (Fig. 7). Mobile medical devices (e.g., wearable sensors, bands, watches) and smart applications facilitate continuous self-monitoring of various vital parameters while Cloud-based architectures enable storing and sharing large amounts of data in an effective and easy manner [19]. Therefore, the presented architecture consists of three basic layers:

- Sensing/perception layer: the most basic layer which key component is sensing device for capturing and presenting the physical in the digital world. The essential data sensing/gathering from sensing devices and some controlling actions and communications are the main functions of this layer.

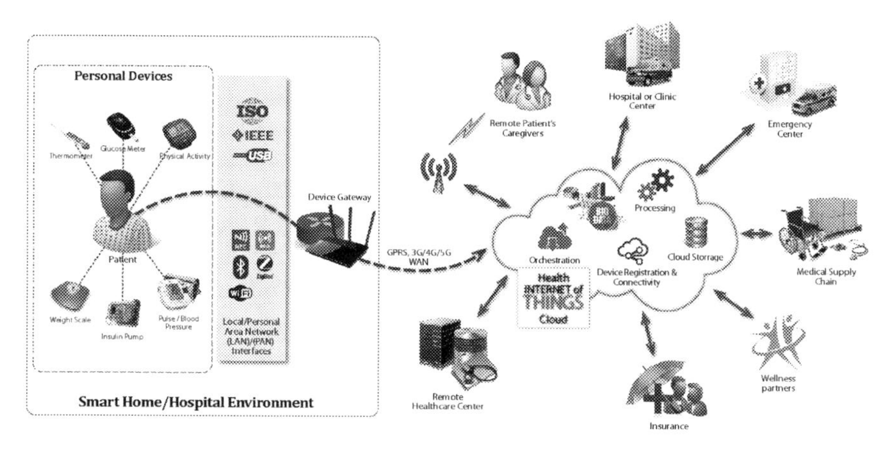

Fig. 7 The IoT-based e-health system architecture

- Network layer: the middle layer which includes all kinds of access networks, protocols, communication devices and routing modules.
- Application layer: includes operating modules for analyzing sensed data, computation, and actions.

Bearing in mind the importance of new healthcare solutions, a variety of recent studies accentuate tendency and challenges for ubiquitous health technologies in the IoT. Over the last years, academic researchers have paid increasing attention to this field, proposing numerous more or less similar solutions, based on the basic three layers IoT architecture, highlighting: the usage of smart, intelligent, wireless sensor devices to perceive utilization of the appliances necessary for daily living and in this way determine the lifestyle of old people living alone [41, 83, 112]; an IoT low-cost technology solution for observing human vital parameter [76, 97, 111, 114]; a simple and secure IoT for creating a general and pervasive Ambient Assisted Living framework to be used by m-health applications [37, 41, 74, 103]; IoT-based e-health solutions, creating a M2M system based on a Cloud computing [102, 110, 123], and more. In addition, one of the most important trends in 2015 became the development of Do It Yourself (DIY) healthcare platforms [24]. With the help of inexpensive hardware and open-source software, a DIY system which satisfies the user's specific needs can be easily created. The created solution can be used to monitor human vital parameters as well as some of the environmental parameters affecting health. Providing techniques and the customizable solutions to the consumers is valuable for both end-users and product developers [76]. Some of the IoT e-health solutions currently present on the market are [105, 115]: *Empatica Embrace* (a sleek watch that collects data regarding to epilepsy, autism and other chronic disorders, makes it available to caregivers and creates alerts in case of emergency); *Lumo Lift* (a discreet lightweight wearable that tracks patient's posture and activity); *Philips Respironics* breathing masks and *SleepMapper* application (an interactive self-management system that tracks user's sleeping patterns); *Chrono*

SmartStop (a wearable lightweight transdermal device that relies on nicotine replacement therapy); *Real Time Healthcare* (a platform that helps the patient follow their medication routines, informs healthcare professionals about important information, including location details if the patient becomes confused and lost); *Scanadu Scout* (an electronic device which enables quickly check of patient's vital signs by placing the device on patient's temple); *iOTOS* (a wireless device which have possibility to be integrated in all kinds of devices used from diagnostics to home monitoring). At the hospital side, it is important to highlight [105]: smart IV pumps (intelligent infusion devices which can preset doses and have ability to communicate with electronic medication administration records); robotic-assisted surgery; wireless capsule endoscopy (as an alternative to the tube-based endoscope where the patient swallows camera in a pill and it moves through the gastrointestinal track taking pictures); tracking medications administered to patients and assets via RFID. Based on currently available IoT-powered healthcare solutions, Islam et al. [59] categorize services (used to develop applications) and applications of IoT in healthcare sector (Fig. 8), where applications are further classified into two groups: single- (a specific disease or infirmity) and clustered-condition applications (a number of diseases or conditions together as a whole).

Despite the way IoT-based e-health systems are realized, they all should provide the effective and efficient healthcare for anyone, anytime and anywhere. Therefore, regarding data, the IoT-driven e-health solution must:

- Collect patient health data from a various types of sensors remotely and in a secure and safe way,
- Apply complex algorithms from a broad scope of pattern recognition and machine learning techniques, to analyze the gathered data, and
- Exchange the data through wireless networks (satisfying privacy and security demands) with who can make real-time feedback.

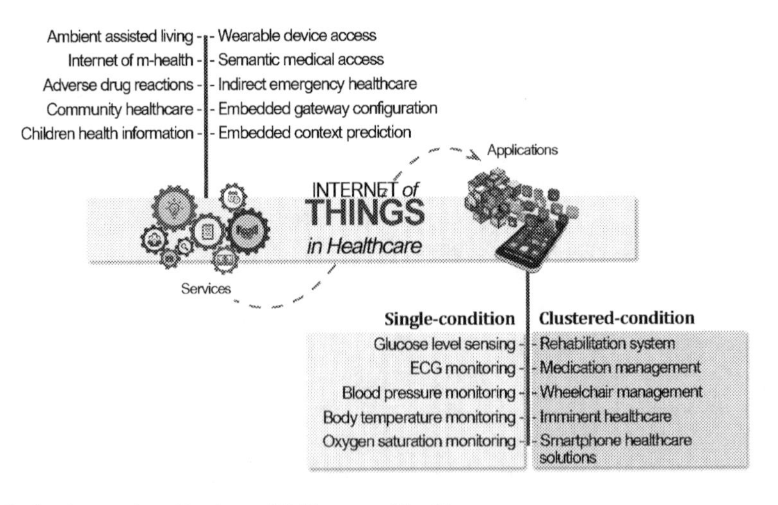

Fig. 8 Services and applications of IoT-powered healthcare

As ICT is used to support the core processes of healthcare, in the first step a prodigious amount of data has been produced. Due to datasets volume, variability, and velocity, there is a need to filter out relevant, differentiating information from the voluminous datasets. This implies a quick growth of Big data analytics, which gives an opportunity to healthcare organizations to improve care and profitability. With the limitless potential to effectively store, process and analyze medical data, the Big data in healthcare are being applied in many prevention and personalization purposes. In other words, successfully dealing with a huge volume of data can improve profits, and effectively reduce the cost of healthcare. Furthermore, the rapid development of IoT healthcare is accompanied with the increased risk of security and privacy. Therefore, security and privacy are crucial design goals that should be taken into consideration. To receive as much as possible benefits of the IoT-based e-health system, devices must connect to networks and the Cloud in ways that are interoperable and secure. It implies that generated, assembled, and shared data must be protected with appropriate authentication methods. The additional important factor is the data access control, which prevents unauthorized accesses to the patient's data. Healthcare providers and patients will be able to experience the advantages of digital modernization for wellness and healthcare only satisfying essential demands for IoT-driven healthcare system development and Quality of Services (QoS) requirements. In order to measure QoS of IoT-based e-health system, various QoS parameters and QoS metrics must be considered. They can be classified according to three layers' structure of IoT [13]:

- Sensing/perception layer: reliability, throughput, real-time, sampling parameters, time synchronization, location/mobility, sensing and actuation coverage.
- Network layer: lifetime of sensing networks, utilization of network resources, bandwidth, delay, packet loss rate, jitter, services perform cost, perform time, load, reliability, fault tolerance.
- Application layer: service issues (time, delay, priority, availability, accuracy, load), information accuracy, costs (network deployment, service usage).

As tracking, identification, authentication, data collection and sensing are essential characteristics of IoT-driven e-health, among various QoS metrics, several of them can be considered as of special interest in IoT healthcare applications: reliability, throughput, delay, energy consumption, system lifetime, network coverage, packet loss rate, scalability. However, QoS support provided in IoT-based e-health systems varies and targets different QoS levels for specific uses (e.g., emergency case, intensive care).

In summary, using smart IoT devices, comprehensive physiological information is collected and shared directly with each other and the Cloud, enabling to gather, store and analyze a mixture of health status indicators faster and more accurately [89]. Therefore, the idea of IoT-based e-health solutions is to accomplish all six goals for health improvements and QoS requirements, by enhancing life quality, providing medical support and life-saving care, decreasing barriers for monitoring important patient health data, reducing the cost of care and providing the on-time and right prevention and treatment.

3.1 Benefits and Expectations

New approaches to the procedures, equipment, and processes by which medical care is delivered have led to impressive achievements in health worldwide during the past few decades. With the power of ICT, healthcare becomes more efficient as well as cheaper and more reliable. In e-health, the IoT's connectivity provides means to monitor, record and transmit health data on a 24/7 basis from a patient home to the healthcare providers (using sensors in mobile devices, within bodies sensors or sensors attached to clothing) and enable the IoT-related data and services to be pervasive and personalized [97].

The IoT-powered e-health systems, using small, lightweight wireless approaches connected through the IoT, have potential to enable remote monitoring and secure capturing of a great wealth of patient health data and fitness information. In other words, medical devices such as wearables and home health monitoring devices (e.g., wirelessly connected thermometers, glucometers, heart rate or blood pressure monitors) can be connected to the IoT technology enabling remote, timely and comfortable monitoring of patient's vital signs from a hospital environment. The device which uses the IoT scheme is unique to the world and identifiable at anytime and anywhere through the Internet. The IoT-powered health devices in distance health monitoring systems, alongside the traditional sensing tasks, can also share health-related data with each other, as well as with hospitals or clinics through the Internet, outstandingly facilitating setup and administration work [49]. The collected health information, stored in a central data server, can be intelligently analyzed to identify patterns and trends and represents a basis for the statistical and epidemiological researches (e.g., disease and epidemic outbreak prediction, tracking and controlling in an efficient manner) [97]. Using gathered information and applying complex algorithms and evidence-based models in order to perform certain actions, significantly improve health by enhancing the access to healthcare and quality of care alongside drastically costs cutting (Fig. 9).

The most promising IoT-based e-health use cases are preventive health actions, proactive monitoring, follow-up care and management of chronic care diseases. The benefits of IoT-driven e-health as a technique to improve the quality of healthcare are recognized worldwide. Opposed to traditional paper-based practice and expensive physical interactions between healthcare givers and patients, the IoT-based e-health solution provides a faster, easier and cost-effective ways to accessing healthcare [119]. The important modifications that IoT has already brought in diverse areas of healthcare are noticeable in [15, 93]:

- Patient tracking, monitoring and diagnostics (e.g., preventive care, monitoring patient's health, chronic disease self-care),
- Sharing and recording health-related data, and collaboration,
- Smart healthcare devices and tools (e.g., smart wheelchair, sensors),
- Cross-organization integration (e.g., connected emergency units, response vehicles, and healthcare institutions).

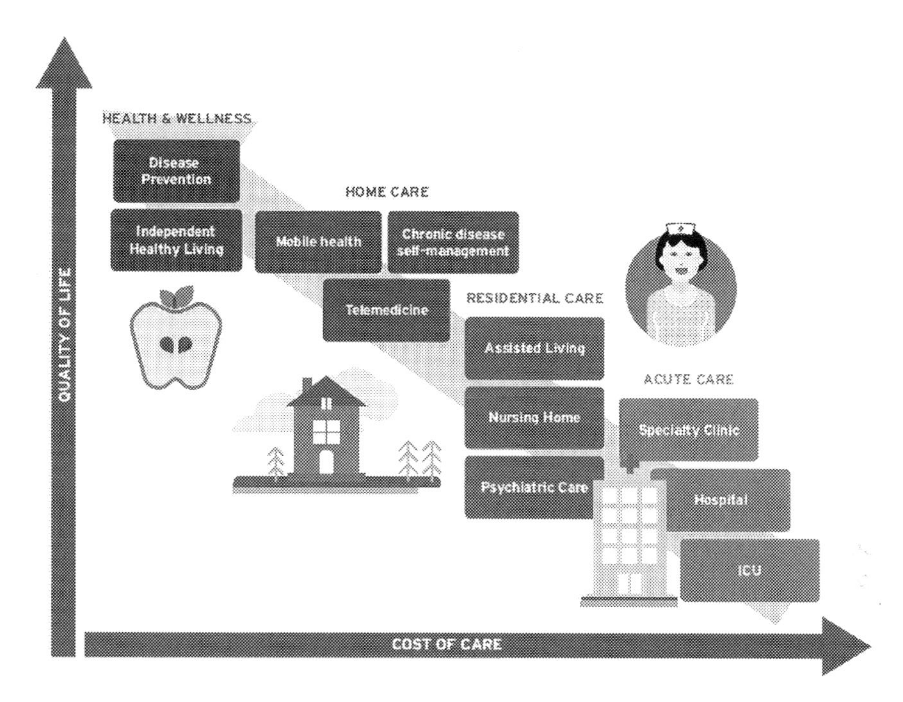

Fig. 9 Improved quality of life followed with reduced cost of care [75]

To develop a successful IoT-driven e-health system, it is necessary to satisfy following demands:

- To effectively manage healthy living, the system must be unobtrusive and comfortable as possible and available 24/7.
- Ubiquitous technology should be used for sensing, monitoring, analyzing, and communicating. Telemedicine advancements, videoconferencing and the IoT, provide means for monitoring patients' health at home, virtually from anywhere. Therefore, using digital communication technologies and virtualization, the appropriate healthcare can be provided anytime and anywhere.
- Any medical device (wearable or portable) must be connected to the Cloud, pulled and be capable of analyzing a vast range of collected health markers of a patient in real time and to identify important signs of possible health risk.
- The connected devices must be able to speak the same language using protocols and collaborate with each other without human involvement. Connected devices should be ubiquitous and a programmable platform.
- Monitoring of vital health indicators collected by portable devices (e.g., smartphones and tablets) must be realized. The data gleaned from the smart IoT devices are used by healthcare professionals to figure out who needs the most hands-on attention and to help diagnose the patient so they can get the best treatment as quickly as possible. Data collected from health monitoring devices

should be visualized in easy understandable charts and diagrams. Thus, providing visualization of the voluminous data and analysis results accessible to healthcare practitioners in an understandable and adjustable format, regardless of the underlying development platform, are essential.
- Shifting reactive treatment towards precise, predictive and preventive should significantly reduce the number of alerts. In the case of emergency (when any abnormality is detected) intelligent notifications must be enabled and sent to a caregiver.
- The growth of medical devices at a hospital and clinical side requires stabilization of existing wired and wireless infrastructure as well as pervasive Wi-Fi connectivity and bandwidth for clinician workflow and communications. Automated and secure provisioning and control of medical devices on the wired/wireless network, staff supporting and consulting, and technical support 24/7 are mandatory.
- Authorization processes, data exchange and privacy must be compliant with EU Data Protection Directive (Europe) or HIPAA (Health Insurance Portability and Accountability Act) in the USA (United States of America) as well as national regulations [88].
- Reduce costly and unnecessary medical services.
- Deliver personalized experiences to users, which meet their specific needs through flexibility, convenience and technologies.
- Scaling sensors down to the nanoscale, and reduce energy consumption.

Remote monitoring, real-time monitoring and online medical consultations are major benefits patients experience in the IoT-driven e-health vision. These benefits are the consequence of growing number of technological solutions aimed to help save lives and improve the health of humans on a global scale. With the help of such IoT-powered e-health systems, patients better understand their health status and much more participate in the healthcare decisions affecting them. An active participation ensures their well-being through access to a summary of their health information (from anywhere), giving them more insight into their health by tracking of their medications, immunizations and allergies. It is believed that web portals, the Internet and social media, improve access to health-related information [19]. Using the IoT-based e-health systems and services the point of care is shifted towards patients, placing the patient in the center of the treatment process followed with the reduced demand for physical contact between patients and healthcare givers [36]. Moreover, in the IoT-based e-health system, where smart (intelligent) devices can bring decisions and perform actions without human intervention, impact of racial bias and any kind of discrimination in healthcare (income, gender, age, education, race, etc.) patient can face with health professionals or anyone else can be minimized [42]. Hence, with the help of the IoT-driven e-health patients can receive better and safer healthcare, anywhere and at any time as needed by them. Fast and more quality healthcare is based on more complete patient information availability. The IoT nature of e-health systems enables data exchange between smart devices as well as between devices and health institutions and professionals automatically through the Internet. Collected and analyzed data facilitate fast and safe treatment decisions. Some of the benefits healthcare professionals achieve are: remote access to the patient chart; identifying necessary laboratory tests; being alerted in case of critical laboratory values or possible medication errors; being reminded to provide preventive care, facilitated direct communications with patients as well as the ability to cope easier with increases in patient numbers. To point out, the IoT has potential to revolutionize how healthcare is delivered and operationalized, by radically reducing costs and improving the availability and quality of healthcare by focusing on the way all participants in healthcare processes, devices and applications are connected and cooperate with each other. Currently applied IoT-driven e-health applications already show the tremendous benefits IoT brings to health services.

Maximization of socioeconomic benefits through the implementation of e-health systems is a goal of the new European e-health Action Plan for the period 2012–2020. It defines the vision for novel healthcare for the 21st Century where physicians will spend more time with their patients and reduce unnecessary administrative tasks. According to the plan, during the period 2014–2020, research and innovation will be supported in the field of IoT in order to develop digital, personalized and predictive, patient-centric and cost-effective healthcare, focusing on the embedded and cyber-physical systems, operating platforms, network technologies, semantic interoperability, and security and privacy issues [30]. Moreover, by 2020, it is expected that shrinking sensors to the nanometer scale will imply nanotechnology widespread use and its involvement in every aspect of life. Embedding nano-devices in the environment creates a new vision—the "Internet of Nano Things" (IoNT). The IoNT in the field of medicine creates a new term—"nanomedicine", which has potential to make diagnoses and treatment less invasive and more intelligent. The elimination of many invasive procedures will be realized with the help of smart pills and nanoscale robotics. Beyond numerous benefits nanomedicine has to offer, big challenges will have to be met: the linkage of the nanoscale networks to the Internet, communication issues between the nano- and micro networks, privacy and safety issues, potential toxic and hazardous effects of nanoparticles, generation of large amounts of data, etc. [91]. Nevertheless, the use of nanotechnology in medicine opens a whole new world of exciting possibilities, and it is expected to revolutionize the healthcare over decades to come.

Beyond the technical/scientific factors, it is important to address and non-technical challenges of different nature, such as socioeconomic challenges during the IoT domains and technologies' progress [36]. Hence, the incredible benefits of the IoT integration into the healthcare system for both an individual and a society will be achieved only when most of these concerns and risks are overcome. Thus, the success of the IoT-powered healthcare depends on the overall ecosystem development, embraced by an adequate regulations and appropriate level of trust. Accomplished identification, privacy and security, confidentiality, trust and semantic interoperability issues can lead to wisely used and widely applied IoT-driven e-health, therefore improving access, availability, and increasing the financial efficiency of healthcare systems in general.

3.2 Challenges, Risks and Concerns

Despite the opportunities and benefits, e-health widespread adoption is facing with numerous barriers. On the other side, the realization of the IoT vision, in order to create adjustable, secure, ubiquitous and non-invasive solution, requires significant modifications of systems, architectures and communications [133]. In general, the challenges IoT faces are: availability of Internet at any place and without costs, development of low-cost smart sensing platforms, scalability, energy consumption, computational capacity, fault tolerance, security and privacy issues and a climate of trust [85]. Alongside technology impacts to the IoT development and usage, it is important to point out and social and economic factors. All these facts make the IoT-driven e-health systems a complex and exciting field. The challenges IoT-based e-health vision deals with may result significantly slower than anticipated adoption of the IoT-powered e-health systems and services as well as nullify any or all of the identified benefits.

In the rest of the chapter main challenges, risks and concerns of modern IoT healthcare system are discussed.

Government action

Governments are responsible for providing fundamental services, such as healthcare and ICTs infrastructure, continuity of funding, accessible education as well to support services around personal health issues including implementation of standards and protecting privacy and security rights.

Technology issues

The technology domains that will provide the IoT practicable and reliable solutions' wider uptake, including healthcare sector, are: (i) identification, (ii) IoT architecture, (iii) communication, (iv) network, (v) network discovery, (vi) software and algorithms, (vii) hardware, (viii) data and signal processing, (ix) discovery and search engine technology, (x) relationship network management technology, (xi) power and energy storage, (xii) security and privacy, and (xiii) standardization [12]. In other words, the experts assume that the progress and mature of IoT technologies will require continuous and intense work in data protection, ethical issues, architecture, identification of networked objects, standards and regulations, and governance [81]. As a consequence, the IoT-driven e-health adoption on a large scale is being hindered by a variety of factors. Successful IoT applications in the area of personalized advanced healthcare require home diagnostic kits, healthcare monitoring and the low-cost collection of medical data shared with the patient's healthcare providers through the Cloud. Medical devices, opposite to office computer systems, are often used in a harsh environment. Therefore, the hardware components of medical devices should have higher physical tolerance against environmental conditions. To prevent wrong measurements or treatment parameters, medical devices often use a dual communication channel design, in order to detect and correct wrong transmission and ensure the totality of the transmitted information [117].

Hence, availability of required data is essential for making right and timely health-related decisions [88]. Therefore, IoT medical devices must: (i) gather data and analyze real-time data, (ii) monitor device operation for faults and prevent malfunctions, (iii) remote control and device configuration, (iv) enable devices to broadcast results and notifications to other devices, (v) maintain an active device inventory and track assets, and (vi) enable remote software/firmware updates. Having in mind that one of the obstacles to healthcare technology embracement is that healthcare professionals and patients often resist technology, the IoT smart medical devices must be easy to handle devices, customized, affordable, powerful, safe and comfortable. With technology advancements, creating hardware and wireless connectivity equipment becomes cheaper and more efficient, enabling connection of a whole range of objects together. As a result, healthcare-related information systems and hardware are now omnipresent. With the help of small, powerful and cheap devices, and medical software applications, people are able to monitor themselves on a daily basis and share their health information with healthcare providers when needed and start to become more responsible for their own care along with a deeper understanding of own illness. To achieve these benefits, interoperability appears as a key challenge. Therefore, an interoperable ecosystem of many heterogeneous sorts of systems (devices, sensors, equipment, etc.), services and applications, to provide the free health-related information stream for accurate and on time decision is crucial.

Human factors

People are key components to the creation and use of e-health products and services. Cognitive, social, and cultural barriers can enable patients and consumers to benefit from rapidly changing and growing e-health systems. These barriers include cultural and language differences, lack of knowledge and access to technology. Even the lack of IT knowledge may be one of the main barriers, the data scandals that regularly occur represents a higher obstacle. Some potential patients of the IoT-driven e-health services, feel their lives are being controlled and therefore have resistance and may reject them. Also, some professionals are mainly focused to give their best to treat the patient and other activities usually consider as a loss of control over their patients' care. Consequently, technology rejection by influential healthcare givers affects other healthcare staffs [35]. One of the ways to deal with these barriers is to give an opportunity for healthcare professionals and customers to participate in designing and adopting technologies, improving system development and facilitating them to control the effects of the information system based on their engagement [95]. Computer and web technology skills, the organizational and managerial competencies and leadership, as well as the awareness of the associated legal, ethical, and economic issues, are necessary for the changes IoT brings in e-health tasks, processes and job roles. Only through the continuous and reactive work on overcoming these barriers e-health strategies can be customized in order to satisfy a wide scope of society demands [47].

Big data and analytics

According to Cisco predictions, by 2020, 50 billion diverse devices will be connected to the Internet [32]. Consequently, the IoT growth will imply the large-volume, complex, growing data sets. Some estimates states that the amount of generated data will be 507.5 ZB (zettabyte = 1 trillion gigabyte) of data per year or 42.3 ZB per month by 2019. It is expected that the data produced by IoT connected devices in 2019 will be 269 times greater than the data being transmitted from end-user devices to data centers and 49 times higher than total data center traffic [27]. Regarding produced healthcare data on a global scale, in 2012 the amount of generated data was 500 petabytes (10^{15} bytes), while 25000 petabytes can be expected in 2020 [34]. Evidently, a voluminous nature of data produced by the IoT-driven e-health systems represents a big challenge. A large, rapidly growing, and mostly unstructured medical data are the consequence of increased digitalization of formerly analogue media (images, reports, lab results, etc.), the continuous optimization of diagnostic laboratory and imaging sensors, increased monitoring with sensors of all kinds, etc. However, voluminous data alone doesn't do much, but IoT collected health data and algorithms together, are exceptionally valuable. Thus, the main question is how to analyze, capture, search, share, store, and visualize data which have a tendency to grow. In the modern approach, a solution can be found in the concept of "Big data", which is primarily used to describe large sets of data. Opposite to traditional datasets, Big data usually encompasses voluminous sets of unstructured data. These data require real time analysis, and any of required operation can't be performed using existing IT and software/hardware tools [22]. Concepts and technologies which are usually closely related to Big data are almost always [22, 101, 107]:

- Cloud computing (provide reliable storage for data),
- IoT (gathering prodigious amount of data from real world—sensors and actuators),
- Data center (acquiring, managing, organizing, and leveraging the data), and
- Hadoop (data storage and processing, system management, and incorporation of variant modules).

One of the essential concepts in Big data is "Not Only Structured Query Language" (NoSQL) which represents a well-known set of non-relational data management systems. Unlike traditional Relational Database Management Systems (RDBMS) which use table-based approach and SQL for accessing data, NoSQL systems are not table-based and do not depend on SQL. Instead, these systems are based on a key-value storage. NoSQL database management systems are useful when working with masses of data which nature does not demand a relational model [7, 33, 43, 113]. Today, there are a various NoSQL database types, such as the Key Value Pairs, Column, Document, and Graph-based databases [107].

Volume, variety, velocity, value and veracity, as the foundational characteristics of Big data, discussed through application in healthcare, justify application of Big data for this purpose [11, 96]:

- *Volume*: As time goes on, a high quantity of health-related data is produced and accumulated, resulting in terabytes and petabytes of data. These systems include medical and healthcare information such as: personal information, radiology images, personal medical records, 3D imaging, genomics, and biometric sensor readings. Nowadays, relying on advances in data management, healthcare systems have the potential for manipulation, storage and use of such a complex data structure by using virtualization and Cloud computing.
- *Variety*: The most challenging aspect of Big data appliance in healthcare consists of joining traditional data with new data forms to get the most closer to the right solution for a specific patient. Structured information, such as clinical data, can be stored, processed and manipulated by machine in an easy way. However, most of health-related data, such as office medical records, doctor handwritten or machine-written notes and prescriptions, images and radiograph films, e-mail messages and attachments are unstructured or semi-structured. From that reason, healthcare applications demand more efficient ways to merge and convert various types of data, in particular to convert structured to unstructured data.
- *Velocity*: Most healthcare data has been traditionally static, but today velocity of data increases with massive data that are the results of continuous regular monitoring. The information stored in healthcare systems is often correct, but not always even if it is updated on a regular basis. Thus, Big data must be retrieved, analyzed and compared to make time and accurate decisions based on real-time data processing, which sometimes can make decision between life and death.
- *Value*: Advances in Big data is process of creating value which can be translated into understanding new diseases and therapies, predicting outcomes at earlier stages, making real-time decisions, promoting patients' health, enhancing medicine, reducing cost and improving healthcare value and quality.
- *Veracity*: Quality of data is of primary concern in health sector because the quality of offered healthcare as well as life or death decisions depends on having the accurate health-related data. In order to achieve effective results with data analytics, it is necessary to provide health-related information of high-quality.

In the summary, Big data analytics, as a top issue in the healthcare industry, are needed to extract useful information from the collected voluminous datasets, and, based on this, adapt the therapy according to the needs. Hence, in the IoT world, health-related data is transmitted to patient' EHR system automatically. The IoT solutions in healthcare enable health practitioners to merge the IoT data from various medical devices. In this way healthcare professionals obtain a complete picture of patient's health status [68]. Possible benefits of Big data application in healthcare include detecting diseases at earlier stages, predicting epidemics, curing disease, avoiding preventable deaths and therefore improving the quality of life and support prevention and personalization. With the help of Big data and analytics, healthcare institutions get an opportunity to create more affordable and better healthcare, moving reactive treatment towards predictive and preventive medicine. However, there are a lot of challenges that hinder the development of Big data in healthcare. Difficulties lie in technical issues (to successfully deal with growing amounts of great variety of data and high speed of data generation and processing—data recording, gathering, analyzing, manipulating and visualization) and security issues (to secure personal data as well as corporate data from unauthorized access or from loss) [45]. So, besides physical sensor development, the IoT-driven e-health system growth relies on the development of Big data analytics tools, interfaces, and systems that will allow healthcare providers to observe and apply the resulting information.

Security and privacy

Matched to the traditional definition of security (which includes secure communication, cryptography and guaranteed privacy), security in the IoT vision involves information integrity, confidentiality of data, availability of services, anti-malware, privacy protection, access control, etc. [72]. Consequently, IoT presents new challenges to network and security architects.

Security, as one of the top challenges IoT faces with, involves the security issues on sensing, communication, and application level as well as overall system security [72]. At the sensing layer, an IoT sensing infrastructure/device/technologies (which have low power and constrained resources, limited connectivity and computing capabilities) don't have the power to provide appropriate security protection. The IoT at middle layers (network and service layers) is based on networking and communications which make easier eavesdropping, interception and Denial of Service (DoS) attacks. The information collection and encryption at the upper (application) layer, which is the topmost and terminal level, help obtaining the security requirements at all layers [66, 72]. In summary, each layer has the ability to provide corresponding security controls, while the security requirements between layers are of the great importance as well. Security threats in IoT layers, as well as those between layers, are shown in Table 1 [72].

The Open Web Application Security Project [92] defines top ten IoT vulnerabilities as:

- Insecure Web interface (e.g., default accounts, SQL injection),
- Insufficient authentication/authorization (e.g., weak passwords, no two-factor authentication),
- Insecure network services (e.g., ports open, DoS attacks),
- Lack of transport encryption/integrity verification (e.g., misconfigured or no use of Transport Layer Security (TLS), custom encryption),
- Privacy concerns,
- Insecure Cloud interface (e.g., default accounts, no lockout),
- Insecure mobile interface (e.g., account enumeration, no account lockout),

Table 1 Security threats in IoT

Sensing/perception layer	Middle layers		Application-interface layer	Between layers
	Network layer	Service layers		
• Unauthorized access • Availability • Spoofing attack • Selfish threat • Malicious code • DoS • Transmission threats • Routing attack	• Data breach • Transmission threats • DoS • Public key and private key • Malicious code • Routing attack	• Privacy threats • Services abuse • Identity masquerade • Service information • Manipulation • Repudiation • DoS • Replay attack • Routing attack	• Remote configuration • Misconfiguration • Security management • Management system	• Sensitive information leakage at border • Identity spoofing • Sensitive information spreads between layers

- Insufficient security configurability (e.g., lack of password security options, no security monitoring and logging),
- Insecure software/firmware (e.g., old device firmware, unprotected device updates), and
- Poor physical security (e.g., accessed or removed data storage media, easily disassembled device itself).

When it comes to healthcare and e-health applications in an IoT environment, there is a need to pay more attention to the security design than in many other IoT networks because the medical data (all data related to a person's health and medical history) are exceptionally sensitive and need to be protected in appropriate way. The exploitation of vulnerabilities mentioned above represents a risk to the safety and effectiveness of IoT-based e-healthcare. The success of healthcare application is determined by the achieved level of patient security and privacy. IoT-based e-health applications operate on a variety of elements: sensor devices, actuators, processing, networking and memory components. The general security level is determined by the weakest element of the system. Therefore, the security must be built into each component, and the overall system (Fig. 10).

With regards to security, data, communication channels and the medical device itself, are the weakest points [69]. In other words, during plugging a large number of diverse connected devices into the IoT system they should be securely identified and have the ability to be discovered. Even most of today's IoT medical devices use secure communication methods, they could still be vulnerable to hackers since communications are mostly wireless (e.g., stealing information, disruption of

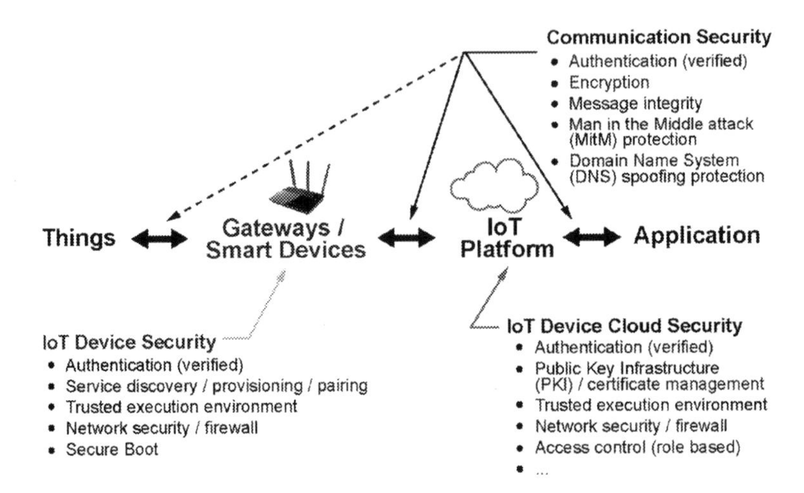

Fig. 10 IoT security points [8]

services like pacemakers, remote hacking of a vehicle control system, remotely unlocking locked door) while unattended elements are mainly unprotected from physical attacks [63]. The additional problem is the fact that execution of complex security-enabling algorithms in IoT devices requires their significant energy, communications, and computation capabilities. Hence, by connecting more intelligent devices to the Internet, the privacy and security issues become critical, representing the major challenges in realization of IoT vision. Considering that the information collected by the IoT system might reveal personal information, the security issues (protection of data and privacy) arise during aggregation of data and their exchange. In other words, with the larger transfer of sensitive data over IoT devices, there is more risk of data to be leaked, falsified or manipulated. Untraceability, unlinkability, unobservability, anonymity and pseudonymity, are mandatory to satisfy privacy issues. Thus, private information from patients, which makes e-health as a highly sensitive yet personal area, appears as an essential component in the widespread adoption of IoT principles in healthcare. The relationship between security and privacy concepts is data protection. Hence, the special interest during the healthcare security architecture design must be given to confidentiality and protection of information. Other factors such as information security, trust, end-to-end personal data privacy and protection should be also systematically and carefully addressed at the conception phase of each component and overall IoT-based e-health system. Figure 11 shows the relationship between information security and present healthcare research problems [9].

The security requirements and challenges of the IoT e-health applications are shown in Fig. 12 [59].

As the first step in the entire health information access procedure, user authentication is essential in healthcare information systems. Some of the authentication mechanisms used to verify the user's identity are: password, PIN (Personal

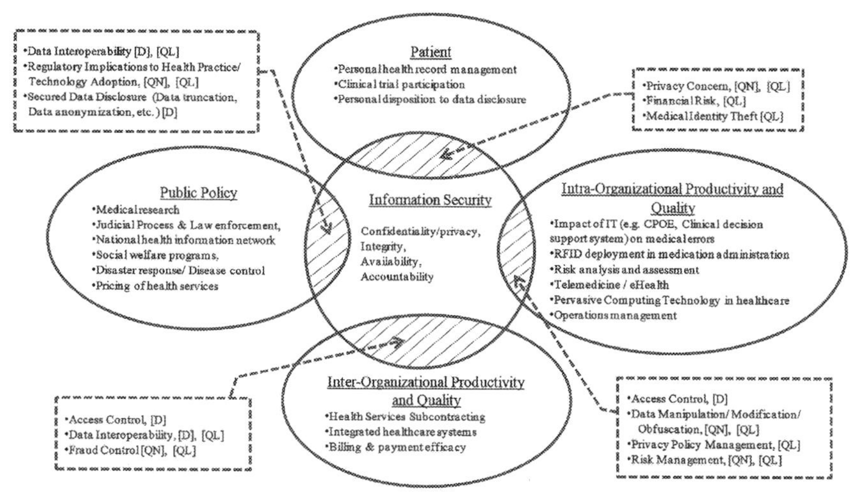

Fig. 11 Research areas in the healthcare information security [9]

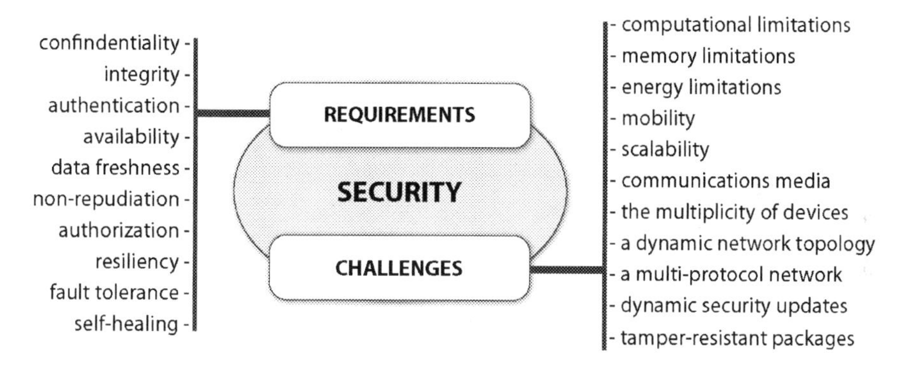

Fig. 12 Security requirements and challenges for the IoT-based healthcare solutions

Identification Number), fingerprint, signature, voice pattern, smart card, token, etc. Only in this way it can be assured that the information is sent by the trusted sender [76]. Moreover, networked devices that exchange data with other IoT devices need to be properly authenticated to avoid security problems. This may need to include certain authentication protocols, and to use integrity-secured or encrypted channels of communication [31]. Interoperability, as an essential characteristic of the IoT-driven e-health system, enables diverse things to better cooperate and integrate in order to produce the desired outcome [18]. In order to make an interoperable system, its elements have to be designed according to standards satisfying their properties on: (i) technical (interoperability achieved using compatible hardware interfaces), (ii) syntactical (compatible data exchange protocols and data containers), and (iii) semantical (the same understanding of the meaning of data) levels [88]. When health-related sensitive data are shared across the network, authentication, availability, confidentiality, and integrity are mandatory in order to realize secure communications in IoT. With patient data integrity, the received medical reports can't be altered in transit. In this way, patient' medical data, transferred to the medical personal, can't be modified, changed or interpreted by any unauthorized source. Additionally, data confidentiality ensures that a patient's health-related records are secured from passive attacks [29]. Availability, as another security requirement (Fig. 12), ensures the continuity of the IoT healthcare services to authorized person upon demand. Due to the sensitive nature of health data, bounded latency and reliability of the IoT-based e-health system are crucial to effective intervention, especially in a case of emergency. It is important to highlight that data or messages sent earlier can't be denied by a node (non-repudiation). Employed system security scheme must protect the data, device and network from any attack as well as to provide respective security services at any moment, even some interconnected health devices are harmed, failed, run out of energy or there is a software glitch [59].

Clearly, to enable at least a minimum level of security, IoT healthcare services are facing with numerous challenges (Fig. 12). Bearing in mind that a typical IoT healthcare system consists of small health-related devices of limited computational performances, memory and battery power, finding a security solution that overcomes these computational, memory and energy limitations and maximizes security performance is a challenging task [59]. To secure devices in sensing layer of IoT, all devices should be produced according to specific security criteria and implement security standards for IoT. A trustworthy data sensing system, ability to detect and identify the source of users and securely designed software or firmware at IoT end-node are mandatory as well [72]. Other serious challenges are focused on develop a mobility-compliant security algorithm and design highly scalable security scheme applicable to the simplest of devices, and be appropriate for dynamic network topology as well. An overall security protocol that has ability to equally deal with both wired and wireless channel characteristics represents important challenges security specialists facing with. Dynamic security updates and tamper-resistant packages of IoT health devices are nothing less challenging to implement [59]. Therefore, to implement the IoT-powered e-health system, using portable health devices to collect, store, and transfer patient health-related sensitive data to a central server, requires secure manners to rapidly transfer recorded data so that patient's personal information can't be compromised at any stage. Only satisfying requirements defined above and successfully dealing with mentioned challenges, this goal can be accomplished. A large number of research is devoted to the integration of enormous streams of real-time data from the IoT with all of existing data, preserving and protecting user security with the help of pervasive sensing and analytics systems and choice of hardware and software which will contribute to development of new intelligent, secure, easy and modern IoT applications. Novel research regarding security topics in IoT-driven e-health are also based on improving several algorithms in medical applications that can be supported by the IoT technology and security issues and on defining new cryptographic protocols that are able to work on tiny, low-power devices [1, 28, 64, 87, 98]. The ways of reducing and solving the risk of security and privacy in an e-health environment are discussed in many works [5, 9, 53, 54, 59, 67, 69, 73, 106, 118, 122, 129].

Nevertheless, protecting privacy and security and assuring fairness in the IoT is a critical, yet complex task. As a very important and full of challenges, security and privacy issues must be taken into account during the whole IoT lifecycle, from the design phase to the services running. To protect privacy, in order to facilitate the overall adoption of the IoT, following tasks must be performed [48, 124]:

- Take into account technical solutions,
- Encompass regulatory considerations,
- Include market-based aspects, and
- Incorporate socio-ethical issues.

However, it has been proven that, regarding privacy, a technical solution is not an unattainable goal. On the contrary, political and economic factors are much greater constraints society is facing with regard the level of privacy [52].

In summary, the security and privacy issues of IoT-powered e-health systems must be threatened on many levels, what is essential for the success of IoT implementation in healthcare. Confidentiality, data integrity, accountability, availability of services and access control are the essential goals that systems have to achieve in order to satisfy certain security and safety demands [88]. Since an IoT-driven e-health system store and process data of special interest, they should be equipped with appropriate mechanisms of their protection. Security should be built hierarchal into the whole healthcare ecosystem. Still, there are many open problems in areas of security and privacy protection, network protocols, standardization, identity management, etc. [72]. Assured privacy, security and consumer trust are the keys to realizing the full potential of the IoT application in healthcare. This highlights the fact that novel security protocols and identification techniques are mandatory, as well as more intelligent security systems that include managed threat detection, anomaly detection, and predictive analysis [23].

Regulations and standardization

The IoT success depends on the standardization issues, which provide secured interoperability, compatibility, reliability, and effective operations on a global level [72]. Therefore, standards, simply put as a list of agreed-upon rules and guidelines, are considered as fundamental for facilitating e-health system interoperability, providing adherence to current privacy and security legislation as well as ensuring the ability to successfully leverage various devices and applications. Not only are they important with regards to traditional e-health systems, standards also playing a role in the success of the novel IoT-based e-health solutions. In other words, taking into account that a patient may necessitate the services of various healthcare providers, uses various devices, many different electronic systems and information systems while used devices and information systems may use disparate (communications) protocols and messaging formats, the IoT-driven e-health must be supported with numerous standards. Lake et al. [69] classify standards used in e-health applications in: data, message, document and process standards. The standards are also classified into syntax, semantics, relationship, purpose and classification based. However, standards for the IoT-based e-health together with technology are key enablers of the transformation and revolutionizing healthcare. To deal with deployments and utilization of diverse products, global interoperability standards are necessary. These standards enable that variety of devices, systems and applications for health monitoring and preventive care talk the same language and intercommunicate. To provide a common methodology for specifying sensor performance and facilitate integration for multi-vendor sensors, the IEEE 2700–2014 "Standard for Sensor Performance Parameter Definitions" has been developed as the result of the IEEE Standards Association and MEMS Industry Group collaboration [10]. Moreover, due to the sensitivity of medical data and required strong legal regulation, healthcare-related systems are significantly harder to develop. Safety and performance of products on the EU market are determined either by Directive 2001/95/EC 11 on general product safety or by specialized medical device directive in case of medical products [36]. Telemedicine, e-health and IoT technologies are advancing rapidly, requiring new generations of communication protocols, provisions for the service layer and interoperability guidelines. Work in standardization of this area is continuous and intense. An IEEE active project P2413 "Draft Standard for an Architectural Framework for the Internet of Things (IoT)," [58] defines an architectural framework proposing cross-domain interaction, system interoperability and functional compatibility for the IoT [10]. As the Cloud is one of the major building blocks of the IoT-based e-health vision, Cloud-related standards at various layers of Cloud infrastructure and services as well as some level of confluence of e-health and Cloud-related standards are essential too. Moreover, the processes and services automation is not feasible without adequate data standards that permit communication through open access Internet-oriented software languages. Some of the common e-health data standards include [69]: ICD (International Classification of Disease)—international standard codes for diagnoses; LOINC (Logical Observation Identifiers Names and Codes)—a universal coding system for the reporting of laboratory and clinical measurements; CPT (Current Procedural Terminology)—standard for coding medical procedures; SNOMED CT (Systematized Nomenclature Of Medicine)—widely used hierarchical healthcare terminology; NDC (National Drug Codes)—Food and Drug Administration's numbering system for medications. It is important to mention and following standards: HL7 (Health Level System 7)—a standard for exchanging integration, sharing, and retrieval information between medical applications; CCR (Continuity of Care Record) and CCD (Continuity of Care Document)—standards for solving the problem of patient-data portability and interoperability; DICOM (Digital Imaging and Communications in Medicine)—the international standard for the communication and management of medical imaging related information; IHE (Integrating the Health Enterprise)—an initiative to improve the way computer systems in healthcare sector exchange information. Furthermore, adequate regulative and standards (necessary to ensure that information systems can exchange and share the patient information in order to provide appropriate and timely care) like the ISO/IEC 27,000-series which encompasses information security standards, must be satisfied [76]. There is also the Federal Information Processing Standard (FIPS 140), a USA government computer security standard, which deals with security in the transmission of information, what is a crucial in the successful deployment of medical IoT applications. The ISO/IEEE 11073 family of standards has potential to provide complete and interoperable health IoT architecture. In this way, the applications in the Cloud are able to supervise and gather health-related information from personal health devices, enabling health professionals to access remotely and directly to the newest measurement values of each patient from the Cloud [77]. A comprehensive review of widely adopted e-health interoperability standards has been presented in [3]. As can be seen, the collection, processing, recording and dissemination of medical patient data are under the control of many laws and regulations. Even these regulations and laws vary greatly between different countries and continents, authorization procedures, data interchange and privacy must be compliant with EU Data Protection Directive (e.g. Directive 2011/24/EU—the application of patients' rights in cross-border healthcare; Directive 2000/31/EC—electronic commerce; Directive 95/46/EC—Data Protection) and the national Patients' Rights Laws (Europe) or the HIPAA in the USA [39].

It is worth to note that the IoT-driven e-health systems create complete new challenges in sense of legislation and policy issues. From a standards perspective, the IoT-based e-health systems represent a huge challenge for standardization. Standardization, as a time-lagged and long-term process, is a complex task that has to involve all participants. Moreover, standards development and implementation lag behind technological development, making this process slow and may require concerted regulatory action. Nevertheless, the success of IoT-powered e-health vision relies mainly on standardization, which provides reliability, compatibility, interoperability, and effectiveness of the operations on a worldwide scale.

Investment

Growing demand for real-time disease management, improved patient care services, effective and efficient treatment outcome implies investors, providers, and developers rising interest in the IoT appliance in the healthcare. The IoT in the healthcare market is segmented based on application, into telemedicine, inpatient monitoring, clinical operations, medication management, and connected imaging. Regardless of the applications, the basic requirement for implementing the IoT e-health services is the access to the Internet. Besides rapid Internet growth, Internet access is not still available to every place in the world. This implies a need to largely invest in IT infrastructure and resources. The private companies will invest only if they can make a profit. Hence, at this point the government comes in play [85]. On the other side, many companies and organizations largely invest in adopting new technologies in order to gain patients' attention and deliver actionable insights for their personalized care. One of the leading trends in the market is the result of high consumerization. Patients want to have insight in their health condition as well as to take control of it [99]. Even BI Intelligence [14] predicts that on a global scale 73 million IoT devices will be installed for the healthcare sector by 2016 and 161 million by 2020, the IoT-based healthcare isn't just about devices. Instead of hardware devices, more investment will be aimed at developing appropriate software and services of IoT healthcare solutions [14]. The development of Big data analytics, Cloud services and artificial intelligence are in the center of healthcare industry's investments. According to multiple market reports, the investments in Big data analytics platforms and tools, the IoT, Cloud computing technologies, and business intelligence tools in healthcare sector will continue their rapid growth. It is anticipated that the healthcare-specific IoT market will expand from $32.47 billion in 2015 to $163.24 billion by 2020 [16]. In other words, the immense interest in completely connected health and supporting devices, sensors, and clinical tools, will imply new and numerous investment in many key market segments that will integrate to create the healthcare-specific IoT [17].

4 Discussion And Concluding Remarks

With the technology-driven developments, people in the 21st Century via more effective and efficient healthcare systems and services are able to have insight and proactively manage their health conditions. The IoT and e-health are keystone technologies which together entirely change person-to-person, human-to-machine and M2M communications, revolutionizing healthcare in all its aspects. IoT smart devices applied in healthcare provide novel and attractive ways to monitor, record patients' data in home and work environments, and automatically transmit gathered information to electronic systems. Data analyzed and delivered in easily understandable formats, enable healthcare practitioners to quick and easy gain insights into the health conditions of patients and start using the collected data in their clinic practice, providing in such way a faster, easier and cost-effective means to accessing healthcare. Even the IoT integration in healthcare is still early in the maturity, it can be expected that connected medical devices will become ubiquitous and programmable, with the possibility to talk to each other while improving quality of care and consequently patients' personal health. In other words, in both hospitals and at home, the possibilities of IoT-based e-health solutions are endless.

With this in mind, it can be pointed out that the advantage of IoT-based e-health system is in possibility of smart objects to continuously monitor the health condition of a patient and exchange information with other devices and health institutions via the Internet, in order to help make correct and personalized treatment decisions. An intelligent infrastructure for personal health management through smart devices and technologies accessible to all citizens, enable omnipresence of many medical applications such as remote health monitoring, fitness and wellness programs, chronic diseases, and care of old and disabled people. Reducing the costs and the time to perform health tasks and processes, more quality health decisions and activities at the operational, managerial and policy levels and dealing with an increasing number of cases without raising staff numbers or associated costs, are the main advantages IoT brings in the healthcare domain.

This chapter, in addition to a performed review of the literature and existing solutions, highlights six objectives for improving the current e-health system. Guided by the improvements' objectives and the new concepts, primarily IoT, Big data and Cloud computing, the IoT-based e-health system architecture that includes key elements of the modern healthcare system is presented as well. The conducted analysis has confirmed that potential outcomes are significant. Still, there is a number of possible challenges, risks and concerns that may prevent the full adoption of IoT-powered healthcare. It is important to note technological, managerial, organizational and ethical challenges, as well as standardization, interoperability, security and privacy issues, and economic factors which all together represent the major challenges and barriers to revolutionize the healthcare processes, increasing the availability and quality of medical care embraced with dramatically lowering costs.

Understanding the IoT-driven e-health may perhaps best be achieved by reviewing a SWOT analysis to evaluate the Strengths, Weaknesses, Opportunities, and Threats of the IoT-based healthcare at the present time.

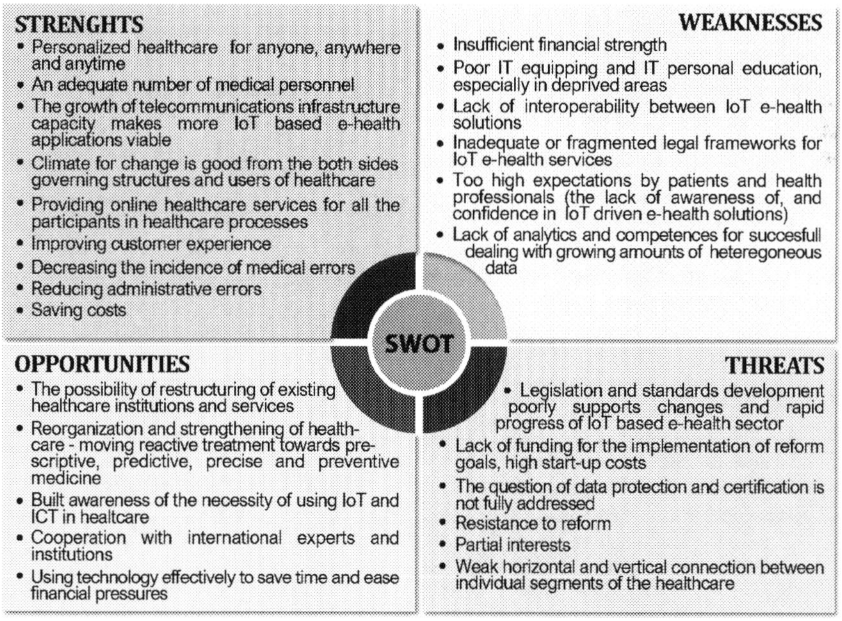

STRENGHTS

- Personalized healthcare for anyone, anywhere and anytime
- An adequate number of medical personnel
- The growth of telecommunications infrastructure capacity makes more IoT based e-health applications viable
- Climate for change is good from the both sides governing structures and users of healthcare
- Providing online healthcare services for all the participants in healthcare processes
- Improving customer experience
- Decreasing the incidence of medical errors
- Reducing administrative errors
- Saving costs

WEAKNESSES

- Insufficient financial strength
- Poor IT equipping and IT personal education, especially in deprived areas
- Lack of interoperability between IoT e-health solutions
- Inadequate or fragmented legal frameworks for IoT e-health services
- Too high expectations by patients and health professionals (the lack of awareness of, and confidence in IoT driven e-health solutions)
- Lack of analytics and competences for succesfull dealing with growing amounts of heteregoneous data

SWOT

OPPORTUNITIES

- The possibility of restructuring of existing healthcare institutions and services
- Reorganization and strengthening of health-care - moving reactive treatment towards pre-scriptive, predictive, precise and preventive medicine
- Built awareness of the necessity of using IoT and ICT in healtcare
- Cooperation with international experts and institutions
- Using technology effectively to save time and ease financial pressures

THREATS

- Legislation and standards development poorly supports changes and rapid progress of IoT based e-health sector
- Lack of funding for the implementation of reform goals, high start-up costs
- The question of data protection and certification is not fully addressed
- Resistance to reform
- Partial interests
- Weak horizontal and vertical connection between individual segments of the healthcare

Hence, to develop and integrate effective ubiquitous IoT-powered healthcare, it is essential to recognize and deal with many ethical concerns, equal rights in accessing to healthcare services and receiving care, accountability, the effectiveness of patient involvement and quantity and quality of online health-related information. Successfully dealing with numerous challenges IoT-based healthcare services are faced with, should enable reduced costs, increased the quality of life, and enrich the both patients and healthcare providers' experience. Even the IoT is immensely changing healthcare, those changes are barely starting. Satisfying essential demands, immensely improving existing healthcare systems and continuously looking for entirely novel ways of monitoring and delivering healthcare will lead to experience the maximal benefits IoT-based e-health has to offer.

References

1. Acharjee, S. et al. (2014) Watermarking in Motion Vector for Security Enhancement of Medical Videos, Control, International Conference on Instrumentation, Communication and Computational Technologies (ICCICCT).
2. Adebesin, F., Kotzé, P., Van Greunen, D. and Foster, R. (2013a) Barriers and Challenges to the Adoption of E-Health Standards in Africa, Health Informatics South Africa (HISA).
3. Adebesin, F., Foster, R., Kotzé, P. and Van Greunen, D. (2013b) A review of interoperability standards in e-Health and imperatives for their adoption in Africa, Research Article – SACJ No. 50, pp. 55–72.
4. Adibi, S. (2015) Mobile Health. A Technology Road Map. Springer International Publishing Switzerland.
5. Agrawal, V. (2014) Security and Privacy Issues in Wireless Sensor Networks for Healthcare. Internet of Things User-Centric IoT. First International Summit, IoT360. Rome, Italy, pp. 223–228.
6. Alliance for Health Policy and Systems Research (2004) Strengthening health systems: the role and promise of policy and systems research, Geneva, Switzerland.
7. Amato, A. and Venticinque, S. (2014) Big Data Management Systems for the Exploitation of Pervasive Environments, Bessis, N. and Dobre, C. (eds.), Big Data and Internet of Things: A Roadmap for Smart Environments, Studies in Computational Intelligence 546, pp 67–90.
8. Andres, R. (2015) Eurotech's Everyware IoT Security Elements Overview, [Online]: http://www.slideshare.net/Eurotechchannel/iot-security-elements.
9. Appari, A. and Johnson, M.E. (2008) Information Security and Privacy in Healthcare: Current State of Research. [Online]: http://www.ists.dartmouth.edu/library/416.pdf.
10. Ash, B. and Bennett, K. (2014) Expanding Wellness Monitoring and Care with e-Health, [Online]: https://www.mdtmag.com/blog/2014/12/expanding-wellness-monitoring-and-care-e-health.
11. Asri, H., Mousannif, H., Moatassime, H. A. and Noel, T. (2015) Big Data in healthcare: Challenges and Opportunities, International Conference on Cloud Technologies and Applications (CloudTech), pp. 1–7.
12. Bandyopadhyay, D. and Sen, J. (2011) Internet of Things - Applications and Challenges in Technology and Standardization, Wireless Personal Communications, Vol. 58, Issue 1, pp 49–69.
13. Bhaddurgatte, R.C. and Kumar, V. (2015) A Review: QoS Architecture and Implementations in IoT Environment, Research & Reviews: Journal of Engineering and Technology, pp. 6–12.

14. BI Intelligence (2016) The global market for IoT healthcare tech will top $400 billion in 2022, [Online]: http://www.businessinsider.com/the-global-market-for-iot-healthcare-tech-will-top-400-billion-in-2022-2016-5.
15. Brasseal, M. (2015) Realtime Technology and the Healthcare Internet of Things, [Online]: https://www.pubnub.com/blog/2015-06-19-realtime-technology-and-the-healthcare-internet-of-things/.
16. Bresnick, J. (2015) Healthcare Big Data Analytics, IoT, Cloud Markets Set for Growth, [Online]: http://healthitanalytics.com/news/healthcare-big-data-analytics-iot-cloud-markets-set-for-growth.
17. Bresnick, J. (2016) Healthcare Internet of Things Investment is Just Getting Started, [Online]: http://healthitanalytics.com/news/healthcare-internet-of-things-investment-is-just-getting-started.
18. Bui, N. and Zorzi, M. (2011) Health Care Applications: A Solution Based on The Internet of Things. Proceedings of the 4th International symposium on Applied Sciences in Biomedical and Communication Technologies – ISABEL 2011.
19. Buzzi, M.C. et al. (2016) Facebook: a new tool for collecting health data? Multimed Tools Appl, Springer Science + Business Media New York.
20. Car, J. et al. (2008) The Impact of eHealth on the Quality & Safety of Healthcare, A Systemic Overview & Synthesis of the Literature, Report for the NHS Connecting for Health Evaluation Programme.
21. Chatterjee, P. and Armetano, R. L. (2015) Internet of Things for a Smart and Ubiquitous eHealth System, International Conference on Computational Intelligence and Communication Networks (CICN - 2015), At Jabalpur, India.
22. Chen, M. et al. (2014) Big Data: Related Technologies, Challenges and Future Prospects, Springer.
23. Cisco (n.d.) Securing the Internet of Things: A Proposed Framework, [Online]: http://www.cisco.com/c/en/us/about/security-center/secure-iot-proposed-framework.html.
24. Comstock, J. (2015) PwC predicts "DIY Healthcare" will be the top trend of 2015. [Online]: http://mobihealthnews.com/39747/pwc-predicts-diy-healthcare-will-be-the-top-trend-of-2015.
25. Conrad, S. K. (1998) Making telehealth a viable component of our national health care system. Prof. Psychol. Res. Pract. 29(6):525–526.
26. Das, R. (2015) Top 10 Healthcare Predictions for 2016, [Online]: http://www.forbes.com/sites/reenitadas/2015/12/10/top-10-healthcare-predictions-for-2016/#146f174c2f63.
27. Daecher, R. and Schmid, R. (2016) Internet of Things: From sensing to doing, Deloitte University Press, [Online]: http://dupress.com/articles/internet-of-things-iot-applications-sensing-to-doing/.
28. Dey, N. et al. (2012) Stationary Wavelet Transformation Based Self-Recovery of Blind-Watermark from Electrocardiogram Signal in the Wireless Telecardiology, Recent Trends in Computer Networks and Distributed Systems Security, Vol., 335 of the series Communications in Computer and Information Science, pp. 347–357.
29. Divi, K., Kanjee, M.R. Liu, H. (2010) Secure Architecture for Healthcare Wireless Sensor Networks. Sixth International Conference on Information Assurance and Security.
30. eHealth Action Plan 2012–2020 - Innovative healthcare for the 21st century (2012), European Commission [Online]: https://ec.europa.eu/digital-single-market/en/news/ehealth-action-plan-2012-2020-innovative-healthcare-21st-century.
31. European Commission (2016) Advancing the Internet of Things in Europe, Commission Staff Working Document accompanying document Communication from the commission to the European parliament, the Council, The European economic and social committee and the committee of the regions, Digitising European Industry - Reaping the full benefits of a Digital Single Market, Brusseless.
32. Evans, D. (2011) The Internet of Things - How the Next Evolution of the Internet Is Changing Everything, Cisco Internet Business Solutions Group (IBSG), [Online]: https://www.cisco.com/c/dam/en_us/about/ac79/docs/innov/IoT_IBSG_0411FINAL.pdf.

33. Feinleib, D. (2014) Big Data Bootcamp - What Managers Need to Know to Profit from the Big Data Revolution, Apress.
34. Feldman, B., Martin, E.M., Skotnes, T. (2012) Big Data in Healthcare, Hype and Hope, Dr. Bonnie 360.
35. Fichman, R.G., Kohli, R. and Krishnan, R. (2011) The Role of Information Systems in Healthcare: Current Research and Future Trends, Information Systems Research, Vol. 22 Issue 3, p 419.
36. Fricker, S.A. et al. (eds.) (2015) Requirements Engineering for Digital Health, Springer International Publishing Switzerland.
37. Forsstrom, S., Kanter, T., Johansson, O. (2012) Real-time distributed sensor-assisted m-health applications on the internet-of-things. In: 2012 IEEE 11th International Conference on Trust, Security and Privacy in Computing and Communications (TrustCom), pp. 1844–1849.
38. Gaddi, A., Capello, F. and Manca, M. (2014) eHealth, Care and Quality of Life, Springer-Verlag Italia.
39. George, C., Whitehouse, D. and Duquenoy, P. (eds.) (2013) eHealth: Legal, Ethical and Governance Challenges, Springer-Verlag Berlin Heidelberg.
40. Georgiadis et al. (2010) An Intelligent Web-based Healthcare Systems: The case of DYMOS. Web-based applications in Healthcare and Medicine (A. Lazadikou (ed.)) Annals of Information System, Vol.7, Springer Science + Business Media LLC.
41. Giaffreda, R. et al. (eds.) (2015) Internet of Things - User-Centric IoT (IoT360 2014), Part I, Lecture Notes of the Institute for Computer Sciences, Social Informatics and Telecommunications Engineering, Springer Cham Heidelberg New York Dordrecht London.
42. Gibbons, M. C. (2008) eHealth Solutions for Healthcare Disparities, Springer Science + Business Media, LLC.
43. Ghavami, P. K. (2015) BIG DATA GOVERNANCE: Modern Data Management Principles for Hadoop, NoSQL & Big Data Analytics, CreateSpace Independent Publishing.
44. Glaser, J. (2014) How The Internet of Things Will Affect Health Care, [Online]: http://www.hhnmag.com/articles/3438-how-the-internet-of-things-will-affect-health-care.
45. Goyen, M. (2016) Big Data and Analytics in Healthcare, Vol. 16, Issue 1, [Online]: https://healthmanagement.org/c/healthmanagement/issuearticle/big-data-and-analytics-in-healthcare.
46. Habib, K., Torjusen, A. and Leister, W. (2015) Security Analysis of a Patient Monitoring System for the Internet of Things in eHealth, eTELEMED 2015: The Seventh International Conference on eHealth, Telemedicine, and Social Medicine, 73–78.
47. Harrison J.P. and Lee A. (2006) The Role of E-Health in the Changing Health Care Environment, Nurs Econ. 24(6):283–288.
48. Hasić, H. and Vujović, V. (2014) Civil law protection of the elements comprising the "Internet of Things" from the perspective of the legal owner of the property in question. Infoteh-Jahorina, Vol. 13. pp. 1005–1011.
49. Hassanalieragh, M. et al. (2015) Health Monitoring and Management Using Internet-of-Things (IoT) Sensing with Cloud-based Processing: Opportunities and Challenges, IEEE International Conference on Services Computing, pp. 285–292.
50. Hillestad, R. et al. (2005) Can Electronic Medical Record Systems Transform Health Care? Potential Health Benefits, Savings, And Costs, Health Affairs 24, no.5 (2005):1103–1117.
51. Hjelm, N.M. (2005) Benefits and drawbacks of telemedicine, J Telemed Telecare. 11(2): 60–70.
52. Hohmann, J. and Benzschawel, S. (2013) Data Protection in eHealth Platforms, R.G. Beran (ed.), Legal and Forensic Medicine,
DOI 10.1007/978-3-642-32338-6_81, # Springer-Verlag Berlin Heidelberg.
53. Hossain, Md. M., Fotouhi, M. and Hasan, R. (2015) Towards an Analysis of Security Issues, Challenges, and Open Problems in the Internet of Things, IEEE World Congress on Services, pp. 21–28.
54. Hu, F. (2016) Security and Privacy in Internet of Things (IoTs): Models, Algorithms, and Implementations, CRC Press, Taylor & Francis Group.

55. Intel (n.d.) The Internet of Things and Healthcare Policy Principles [Online]: http://www.intel.eu/content/dam/www/public/emea/xe/en/documents/iot-healthcare-policy-principles-paper.pdf.
56. Internet Society (2015) The Internet of Things: An Overview, Understanding the Issues and Challenges of a More Connected World, [Online]: https://www.internetsociety.org/sites/default/files/ISOC-IoT-Overview-20151014_0.pdf.
57. Institute of Medicine (2001) Crossing the Quality Chasm: A New Health System for the 21st Century, Academies Press.
58. IoT Architecture (2016) P2413 - Standard for an Architectural Framework for the Internet of Things (IoT), [Online]: http://standards.ieee.org/develop/project/2413.html.
59. Islam, S.M.R. et al. (2015) The Internet of Things for Health Care: A Comprehensive Survey, IEEE Access (Vol. 3), pp. 678–708, ISSN: 2169-3536.
60. Jog, Y. et al. (2015) Internet of Things as a Solution Enabler in Health Sector, International Journal of Bio-Science and Bio-Technology, Vol.7, No.2, pp. 9–24.
61. Kabene, S. M. (2010) Healthcare and the Effect of Technology: Developments, Challenges and Advancements, Premier Reference Source.
62. Kang, H. et al. (2015) A conceptual device-rank based resource sharing and collaboration of smart things, Multimed Tools Appl, Springer Science + Business Media New York.
63. Kansal, S. and Kaur, N. (2016) Multi-level Authentication for Internet of Things to Establish Secure Healthcare Network –A Review, International Journal of Advance Research, Ideas and Innovations in Technology, Vol. 2., Issue. 3, pp. 1–5.
64. Katagi, M. and Moriai, S. (n.d.) Lightweight Cryptography for the Internet of Things [Online]: https://www.iab.org/wp-content/IAB-uploads/2011/03/Kaftan.pdf.
65. Kendler, P.B. (n.d.) Trends in e-health, Wipro Technologies, [Online]: http://www.ehealthnews.eu/images/stories/pdf/trends_in_ehealth.pdf.
66. Keoh, S.L., Kumar, S.S., Tschofenig, H. (2014) Securing the Internet of Things: A Standardization Perspective, IEEE Internet of things Journal, 1(3), 265–275.
67. Kim, J. T. (2014) Privacy and Security Issues for Healthcare System with Embedded RFID System on Internet of Things. Advanced Science and Technology Letters. Vol.72. (Healthcare and Nursing). pp. 109–112.
68. Kirk, S. (2015) Healthcare: A $117B opportunity for the Internet of Things [Online]: https://www.ariasystems.com/blog/healthcare-a-117b-opportunity-for-the-internet-of-things/#sthash.VByNaXsz.dpuf.
69. Lake, D. et al. (2013) Internet of Things: Architectural Framework for eHealth Security, Journal of ITC Standardization.
70. Laxman, K., Krishnan and S.B., Dhillon, J.S. (2015) Barriers to Adoption of Consumer Health Informatics Applications for Health Self Management, Health Science Journal, Vol. 9, No. 5:7.
71. Li, J. et al. (2013) Health Care Provider Adoption of eHealth: Systematic Literature Review, Interact J Med Res. 2013 Jan-Jun; 2(1): e7.
72. Li, S., Tryfonas, T., and Li, H. (2016) The Internet of Things: A Security Point of View. Internet Research, 26(2), 337–359. 10.1108/IntR-07-2014-0173.
73. Löhr, H., Sadeghi, A.-R. and Winandy, M. (2010) Securing the E-Health Cloud. Proceedings of the 1st ACM International Health Informatics Symposium.
74. Lv, Z., Chirivella, J. and Gagliardo, P. (2016) Big data Oriented Multimedia Mobile Health Applications, J Med Syst, 40: 120.
75. MacIntosh, E., Rajakulendran, N. and Salah, H. (2014) Transforming Health: Towards Decentralized and Connected Care, MaRS Market Insights.
76. Maksimović, M., Vujović, V. and Perišić, B. (2016) Do It Yourself solution of Internet of Things Healthcare System: Measuring body parameters and environmental parameters affecting health, Journal of Information Systems Engineering & Management, Vol. 1, No. 1, pp. 25–39.

77. Martins, A.F. (2014) IEEE 11073 and Connected Health: Preparing Personal Health Devices for the Internet, IEEE International Conference on Consumer Electronics (ICCE), pp. 274–275.
78. Matusitz, J., and Breen, G. M. (2007) Telemedicine: Its effects on health communication. Health. Commun. 21(1):73–83.
79. McGrath, M. J., Scanaill, C. N. (2013) Sensor Technologies, Healthcare, Wellness and Environmental Application, Apress.
80. McKinsey Global Institute (2013) Big Data at Center of Disruptive Technologies [Online]: http://www.mckinsey.com/insights/business_technology/disruptive_technologies.
81. Meier-Hahn, U. (2013) European Commission publishes report on Internet of Things, [Online]: http://policyreview.info/articles/news/european-commission-publishes-report-internet-things/114.
82. Mukherjee, S., Dolui, K. and Datta, S. K. (2014) Patient Health Management System using e-Health Monitoring Architecture. IEEE International Advance Computing Conference (IACC). pp. 400–405.
83. Mukhopadhyay, S. C. and Leung H. (2010) Advances in Wireless Sensors and Sensor Networks. Springer-Verlag Berlin Heidelberg.
84. Mukhopadhyay, S. C. and Lay-Ekuakille, A. (2010) Advances in Biomedical Sensing, Measurements, Instrumentation and Systems. Springer-Verlag Berlin Heidelberg.
85. Mukhopadhyay, S. C. (2014) Internet of Things Challenges and Opportunities, Smart Sensors, Measurement and Instrumentation, Vol. 9, Springer International Publishing Switzerland.
86. Nakashima, H., Aghajan, H. and Augusto, J. C. (2010) Handbook of Ambient Intelligence and Smart Environments. Springer Science + Business Media.
87. Nandi, S. et al. (2014) Cellular Automata based Encrypted ECG-hash Code Generation: An Application in Inter-Human Biometric Authentication System, I.J. Computer Network and Information Security, 11, 1–12.
88. Neuhaus, C., Polze, A. and Chowdhuryy, M.M.R. (2011) Survey on Healthcare IT Systems: Standards, Regulations and Security, Hasso-Plattner-Instituts für Softwaresystemtechnik an der Universität Potsdam.
89. Niewolny, D. (2013) How the Internet of Things Is Revolutionizing Healthcare - White Paper, [Online]: https://cache.freescale.com/files/corporate/doc/white_paper/IOTREVHEALCARWP.pdf.
90. Nugent C., Coronato, A. and Bravo, J. (2013) Ambient Assisted Living and Active Aging. 5th International Work-Conference, IWAAL 2013 Carrillo, Costa Rica.
91. Omanović-Mikličanin, E., Maksimović, M. and Vujović, V. (2015) The Future of Healthcare: Nanomedicine and Internet of Nano Things, Folia Medica, Facultatis Medicinae, Universitatis Saraeviensis, Vol. 50, No. 1.
92. OWASP (2014) Internet of Things Top ten [Online]: https://www.owasp.org/images/7/71/Internet_of_Things_Top_Ten_2014-OWASP.pdf.
93. Pang, Z. (2013) Technologies and Architectures of the Internet-of-Things (IoT) for Health and Well-being, PhD Thesis in Electronic and Computer Systems, KTH – Royal Institute of Technology, Stockholm, Sweden.
94. Pitsillides, A. et al. (2006) DITIS: Virtual Collaborative Teams for Home Healthcare, Journal of Mobile Multimedia, Vol. 2, No.1, pp. 023–036, Rinton Press.
95. Qureshi, Q. A. et al. (2013) Infrastructural Barriers to e-Health Implementation in Developing Countries, European Journal of Sustainable Development (2013), 2, 1, 163–170.
96. Raghupathi, W. and Raghupathi, V. (2014) Big data analytics in healthcare: promise and potential, Health Information Science and Systems.
97. Rahmani, A.M. et al. (2015) Smart e-Health Gateway: Bringing Intelligence to Internet-of-Things Based Ubiquitous Healthcare Systems, 12th Annual IEEE Consumer Communications and Networking Conference (CCNC), 826–834.
98. Raza, S. (2013) Lightweight security solutions for the Internet of Things, PhD thesis, School of Innovation, Design and Engineering, Malardalen University, Sweden.

99. Research and Markets (2016) IoT in Healthcare - Types, Technologies & Services, Applications, By Regions, Global Market Drivers, Opportunities, Trends, and Forecasts, 2016–2022, [Online]: http://www.researchandmarkets.com/research/8pjcct/iot_in_healthcare.
100. Rezvan, M. and Barekatain, M. (2015) The Sensors Are Innovative in Internet of Things, S. Mumtaz et al. (eds.): WICON 2014, LNICST 146, pp. 253–261, Springer Cham Heidelberg New York Dordrecht London.
101. Rodríguez-Mazahua, L. et. al. (2015) A general perspective of Big Data: applications, tools, challenges and trends, The Journal of Supercomputing, vol. 2, no. 8, pp. 3073–3113.
102. Said, O. and Tolba, A. (2012) SEAIoT: Scalable E-Health Architecture based on Internet of Things, International Journal of Computer Applications (0975–8887) Volume 59– No.13.
103. Santos, A., Macedo, J., Costa, A., Nicolau, M.J. (2014) Internet of Things and Smart Objects for M-Health Monitoring and Control, CENTERIS 2014 - Conference on ENTERprise Information Systems/ ProjMAN 2014 - International Conference on Project MANagement/ HCIST 2014 - International Conference on Health and Social Care Information Systems and Technologies, Procedia Technology 16:1351–1360.
104. Salvi, D., Villalba Mora, E. and Arredondo Waldmeyer, M. T. (2010) An architecture for secure e-Health systems. Universidad Politecnica de Madrid, Spain. Vol.1, pp. 2–4.
105. Sharp, J. (2013) Health Start-Ups! - The Internet of Things Creeps into Healthcare, [Online]: http://www.healthworkscollective.com/sharpjw1/112411/health-start-ups-internet-things-creeps-healthcare.
106. Shih, F. and Zhang, M. (2010) Towards Supporting Contextual Privacy in Body Sensor Networks for Health Monitoring Service. [Online]: http://www.w3.org/2010/policy-ws/papers/09-Shih-Zhang-MIT.pdf.
107. Stackowiak, R., Licht, A., Mantha, V. and Nagode, L. (2015) Big Data and The Internet of Things, Enterprise Information Architecture for a New Age, Apress.
108. Stein, J. (2015) The Emergence of the 'Internet of Medical Things'. Huffpost Tech. [Online]: http://www.huffingtonpost.com/josh-stein/the-emergence-of-the-inte_b_6801714.html.
109. Steinwachs, D. M. and Hughes, R.G. (2008) Patient Safety and Quality: An Evidence-Based Handbook for Nurses: Health Services Research: Scope and Significance (Chapter 8), Agency for Healthcare Research and Quality (US).
110. Suciu, G. et al. (2015) Big Data, Internet of Things and Cloud Convergence – An Architecture for Secure E-Health Applications, J Med Syst 39:141.
111. Suryadevara, N. K., Kelly, S. and Mukhopadhyay, S. C. (2014) Internet of Things Challenges and Opportunities: Ambient Assisted Living Environment Towards Internet of Things Using Multifarious Sensors Integrated with XBee Platform, Springer International Publishing Switzerland.
112. Suryadevara, N. K. and Mukhopadhyay S. C. (2015) Smart Homes, Design, Implementation and Issues, Smart Sensors, Measurement and Instrumentation, Volume 14, Springer International Publishing Switzerland.
113. Ta, V.-D., Liu, C.-M., Nkabinde, G. W. (2016) Big Data Stream Computing in Healthcare Real-Time Analytics, International Conference on Cloud Computing and Big Data Analysis, pp. 37–42.
114. Takpor, T.O. and Atayero, A.A. (2015) Integrating Internet of Things and EHealth Solutions for Students' Healthcare, Proceedings of the World Congress on Engineering Vol I WCE 2015, London, U.K.
115. Telefónica IoT Team (2015) 5 Amazing Things come true thanks to the IoT: eHealth Edition, [Online]: https://iot.telefonica.com/blog/5-amazing-things-come-true-thanks-to-the-iot-ehealth-edition.
116. Theodoropoulos, S. (n.d.) On the effectiveness of Publicly or Privately produced Health care services, [Online]: www.vsfs.cz/…/1_ws_3_1_theodopulos.doc.
117. Ting, D. (2015) The Internet of Things Can Revolutionize Healthcare, But Security is Key. [Online]: http://histalk2.com/2015/05/28/readers-write-the-internet-of-things-can-revolutionize-healthcare-but-security-is-key/.

118. Tsai, F. S. (2010) Security Issues in E-Healthcare, Journal of Medical and Biological Engineering, 30(4): 209–214.
119. Turner, J.W., Thomas, R. J., and Reinsch, N. L. (2004) Willingness to try a new communication technology: Perpetual factors and task situations in a health care context. J. Bus. Comm. 41(1):5–26.
120. Uniyal, D. and Raychoudhury, V. (2014) Pervasive Healthcare: A Comprehensive Survey of Tools and Techniques, arXiv:1411.1821 [cs.CY].
121. Vermesan, O. and Friess, P. (2014) Internet of Things – From Research and Innovation to Market Deployment, Rivers Publishers Series in Communication.
122. Waegemann, C. P. (n.d.) Confidentiality and Security for e-Health. CEO, Medical Records Institute (MRI). [Online]: https://www.itu.int/itudoc/itu-t/workshop/e-health/s5-05.pdf.
123. Wang, L. et al. (2012) Technology Enabled Knowledge Translation for eHealth: Principles and Practice, Healthcare Delivery in the Information Age (K. Ho et al. (eds.),) - Chapter 23: Low-Cost Health Care: Improving Care to Rural Chinese Communities Through the Innovations of Integrated Diagnostic Terminals and Cloud Computing Platforms, Springer Science + Business Media.
124. Weber, R. H and Weber, R. (2010) Internet of Things: Legal Perspectives. Springer-Verlag Berlin Heidelberg.
125. Weerasinghe, D. (ed.) (2009) eHealth - Lecture Notes of the Institute for Computer Sciences, Social Informatics and Telecommunications Engineering, Germany.
126. West, D. M. (2016) How 5G technology enables the health Internet of Things, Center for technology innovation at Brookings.
127. Wickramasinghe, N. et al. (eds.) (2012) Critical Issues for the Development of Sustainable E-health Solutions, Healthcare Delivery in the Information Age, Springer Science + Business Media, LLC.
128. Wiecha, J. and Pollard, T. (2004) The Interdisciplinary eHealth Team: Chronic Care for the Future, J Med Internet Res 2004; 6(3): e22.
129. Wilkowska, W. and Ziefle, M. (2012) Privacy and data security in E-health: Requirements from the user's perspective. Health Informatics Journal 18(3) pp. 191–201.
130. Wilson, D.H. and Atkenson, C. (2005) Simultaneous Tracking and Activity Recognition (STAR) Using Many Anonymous, Binary Sensors. In Proceedings of the Springer Berlin Heidelberg, Pervasive computing, pp. 62–79.
131. Wootton, R. (2001) Telemedicine. Br. Med. J. 323:557–560.
132. Wright, D. (1998) Telemedicine and developing countries. J. Telemed. Telecare. 4(2) L2–37.
133. Yan, L. et al. (2008) The Internet of Things, From RFID to the Next-Generation Pervasive Networked Systems. Auerbach Publications, Taylor & Francis Group.
134. Yang, G. et al. (2014) A Health-IoT Platform Based on the Integration of Intelligent Packaging, Unobtrusive Bio-Sensor and Intelligent Medicine Box, IEEE Transactions on Industrial Informatics.
135. Zhang, X., Yu, P. and Yan, J. (2014) Patients' adoption of the e-appointment scheduling service: A case study in primary healthcare, Investing in E-Health: People, Knowledge and Technology for a Healthy Future, H. Grain et al. (eds.), pp. 176–181, The authors and IOS Press.

Fog Computing in Medical Internet-of-Things: Architecture, Implementation, and Applications

Harishchandra Dubey, Admir Monteiro, Nicholas Constant, Mohammadreza Abtahi, Debanjan Borthakur, Leslie Mahler, Yan Sun, Qing Yang, Umer Akbar and Kunal Mankodiya

Abstract In the era when the market segment of Internet of Things (IoT) tops the chart in various business reports, it is apparently envisioned that the field of medicine expects to gain a large benefit from the explosion of wearables and internet-connected sensors that surround us to acquire and communicate unprecedented data on symptoms, medication, food intake, and daily-life activities impacting one's health and wellness. However, IoT-driven healthcare would have to overcome many barriers, such as: (1) There is an increasing demand for data storage on cloud servers where the analysis of the medical big data becomes increasingly complex; (2) The data, when communicated, are vulnerable to security and privacy issues; (3) The communication of the continuously collected data is not only costly but also energy hungry; (4) Operating and maintaining the sensors directly from the cloud servers are non-trial tasks. This book chapter defined Fog Computing in the context of medical IoT. Conceptually, Fog Computing is a service-oriented intermediate layer in IoT, providing the interfaces between the sensors and cloud servers for facilitating connectivity, data transfer, and queryable local database. The centerpiece of Fog

H. Dubey (✉)
Center for Robust Speech Systems, Erik Jonsson School of Engineering and Computer Science, The University of Texas at Dallas, Richardson, TX 75080, USA
e-mail: harishchandra.dubey@utdallas.edu

A. Monteiro · N. Constant · M. Abtahi · D. Borthakur · Y. Sun · Q. Yang · K. Mankodiya
Department of Electrical, Computer, and Biomedical Engineering, University of Rhode Island, Kingston, RI, USA

K. Mankodiya
e-mail: kunalm@uri.edu

L. Mahler
Department of Communicative Disorders, University of Rhode Island, Kingston, RI, USA

H. Dubey · A. Monteiro · N. Constant · M. Abtahi · D. Borthakur · K. Mankodiya
Wearable Biosensing Lab, University of Rhode Island, Kingston, RI, USA

U. Akbar
Movement Disorders Program, Rhode Island Hospital, Providence, RI, USA

© Springer International Publishing AG 2017

S.U. Khan et al. (eds.), *Handbook of Large-Scale Distributed Computing in Smart Healthcare*, Scalable Computing and Communications,
DOI 10.1007/978-3-319-58280-1_11

computing is a low-power, intelligent, wireless, embedded computing node that carries out signal conditioning and data analytics on raw data collected from wearables or other medical sensors and offers efficient means to serve telehealth interventions. We implemented and tested an fog computing system using the Intel Edison and Raspberry Pi that allows acquisition, computing, storage and communication of the various medical data such as pathological speech data of individuals with speech disorders, Phonocardiogram (PCG) signal for heart rate estimation, and Electrocardiogram (ECG)-based Q, R, S detection. The book chapter ends with experiments and results showing how fog computing could lessen the obstacles of existing cloud-driven medical IoT solutions and enhance the overall performance of the system in terms of computing intelligence, transmission, storage, configurable, and security. The case studies on various types of physiological data shows that the proposed Fog architecture could be used for signal enhancement, processing and analysis of various types of bio-signals.

Keywords Big data · Body area network · Body sensor network · Edge computing · Fog computing · Medical cyber-physical systems · Medical internet-of-things · Telecare · Tele-treatment · Wearable devices

1 Introduction

The recent advances in Internet of Things (IoT) and growing use of wearables for the collection of physiological data and bio-signals led to an emergence of new distributed computing paradigms that combined wearable devices with the medical internet of things for scalable remote tele-treatment and telecare [11, 14, 36]. Such systems are useful for wellness and fitness monitoring, preliminary diagnosis and long-term tracking of patients with acute disorders. Use of Fog computing reduces the logistics requirements and cut-down the associated medicine and treatment costs (See Fig. 1). Fog computing have found emerging applications into other domains such as geo-spatial data associated with various healthcare issues [4].

This book chapter highlights the recent advancements and associated challenges in employing wearable internet of things (wIoT) and body sensor networks (BSNs) for healthcare applications. We present the research conducted in Wearable Biosensing Lab and other research groups at the University of Rhode Island. We developed prototypes using Raspberry Pi and Intel Edison embedded boards and conducted case studies on three healthcare scenarios: (1) Speech Tele-treatment of patients with Parkinson's disease; (2) Electrocardiogram (ECG) monitoring; (3) Phonocardiography (PCG) for heart rate estimation. This book chapter extends the methods and systems published in our earlier conferences papers by adding novel system changes and algorithms for robust estimation of clinical features.

This chapter made the following contributions to the area of *Fog Computing for Medical Internet-of-Things*:

- **Fog Hardware**: Intel Edison and Raspberry Pi were leveraged to formulate two prototype architectures. Both of the architectures can be used for each of the three case-studies mentioned above.

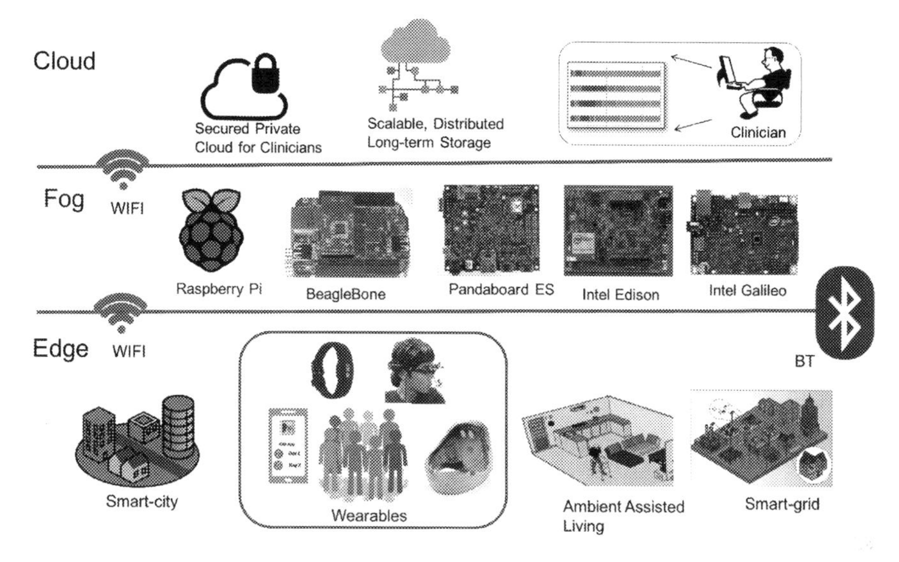

Fig. 1 Fog computing as an intermediate computing layer between edge devices (wearables) and cloud (backend). The Fog computer enhances the overall efficiency by providing computing near the edge devices. Such frameworks are useful for wearables (employed for healthcare, fitness and wellness tracking), smart-grid, smart-cities and ambient-assisted living etc.

- **Edge Computing of Clinical Features**: The Fog devices executed a variety of algorithms to extract clinical features and performed primary diagnosis using data collected from wearable sensors;
- **Interoperability**: We designed frontend apps for body sensor network such as android app for smartwatch [22], PPG wrist-band, and backend cloud infrastructure for long-term storage. In addition, transfer, communication, authentication, storage and execution procedures of data were implemented in the Fog computer.
- **Security**: In order to ensure security and data privacy, we built an encrypted server that handles user authentication and associated privileges. The rule-based authentication scheme is also a novel contribution of this chapter where only the individuals with privileges (such as clinicians) could access the associated data from the patients.
- **Case Study on Fog Computing for Medical IoT-based Tele-treatment and Monitoring**: We conducted three case studies: (1) Speech Tele-treatment of patients with Parkinson's disease; (2) Electrocardiogram (ECG) monitoring; (3) Phonocardiography (PCG) for heart rate estimation. Even if we conducted validation experiments on only three types of healthcare data, the proposed Fog architecture could be used for analysis of other bio-signals and healthcare data as well.
- **Android API for Wearable (Smartwatch-based) Audio Data Collection**: The EchoWear app that was introduced in [12] is used in proposed architecture for collecting the audio data from wearables. We have released the library to public at: https://github.com/harishdubey123/wbl-echowear.

2 Related and Background Works

In this section, we present recent emergence of wearables and fog computing for enhancement processing of physiological data for healthcare applications (Fig. 2).

2.1 Wearable Big Data in Healthcare

The medical data is collected by the intelligent edge devices such as wearables, wrist-bands, smartwatches, smart textiles etc. The intelligence refers to knowledge of analytics, devices, clinical application and the consumer behavior. Such smart data is structured, homogeneous and meaningful with negligible amount of noise and meta-data [28]. The big data and quiet recently smart data trend had revolutionized the biomedical and healthcare domain. With increasing use of wireless and wearable body sensor networks (BSNs), the amount of data aggregated by edge devices and synced to the cloud is growing at enormous rate [30]. The pharmaceutical companies are leveraging deep learning and data analytics on their huge medical databases. These databases are results of digitization of patient's medical records. The data obtained from patient's health records, clinical trials and insurance programs provided an opportunity for data mining. Such databases are heterogeneous, unstructured, scalable and contain significant amount of noise and meta-data. The noise and meta-data have low or no useful information. Cleaning and structuring the real-world data is another challenge in processing medical big data. In recent years, the big data trend had transformed the healthcare, wellness and fitness industry. Adding value and innovation in data processing chain could help patients and healthcare stakeholders accomplish the treatment goals in lower cost with reduced logistic requirements [30]. Authors in [45] presented the smart data as a result of using semantic web and data analytics on structured collection of big data. Smart data attempts to provide

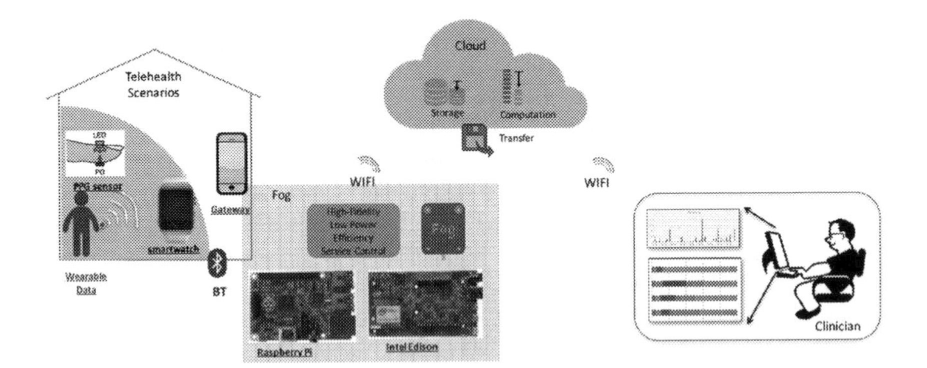

Fig. 2 The conceptual overview of the proposed Fog architecture that assisted Medical Internet of Things framework in tele-treatment scenarios

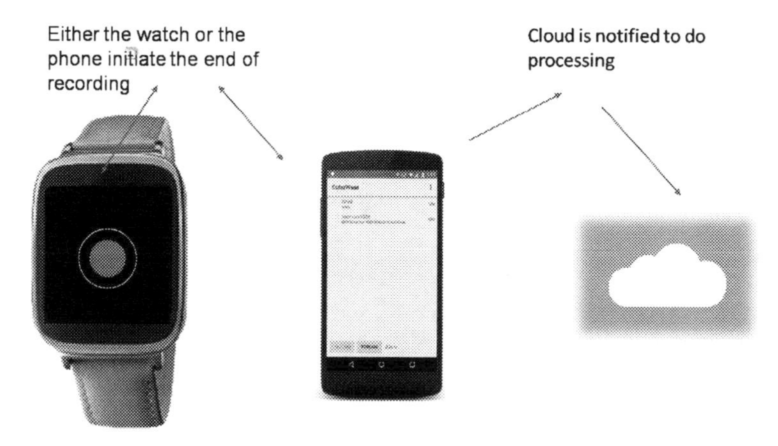

Fig. 3 The flow of information and control between three main components of the medical IoT system for smartwatch-based speech treatment [12]. The smartwatch is triggered by the patients with Parkinson's disease. At fixed timings set by patients, caregivers or their speech-language pathologist (SLPs), the tablet triggers the recording of speech data. The smartwatch interacts with the tablet via Bluetooth. Once tablet gets the data from smartwatch, it send to the Fog devices that process the clinical speech. Finally, the features were sent to the cloud from where those could be queried by clinicians for long-term comparative study. SLPs use the final features for designing customized speech exercises and treatment regime in accordance with patient's communications deficits

a superior avenue for better decision and inexpensive processing for person-centered medicine and healthcare. The medical data such as diagnostic images, genetic test results and biometric information are getting generated at large scale. Such data has not just the high volume but also a wide variety and different velocity. It necessitates the novel ways for storing, managing, retrieving and processing such data. The smart medical data demand development of novel scalable big data architecture and applicable algorithms for intelligent data analytics. Authors also underlined the challenges in semantic-rich data processing for intelligent inference on practical use cases [45] (Figs. 3 and 4 and Table 1).

2.2 *Speech Treatments of Patients with Parkinson's Disease*

The patients with Parkinson's Disease (PD) have their own unique set of speech deficits. We developed EchoWear [12] as a technology front-end for monitoring the speech from PD patients using smartwatch. The speech-language pathologists (SLPs) had access to such as system for remote monitoring of their patients. The rising cost of healthcare, the increase in elderly population, and the prevalence of chronic diseases around the world urgently demand the transformation of healthcare from a hospital-centered system to a person-centered environment, with a focus on patient's disease management as well as their wellbeing.

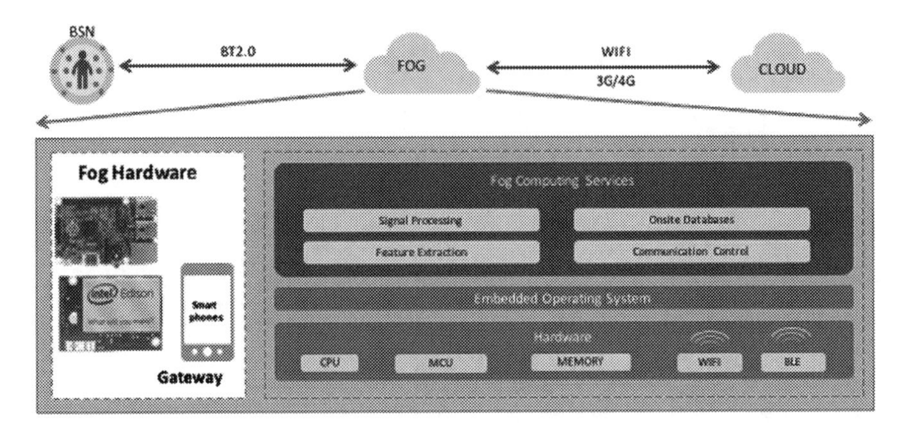

Fig. 4 The proposed Fog architecture that acquired the data from body sensor networks (BSNs) through smartphone/tablet gateways. It has two choices for fog computers: Intel Edison and Raspberry Pi. The extraction of clinical features was done locally on fog device that was kept in patient's home (or near the patient in care-homes). Finally, the extracted information from bio-signals was uploaded to the secured cloud backend from where it could be accessed by clinicians. The proposed Fog architecture consists of four modules, namely BSNs (e.g. smartwatch), gateways (e.g. smartphone/tablets), fog devices (Intel Edison/Raspberry Pi) and cloud backend

Table 1 A comparison between Fog computing and cloud computing (adopted from [7])

Criterion	Fog nodes close to IoT devices	Fog aggregation nodes	Cloud computing
Response time	Milliseconds to sub-second	Seconds to minutes	Minutes, days, weeks
Application examples	Telemedicine and training	Visualization simple analytics	Big data analytics graphical dashboards
How long IoT data is stored	Transient	Short duration: perhaps hours, days or weeks	Months or years
Geographic coverage	Very local: for example, one city block	Regional	Global

Speech Disorders affected approximately 7.5 million people in US [40]. Dysarthria (caused by Parkinson's disease or other speech disorders) refers to motor speech disorder resulting from impairments in human speech production system. The speech production system consists of the lips, tongue, vocal folds, and/or diaphragm. Depending on the part of nervous system that is affected, there are various types of dysarthria. The patients with dysarthria posses specific speech characteristics such as difficult to understand speech, limited movement in lips, tongue and jaw, abnormal pitch and rhythm. It also includes poor voice quality, for instance, hoarse, breathy or nasal voice. Dysarthria results from neural dysfunction. It might happen at birth (cerebral palsy) or developed later in person's life. It can be due to variety of ailments in the nervous system, such as Motor neuron diseases, Alzheimer's disease, Cerebral Palsy (CP), Huntington's disease, Multiple Sclerosis, Parkinson's disease (PD), Traumatic brain injury (TBI), Mental health issues, Stroke, Progressive neurological conditions, Cancer of the head, neck and throat (including laryngectomy). The patients with dysarthria are subjectively evaluated by the speech-language pathologist (SLP) who identifies the speech difficulties and decide the type and severity of the communication deficit [16].

Authors in [48] compared the perceived loudness of speech and self-perception of speech in patients with idiopathic Parkinson's disease (PD) with healthy controls. Thirty patients with PD and fourteen healthy controls participated in the research survey. Various speech tasks were performed and nine speech and voice characteristics were used for evaluation. Results showed that the patients with PD had significant reduction in loudness as compared to healthy controls during various speech tasks. These results furnished additional information on speech characteristics of patients with PD that might be useful for effective speech treatment of such population [48]. Authors in [24] studied the acoustic characteristics of voice in patients with PD. Thirty patients with early stage PD and thirty patients with later stage PD were compared with thirty healthy controls for acoustic characteristics of the voice. The speech task included sustained /a/ and one minute monologue. The voice of patients with early as well as later stage PD were found to have reduced loudness, limited loudness and pitch variability, breathiness, and harshness. In general, the voice of patients with PD had lower mean intensity levels and reduced maximum phonational frequency range as compared to healthy controls [24].

Authors in [50] studied and evaluated the voice and speech quality in patients with and without deep brain stimulation of the subthalamic nucleus (STN-DBS) before and after LSVT LOUD therapy. The goal of the study was to do a comparative study of improvement in surgical patients as compared to the non-surgical ones. Results showed that the LSVT LOUD is recommended for voice and speech treatment of patients with PD following STN-DBS surgery. Authors in [18] performed acoustic analysis of voice from 41 patients with PD and healthy controls. The speech exercises included in the study were the sustained /a/ for 2 s and reading sentences. The acoustic measures for quantifying the speech quality were fundamental frequency, perturbation in fundamental frequency, shimmer, and harmonic to noise ratio of the sustained /a/, phonation range, dynamic range, and maximum phonation time. Authors concluded that the patients with PD had higher jitter, lower harmonics to noise ratio, lower frequency and intensity variability, lower phonation range, the presence of low voice intensity, mono pitch, voice arrests, and struggle irrespective of the severity of the PD symptoms.

People suffering from Parkinson's disease experience speech production difficulty associated with Dysarthria. Dysarthria is characterized by monotony of pitch, reduced loudness, an irregular rate of speech and, imprecise consonants and changes in voice quality [34]. Speech-language pathologists do the evaluation, diagnosis and treat communication disorders. Literature suggests that Lee Silverman Voice Treatment (LSVT) has been most efficient behavioral treatment for voice and speech disorders in Parkinson's disease. Telehealth monitoring is very effective for the speech-language pathology, and smart devices like EchoWear [12] can be of much use in such situations. Several cues indicate the relationship of dysarthria and acoustic features. Some of them are,

1. Shallower F2 trajectories in male speakers with dysarthria is observed in [31].
2. Vowel space area was found to be reduced relative to healthy controls for male speakers with amyotrophic lateral sclerosis [31].
3. Shimmers as described in [13] as a measure of variation in amplitude of the speech and it is an important speech quality metric for people with speech disorders.
4. Like shimmers, Jitters (pitch variations) and loudness and sharpness of the speech signal can be used as a cue for speech disorders [13].
5. In ataxic dysarthria, patients can produce distorted vowels and excess variation in loudness, so speech prosody and acoustic analysis are of much use.
6. Multi dimensional voice analysis as stated in [31] plays an important role in motor speech disorder diagnosis and analysis. Parameters that can effectively used are relative perturbation (RAP), pitch perturbation quotient (PPQ), fundamental frequency variation (vF0), shimmer in dB (ShdB), shimmer percent (Shim), peak amplitude variation (vam) and amplitude tremor intensity index (ATRI).
7. Shrinking of the F0 range as well as vowel space are observed in dysarthria speech. Moreover, from the comparison of F0 range and vowel formant frequencies, it is suggested that speech effort to produce wider F0 range can influence vowel quality as well.

EchoWear [12] is a smartwatch technology for voice and speech treatments of patients with Parkinson's disease. Considering the difficulties associated with the patients in following prescribed exercise regimes outside the clinic, this device remotely monitors speech and voice exercise as prescribed by speech-language pathologists. The speech quality metrics used in EchoWear presently as stated in [12] were average loudness level and average fundamental frequency (F0). Features were derived from the short-term speech spectrum of a speech signal. To find the fundamental frequency, EchoWear uses SWIPE pitch estimator, whereas other methods such as cepstral analysis and autocorrelation methods are also extensively used for estimation of the pitch. The software Praat is designed for visualizing the spectrum of a speech signal for analysis. Fundamental frequency (F0) variability is associated with the PD speech. There is a decrease variation in pitch, i.e. Fundamental frequency associated with PD speech.

3 Proposed Fog Architecture

In this section, we describe the implementation of the proposed Fog architecture. Figure 5 shows the overall architecture of proposed system in the context of frontend and backend services. It shows the information flow from the patients to SLPs through the communication and processing interfaces. Instead of layers, we describe

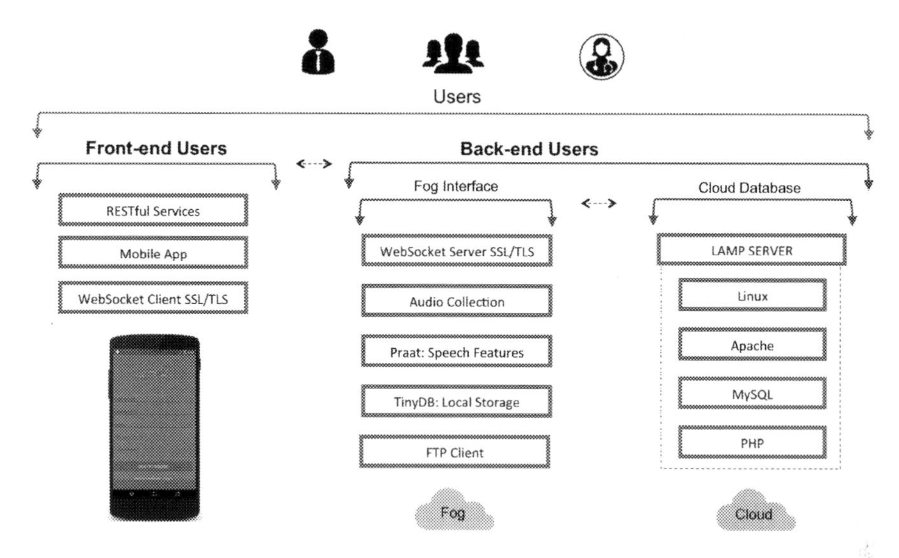

Fig. 5 Overall architecture of the proposed Fog architecture in the context of frontend and backend services. It shows the information flow from patients to clinicians through the modular architecture

the implementation using three modules namely, (1) Fog device; (2) Backend Cloud Database; and (3) Frontend App Services. These three modules gave a convenient representation for describing the multi-user model of the proposed Fog architecture.

3.1 Fog Computing Device

To transfer the audio file/other data file from a patient, we used socket streaming using TCP wrapped in Secure Socket Layer/Transmission Layer Security (SSL/TLS) sockets to ensure the secure transmission. Sockets provide communication framework for devices using different protocols such as TCP and UDP that could then be wrapped in secured sockets. Next, we describe these protocols and their usage in the proposed architecture.

- **Transmission Control Protocol (TCP)** is a networking protocol that allows guaranteed and reliable delivery of files. It is a connection-oriented and bi-directional protocol. In other words, both devices could send and receive files using this protocol. Each point of the connection involved Internet Protocol (IP) address and a port number so the connection could be made with a specific device. Furthermore, we wrapped the TCP sockets in SSL Sockets for ensuring the security and privacy of the data collected from the users/patients.

- **Secure Sockets Layer (SSL)** is a network communication protocol that allows encrypted authentication for network sockets from the server and client sides. To implement it in the proposed Fog architecture, we used two python modules, namely *SSL* and *socket*. To create the certifications for the server and client, we also used the command line program called *OpenSSL* [41]. *OpenSSL* is an open-source project that provides a robust, commercial-grade, and full-featured toolkit for the Transport Layer Security (TLS) and Secure Sockets Layer (SSL) protocols.

Once all the SSL certification keys were built for client (the Android gateway devices/wearables) and server (Fog computer e.g. Intel Edison or Raspberry Pi), we ran the secure sockets on the server and continuously listened for a connection for file transfer. We renamed the file with date and time stamps before it could be used for further processing. As soon as the audio file was completely transferred, the connection was closed and the processing began. We used the python based *Praat* and *Christian's Library* described for processing and analysis of audio data. For other healthcare data such as Phonocardiography (PCG) data and Electrocardiogram (ECG) data etc., we implemented the associated methods using Python, C and GNU Octave.

3.2 Frontend App Services

For the frontend users, including patients and clinicians (SLPs), we designed Android applications and web applications that could be used to log-into the system and access clinical features. Also, front-end apps were running on wearable devices are facilitating the data collection. Our app, *IoT PD*, took advantage of the REST protocol. We used REST protocol for simplicity of implementation. For every REST request of data information gathering, we returned a JSON (JavaScript Object Notation), a format of data-interchange between programs [25]. The *IoT PD* app is based on software engine Hermes. We open-source the URI library for audio data collection from wearable devices.

The app allowed access to two categories of users as shown in Fig. 6. Both the patients and healthcare providers were allowed to login and view their profile; however their profiles were different, only the clinicians could give permission to their patients for app registration. Further, the physician could setup personalized notifications for their patients. For example, the physician could schedule a personalized exercise regime for a given patient so that their speech functions could be enhanced. On the other hand, patients could only view their information and visual data.

3.3 Backend Cloud Database

To support the centralized storage of clinical features and analytics, we implemented a backend cloud database using *PHP* and *MySQL*. Firstly, we set up a *Linux, Apache,*

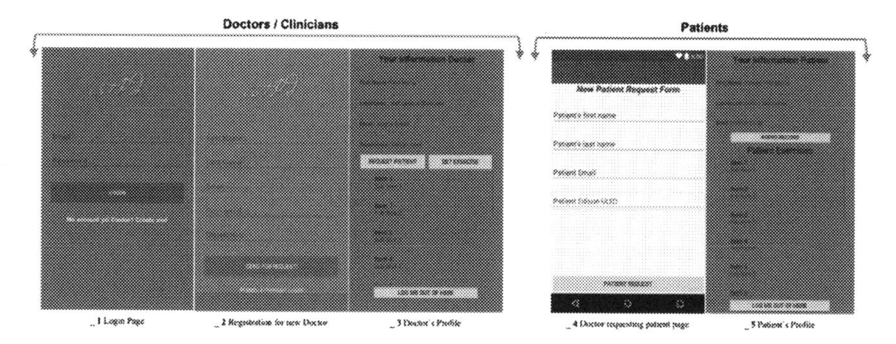

Fig. 6 The interface view of the IoT PD Android app for frontend users such as clinicians, caregivers and patients. Different categories of users have different privileges. For example, a patient can register with the app only upon receiving the clinician's approval

MySQL, PHP (LAMP) server, an open-source web platform for development on *Linux* systems using *Apache* for web servicing, *MySQL* as database system for management and storage, and *PHP* as the language for server interaction with applications [49]. The main component of the backend was the relational database development. We designed a database revolving around the users and Fog computers that could easily engage with the database. It created three tables that were used for the users (patients and healthcare providers such as clinicians). The fourth table was created for the information extracted from the patient's data. The extracted features obtained from the Fog computer were entered in the data table.

3.4 Pathological Speech Data Collection

Earlier, we described our implementation of EchoWear that was used in an in-clinic validation study on six patients with Parkinson's disease (PD). We received an approval (no: 682871-2) of the University of Rhode Island's Institutional Review Board to conduct human studies involving the presented technologies including *IoT PD* and proposed Fog architecture. First, the six patients were given an intensive voice training in the clinic by Leslie Mahler, a speech-language pathologist, who also prescribed home speech tasks for each patient. Patients were given a home kit consisting of a smartwatch, a companion tablet and charging accessories. Patients were recommended to wear the smartwatch during the day. Patients chose their preferred timings for speech exercise. A tactile vibration of the smartwatch was used as a notification method to remind the patients to perform speech exercises. The *IoT PD* app took the timings to set the notifications accordingly. Home exercise regime had six speech tasks. The six speech tasks assigned to patients with PD are given in Table 2.

Table 2 List of speech exercises performed by the patients with Parkinson's disease

Task	Exercise name	Description
t_1	Vowel prolongation	Sustain the vowel /a/ for as long as possible for three repetitions
t_2	High pitch	Start saying /a/ at talking pitch and then go up and hold for 5 s (three repetitions)
t_3	Low pitch	Start saying /a/ at talking pitch and then go down and hold for 5 s (three repetitions)
t_4	Read sentence	Read 'The boot on top is packed to keep'
t_5	Read passage	Read the 'farm' passage
t_6	Functional speech task	Read a set of customized sentences
t_7	Monologue	Explain happiest day of your life

Speech-language pathologists (SLPs) use extensive number of speech parameters in their diagnosis. We skip the clinical details of prescription as it is out-of-the-scope of this book chapter.

3.5 *Dynamic Time Warping*

Dynamic time warping (DTW) is an algorithm for finding similar patterns in a time-series data. DTW has been used for time-series mining for a variety of applications such as business, finance, single word recognition, walking pattern detection, and analysis of ECG signals. Usually, we use Euclidean distance to measure the distance between two points. For example, consider two vectors, $x = [x_1, x_2, \ldots, x_n]$ and $y = [y_1, y_2, \ldots, y_n]$

$$d(x, y) = \sqrt{(x_1 - y_1)^2 + (x_2 - y_2)^2 + (\cdot x_n - y_n)^2} \quad (1)$$

Euclidean distance works well in many areas. But for some special case where two similar and out-of-phase series are to be compared, Euclidean distance fails to detect similarity. For example, consider two time series A = [1, 1, 1, 2, 8, 1] and B = [1, 1, 1, 8, 2, 1], the Euclidean distance between them is $\sqrt{72}$. Thus, DTW is an effective algorithm that can detect the similarity between two series regardless of different length, and/or phase difference. The example vectors are similar but the similarity could not be inferred by Euclidean distance metric while DTW can detect the similarity easily. DTW is based on the idea of dynamic programming (DP). It builds an adjacency matrix then finds the shortest path across it. DTW is more effective than Euclidean distance for many applications [10] such as gesture recognition [19], fingerprint verification [32], and speech processing [39] (Figs. 7 and 8).

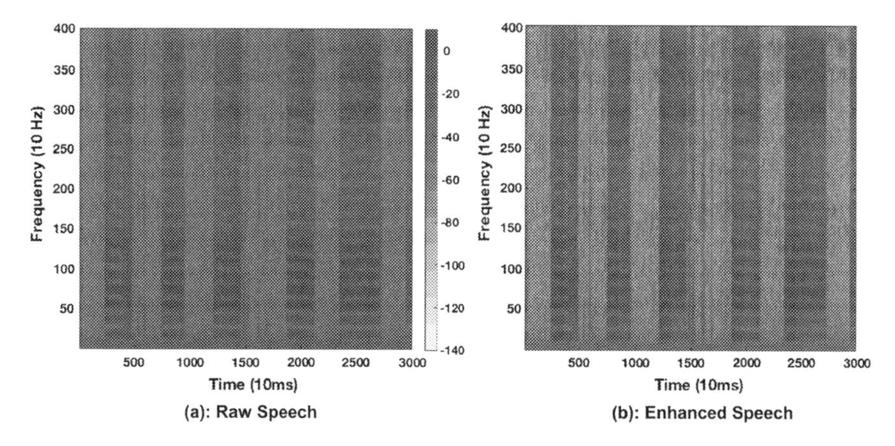

Fig. 7 **a** Spectrogram of acquired speech signal. The frequency sampling rate is 8000 Hz. Time-windows of 25 ms with 10 ms skip-rate were used. **b** Spectrogram of enhanced speech signal

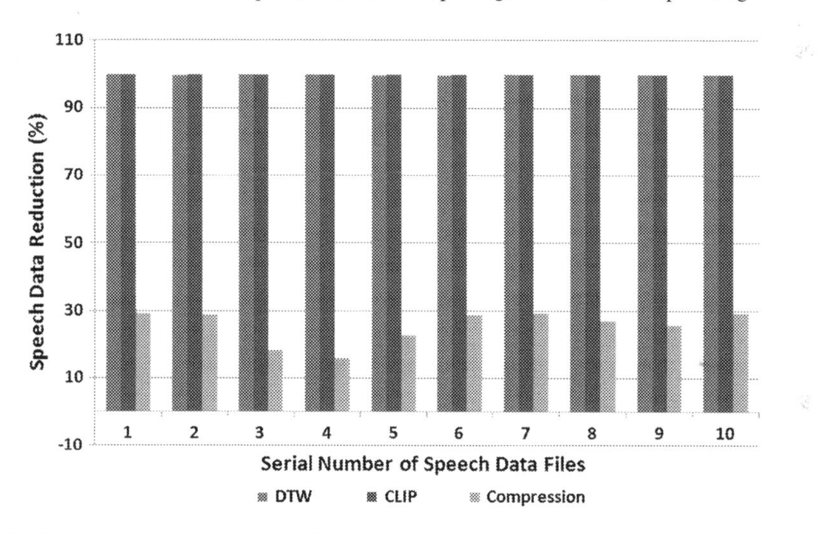

Fig. 8 Bar chart depicting the data reduction achieved by using dynamic time warping (DTW), clinical speech processing (CLIP) and GNU zip compression on ten sample speech files collected from in-home trails of patients with Parkinson's disease (PD)

4 Case Studies Using Proposed Fog Architecture

4.1 Case Study I: Speech Tele-treatment of Patients with Parkinson's Disease

A variety of acoustic and spectral features were derived from the speech content of audio file acquired by wearables. In proposed Fog architecture, noise reduction, automated trimming, and feature extraction were done on the Fog device. In our earlier studies [9, 12, 15, 38], trimming was done manually by human annotator and feature extraction was done in the cloud. In addition, there were no noise reduction done in previous studies [12, 15]. The Fog computer syncs the extracted features and preliminary diagnosis back in the secured cloud backend. Fog was employed for in-home speech treatment of patients with Parkinson's disease. The pathological features were later extracted from the audio signal. Figure 14 shows the block diagram of pathological speech processing module. In our earlier studies, we computed features from the controlled clinical environment and performed Fog device trails in lab scenarios [15]. This paper explored the in-home field application. In-clinic speech data was obtained in quiet scenarios with negligible background noise. On the other hand, data from in-home trials had huge amounts of time-varying non-stationary noise. It necessitated the use of robust algorithms for noise reduction before extracting the pathological features. In addition to previously studied features such as loudness and fundamental frequency, we developed more features for accurate quantification of abnormalities in patient's vocalization. The new features are jitter, frequency modulation, speech rate and sensory pleasantness. In our previous studies, we use just three speech exercises (tasks t_1, t_2 and t_3) for analysis of algorithms. In this paper, we incorporated all six speech exercises. The execution was done in real-time in patient's home unlike pilot data used in our previous studies [15, 38]. Thus, Fog speech processing module is an advancement over earlier studies in [12, 15, 38].

The audio data was acquired and stored in *wav* format. Using perceptual audio coding such as *mp3* would have saved transmission power, storage and execution time as the size of mp3 coded speech data is lower than corresponding wav format. The reason for not using mp3 or other advanced audio codecs is to avoid loss of information. Perceptual audio codes such as mp3 are lossy compression scheme that removes frequency bands that are not perceptually important. Such codecs have worked well for music and audio streaming. However, in pathological speech analysis, patients have very acute vocalizations such as nasal voice, hypernasal voice, mildly slurred speech, monotone voice etc. Clinicians do not recommend lossy coding for speech data as it can cause confusion in diagnosis, monitoring, and evaluation of pathological voice. Since we use the unicast transmission from BSNs to fog computers, we employed Transmission Control Protocol (TCP). The data have to be received in the same order as sent by BSNs. We did not use User Datagram Protocol (UDP) that is more popular for audio/video streaming as UDP does not guarantee receipt of packets. For videos/audios that are perceptually encoded and decoded, small losses lead to temporary degradation in received audio/video. We do not have that luxury in pathological speech or PCG data that have to be guaranteed delivery even if delayed and/or have to be re-transmitted. The pathological data was saved as mono-channel audio sampled at 44.1 kHz with 16-bit precision in .wav format.

4.1.1 Background Noise Reduction

The audio signals from in-home speech exercises are highly contaminated with time-varying background noise. Authors developed a method for reducing non-stationary noise in speech [8]. The audio signal is enhanced using noise estimates obtained from minima controlled recursive averaging. We performed a subjective evaluation for validating the suitability of this algorithm for our data. The enhanced speech was later used for extracting perceptual speech features such as loudness, fundamental frequency, jitter, frequency modulation, speech rate and sensory pleasantness (sharpness). We used the method developed in [8] for reducing non-stationary background noise in speech. It optimized the log-spectral amplitude of the speech using noise estimates from minima-controlled recursive averaging. Authors used two functions for accounting the probability of speech presence in various sub-bands. One of these functions was based on the time frequency distribution of apriori signal-to-noise ratio (SNR) and was used for estimation of the speech spectrum. The second function was decided by the ratio of the energy of noisy speech segment and its minimum value within that time window. Objective, as well as subjective evaluation, illustrated that this algorithm could preserve the weak speech segments contaminated with a high amount of noise [8]. Figure 7 shows the spectrogram of acquired speech signal from in-home trials and the spectrogram of corresponding enhanced speech signal. Speech enhancement is clearly visible in the darker regions (corresponding to speech) and noise reduction in lighter regions (corresponding to silences/pauses).

4.1.2 Automated Trimming of the Speech Signal

We used the method developed in [52] for automated trimming of audio files by removing the non-speech segments. This method was validated to be accurate even at low SNRs that is typical for in-home audio data. The low computational complexity of this algorithm qualifies it for implementation on Fog device with limited resources. After applying the noise reduction method on acquired speech signal, we used voice activity detection (VAD) algorithm for removing the silences. Authors in [52] proposed a simple technique for VAD based on an effective selection of speech frames. The short time-windows of a speech signal are stationary (for 25–40 ms windows). However, for an extended time duration (more than 40 ms), the statistics of speech signal changes significantly rendering unequal relevance of speech frames. It necessitates the selection of effective frames on the basis of posteriori signal-to-noise ratio (SNR). The authors used energy distance as a substitute to the standard cepstral distance for measuring the relevance of speech frames. It resulted in reduced computational complexity of this algorithm. Figure 9 illustrates automated trimming of a speech signal for removing the pauses present in the audio files. We used time-windows of size 25 ms with 10 ms skip-rate between successive windows.

4.1.3 Fundamental Frequency Estimation

We used the method proposed in [23] for estimation of the fundamental frequency. It was found to be effective even at very low SNRs. It is a frequency-domain method referred as Pitch Estimation Filter with Amplitude Compression (PEFAC). We used

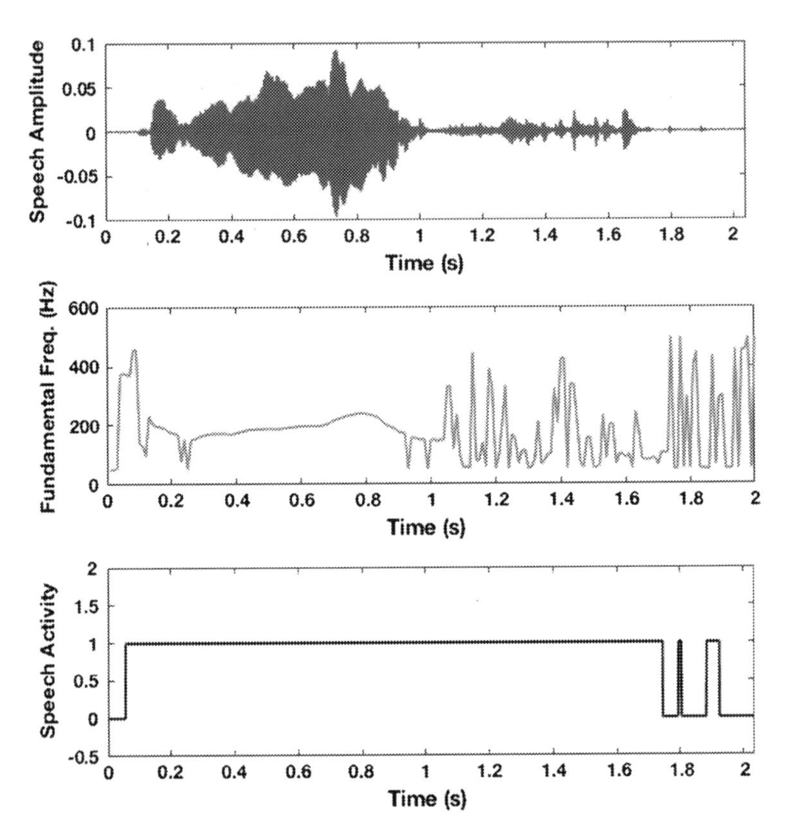

Fig. 9 *Top sub-figure* shows time-domain enhanced speech signal. The *middle sub-figure* depicts corresponding fundamental frequency contour. The *bottom sub-figure* shows the speech activity labels where '1' stands for speech and '0' for silence/pauses. We used speech activity detection proposed in [52]. This is effective and has low computational expense

25 ms time-windows with 10 ms skip-rate for estimation of the fundamental frequency. In the first step, noise components were suppressed by compressing the speech amplitude. In the second step, the speech was filtered such that the energy of harmonics was summed. It involved filtering of power spectral density (PSD) followed by picking the peaks for estimation of the fundamental frequency (in Hz). Figure 9 shows the time-domain speech signal along with automatic trimming decision and pitch estimates for each overlapping windows.

Another method we implement for fundamental frequency estimation is based on harmonic models [2]. Voiced speech is not just periodic but also rich in harmonic, so voiced segments are modeled by adopting harmonic models.

4.1.4 Perceptual Loudness

Speech-language pathologists (SLPs) use loudness as an important speech feature for quantifying the perceptual quality of clinical speech. It is a mathematical quantity computed using various models of the human auditory system. There are different models available for loudness computation valid for specific sound types. We used Zwicker model for loudness computation valid for time-varying signals [56]. The loudness is perceived intensity of a sound. The human ears are more sensitive to some frequencies than the other. This frequency selectivity is quantified by the Bark-scale. The Bark scale defines the critical bands that play an important role in intensity sensation by the human's ears. The specific loudness of a frequency band is denoted as L_0 and measured in units of Phon/Bark. The loudness, L, (in unit Phon) is computed by integrating the specific loudness, L_0, over all the critical-band rates (on bark scale). Mathematically, we have

$$L = \sum_{0}^{24Bark} L_0 \cdot dz \tag{2}$$

Typically, the step-size, dz, is fixed at 0.1 [56]. We used Phon (in dB) as the unit of loudness level. Figure 10 shows a time-domain speech signal and corresponding instantaneous loudness in dB Phon. It depicts the dependence of loudness on speech amplitude.

4.1.5 Jitter

Jitter (J_1) quantifies changes in the vocal period from one cycle to another. Instantaneous Fundamental frequency was used for computing the jitter [53]. J_1 was defined as the average absolute difference between consecutive time-periods. Mathematically, it is given as:

$$J_1 = \frac{1}{M} \sum_{j=1}^{M-1} |F_j - F_{j+1}| \tag{3}$$

where F_j was the j-th extracted vocal period and M is the number of extracted vocal periods.

Figure 11 shows the comparison of jitter of six patients with PD from home-trials. Three patients used the Fog for first week and third week of the trial-month. Another three patients used Fog for second and fourth week. This swapping was done to see the effect of Fog architecture. In absence of Fog device, data was stored in android tablet (gateway) device and later was processed in offline mode. In presence of Fog, the data was processed online. Since same program produced these results, we can compare them. Figure 11 shows the Jitter (in ms) for all cases. We can see that the change in jitter from first/second to third/fourth week is complicated. In some cases

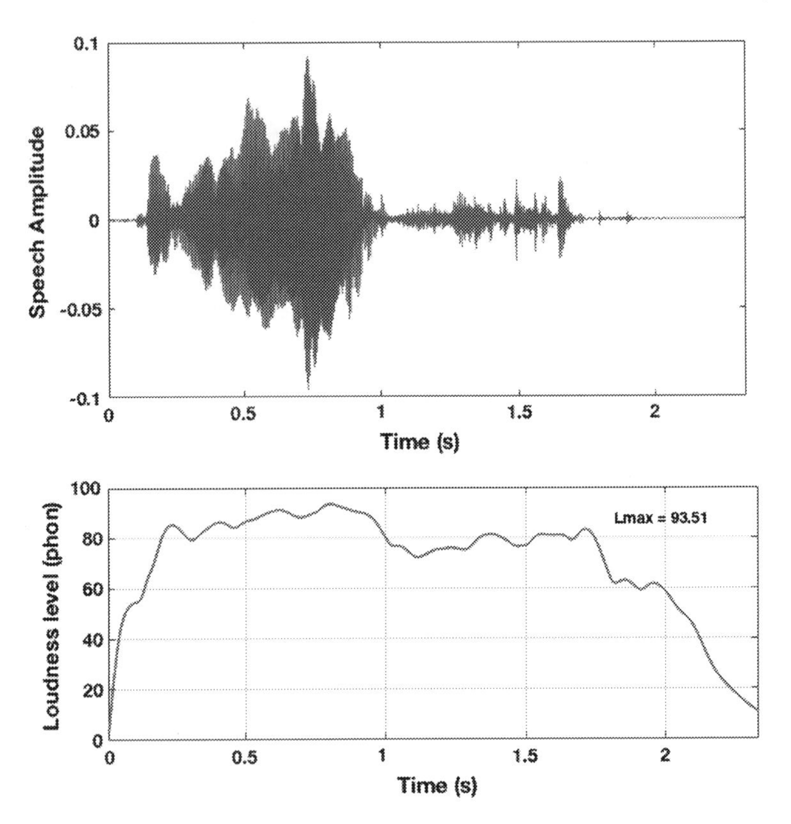

Fig. 10 The time-domain speech signal and corresponding instantaneous loudness *curve*. Loudness was computed over short windows of 25 ms with 10 ms skip-rate

it increases while in other it decreases. Only specialized clinicians can interpret such variations. The Fog architecture facilitate the computation of jitter and sync it to cloud backend. Speech-language pathologists (SLPs) can later access these charts and correlated it with corresponding patient's treatment regime.

4.1.6 Frequency Modulation

It quantifies the presence of sub-harmonics in speech signal. Usually, speech signals with many sub-harmonics lead to a more complicated interplay between various harmonic components making it relevant for perceptual analysis. Mathematically, it is given as [51]:

$$F_{mod} = \frac{\max\left(F_j\right)_{j=1}^{M} - \min\left(F_j\right)_{j=1}^{M}}{\max\left(F_j\right)_{j=1}^{M} + \min\left(F_j\right)_{j=1}^{M}} \quad (4)$$

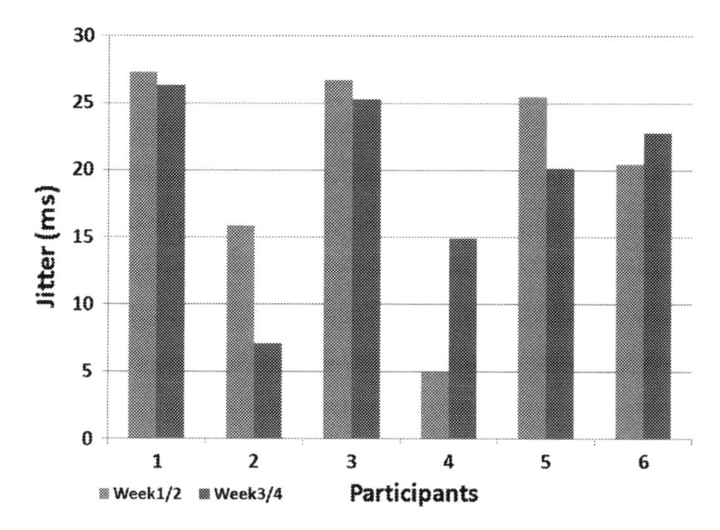

Fig. 11 The average jitter, J_1 (ms) computed using speech samples from six patients with Parkinson's disease who participated in field-trial that lasted 4 weeks. Three patients used Fog for first and third week while other three patients used it for second and fourth week. We are comparing weeks where Fog was used

where F_{mod} is frequency modulation, and F_j is the fundamental frequency of j-th speech frame.

4.1.7 Frequency Range

The range of frequencies is an important feature of speech signal that quantifies its quality [3]. We computed the frequency range as the difference between 5-th and 95-th percentiles. Mathematically, it becomes:

$$F_{range} = F_{95\%} - F_{5\%} \tag{5}$$

Taking 5-th and 95-th percentiles helps in eliminating the influence of outliers in estimates of fundamental frequency that could be caused by impulsive noise and other interfering sounds.

4.1.8 Harmonics to Noise Ratio

Harmonics to Noise Ratio (HNR) quantifies the noise present in the speech signal that results from incomplete closure of the vocal folds during speech production process [53]. We used method proposed in [5] for HNR estimation. The average and standard deviation of the segmental HNR values are useful for perceptual analysis by speech-language pathologist. Lets assume that R_{xx} is normalized autocorrelation and $l_{\max}$ is the lag (in samples) at which it is maximum, except the zero lag. Then, HNR is mathematically given by [5]:

$$HNR_{dB} = 10 \log 10 \left(\frac{R_{xx}(l_{\max})}{1 - R_{xx}(l_{\max})} \right) \tag{6}$$

4.1.9 Spectral Centroid

It is the *center of mass* of spectrum. It measure the *brightness* of an audio signal. Spectral centroid of a spectrum-segment is given by average values of frequency weighted by amplitudes, divided by the sum of amplitudes [43]. Mathematically, we have

$$SC = \frac{\sum_{n=1}^{N} kF[k]}{\sum_{n=1}^{N} F[k]} \tag{7}$$

where SC is the spectral centroid, and $F[k]$ is amplitude of k-th frequency bin of discrete Fourier transform of speech signal.

4.1.10 Spectral Flux

It quantifies the rate of change in power spectrum of speech signal. It is calculated by comparing the normalized power spectrum of a speech-frame with that of other frames. It determines the timbre of speech signal [55] (Fig. 12).

4.1.11 Spectral Entropy

We adopted it for speech-language pathology in this chapter. It is given by:

$$SE = \frac{-\sum P_j log(P_j)}{log(M)} \tag{8}$$

where SE is the spectral entropy, P_j is the power of j-th frequency-bin and M is the number of frequency-bins. Here, $\sum P_k = 1$ as the spectrum is normalized before computing the spectral entropy.

4.1.12 Spectral Flatness

It measures the flatness of speech power spectrum. It quantifies how similar the spectrum is to that of a noise-like signal or a tonal signal. Spectral Flatness (SF) of white

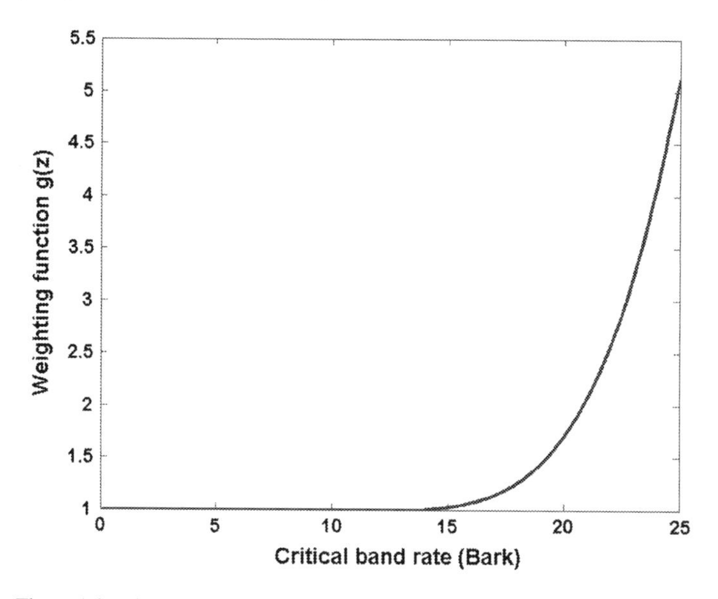

Fig. 12 The weights that were used for computing sharpness based on [56]. Sharpness quantifies perceptual pleasantness of the speech signal. We can see that the higher critical band rates use lower weights for computing the sharpness

noise is 1 as it has constant power spectral density (PSD). A pure sinusoidal tone has SF close to zero showing the high concentration of power at a fixed frequency. Mathematically, SF is ratio of geometric mean of power spectrum to its average value [26].

4.1.13 Sharpness

Sharpness is a mathematical function that quantifies the sensory pleasantness of the speech signal. High sharpness implies low pleasantness. It value depends on the spectral envelope of the signal, amplitude level and its bandwidth. The unit of sharpness is acum (Latin expression). The reference sound producing 1 acum is a narrowband noise, one critical band wide with 1 kHz center frequency at 60 dB intensity level [17]. Sharpness, S is mathematically defined as

$$S = 0.11 \frac{\sum_{0}^{24Bark} L_0 \cdot g(z) \cdot z \cdot dz}{\sum_{0}^{24Bark} L_0 \cdot dz} acum \tag{9}$$

However, its numerator is weighted average of specific loudness (L_0) over the critical band rates. The weighting function, $g(z)$, depends on critical band rates. The $g(z)$ could be interpreted as the mathematical model for the sensation of sharpness shown in Fig. 16.

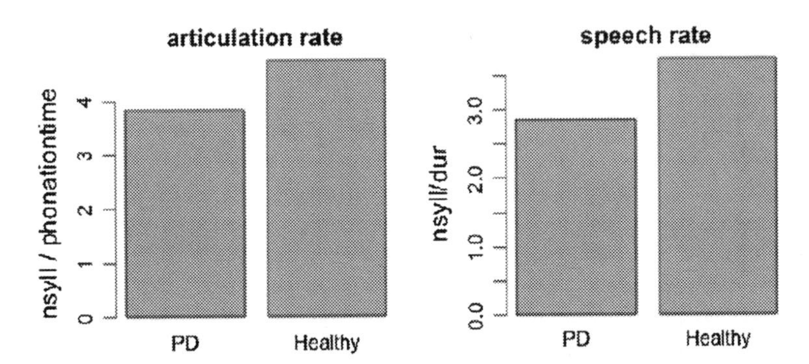

Fig. 13 The *left sub-figure* **a** shows the articulation rate (nsyll/phonation time) for the patients with PD and healthy controls. It shows that the healthy controls exhibit significantly higher articulation rate as compared to the patients with PD that is in accordance with the findings in [37]. The *right sub-figure* depicts speech rate for the same case. The y-axis represents the speech rate (number of syllables/duration) for the healthy controls and the patients with PD. The findings were that, Healthy control showed a higher speech rate as compared to the patients with Parkinson's disease. Speech rate for the healthy control was, 3.74 and for the PD subject 2.86. The analysis is done using Praat [46] and the bar graph plots were generated using R statistical analysis software

4.1.14 Speech Rate and Articulation Rate

Praat scripting is extensively used in speech analysis. Some analysis were done using Praat scripting language. Slurred speech, breathy and hoarse speech, difficulty in fast-paced conversations are some of the symptoms of Parkinson's disease. The progressive decrease in vocal sonority and intensity at the end of the phonation is also observed in patients with PD [37]. Literature suggests that speech and articulation rates decrease in PD, and there is a causal link between duration and severity of PD with this decrease in articulation rate [37]. Articulation rate is a prosodic feature and is defined as a measure of rate of speaking excluding the pauses. Speech rate is usually defined as the number of sounds a person can produce in a unit of time [37]. As illustrated in [46], Speech rate is calculated by detecting syllable nuclei. We used Wempe's algorithm for estimating the speech rate [46]. For analysis of speech rate and articulation rate, Praat scripts were used. Two sound samples were chosen for comparative analysis. Samples comprised of healthy control and the patients with PD. Figure 13 shows the bar-chart for articulation rate and speech rate (Fig. 14).

4.2 Case Study II: Phonocardiography (PCG)-Based Heart Rate Monitoring

Phonocardiography refers to acquisition of heart sounds that contains signatures of abnormalities in cardiac cycle. There are two major sound, S1 and S2 associated with cycle of cardiac rhythm. Traditionally, specialized clinicians listen heart sound using

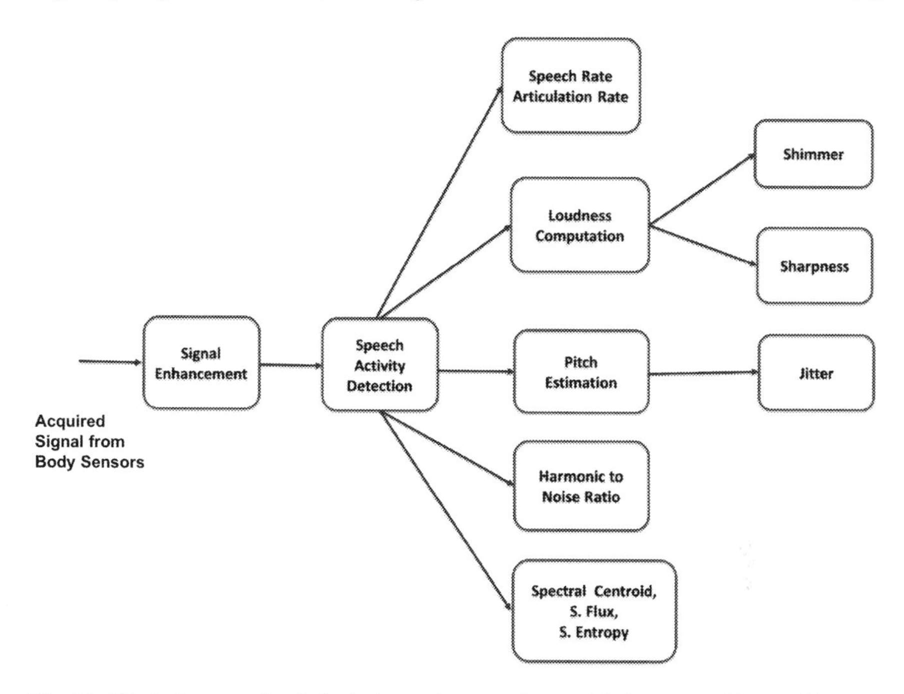

Fig. 14 Block diagram of pathological speech processing module in proposed Fog architecture. The speech signal is first enhanced to reduce the non-stationary background noise. Next, speech activity is detected to identify the speech regions and discard pauses/silences. Speech activity detection reduces the computation by ignoring non-speech frames. Finally, the speech is used for computing clinically relevant features using mathematical models of auditory perception

devices such as stethoscopes for cardiac diagnosis. Such examination need specialized training [20]. Authors developed a computationally inexpensive method for preliminary diagnosis of heart sound [47]. Segmentation of PCG signals and estimation of heart rate from it has been done primarily using two approaches. Segmentation of PCG signals and estimation of heart rate from it has been done primarily using two approaches. The first approach uses ECG as a reference for synchronization of cardiac cycles. Second approach relies solely on PCG signal and is appropriated for wearable devices that relies on smaller number of sensors (Figs. 15 and 16).

In this paper, we integrated the analysis method into Fog framework for providing local computing on Fog device. With the growing use of wearables [6] for acquiring PCG data, there is need of processing such data for preliminary diagnosis. Such preliminary diagnosis refers to segmentation of PCG signal into heart sounds S1 and S2 and extraction of heart rate. Figure 17 shows the proposed scheme for analysis of PCG data for extracting the heart rate. We detect the time-points for heart sounds S1 and S2. Later, these were used for extracting the heart rate. The development and execution of a robust algorithm on Fog device is novel contribution of this chapter.

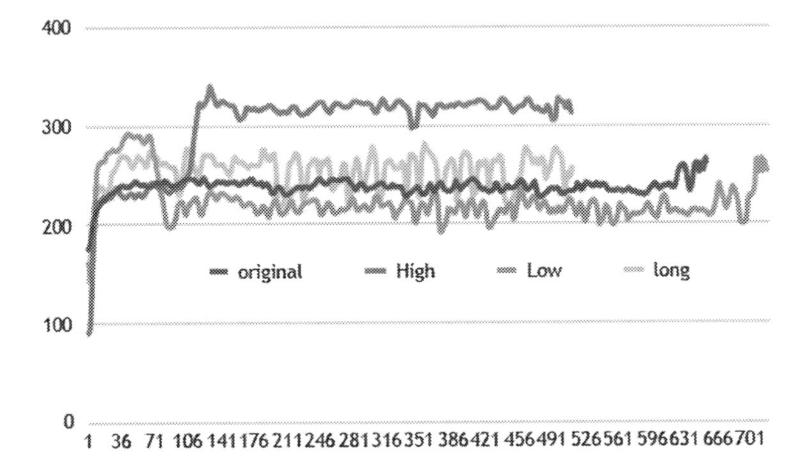

Fig. 15 Depicting the variations in frequency in sustained /a/ (task t_1), HIGHS (task t_2), and LOWS (task t_3) for several speech samples

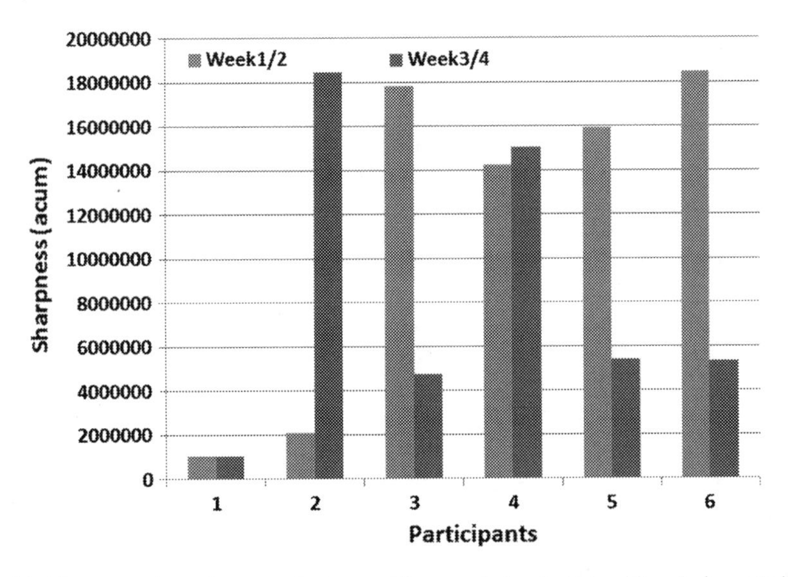

Fig. 16 The comparison of average sharpness of the speech signal obtained from in-home trails of a patient. The 6 days of 2 weeks are compared with respect to average sharpness (in acum). These 2 weeks are separated by 1 week. Low sharpness shows high sensory pleasantness in a speech signal. We can see that the evolution of sharpness on different days is very complicated even during the same week. It is because the speech disorders are unique for each patient with PD

4.2.1 PCG Data Acquisition

PCG signals were acquired using a wearable microphones kept closer to the chest. Such wearable devices could send data to a nearby placed fog device through a smart-

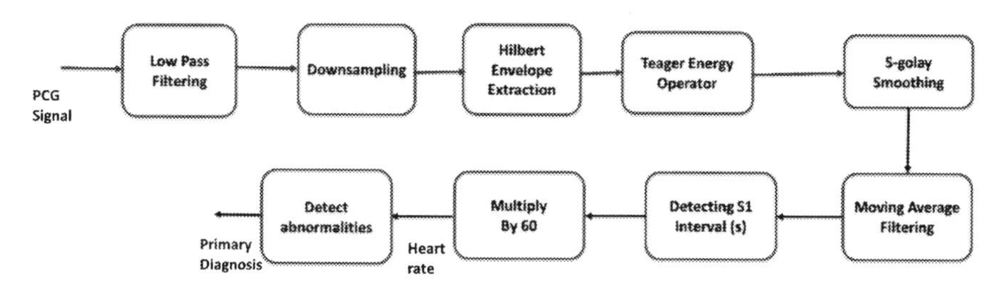

Fig. 17 Proposed method for estimation of heart rate from PCG signal. We first do low pass filtering for reducing the high frequency noise. It is followed by downsampling for reducing the computational complexity. Next, Hilbert envelope is extracted and envelope is processed with Teager energy operator (TEO). The output of TEO is smoothed by Savitzky–Golay filtering. We performed moving averaging for further enhancement of peaks corresponding to heart sound S1. The time-period of heart sound S1 (in seconds) is multiplied with 60 get the heart rate in Beats per minute (BPM). The normal heart rate lies in range 70–200 BPM. Significant deviation from this range shows abnormality in cardiac cycle. This method was implemented in Python and executed in the Fog computer

phone/tablet (gateway). Fog saves the PCG data in .wav format sampled at 800 Hz with 16 bit resolution. The microsoft wav format is lossless format and is widely used for healthcare sound data. We are not discussing the hardware details as our primary goal is computing signal features on Fog device. The segmentation step (see block diagram in Fig. 17) separated the heart sounds S1 and S2 from the denoised PCG signal. The heart sounds S1 and S2 captures the acoustic cues from cardiac cycle. The peak-to-peak time-distance between two successive S1 sounds make one cardiac cycle. Thus, time-distance between two S1 sound determines the heart rate.

We used the data from four scenarios of cardiac cycles namely, normal, asd, pda, and diastolic. The 'normal' refers to normal heartbeat from an healthy person. The 'asd' refers to PCG data induced by an atrial septal defect (a hole in the wall separating the atria). The 'pda' refers to PCG signal induced by patent ductus arteriosus (a condition wherein a duct between the aorta and pulmonary artery fails to close after birth). The last one, 'diastolic' refers to PCG signal corresponding to a diastolic murmur (leakage in the atrioventricular or semilunar valves). Figure 18 shows the time domain PCG signals corresponding to these scenarios. We can see that PCG signal contain signatures of cardiac functioning and clear distinction is portrayed by these time-domain signals. Figure 19 shows the enveloped of these signals (see Fig. 17). We can see that envelope shows the better track of time-domain variations.

4.2.2 Noise Reduction in PCG Data

The PCG signal was acquired at 800 Hz for capturing high fidelity data. Some noise is inherently present in data collected using wearable PCG sensors. We do low pass filtering using a sixth-order Butterworth filter with a cutoff frequency of 100 Hz. It reduces the noise leaving behind spectral components of cardiac cycle. We downsampled the low-pass filtered signal to reduce the computational complexity.

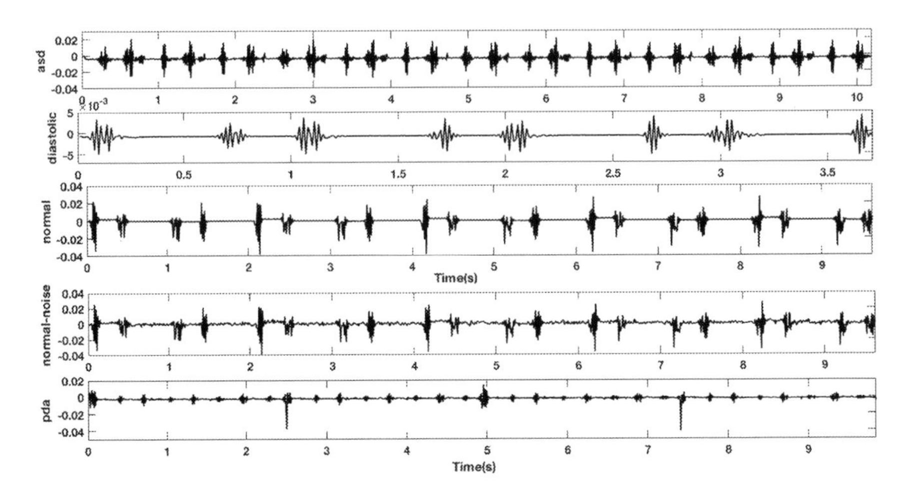

Fig. 18 Time-domain PCG signal for four conditions namely normal, asd, pda, diastolic. The variations in these signals reflect the corresponding cardiac functions

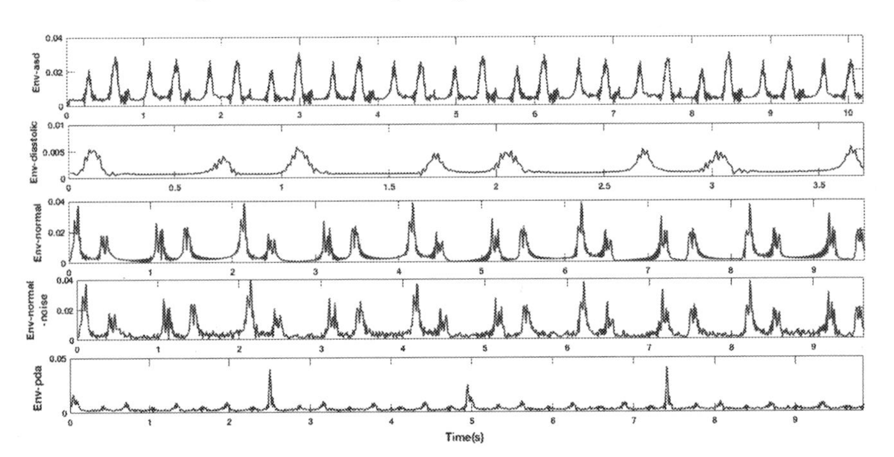

Fig. 19 Envelope of the PCG signal using procedure shown in block diagram (see Fig. 17) for four conditions namely normal, asd, pda, diastolic. The envelope shows clear transitions in PCG signal that can be further processed for localizing the fundamental sound S1 and hence estimation of heart rate in Beats per minute (BPM)

4.2.3 Teager Energy Operator for Envelope Extraction

Teager Energy Operator (TEO) is a nonlinear energy function [29]. TEO captures the signal energy based on physical and mechanical aspects of signal production. It has been successfully in various applications [33, 35]. For a discrete signal $x[n]$, it is given by

$$\Psi(x[n]) = x[n] * x[n] - x[n+1] * x[n-1] \tag{10}$$

where $\Psi(x[n])$ is the TEO corresponding to the sample $x[n]$. We applied TEO on the downsampled signal (see Fig. 17) to extract the envelope. The TEO output is further smoothed using Savitzky–Golay filtering. Savitzky–Golay filters are polynomial filters that achieve least-squares smoothing. These filters performed better than standard finite impulse response (FIR) smoothing filters [42]. We used fifth-order Savitzky–Golay smoothing filters with a frame-length of 11 windows. Next, we perform moving-average filtering on smoothed TEO envelope. The window-length of 11 was used for moving averaging. In next step, the output of moving-average filter is mean and variance normalized to suppress the channel variations.

4.2.4 Heart Rate Estimation by Segmentation of Heart Sounds S1

The heart sound S1 marks the start of the systole. It is generated by closure of mitral and tricuspid valves that cause blood flow from atria to ventricle. It happens when blood has returned from the body and lungs. The heart sound S2 marks the end of systole and the beginning of diastole. It is generated upon closure of aortic and pulmonary valves following which the blood moves from heart to the body and lungs. Under still conditions, the average heart-sound duration are S1 (70–150 ms) and S2 (60–120 ms). The cardiac cycle lasts for 800 ms where systolic period is around 300 ms and diastolic period being 500 ms [54] (Fig. 20).

The mean and variance normalized envelope is used for detecting the fundamental heart sound (S1). Since S1 marks the span of cardiac cycle, we compute time-distance between two S1 locations. It gives the length of cardiac cycle (in seconds). This is multiplied by 60 (see Fig. 17) to get the heart rate in Beats per minute (BPM). Under normal cardiac functioning heart rate lies in range 70–200 BPM. In case, where estimated heart rate is significantly large than this range over a long duration of time, it shows some abnormality in health. It is worth to note that intense exercises such as running on treadmill, cycling etc. can also cause increase in heart rate. The Fog computer receives the PCG signals from wearable sensors and extract heart rate in BPM for each frame. We choose a time-windows of size 2 s with 70% overlap between successive windows.

4.3 Case Study III: Electrocardiogram (ECG) Monitoring

Heart diseases are one of the major chronic illness with a dramatic impact on productivity of affected individuals and related healthcare expenses. An ECG sub-system is considerably for more out-of-hospital applications, manufacturers face continued pressure to reduce system cost and development time while maintaining or increasing performance levels. The electrocardiogram (ECG) is a diagnostic tool to assess the electrical and muscular functions of the heart. The ECG signal consists of components such as P wave, PR interval, RR interval, QRS complex, pulse train, ST segment, T wave, QT interval and infrequent presence of U wave. Presence of arrhyth-

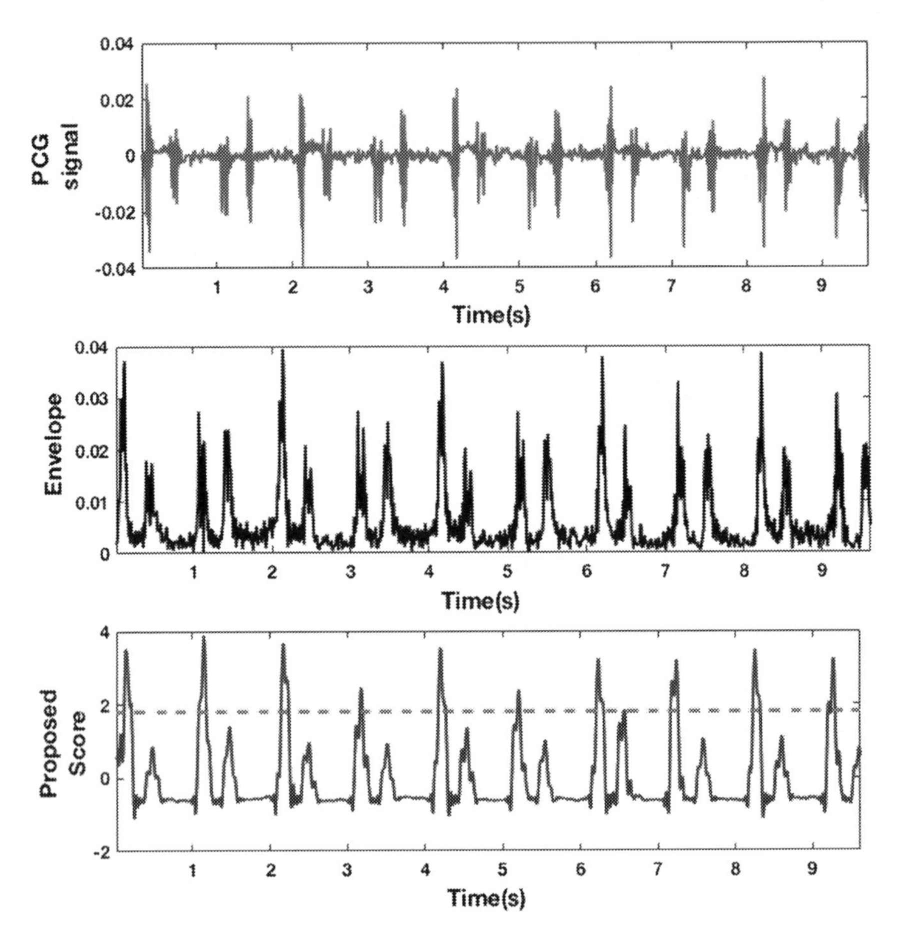

Fig. 20 Detecting heart sound S1 and using it for heart rate estimation in units of beats per minute (BPM). The *top-figure* shows the low pass and downsampled PCG signal. The *middle figure* shows the envelope by procedure shown in block diagram of Fig. 17. The *bottom sub-figure* shows the final post-processed envelope. It is clear that by choosing a suitable threshold, we can detect the S1 sound from PCG signal. Since the cardiac cycle time-length (in seconds) is same as time-difference between two S1 sound (in seconds), we can estimate heart rate by multiply it with 60

mias changes QRS complex, RR interval and pulse train. For instance a narrow QRS complex (<120 ms) indicates rapid activation of the ventricles that in turn suggests that the arrhythmia originates above or within the his bundle (supraventricular tachycardia) and a wide QRS (greater than 120 ms) occurs when ventricular activation is abnormally slow. The most common reason for a wide QRS complex is arrhythmia of the ventricular myocardium (e.g. ventricular tachycardia) [1]. Figure 21 shows ECG time series with P wave, T wave and QRS complex. These three patterns are search using DTW for a large number of ECG data sets. The last section of this case study will discuss the data reduction using DTW and GNU zip compression on ECG data.

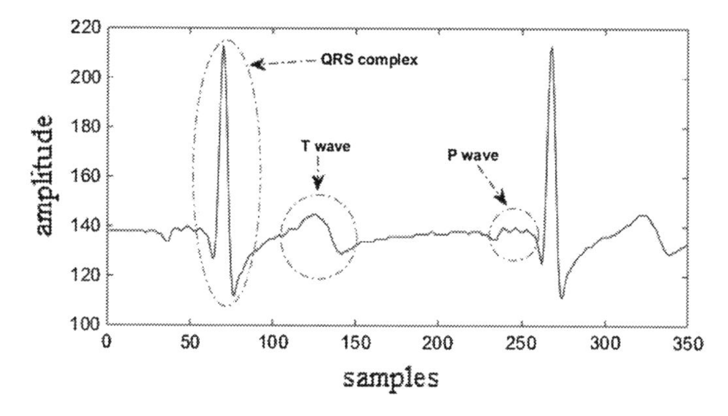

Fig. 21 An example typical time-domain ECG waveform showing phases P, QRS complex and T

The goal of our experiment is to detect arrhythmic ECG beats or QRS changes using QRS complex and the RR interval measurements. The ECG data is fed to the Fog computer from Internet-based database. The Fog computer extracts QRS complex from ECG signals using real-time signal processing implemented in Python on Intel Edison. The Pan–Tompkins algorithm is used for detection of QRS complex [44]. Pan–Tompkins algorithm consists of five steps:

4.3.1 Band Pass Filtering

The energy contained in QRS complex is approximated in 5–15 Hz range [1]. We apply a band pass filter for extracting 5–15 Hz content of ECG signals. The band pass filter reduces muscle noise, 60 Hz power-line interference, baseline wandering and T wave interference. This filter achieve a 3 dB pass-band from about 5–12 Hz. The high-pass filter is designed by subtracting the output of first-order low-pass filter from an all-pass filter with delay of 16 samples (80 ms) [44].

4.3.2 Derivation

The output of band-pass filter is differentiated to get the slope. It uses a five-point derivative. After differentiation, the output signal is squared to get only positive values. It performs non-linear amplification of the output suppressing the values lower than 1 A moving-window integration is applied on output of last step. It smoothens the output resulting in multiple peaks within duration of QRS complex. It adapts to changes in the ECG signal by estimating the signal and noise peaks for finding the R-peaks (Fig. 22). The Pan–Tompkins based QRS detection is implemented on ECG signals obtained from MIT-BIH Arrhythmia Database [27]. Figure 22 illustrates the QRS detection using Pan–Tompkins algorithm on Intel Edison using MIT-BIH Arrhythmia data. The ECG signal containing 2160 samples take 1 s of process-

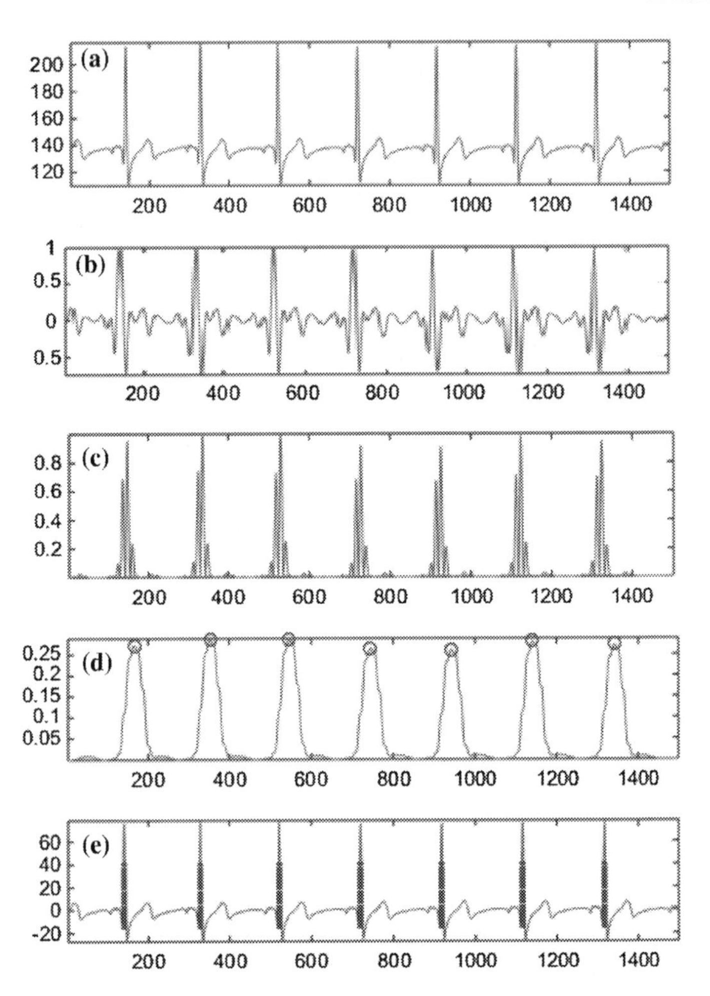

Fig. 22 Illustration of QRS detection using Pan–Tompkins algorithm; **a** Raw ECG data; **b** ECG signal after band-pass filtering and derivation; **c** Squaring the data; **d** Integration and thresholding to detect QRS; **e** Pulse train of ECG signal

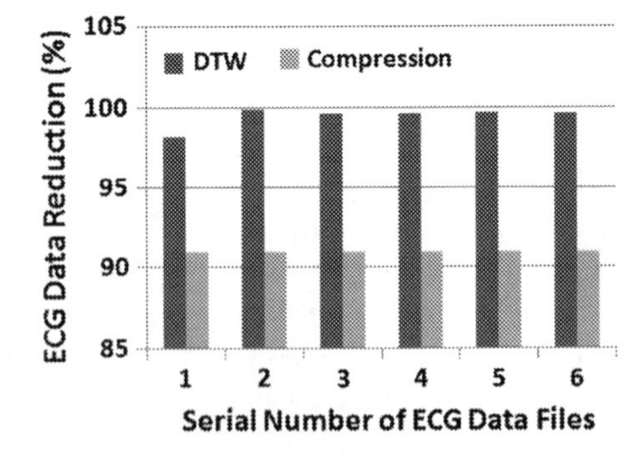

Fig. 23 Comparison of data reduction resulting from DTW based pattern mining and GNU zip based compression for ECG data obtained from MIT-BIH Arrhythmia Database [27]

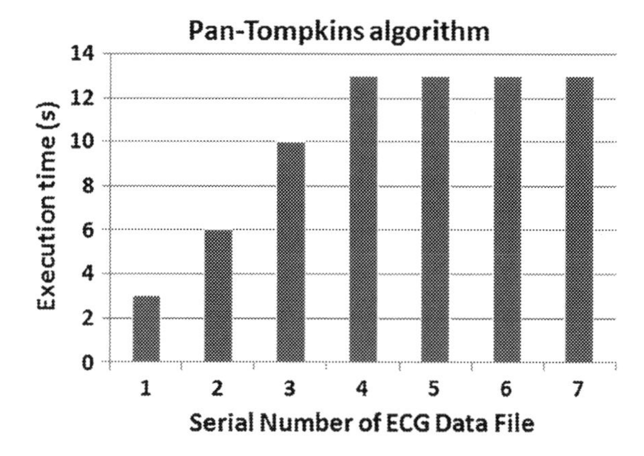

Fig. 24 Execution time (in seconds) for Pan–Tompkins based QRS detection on Inter Edison Fog computer for ECG data from MIT-BIH Arrhythmia Database [27]

ing time on Intel Edison Fog computer. It shows that proposed Fog architecture is well suited for real-time ECG monitoring.

We used DTW based pattern mining for P wave, T wave and QRS complex in ECG data. The DTW indices showing the location of these pattern in ECG time-series is sent to the cloud. Similarly, we use GNU zip program to compress the original ECG time series. The compressed ECG data files are then send to the cloud. Figure 23 shows the data reduction resulting from DTW based pattern mining with compression. Similar to speech data, DTW reduces ECG data by more than 98% in most of the cases while compression reduces around 91%. Figure 24 shows the execution time (in seconds) for Pan–Tompkins based QRS detection implemented in Python on Intel Edison Fog computer. The data sets from MIT-BIH Arrhythmia Database are used. The size of the data sets range from 16.24 to 36.45 kB. The execution time increases with increase in file size. The time taken is always less than 15 s. This validates the efficacy of Fog Data architecture for real-time ECG monitoring (Figs. 25 and 26).

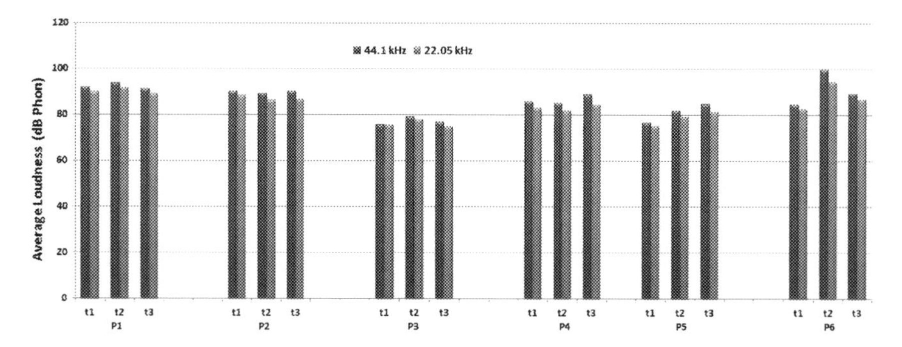

Fig. 25 Comparing loudness computed from speech signal recorded by smartwatch at sampling rate of 44.1 kHz and half of it. We can see the variations are low. The mean change with respect to 44.1 kHz is 2.86% with a standard deviation of 1.26%

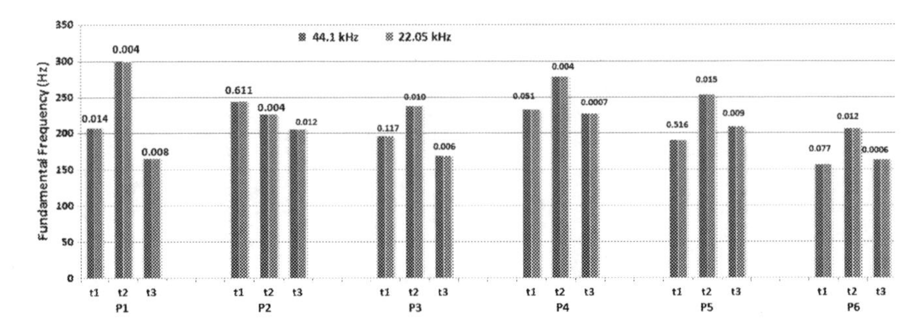

Fig. 26 Comparing fundamental frequency (in Hz) computed from speech signal recorded by smartwatch at sampling rate of 44.1 kHz and half of it. We can see the variations are low. The mean change with respect to 44.1 kHz is 0.0818 % with a standard deviation of 0.1786%

5 Experiments and Results

5.1 Intel Edison Description

The Intel Edison platform used in this application was designed with a core system consisting of dual-core, dual-threaded Intel Atom CPU at 500 MHz and a 32-bit Intel Quark microcontroller at 100 MHz, along with connectivity interfaces capable of Bluetooth 4.0 and dual-band IEEE 802.11a/b/g/n via an on-board chip antenna. This platform came with a Linux environment called Yocto, which is not an embedded distribution of Linux itself, its true purpose is to provide an environment to develop a custom Linux distribution. We did not create a Linux distribution, instead we deployed a prebuilt distribution of Debian/Jessie for 32-bit systems. This decision was made such that we could deploy the same environment on both the Intel Edison and the Raspberry Pi.

5.2 Raspberry Pi Description

The Raspberry Pi Model B platform used in this application was designed with a core system consisting of a 900 MHz 32-bit quad-core ARM Cortex-A7 CPU, and 1 GB RAM. Since the Raspberry Pi does did not have WIFI connectivity built-in a WIFI dongle based on the Realtek RTL8188CUS chipset was installed. This platform came with a custom Linux distribution called Raspbian. Since Raspbian would provide a slightly different environment it was replaced with the Debian/Jessie distribution used on the Intel Edison.

5.3 *Fog Computing: Feature Extraction on Fog Devices*

The fog devices, the Intel Edison and Raspberry Pi, were both configured to run the same Debian/Jessie i386 distribution. Once the distribution was setup, both devices installed the same version of Octave 3.8.2-4, along with the additional packages required to perform the processing required by our algorithms. We also ensured that both gateway devices tracking system performance using the same tools. The tools we used included the Linux program *top* and the Octave function *Profiler*. The *top* program provided real-time insights into CPU Load, Memory Usage, and run-times for processes or threads being managed by the Linux kernel. This was used later to provide use with benchmarking for the system overall. The Octave function *Profiler* provided insights into the run-times for each of section of the algorithm. This was used later determine which parts of the algorithm required more time to complete.

5.4 *Benchmarking and Program Setup*

The gateway devices where remotely logged into via the SSH protocol. From here we ran the same benchmarking scripts for both devices. The scripts would start Octave and load it with the data and use-case based algorithm, while top was started in parallel. The script searched top for the process ID (PID) for this new instance of Octave. Once determined it would extract all the information top provided about the systems performance and the load imposed on the system by this instance of Octave. The extracted information was logged into a csv file and saved for analysis after the algorithm ran its course. Once the instance of Octave was ready to run the algorithm it started the Profiler function in the background. At the conclusion of the algorithm the Profilers set of data was stored into a .mat file for later analysis.

5.5 *Bandwidth and Data Reduction*

We conducted an experiment to measure the percentage by which Fog could reduce the data by processing the audio files using proposed Fog architecture. In our previous studies [12], we developed a clinical speech processing chain (CLIP), a series of filtering operations applied on the speech data for computing the clinical features such as loudness and fundamental frequency. We incorporated several new features in present chapter in addition to loudness and fundamental frequency used in [12]. We took 20 audio files and processed them with two methods;

1. Conventional method of compressing the files using GNU zip [21] and sending them to the cloud server for further processing;
2. Extracting the clinical features on the fog computer (proposed Fog architecture).

Table 3 Latency measurements of Fog for computing the clinical speech features namely zero crossing rate (ZCR), special centroid (SC), and short-time energy (STE)

Speech tasks	Processing time (s)	File duration (s)	Size (kB)
Task 1	2.34	6.24	551
Task 2	2.33	6.18	545
Task 3	2.12	5.62	496
Task 4	2.28	6.08	537
Task 5	1.86	4.96	438
Total	10.94	29.08	2567

Table 3 lists the performance of Fog computer with respect to computation of clinical features. Figure 8 shows the percentage reduction in data size achieved by clinical speech processing and GNU zip compression. We can see that there is huge gains by processing data on Fog computer and sending only the features to cloud as compared to sending the original files to the cloud.

5.6 *Engineering Perspectives*

Charging the wearables such as smartwatches etc. and gateways such as (smartphones/tablets) was necessary at least once in a day. In case patients want to do exercise while being away from home, they need to carry the tablet along with them. Patients were asked to do exercise in a quiet place where the noise is very low or negligible. The patients could wear the smartwatch all the time. The tablet and the smartwatch need to be within a range of 50 m. The speech recordings were saved with date and time stamp that helped in sorting and query-ing them in cloud database. The participants have the choice to switch-on the recording system using smartwatch when they want to perform their vocal and other exercises. Similar procedures for other wearables.

5.7 *Medical Data Analytics and Visualization*

The part (a) of Fig. 27 shows the size of speech data collected from one of the patients for 8 days. We can see that the least amount of data (24 MB) was collected on the first day. On later days, the data size had been increasing. The part (b) of Fig. 27 shows the patients feedback on using the *IoT PD* technology for facilitating the remote monitoring of their vocal and speech exercises. Five out of six participants of in-home trials express a pleasant experience in using it. One participants had problems in using it for the first week. This patient had severe movement disorders in addition to speech disorder that made it difficult to switch ON/OFF the smartwatch. One week later, we

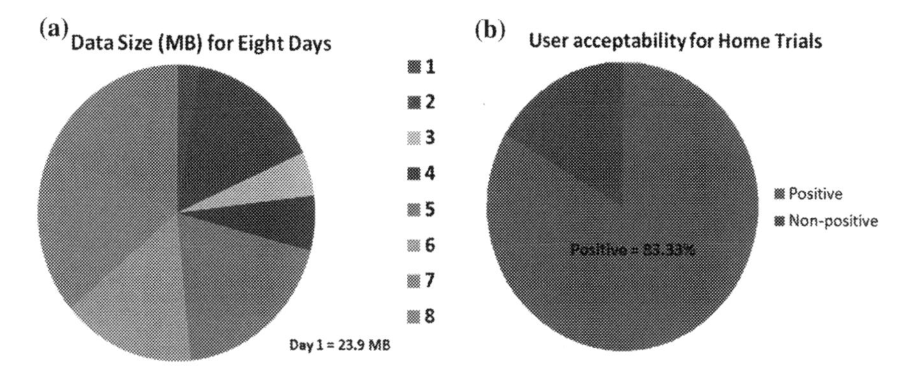

Fig. 27 **a** The data collected from one of the patients for 8 days. The speech data collected was well structured with date and time stamps. **b** The pie chart shows the user acceptability of the proposed system during in-home trials. By non-positive, we mean neither a positive nor a negative inclination towards proposed system. For one participant with severe motor disorders, using smartwatch needed some effort and hence had neither a positive or negative inclination

made a software update allowing easier mechanism for switching ON/OFF. After using the updated *IoT PD*, the patient reported that it was easy to use it. Accounting one feedback out of six as neutral, we depict the user experience as the pie chart shown in Fig. 27b.

6 Practical Insights

6.1 Data Versus Fog Data for Cloud Storage

Table 4 shows approximation on the cloud storage requirement when we compare the conventional model of raw data transfer with the presented Fog Data. It is clear that for the long-term continuous data including speech and ECG, Fog Data architecture reduces the storage requirements tremendously and ultimately cuts the storage and maintenance cost as well as power demand on the cloud. Moreover, the reduced storage reduces the complexity of Big Data Analytics (Figs. 28 and 29).

Figure 30 shows the loudness computed by capturing pathological speech data at 44.1 kHz and downsampling it half the rate. It is clear that downsampling degrades

Table 4 Cloud storage requirement for 100 patients undergoing speech tele-therapy at home

Time	Raw data (GB)	Fog data (GB)
1 Day	12	0.0012
1 Week	84	0.84
1 Month	360	3.6
1 Year	4079	43.8

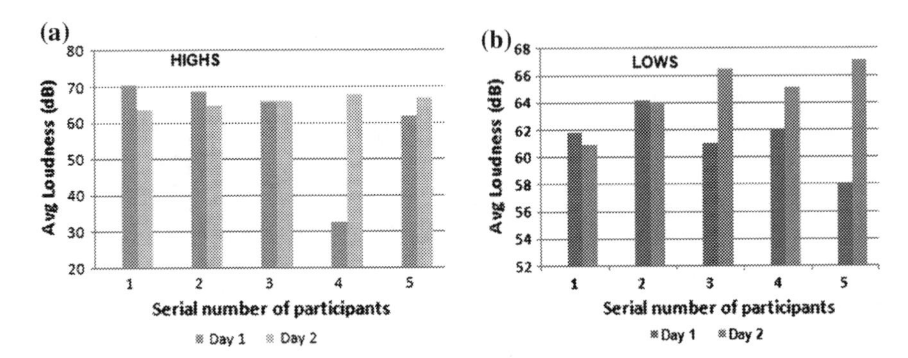

Fig. 28 The average loudness for 2 days on task "Highs" (task t_2) and "Lows" (task t_3) for six patient doing speech exercises at home. The data was processed with Fog in real-time. It illustrates the Fog functionality to compute these features

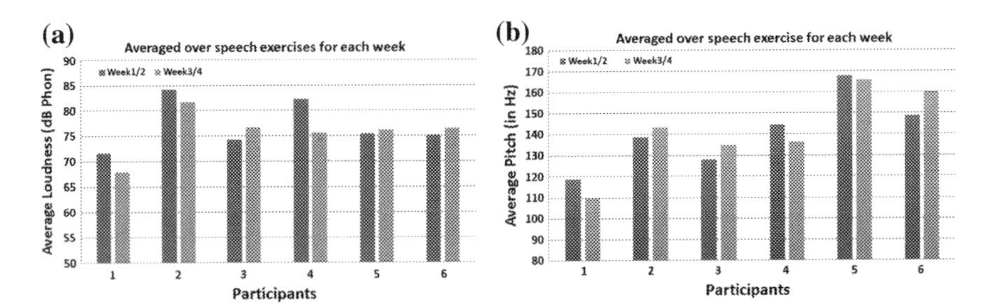

Fig. 29 Showing average loudness and pitch for each day for in-home trials for six patients. The patients used Fog for alternate weeks. We can see that each patient has a different trend for change in loudness and pitch. Interpretation of these variations is done by trained clinicians such as speech-language pathologists (SLPs). Fog compute these features and sync it to the secured cloud backend from where it can be accessed by SLPs, caregivers

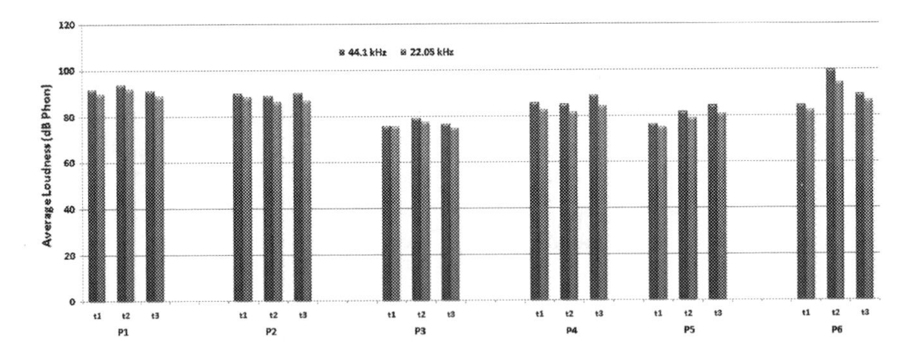

Fig. 30 Showing effect of downsampling on loudness. We can see that by capturing pathological speech at lower sampling rate, we are still approximately at same loudness level. The lower sampling rate would lead to lower power consumption in battery-operated wearable devices

Table 5 Various resources required to develop Fog architecture

Languages	Tools	Usage
MySQL	SequelPro, DataGrip	Run queries and check database tables for testing purposes
PHP	PhpStorm, Postman	Code the server to return the data and information to the mobile application
Python	PyCharm	Code the data processing, storage, transmission, and interfacing with database
Android	IntelliJ, Android Studio	Coded the client transfer code and the complete mobile application
All languages	Atom, Sublime Text2	Editors which can code all languages

the perceptual quality of pathological speech at the advantage of lower power consumption. This graph shows that if needed lower sampling rate can still be a useful in situations where power consumption on wearable devices is an issue.

System Complexity: Our experiences with Fog provide evidence that establishing an intelligent computing resource in remote settings where the patients were located was not only challenging in terms of hardware development and programming, but also required the interdependence of many tools and libraries to build automated exchange of information among various elements of telemedicine. For example, Table 5 shows the various tools needed to bring autonomy, configurability, security, and smart computing on the Intel Edison. We spent months to pursue a systematic survey of what was available and what was useful. Surveying the useful tools was time consuming yet rewarding.

6.2 Compatibility Issues

There were countless instances when we had to find unconventional ways to establish intelligence in Fog. For example, installing Praat python library on the Intel Edison was extremely difficult.

6.3 Security and Privacy

In this work, we presented how the fog computer could be configured for computation and database access. We also touched upon Fog security from the authenticated access point-of-view. However, we believe that security needs can be addressed more rigorously since Fog allows us to configure the fog computing node remotely and inject algorithms that could make the communication and storage more secure.

6.4 Challenges in Using Fog Computing for Telemedicine

No system is perfect and fog computing is no exception. There are difficulties in deploying Fog architecture for telemedicine applications. Although the fog computing provides the data computation on the edge, reducing the data significantly, the data becomes non-reversible when only analytics are communicated to the cloud. The fog has a limited storage space such that it can only store data for days or weeks, depending on the type of data. In our case, the data were audio files that could easily exceed the storage limit on the fog within a few days. An alternative is to create a query mechanism to access the data on fog when the clinicians want to listen to the audio files. Furthermore, since the raw data was not communicated to the cloud, there was no way to perform additional analysis in the cloud. In other words, it is necessary to ensure the reliability of the computational models used for analysis of the data before they are injected into the fog computing resources.

7 Conclusions

We presented a multi-layer telemedicine architecture of the fog-assisted Medical Internet-of-things that was implemented on Intel Edison with layers for hardware, middleware (communication and software), and application (with security services). The Fog framework achieves intelligent gateway functions by processing audio files using signal processing algorithms such as psychoacoustic analysis to extract the clinical features; storage of raw data and features that are on-demand queryable by the cloud as well as the Fog interface. We also implemented Android apps for stakeholders such as patients, healthcare providers and administrators who require access to the backend database. This enabled speech-language pathologists (SLPs) to query the data showing daily progress of their patients. Our case study demonstrated that managing computations on Intel Edison (fog computer) reduces the data by 99%; though less data reduction would occur if more features were analyzed. Our study also showed that it is possible to perform high-fidelity signal processing on the fog device to extract pathological speech features and communicate them to the cloud database.

Moreover, the paper not only provides a high level understanding of the fog-based IoT system, but also provides details of how each layer was implemented including the tools and libraries used in the development. If implemented appropriately, Fog has a great potential to provide more autonomy and reliability in telemedicine applications driven by IoT. In future, we plan to deploy Fog in patient's homes. This will help us face operational challenges when the fog computer is located remotely in a different network.

Acknowledgements Authors would like to thank the patients with Parkinson's disease for their co-operation during validation studies reported in this chapter. This work was supported by a grant (No: 20144261) from Rhode Island Foundation Medical Research and NSF grants CCF-1421823,

CCF-1439011 and NSF CAREER CPS 1652538. Any opinions, findings, and conclusions or recommendations expressed in this material are those of the author(s) and do not necessarily reflect the views of the National Science Foundation or Rhode Island Foundation Medical Research. Authors would like to thank Alyssa Zisk for proofreading the manuscript. Authors would like to thank Manob Saikia, and Dr. Amir Mohammad Amiri for helpful discussions and suggestions for preparation of this chapter.

References

1. Alzand, B.S., Crijns, H.J.: Diagnostic criteria of broad QRS complex tachycardia: decades of evolution. Europace 13(4), 465–472 (2011)
2. Asgari, M., Shafran, I., Bayestehtashk, A.: Robust detection of voiced segments in samples of everyday conversations using unsupervised hmms. In: IEEE Spoken Language Technology Workshop (2012)
3. Banse, R., Scherer, K.R.: Acoustic profiles in vocal emotion expression. Journal of personality and social psychology 70(3), 614 (1996)
4. Barik, R.K., Dubey, H., Samaddar, A.B., Gupta, R.D., Ray, P.K.: FogGIS: Fog Computing for Geospatial Big Data Analytics. In: 3rd IEEE Uttar Pradesh Section International Conference on Electrical, Computer and Electronics Engineering, India (2016)
5. Boersma, P.: Accurate short-term analysis of the fundamental frequency and the harmonics-to-noise ratio of a sampled sound. In: Proceedings of the institute of phonetic sciences. vol. 17, pp. 97–110. Amsterdam (1993)
6. Brusco, M., Nazeran, H.: Development of an intelligent pda-based wearable digital phonocardiograph. In: Proceedings of the 27th IEEE Annual Conference on Engineering in Medicine and Biology. vol. 4, pp. 3506–3509 (2005)
7. Cisco: White paper published by cisco. fog computing and the internet of things: Extend the cloud to where the things are. (2015)
8. Cohen, I.: Noise spectrum estimation in adverse environments: Improved minima controlled recursive averaging. IEEE Transactions on audio, speech and language processing 11(5), 466–475 (2003)
9. Constant, N., Borthakur, D., Abtahi, M., Dubey, H., Mankodiya, K.: Fog-Assisted wIoT: A Smart Fog Gateway for End-to-End Analytics in Wearable Internet of Things. In: The 23rd IEEE Symposium on High Performance Computer Architecture HPCA, Austin, Texas, USA (2017)
10. Ding, H., Trajcevski, G., Scheuermann, P., Wang, X., Keogh, E.: Querying and mining of time series data: experimental comparison of representations and distance measures. Proceedings of the VLDB Endowment 1(2), 1542–1552 (2008)
11. Dubey, H., Mehl, M.R., Mankodiya, K.: BigEAR: Inferring the Ambient and Emotional Correlates from Smartphone-Based Acoustic Big Data. In: IEEE First International Conference on Connected Health: Applications, Systems and Engineering Technologies (CHASE), Washington DC, USA (June 2016)
12. Dubey, H., Golberg, C., Abtahi, M., Mahler, L., Makodiya, K.: EchoWear: Smartwatch Technology for Voice and Speech Treatments of Patients with Parkinson's Disease. In: Proceedings of the Wireless Health 2015, National Institutes of Health, Baltimore, MD, USA. ACM (2015)
13. Dubey, H., Goldberg, J.C., Makodiya, K., Mahler, L.: A multi-smartwatch system for assessing speech characteristics of people with dysarthria in group settings. In: Proceedings IEEE 17th International Conference on e-Health Networking, Applications and Services (Healthcom), Boston, USA (2015)
14. Dubey, H., Kumaresan, R., Mankodiya, K.: Harmonic sum-based method for heart rate estimation using PPG signals affected with motion artifacts. "Journal of Ambient Intelligence and Humanized Computing" pp. 1–14 (2016), doi:10.1007/s12652-016-0422-z

15. Dubey, H., Yang, J., Constant, N., Amiri, A., Yang, Q., Makodiya, K.: Fog Data: Enhancing Telehealth Big Data Through Fog Computing. In: Proceedings of The Fifth ASE International Conference on BigData, Kaohsiung, Taiwan. ACM (2015)
16. Dysarthria: http://www.asha.org/public/speech/disorders/dysarthria/. accessed: 2015-10-21
17. Fastl, H., Zwicker, E.: Psychoacoustics: Facts and models, vol. 22. Springer Science & Business Media (2007)
18. Gamboa, J., Jiménez-Jiménez, F.J., Nieto, A., Montojo, J., Ortí-Pareja, M., Molina, J.A., García-Albea, E., Cobeta, I.: Acoustic voice analysis in patients with parkinson's disease treated with dopaminergic drugs. Journal of Voice 11(3), 314–320 (1997)
19. Gavrila, D., Davis, L., et al.: Towards 3-d model-based tracking and recognition of human movement: a multi-view approach. In: International workshop on automatic face-and gesture-recognition. pp. 272–277 (1995)
20. Geddes, L.: Birth of the stethoscope. IEEE Engineering in Medicine and Biology Magazine 24(1), 84–86 (2005)
21. GNU compression and decompression methods: https://www.gnu.org/software/gzip/gzip.html, year=2015,
22. Goldberg, J.C., Dubey, H., Mankodiya, K.: https://github.com/harishdubey123/wbl-echowear. online (2016), API for Hermes
23. Gonzalez, S., Brookes, M.: Pefac-a pitch estimation algorithm robust to high levels of noise. IEEE Transactions on Audio, Speech, and Language Processing 22(2), 518–530 (2014)
24. J Holmes, R., M Oates, J., J Phyland, D., J Hughes, A.: Voice characteristics in the progression of parkinson's disease. International Journal of Language & Communication Disorders 35(3), 407–418 (2000)
25. JavaScript Object Notation: http://www.json.org/ (2015)
26. Johnston, J.D.: Transform coding of audio signals using perceptual noise criteria. IEEE Journal on Selected Areas in Communications 6(2), 314–323 (1988)
27. http://www.physionet.org/physiobank/database/mitdb. online (2016), accessed
28. http://www.siemens.com/innovation/en/home/pictures-of-the-future/digitalization-and-software/from-big-data-to-smart-data-infographic.html. accessed: 2015-10-21
29. Kaiser, J.F.: Some useful properties of teager's energy operators. In: IEEE International Conference on Acoustics, Speech, and Signal Processing (ICASSP) (1993)
30. Kayyali, B., Knott, D., Van Kuiken, S.: The big-data revolution in us health care: Accelerating value and innovation. Mc Kinsey & Company (2013)
31. Kent, R.D., Weismer, G., Kent, J.F., Vorperian, H.K., Duffy, J.R.: Acoustic studies of dysarthric speech: Methods, progress, and potential. Journal of communication disorders 32(3), 141–186 (1999)
32. Kovacs-Vajna, Z.M.: A fingerprint verification system based on triangular matching and dynamic time warping. IEEE Transactions on Pattern Analysis and Machine Intelligence 22(11), 1266–1276 (2000)
33. Kvedalen, E.: Signal processing using the teager energy operator and other nonlinear operators. Master, University of Oslo Department of Informatics 21 (2003)
34. Lansford, K.L., Liss, J.M.: Vowel acoustics in dysarthria: Speech disorder diagnosis and classification. Journal of Speech, Language, and Hearing Research 57(1), 57–67 (2014)
35. Li, F., Gao, Y., Cao, Y., Iravani, R.: Improved teager energy operator and improved chirp-z transform for parameter estimation of voltage flicker. IEEE Transactions on Power Delivery 31(1), 245–253 (2016)
36. Mahler, L., Dubey, H., Goldberg, C., Mankodiya, K.: Use of smartwatch technology for people with dysarthria. In: Motor Speech Conference at. Madonna Rehabilitation Hospital, Newport Beach, CA, USA. (2016)
37. Martínez-Sánchez, F., Meilán, J., Carro, J., Gómez, Í.C., Millian-Morell, L., Pujante, V.I., López-Alburquerque, T., López, D.: Speech rate in parkinson's disease: A controlled study. Neurologia (Barcelona, Spain) (2015)
38. Monteiro, A., Dubey, H., Mahler, L., Yang, Q., Mankodiya, K.: FIT: A Fog Computing Device for Speech TeleTreatments. 2nd IEEE International Conference on Smart Computing (SMARTCOMP), Missouri, USA (2016)

39. Myers, C., Rabiner, L., Rosenberg, A.: Performance tradeoffs in dynamic time warping algorithms for isolated word recognition. IEEE Transactions on Acoustics, Speech, and Signal Processing 28(6), 623–635 (1980)
40. National institute of deafness and other communication disorders, https://www.nidcd.nih.gov/health/statistics/statistics-voice-speech-and-language (2015)
41. OpenSSL: https://www.openssl.org/ (2015)
42. Orfanidis, S.J.: Introduction to signal processing. Prentice-Hall, Inc. (1995)
43. Paliwal, K.K.: Spectral subband centroid features for speech recognition. In: Proceedings of IEEE International Conference on Acoustics, Speech and Signal Processing (1998)
44. Pan, J., Tompkins, W.J.: A real-time QRS detection algorithm. IEEE transactions on biomedical engineering (3), 230–236 (1985)
45. Panahiazar, M., Taslimitehrani, V., Jadhav, A., Pathak, J.: Empowering personalized medicine with big data and semantic web technology: Promises, challenges, and use cases. In: IEEE International Conference on Big Data. pp. 790–795 (2014)
46. Python script for PRAAT, https://github.com/JoshData/praat-py (2015)
47. Reed, T.R., Reed, N.E., Fritzson, P.: Heart sound analysis for symptom detection and computer-aided diagnosis. Simulation Modelling Practice and Theory 12(2), 129–146 (2004)
48. Sapir, S., Ramig, L., Fox, C.: Speech and swallowing disorders in parkinson disease. Current opinion in otolaryngology & head and neck surgery 16(3), 205–210 (2008)
49. Sobell, M.G.: A Practical Guide to Fedora and Red Hat Enterprise Linux. Pearson Education (2013)
50. Spielman, J., Mahler, L., Halpern, A., Gilley, P., Klepitskaya, O., Ramig, L.: Intensive voice treatment (lsvt® loud) for parkinson's disease following deep brain stimulation of the subthalamic nucleus. Journal of communication disorders 44(6), 688–700 (2011)
51. Sun, X.: A pitch determination algorithm based on subharmonic-to-harmonic ratio (2000)
52. Tan, Z.H., Lindberg, B.: Low-complexity variable frame rate analysis for speech recognition and voice activity detection. IEEE Journal of Selected Topics in Signal Processing 4(5), 798–807 (2010)
53. Tsanas, A.: Accurate telemonitoring of Parkinson's disease symptom severity using nonlinear speech signal processing and statistical machine learning. Ph.D. thesis, University of Oxford (2012)
54. Varghees, V.N., Ramachandran, K.: A novel heart sound activity detection framework for automated heart sound analysis. Biomedical Signal Processing and Control 13, 174–188 (2014)
55. Yang, Y.H., Lin, Y.C., Su, Y.F., Chen, H.H.: A regression approach to music emotion recognition. IEEE Transactions on Audio, Speech, and Language Processing 16(2), 448–457 (2008)
56. Zwicker, E., Fastl, H.: Psychoacoustics: Facts and models, vol. 22. Springer Science & Business Media (2013)

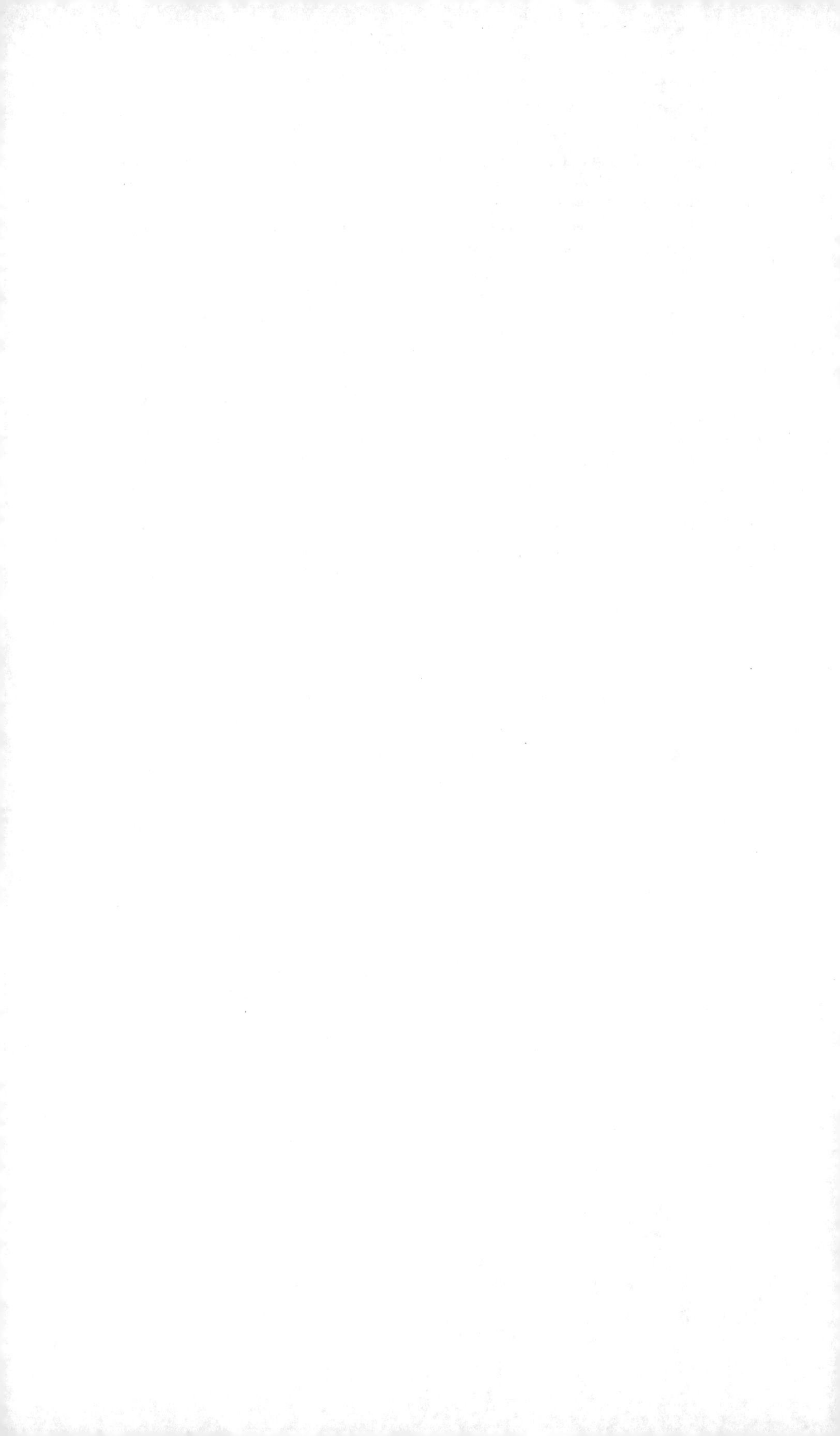

Technologies and Practices: Mobile Healthcare Based on Medical Image Cloud and Big Data (in China)

Jianzhong Hu, Weihong Huang and Yedong Huang

Abstract Modern information technologies such as mobile computing, cloud computing and big data have brought new possibilities for modern healthcare services. In developing countries such as China where the vast majority of healthcare has been delivered in hospitals, mobile healthcare is of great significance to provide easy and quality care for everyone in and out of hospitals. In response to China's national strategy "Healthy China 2030", a nationwide hierarchical medical system needs to be established in due course. Featuring ubiquitous access with quality guarantee and consistent user experience on different terminals anytime anywhere, mobile healthcare has been regarded as one of the most important means to support the grand mission of hierarchical medical system. In the process of implementing mobile healthcare, all types of medical data (e.g. patient information, medical records, medical images, health check data, etc.) are to be shared across hospitals boarders. From the computing perspective, mobile medical imaging is regarded as the most challenging issue as medical image processing is the most network and computation resource consuming. Based on systematic requirement analysis, this chapter presents an innovative mobile medical image cloud system. The system enables seamless integration of multiple types of medical data especially medical image data from different vendors globally, and forms the basis for Big Data analysis for smarter healthcare in the future. A real-world case study of cloud teleconsultation using medical image cloud and big data technologies is also presented to prove its technical feasibility and replicability in practice in China.

Keywords Mobile healthcare · Mobile image cloud (MIC) · Big data

J. Hu · W. Huang
Xiangya Hospital Central South University, Changsha, China

J. Hu · W. Huang (✉)
"Mobile Health" Ministry of Education – China Mobile Joint Laboratory, Changsha, China
e-mail: whuangcn@qq.com

Y. Huang
AccuRad Healthcare Technology Co., Xi'an, China

© Springer International Publishing AG 2017

S.U. Khan et al. (eds.), *Handbook of Large-Scale Distributed Computing in Smart Healthcare*, Scalable Computing and Communications,
DOI 10.1007/978-3-319-58280-1_12

1 Introduction and Background

1.1 Introduction of Modern Healthcare Information Technologies

With the fast development and popular use of Information and Communication Technology (ICT), healthcare services provided by general hospitals are now in good use of information technologies for acute care. The digitalised healthcare is usually called eHealth, and its typical systems include Hospital Information System (HIS), Electronic Medical Record (EMR) system, Picture Archiving and Communication Systems (PACS), Laboratory Information Systems (LIS) and related medical emergency services (e.g. 999 in the United Kingdom, 119 in the United States, 112 in China). Mobile healthcare (mHealth) is commonly regarded as an extension of eHealth, a term used for the practice of medicine and public health supported by mobile devices [11]. The term is used in reference to using mobile communication devices, such as mobile phones, tablet computers and PDAs, for health services and information. A lot of mobile devices are now widely adapted in community and rural healthcare contexts, where patients or health professionals might have difficulties in travelling or short in time to get prompt results and right information, smart mobile devices could help to provide flexible communication among consultants, general practitioners and patients in care process. In most cases, mobile healthcare features real-time monitoring of patient vital signs (e.g. heart rate, blood pressure, blood oxygen, blood glucose, etc.), viewing medical images such as X-Ray, Computed Tomography (CT), Magnetic Resonance Imaging (MRI), ultrasound, and pathology images, and video/audio conferencing. These on-demand mobile healthcare services could be provided based on networking and computing capacities conditions where mobile imaging is the most challenging and complex among these mobile services.

Mobile computing is not the only new technology that modern healthcare embraces, cloud computing [20] is another important emerging healthcare information technology and gradually got matured in the past several years. Cloud computing is a model for enabling ubiquitous, on-demand access to a shared pool of configurable computing resources (e.g., computer networks, servers, storage, applications and services), which can be rapidly provisioned and released with minimal management effort. Traditionally medical images are accessed and managed through PACS in hospitals using proprietary formats, patient care and services outside the hospital may be compromised without support. By introducing the cloud technology into medical imaging, the medical imaging service could offer global storage of image generated by different devices and global access on different terminals including mobile phones and tablets anytime anywhere with consistent user experience. The ubiquitous storage and access model of medical images eliminates the barrier between hospitals and saves the hassle of carrying large scale printed copy around.

In addition to medical images from PACS, there are many other types of data in healthcare generated by all kinds of systems such as HIS/EMR/LIS in hospitals. To analyse and understand the huge amount of data better, this intersection of technology and healthcare sometimes is called "Big Data" [19]. The utilisation of Big Data technology from traditional management perspective could help to improve profits and cut down on wasted overhead, Big Data in healthcare means more than that. It is expected to help predicting epidemics, curing disease, improving quality of life and avoiding preventable deaths. However the bright future of Big Data in healthcare is yet to arrive. One of the reasons is because most IT systems in hospitals built in the past mainly work in proprietary ways and don't talk/interact to other systems within the same hospital easily, not to mention other hospitals. This has caused a typical "information island" problem which not only creates difficulties for doctors and nurses in practices, but also brings extra hassles to patients particularly in referral. From practical point of view, it is critical to enable flexible data and information sharing among clinical settings and to offer simple and clear healthcare pathways for patients with good user experience in order to welcome the new era of Big Data.

1.2 Background of Healthcare Information Technology Development in China

The majority of hospitals in China started their digitalisation process using information technologies in 1990s. At present time, most referral hospitals in China in secondary care have established essential information systems such as HIS, EMR and PACS. But in contrast to those in developed countries such as the UK and USA, the digitalisation level of primary care in China is rather poor. With limited resources in hardware and personnel, the traditional model of healthcare service provided by hospitals and within hospitals has met the biggest challenge ever in history to cope with the 1.4 billion people's ever-growing demand of healthy living. In order to address the general care and health issues in the long run, China published its national strategy of "Healthy China 2030" in August 2016. It is now a national policy and demand to improve medical care as high quality as possible for everybody around the country. Notified challenging issues in the national policy include public hospitals reform, national health insurance system, drug supply assurance mechanism and many others. Among these topics, a pragmatic hierarchical medical system [6] is considered the top priority to be addressed immediately.

There are several tangible targets to be met for a hierarchical medical system in China: bidirectional patient transfer between hospitals (70% cities to pilot test), resident registration to general practitioners (200 cities to pilot test), and primary hospital service capacity improvement (90% patients cared in local districts). In order to meet those targets and to balance the service and quality of care gap between big hospitals and primary level hospitals/surgeries, great efforts will be needed in both technology and clinical practices. To some extent, the blueprint of hierarchical medical system in China [6] is similar to the NHS system in the UK.

Apart from building more and closer links between top hospitals and primary hospitals, consultants in hospitals and general practitioners in communities, technical assistance by mobile telemedicine services could be very helpful and easy to adapt to build the hierarchical medical system [6]. However, after over 10 years of introduction of telemedicine [17], it is not frequently used due to various reasons in China. Since telemedicine is actually an advancement of health information technology at the time of invention, its use by doctors has been limited by their fixed locations of communication and high costs of terminal installation, these drawbacks appeared to be even worse when almost everyone gets a mobile phone in China where the total population of mobile user has reached 1.306 billion in January 2016 [21].

With new mobile computing and cloud computing technologies, the concept of telemedicine has now been redefined. Mobile imaging technology is now practically available for patients and doctors to access medical images such as MRI, CT and X-ray on their smart phones and tablets anytime anywhere, and the operation and quality of images are similar to PACS desktop applications in Intranets within hospitals.

1.3 Major Contribution of This Chapter

There are two approaches in implementation of mobile medical imaging applications [23]. The first approach features moving traditional desktop PACS applications onto mobile terminals by transferring image data to tablets and smart phones, where data is still stored in PACS systems within hospitals and transcoded onto mobile devices for access. The advantage of this approach is being straightforward and leaving existing system architecture and data flow unaffected, where its weakness is limited access and performance due to restriction on computation resources and extra costs for extension. The second approach features reconstructing and storing image data on cloud for universal mobile access. The advantage of this approach is high flexibility of universal access, good image quality and user experience in clinical practice where its disadvantage is in need of new establishment of image data flow for cloud operation. Apparently the second approach is more practical despite it may require dedicated system design and implementation as its major computing work is done on the cloud.

Following the second approach, this chapter systematically presents an innovative medical image cloud (MIC) system which enables universal mobile image storage and access on various cloud terminals. The system also enables seamless integration of multiple types of medical data from different hospitals over the Internet, and forms the basis for Big Data analysis for smarter medical care in the future. A case study of regional medical imaging centre is presented to demonstrate its technical feasibility with evaluation of system operational metrics in comparison with traditional PACS services, and to prove its replicability in practice in China.

2 Why Medical Image Cloud?

2.1 Demands for MIC in Operations

With the wide deployment of advanced medical imaging equipment such as MRI/CT/X-Ray/Ultrasound in recent years, hospital generates vast amounts of medical image data every day [13]. The average total volume of medical image data of a tertiary referral hospital is about 100 GB per day (equivalent to about 500 CT scans), while a basic level primary hospital could have 5 GB data per day (equivalent to 25 CT scans). With such large volume of data in size and quantity, manging such a vast amount of medical image data becomes the most resource consuming task for the IT department in hospitals. Also traditional PACS only works within the intranet, it is impractical for doctors to access and share quality medical images over the Internet securely for both clinical practice and research. A cloud solution of mobile medical imaging could help in this case.

Firstly, image cloud could ease the burden of hospital networks. Massive volume of medical image has great impact on hospital intranets. In the networks and databases of a hospital, medical image data accounts for almost 95% of the total volume. If this large volume of medical image data transmits across hospital networks, the shared bandwidth naturally takes very high load, and affects other network applications, which might risk into safety and stability issues. With the fast development of science and technology in big data, more and more advanced medical devices and systems produce much more data, for example, Positron Emission Tomography/Computed Tomography (PET-CT) aims at showing tumour as small as 0.2 mm, while the finest CT/MRI does the check at 0.8 mm [9]. Finer granularity means more levels of scans and more pieces of image data. The exponential growth of medical image data will bring great impact on hospital network. By diverting the medical image data flow to the cloud and only stream down to terminals on demand, it could release the bottleneck of hospital networking at all times.

Secondly, image cloud could support flexible and affordable new functional upgrades. Traditional PACS system usually works in client/server mode, and new functional requirements are not easily updatable and upgrades usually cost a lot of money. Most old PACS systems built many years ago in small hospitals only came with simple functions such as 2D image processing and adjustments. New image processing technologies such as intensity projection, 3D reconstruction, interface to

3D printing, and new requirements in practices such as Multi-Disciplinary Team (MDT) consultation [25] would be very interesting to doctors and radiologists, but the financial, time and personnel costs of upgrading the whole PACS hardware and software system sometimes are too expensive to afford by hospitals, and sadly the upgrades could never catch up the pace of technology advancements. By pushing the medical imaging services on to the cloud, upgrading in functionality would not be an awkward issue anymore and also more affordable to hospitals especially small hospitals.

Thirdly, image cloud could support universal practice by clinicians. Traditional PACS and other healthcare information systems only work within the hospital, which creates a nature barrier for universal practice. Despite the adoption of mobile technologies has enabled various types of mobile healthcare services such as mobile clinical rounds and PDA-based mobile nursing, proven with good user experiences to doctors, nurses and patients [26]. In the context of telemedicine and hierarchical medical care, doctors require easy communication on mobile phones, tablets, and networked computers for consultation, education, diagnosis and treatment and many more. Traditionally restricted service model would not meet the growing demand. Having the clinical pathway and required medical data enabled on the cloud could eliminate the barriers and bring the freedom for clinicians in practice, but also forms a good basis for future Big Data analysis with coverage of more and more cases and medical records.

2.2 Roles and Problems Faced in MIC

There are four categories of users (roles) in a regional medical image cloud:

(1) Health administrative departments (i.e. different levels of Health and Family Planning Commission offices in China);
(2) Healthcare service organisations (i.e. hospitals and community health centres);
(3) Medical experts (i.e. doctors, radiologists, pathologists, lab technicians);
(4) Customers (i.e. patients).

Different roles face different problems in the context of mobile healthcare and MIC.

(1) Problems faced by health administrative departments
Resource equal distribution: care quality and professional excellence are the core resources of medical services, and these core resources are currently centralised in good hospitals in China. It is under the top priority of the administrative department to share and distribute valuable resources across regions, which means remote out-patients with complex conditions are expected to have the same consultation of their examinations, diagnosis just like the quality services they could get as in-patients in top hospitals.

Homogenization of medical examinations: the quality of medical report not only relies on equipment but also experience and expertise of clinicians. Without quality control of diagnostic practices and assessment standards, it is hard to mutually approve the examination results across hospitals, and this may lead to unnecessary troubles in administration and resource waste in repeated examinations. A standard of practice in similar context would help to assure the quality in medical examinations.

Practices of distance health education: Every year there are about 600 thousands medical students graduate from universities in China, but there is still a long way ahead when these graduates get their licenses to work as formal physicians. Continuous education and distance learning has always been an important matter on the health regulatory authorities' agendas, unfortunately they still lack of feasible solutions in practice.

Real-time disease statistics: without regional centres of medical imaging and examination reporting, it is hard for the regional health regulatory authorities to get accurate real-time statistics as hospitals work independently on their own health information technology systems. It would be good to have a centralised platform of raw data and reports across the region for future Big Data analysis, and to provide a scientific basis for decision making in disease control and prevention.

(2) Problems faced by healthcare service organisations

Tertiary referral hospitals: Medical image data volume increases constantly, but the hardware computing capacity of existing PACS system is always limited and system can be slowed down if the data volume gets bigger and bigger. In order to maintain the operation speed of PACS system in daily use, it is reasonable to put some historical medical image data stored offline for archive and only leave certain period of image data online (e.g. 2 years). This compromised solution may lead to two potential risks: safety of historical data in offline disk storage and difficulty in accessing historical data when it comes to clinical research and data analysis.

Secondary and primary level hospitals: traditional PACS system requires certain level of IT support, but the information departments of these hospitals are relatively weak in personnel. The workload of general maintenance has somehow constrained the adoption and upgrade of traditional PACS in these hospitals. On the other hand, there is a shortage of qualified radiologist in these hospitals due to various reasons such as income level and career development, but it is relatively easy to recruit a technician to operate the medical equipment.

(3) Problems faced by medical experts
With the wide adoption of mobile technology, people work and communicate everywhere with their tablets and smart phones, it is naturally expected by medical experts (including clinicians, radiologist, pathologist, and so on) to have access to high quality medical image when they are not in front of office desktop computers. Without a cloud-based secure solution, doctors can only share images by re-taking photos with their phone cameras and transmit over public social networks e.g. mobile Apps like WeChat in China [27].

(4) Problems faced by customers
Most top medical experts work in good hospitals in China, which means majority residents in urban and rural areas may not have the opportunity to be cared by top experts. The demand of care mainly shows in the following aspects: firstly, cared at the nearest clinic to save time and money involved in travelling and queuing for consultation. This is actually one of the targets defined in the national health reform strategy: minor illness cared in communities, serious and complex diseases treated in hospitals. Secondly, accessible to assured quality care with affordable cost by having the same quality diagnosis remotely by experts on the cloud. Thirdly, universal access of personal health records especially medical images and reports on regional cloud would help to manage full lifecycle health information of patients.

3 Objectives of Building a Medical Image Cloud

3.1 Administrative Objectives of MIC

To resolve the problems faced by different stakeholders in the hierarchical medical system, a regional medical image cloud is set to achieve the following objectives from technical and operational perspectives:

(1) To offer quality imaging services in secondary and primary level hospitals
Without costly investments in money, time and human resources, secondary and primary hospitals could be connected to a cloud PACS system and assisted by experts on the Internet, carrying out medical imaging diagnosis and reporting service in full with quality control. Other business extensions such as two-way patient referral could improve the overall healthcare service level locally.

(2) To achieve mobile medical imaging services
Based on cloud computing technologies, doctors and patients could share the same quality medical image, communicate in real-time, anywhere anytime on any available terminal devices. Mobile phones with large screen and tablets could be used to access image for viewing and analysis, which makes for teleconsultation and tele-diagnosis and discussion convenient and effective at very low cost.

(3) To achieve the integration of medical resources regionally
In China, first-hand medical data and resources are managed independently by individual hospitals. By pushing doctor-doctor collaboration onto medical cloud platforms (e.g. regional imaging and examination cloud centre), originally centralised resources in top hospitals could be shared across the region in low cost, and related education and quality control could be achieved in a relatively easy way.

(4) To reduce the cost of medical care
By having centrally controlled quality medical imaging services on cloud, raw images and reports could be recognised and accepted in different hospitals in the region. This is a very direct and important factor to avoid duplicated and over examinations. On one hand it reduces the radiation damage to patients, and on the other hand it reduces the cost of medical care when transfer happens between hospitals.

3.2 *Technological Objectives of MIC*

In order to fulfil the requirements above, a medical image cloud system should also meet the technological objectives as follows:

(1) To adapt to regular routines of radiology department including workflow management, collaboration, communication and interaction over the same platform;
(2) To enable paperless and filmless medical mobile image services;
(3) To achieve minimum maintenance over the Internet with ultimate aim of training-free and support-free after sales;
(4) To support universal access (server: Windows, Mac, Linux, client: iOS, Android, Windows Phone);
(5) To enable mobile healthcare services (e.g. multimedia tele-consultation, online doctor-patient triage, history electronic medical records review, etc.);
(6) To support further medical Big Data analysis.

4 Requirement Analysis of Medical Image Cloud

4.1 Process Requirement Analysis of MIC

The medical image cloud system mainly addresses two functional issues: storage and transmission of large volume of medical image data and medical image front-end processing. Ultimately full scale and quality images should be presented on tables and mobile phones over mobile networks just like that on desktops. Normal PACS operational functions (e.g. image zooming and marking, advanced image processing, image segmentation and analysis, and smart decision support) should also be supported on all types of mobile terminals.

There are several important modules of function involved in regional cloud medical image services: cloud PACS with full process support, doctor-to-doctor teleconsultation and tele-diagnosis, remote video/image education, patient referral, mobile imaging application.

(1) Cloud PACS with full process support
To simplify the overall process of PACS in secondary and primary level hospitals, most IT maintenance work could be done directly on cloud. After the medical equipment such DR X-Ray, ultrasound, CT were install locally, the rest processes could be done on the cloud rather than buying an expensive and complex set of PACS software and storage facility. Processes in its typical workflow include patient registration, examination appointments, image processing, report generation and distribution, image storage and searching [18]. This means least requirements on IT support, least requirements on radiologist, but same quality of imaging assessment and report as that of referral hospitals.

(2) Doctor-to-doctor teleconsultation and tele-diagnosis
Teleconsultation [8] processes are fully supported on cloud, which include tele-consultation request, request acceptance, tele-diagnosis, cloud-based reporting. Normally a teleconsultation process involves two parties, and more parties are also supported without any problem based on the extensible cloud computing architecture. By enabling the universal electronic medical record sharing and medical image presentation, doctors from different hospitals could work seamlessly as a team on cloud.

(3) Remote multimedia medical education
The image cloud should also support live/on-demand multimedia (video/audio/image) medical education which is quite useful rural areas [10]. Alongside medical images, other demonstration video/audio and education contents could also be shared online, which could be of great help for young doctors learn from senior experts anytime.

(4) Two-way patient referral support

As the cloud connects many hospitals in the region, with patient electronic medical records, medical images and reports, it is easy to implement a two-way referral system between any two hospitals (mainly between a secondary hospital or community health centre and a tertiary hospital) or at least to provide necessary information for referral without information loss or distortion.

The two-way patient referral system is one of the targets set in the hierarchical medical system [3]. It is of great importance to coordinate resources among public hospitals at different levels, chronic and common diseases and post-operation re-habitation could be cared in community health centre and primary hospitals, while serious and emergencies could be treated in referral hospitals with better resources. To get the referral process done smoothly, ideally all hospitals in the region should have the same access to patients' medical data rather than asking patients to wait and carry hardcopies from one hospital to another.

(5) Mobile imaging application

Based on cloud computing and mobile Internet technology, the system platform provides mobile imaging applications across different platforms. Mobile terminals such as smart phones and tablets could access original standard DICOM [24] images anytime anywhere. Advanced features are also supported to resolve real-time high quality mobile imaging requirements, including 3D reconstruction, virtual scalpel function, coronary segmentation and analysis, vessel analysis, lung segmentation analysis, 1:1 operation mode and other advanced imaging capabilities, which is particularly useful in emergencies.

4.2 Technical Requirements Analysis of MIC

To build a successful medical image cloud, technical solutions should not only consider the advancements of new technologies, but also the maturity, practicality and scalability of technologies used, so that data processing sharing between connected systems and other functional information systems could meet future extension requirements.

The overall system architectural design and development should:

(1) Use mainstream technology in accordance with international standards, national standards, regulations in related technical requirements and management practices;

(2) Use advanced architecture to build a powerful system with distinctive features; it should integrate various information resources in medical imaging and structured/semi-structured medical record information under reliable networking environments;
(3) Construct secure and fast medical image cloud for storage and indexing, breaking the traditional medical information "isolated island" effect;
(4) Achieve the shared standard image data exchange, and consequently support all kinds of cloud applications and get ready for future research in medical big data applications.

The system should be component-based, modularised, object-oriented, and flexible enough for future extension [7]. Its basic technical requirements are as follows:

Standardization: the entire cloud system is to meet the related practice codes and regulations issued by the National Health and Family Planning Commission in China, and to be compatible to relevant national and international standards.

Reliability: as the cloud works on the Internet, it requires top reliability to guarantee the operation 24/7, to some extend it should be more reliable than a local PACS and eventually treated as a new technical alternative to traditional PACS solutions.

Usability: the client user interface UI on different platforms and terminals should be universally accessible, user-friendly and consistent in design. The system should be easy to operate, and no need for complicated professional training to use the system.

Scalability: the system operation, storage and indexing capacities should not be affected when medial data volume grows, the overall performance should show excellent scalability.

Modularity: it is expected to have more types of equipment and devices to the cloud, and new functions will be developed to fulfil specific tasks. System design and implementation should support modular extension and work in cloud architecture.

Data interface: the medical image cloud database should support standard data interface for exchange, backup and recovery. It is also expected to provide superior query performance guaranteed security mechanism over mass.

Adaptability: system should be adaptable to different operational environments such as terminal processing capability, network connection speed, browser and operating system variety etc.

Performance: system shall provide 7 × 24 h of continuous operation, the average annual downtime should be less than 1 day and the Mean Time to Restoration should be less than 30 min. System should not run into fatal errors in daily use and affect daily routines.

Security: it should technically meet the security requirements in physical security, network security, host security, application security, and data security. There should also be unified authentication centre for identification and role-based authorisation control. Access control is down to the page level and to ensure encryption in transmission for secure transmission without leakage of sensitive data.

4.3 Information Security Requirement Analysis of MIC

In addition to the basic physical and networking and security mechanisms, extra care should be taken consideration for the privacy and information security in MIC.

(1) Privacy protection of patient personal information
When data flows on regional medical image cloud, patient personal information needs to be protected, particularly identification and contact information contained in DICOM images, reports, and teleconsultation and health history in diagnosis and records [22]. Leak of patient data without authorisation will directly violate the privacy of patients, and affect the reputation of the hospital. The information might leaked in transmission, be tampered, damaged or even lost in storage, which could affect the consultation result, and might even lead to medical accidents. It is required to have overall data transmission and storage being secured on integrity, confidentiality, safety, recoverable and traceable.

(2) Protection of internal information of hospitals
Regional medical image cloud contains medical data from various hospitals. This connection brings new challenges to hospital IT systems when data exchanges between the hospital Intranet and Extranet. It is important to assure other information on network not to be compromised, and the information gateway needs to be robust enough to assure leak-free and anti-intrusion. To do that, domain division needs to be in place clearly, and firewalls should have control measures such as malicious code attack protection, border integrity protection, intrusion detection and so on.

(3) Safety in medical information service processes
Regional medical image cloud not only stores massive volume of medical examination data, but also contains a large number of telemedicine, two-way referral, the doctor-patient interaction and other medical service process information. Therefore it is important to maintain the continuity and completeness of information across multiple hospitals [16]. If the information on cloud is leaked, damaged or lost due to external attacks, the care business will be affected adversely and immeasurably.

(4) Safety in hospital operational management
The regional medical image cloud platform is operated by people just like other information systems, but it involves much more parties, therefore it is important to have regulations in place to ensure role-authorisation access mechanism well in place, and try to avoid security risks caused by human factors such as abuse of authority that may lead to excessive use of system resources, abnormal changes to the system configuration that affects performance, maintenance error made by IT staff and so on [12].

5 System Architecture of Medical Image Cloud

5.1 Mobile Healthcare System

Figure 1 shows a typical modern mobile healthcare eco-system in China. The lead hospital Xiangya Hospital Central South University is located in Changsha, Hunan Province, China. It is a top class hospital in China as being one of the 44 comprehensive public hospitals under direct administration of the National Health and Family Planning Commission of China (The Ministry of Health). It serves about 100 million people across 3 provinces in southern China. Its mobile healthcare network runs across a large regional medical collaboration network, which includes 1 lead hospital (Xiangya Hospital), 19 general hospitals in 12 provinces, 20 community hospitals in Changsha, 51 primary hospitals in Hunan Province, and 138 remote networking hospitals nationwide. Major network collaboration activities include staff training, practice supervision, research collaboration, telemedicine, and bi-directional referral (as shown in Fig. 2).

A typical mobile healthcare system reference architecture is illustrated in Fig. 3. There are two versions of mobile applications to be delivered on the client side, one for patient and one for clinician. The patient version client features an interface connected with sensors for home care. On the server side, the mobile healthcare platform contains necessary modules to connect and management data for operation and user accounts. A security gateway is normally in use to ensure necessary security mechanisms in place while other operational modules such as configuration management, session management, service management, and help desk are to assist the access of medical data based on account management (sometimes including billing function if required). The medical data management module then connects to the traditional healthcare information systems such as HIS/EMR/LIS/PACS in different hospitals. As mentioned before the most challenging issue in traditional mobile healthcare information services is medical imaging, which requires high computation capacity and high bandwidth in operation. The challenge should be addressed in a systematic way if mobile healthcare services go onto cloud.

5.2 Construction Principles of MIC

There are several principles to be considered in design and development of a medical image cloud.

(1) Comprehensive planning, gradual implementation

Normally a regional medical image is formed by a number of hospitals and health centres, it is important to have an overall planning with all social, economic, technological, and political aspects considered from the beginning. In the process of

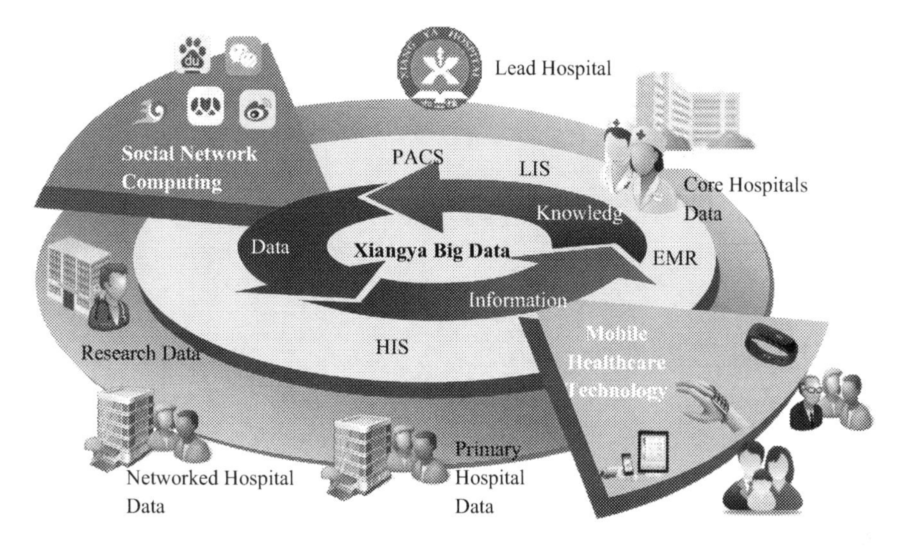

Fig. 1 Mobile healthcare eco-system of Xiangya hospital

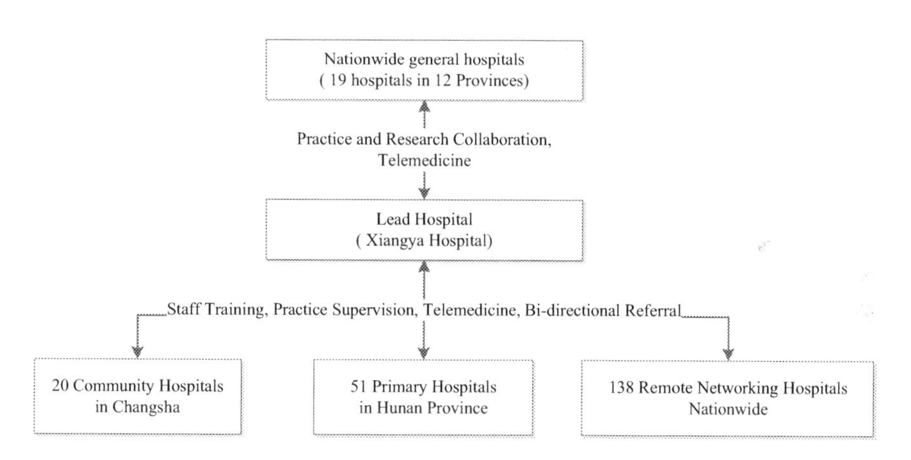

Fig. 2 Regional medical collaboration network

implementation, apart from building the centralised cloud for the whole region, pilot tests and experiments in departments and hospitals are to be carried out individually and regionally before the whole platform is rolled out in full scale action.

(2) Standardised interface, connected process

To achieve smooth universal medical imaging operation across tens of hospitals and hundreds of different medical equipment from different manufactures, it is critical to ensure raw data and information exchange interfaces are standardised (e.g. DICOM

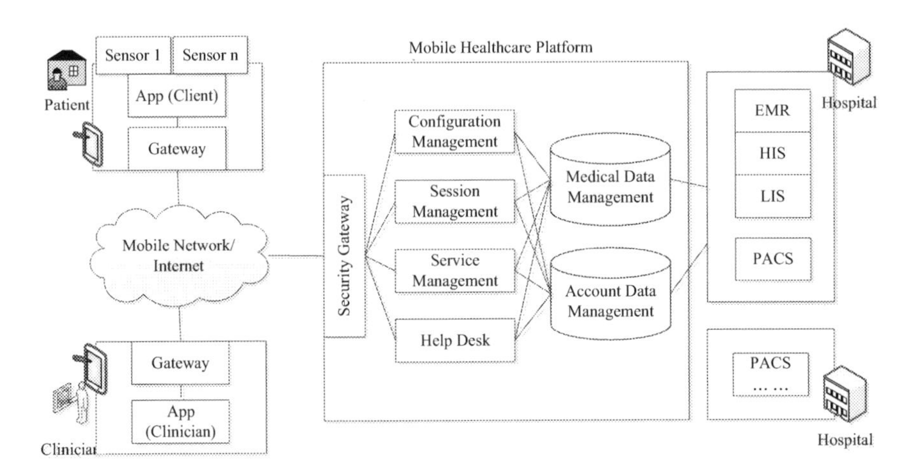

Fig. 3 Mobile healthcare system reference architecture

for medical images). Other business processes other than image processing such as referral and teleconsultation processes should also be tested in workflow and connected to existing hospital information systems.

(3) Collaborative service, improved performance
One of the objectives to build a regional medical image is to enable more collaboration between hospitals and doctors, and under the same quality control framework in the region, it is expected improve the overall performance of care services by enlarging the service coverage, improving information sharing, reducing resource waste and enhanced service administration.

(4) Extensible architecture, secured protection
Cloud system should support constant data growth and new application developments, therefore should follow open architecture for scalable and sustainable future extension. Its built-in security mechanisms should be effective and reliable in trust management, access control, network security, storage and recovery to guarantee the safe operation of regional medical care and patient information privacy.

5.3 System Components of MIC

A medical image cloud normally includes the following important components: the medical image cloud centre is responsible for storage of medical image data on the large image cloud pool provided by cloud service provider (e.g. China Telecom or other mobile network providers offering similar service). The front-end gateway is normally a hardware device similar to the size of a set-top box or a blade server in large scale applications in core hospitals. The cloud PACS system for hospitals refers to the full PACS workflow process management for radiology department, just like a traditional PACS on cloud for better understanding by radiologists. There are also two major types of image viewing/diagnosis applications, one is mobile (Android & iOS) and the other is a typical application on desktop OS. As the cloud computing relies heavily on network bandwidth, it is always recommended to have high-speed dual fibre connection to ensure major data flow between hospitals and the cloud, note the viewing client network doesn't require such.

Module	System and resources	Description
Medical image cloud centre	Mobile network operator medical image cloud	Reginal cloud PACS centre storage management system
	Image storage pool	Storage resource pool for medical images for the region
Front-end gateway	M-Box (hardware)	Hardware gateway to enable medical equipment directly connected to the regional cloud PACS
Cloud PACS system for hospitals	Mobile network operator Cloud PACS platform	Offer full PACS workflow process management for radiology department including 2D/3D image processing capacity on cloud
Medical image diagnosis mobile application	Mobile Apps for medical imaging	iOS and Android applications on smartphone and tablets to support full image review and diagnosis operations
Medical image diagnosis desktop application	Desktop application for medical imaging	Client application on desktop to load, read, save, process and report on medical images just like traditional PACS clients
Network connection	Fibre Internet/Gigabit Intranet	Dual fibre connection if available to support reliable connection from hospital to regional cloud

5.4 System Architecture of MIC

There are two major parts in the regional imaging cloud system: hospitals and cloud of regional centre. To ensure the best speed, quality and capacity of massive medical image processing, system architecture should work a guaranteed service provider on the network. In this case, the image cloud computing service provider is China Telecom. The overall system architecture is illustrated as Fig. 4.

Local medical image data generated by medical equipment like CT/X-Ray will be uploaded to cloud in real-time via the gateway M-Box in a secured channel. After the image raw data is stored and processed instantly by the powerful cloud

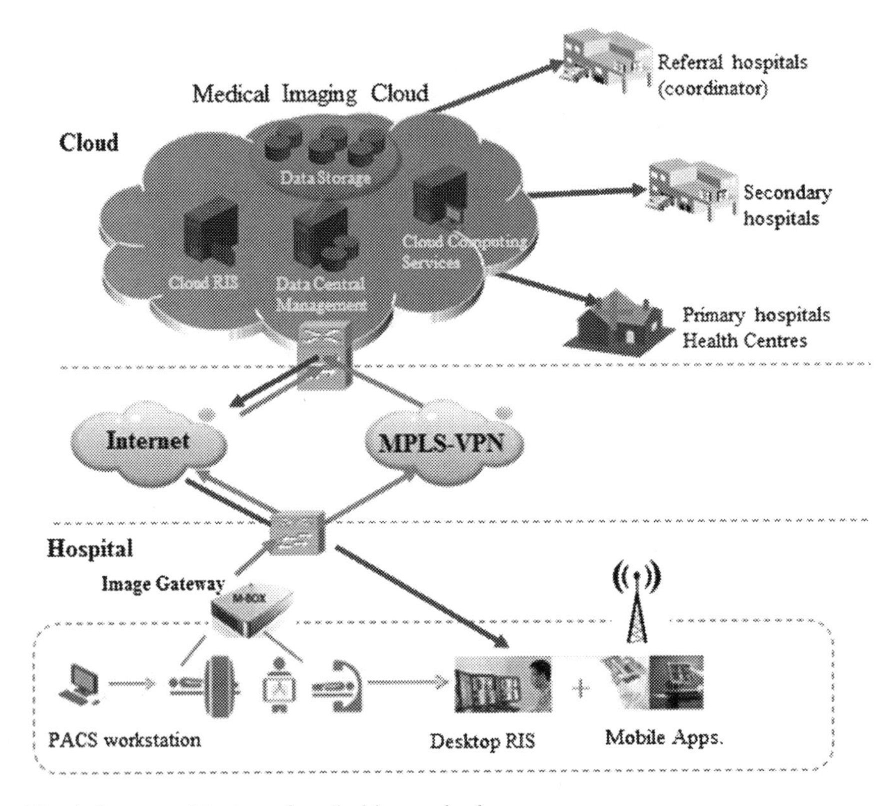

Fig. 4 System architecture of medical image cloud

computing centre, doctor could review and process the image data on desktop computers and mobile terminals without delay, and diagnosis and reporting could be done afterwards.

5.5 *Data Logic Architecture of MIC*

In accordance with the system architecture, the data generated from the hospital will be uploaded and stored in the cloud and processed for cloud access later. The overall data flow process involves several steps (as shown in Fig. 5):

(1) Medical equipment pushes raw data to gateway;
(2) Gateway preprocesses data upload to the cloud;
(3) Cloud receives data and processes it for storage on cloud Object-Oriented Storage (OOS) [15];

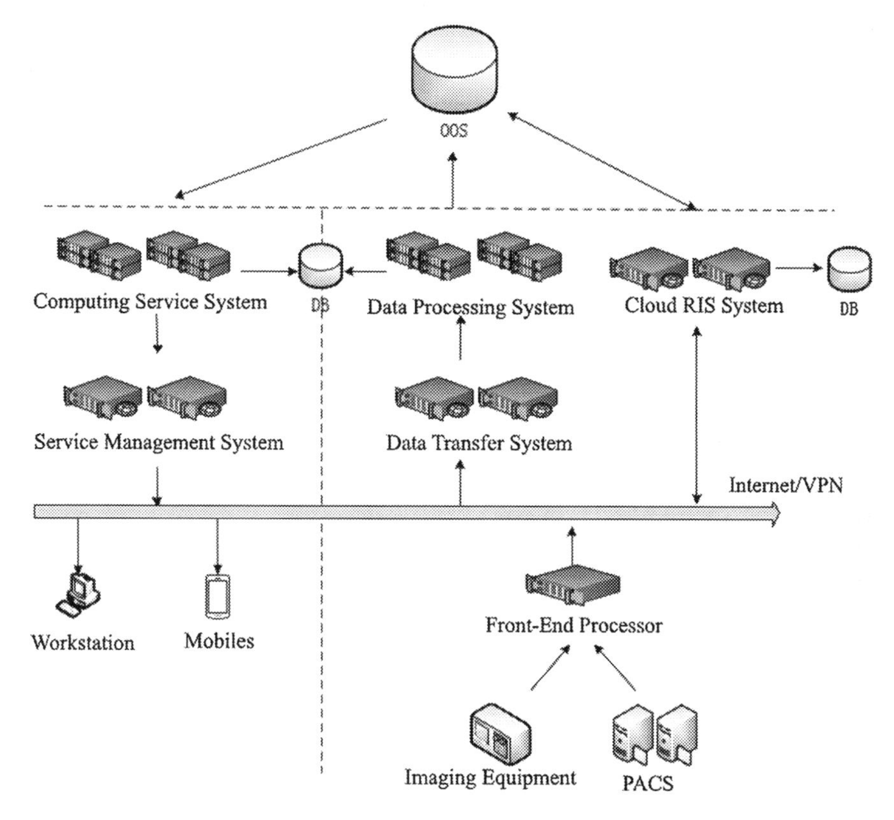

Fig. 5 Data logic architecture of medical image cloud

(4) Cloud offers service management and cloud PACS and Radiology Information System (RIS) for universal access (e.g. desktop and mobile applications) over the Internet.

5.6 *Software Architecture of MIC*

The medical image cloud system consists of three parts: computing service system, data management system and OOS cloud storage system. Computing service system and data management system are constructed in clustering architecture, which supports linear scalability, can be extended from a single server to multiple servers according to the volume of business volume. Gigabit network is in place to support internal data exchange within the cloud system.

(1) Computing service architecture

The computing service system architecture is shown as Fig. 6.

The computing service system architecture consists of four layers:

(1) Data Layer: designed for medical image processing and computing, consists of multiple servers. These arrays do not need to face external access directly, and only communicate with the Process Layer via different functional centres such as patient centre, filming centre and image centre. Its scale of computing could grow depending on the computation demand, and the overall elastic increment on cloud would assure the smooth capacity upgrade and guarantee the performance for medical imaging operations online.
(2) Process Layer: designed for data process workload distribution and balancing, consists of multiple provider groups where each group contains one or more providers. Each provider connects functional centres in the data layer. Each server requires an independent external network IP for data exchange. Network bandwidth is to be allocated depending on data volume from external.
(3) Access Layer: designed for account management for user identification and verification, consists of two servers, one for disaster recovery redundancy, and these two servers do not need to have public network IP address.
(4) Device Layer: generally refers to terminal devices over the Internet and connected to the cloud via Network Address Translation (NAT) from Intranet,

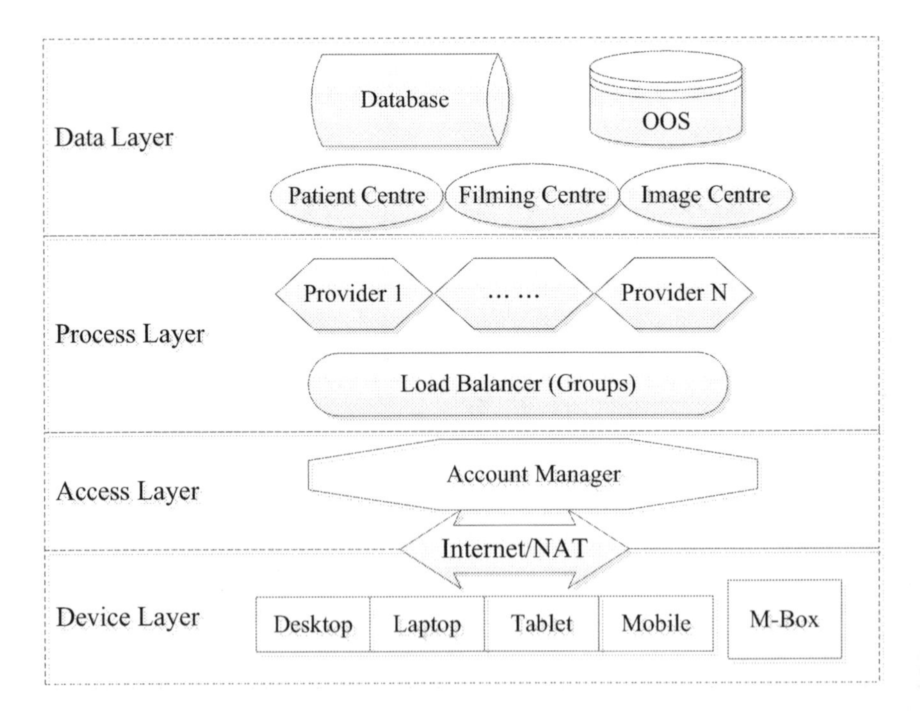

Fig. 6 Software architecture of medical image cloud

which include designated M-Box from medical devices, Laptops, desktops, tablets, and smart phones with applications.

5.7 Data Management System Architecture of MIC

The data management system architecture is shown as Fig. 7.

Data management system architecture consists of three parts on top of devices:

(1) Storage Arrays: consists of multiple servers for medical image storage. These arrays do not need to face external access directly, and only communicate with the transfer servers. Its scale of computing could grow depending on the computation demand, and the overall elastic increment on cloud would assure the smooth capacity upgrade and guarantee the performance for medical imaging operations online.

(2) Transfer Servers: consists of multiple servers for receiving and sending the medical image data from clients, user identification and verification. Each

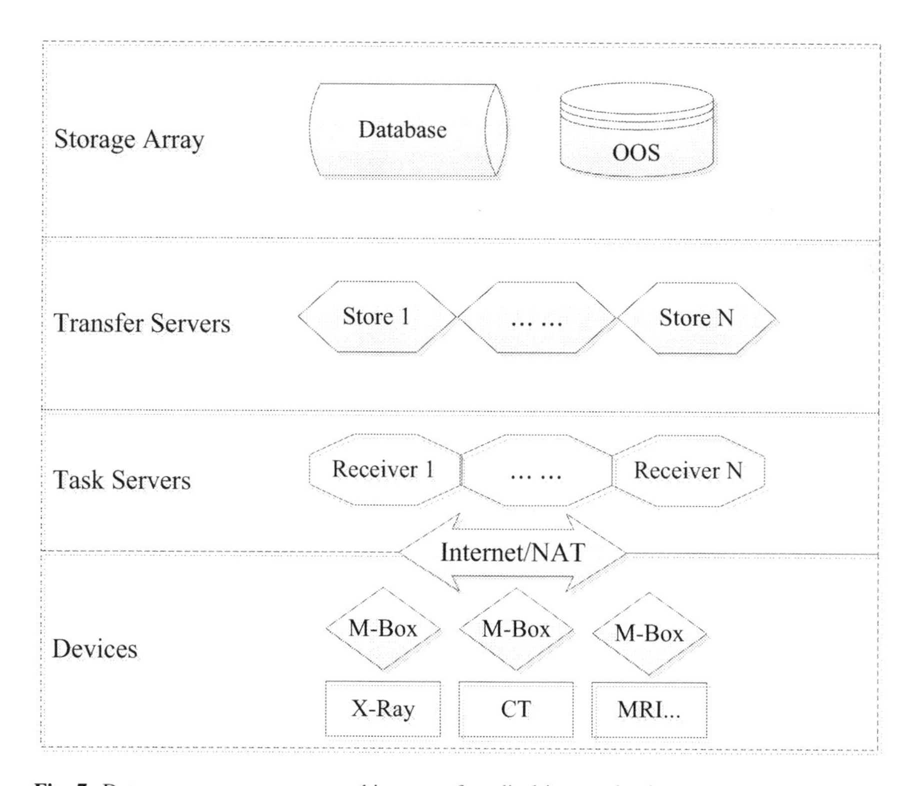

Fig. 7 Data management system architecture of medical image cloud

server requires an independent external network IP for data exchange. Network bandwidth is to be allocated depending on data volume from external.

(3) Task Servers: consists of two servers for task access and distribution with including one as disaster recovery redundancy, and these two servers share a single network IP address for users to access from external.

5.8 Standards and Interfaces of MIC

(1) Medical image standard

In order to work with different medical devices and equipment from different vendors, it is important to have the whole system data for storage and processing be compliant with international standard in medical image, which currently is DICOM3.0 [14].

(2) Interface with hospital

The interface between a hospital and the medical image cloud is implemented by Front-end Processor (FEP). There are two types of FEPs for different scenarios. One is blade server on rack in top hospitals that connects multiple CT/MRI/X-Ray machines, and the other is a small box at the size of a set-top-box that deals with one single medical imaging device. Both machines work in Linux. It is quite simple and easy to setup for interface, a normal installation process of FEP takes only about 30 min (Fig. 8).

The major functions of FEP include:

(1) Receiving/pulling device from local PACS or medical imaging device workstation;
(2) Uploading data to cloud with automatic routing;
(3) Data returning and synchronization of image data;
(4) Medical image data encryption and compression.

FEP gets data from local PACS in two different modes:

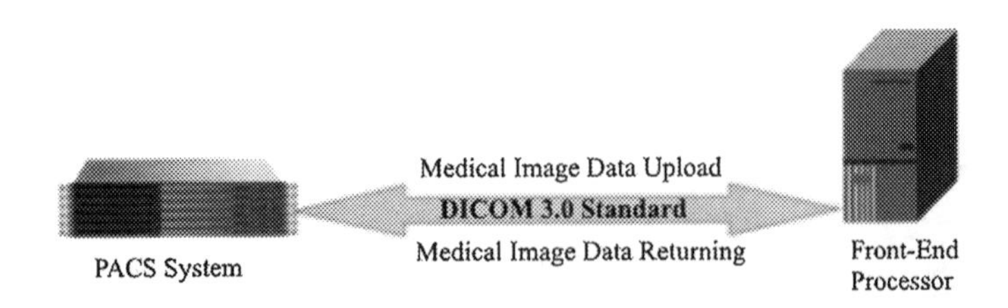

Fig. 8 DICOM3.0 and front-end processor

The first mode is use of PACS image data automatically routing. Automatic routing means is a basic file transfer function of a PACS system [2]. By predefining the destination machine's IP address for image transfer, this function automatically transfers the image files to the destination (usually a radiologist's computer) once the image files are generated. It saves time for radiologist to pull the data from the device to their computers. To route the image data to the FEP, just need to add data receiving terminal's IP, Port, AETitle in the system, and on the FEP, just need to add DICOM parameters (i.e. FEP IP, Port, AETitle, PACS etc.), then the data received from PACS will be uploaded automatically to the cloud.

The second mode is DICOM Query PACS image data. This query function is also another basic function of PACS, supported by all PACS vendors [4]. The only difference here is the FEP fetches data from PACS or workstation automatically, and only the PACS or workstation needs to set related parameters (e.g. IP, Port, AETitle) to allow FEP fetch the data, and rest process of upload to the cloud is the same as that in the first mode.

In order to maintain the data consistency, the FEP also supports data returning and synchronization. After the data from hospital PACS is uploaded to the cloud, whenever it is requested, the local hospital PACS could acquire the same raw data from the cloud down to PACS, only in a reversed order to the upload process.

6 Cloud-Based Mobile Healthcare Services

The medical image cloud provides three different front-end entries: Yizhen website [28], a mobile app (for iPad, iPhone and Android), and a desktop application. The website is mainly used for business services such as registration and teleconsultation, while the standalone applications are used to execute the image processing tasks.

6.1 Services Enabled on Applications in MIC

Both basic and advanced functions are supported in medical image processing services on desktop and mobile applications.

Types	Function descriptions
Basic functions	Mobile medical image review
	2D image processing (grayscale adjustment, measurement, tag and annotation)
	Ultrasound application module
	3D image processing (density projection, surface reconstruction, volume reconstruction, etc.)
	2D image chord processing, DSA subtraction angiography
	Full lung reconstruction, coronary extraction

(continued)

(continued)

Types	Function descriptions
Advanced functions	Automatic boning
	Stenosis analysis
	Operation mode (1:1), virtual operation
	Stereoscopic display, 3D printing interface (3D printers needed)

6.2 Care Services Enabled on the Website

The website actually enables a full workflow in RIS for radiology department. The processes enabled on the website are listed as follows:

No.	Processes	Process descriptions
1	Registration and booking	Automatically or manually arrange booking according to requirements
2	Queuing and number calling	Queue management and supporting queue number calling when connects to big screens with speakers
3	Medical image examination	Get ready to operate the medical equipment and transfer the image data to cloud
4	Medical image review	Viewing the image cloud with advanced features in processing
5	Tele-consultation and tele-diagnosis	Initiate and manage group consultation, filing report online
6	Report review and audit	The final reports on medical images could be reviewed and audited online before released to patients

The external and internal processes are described as Figs. 9 and 10.

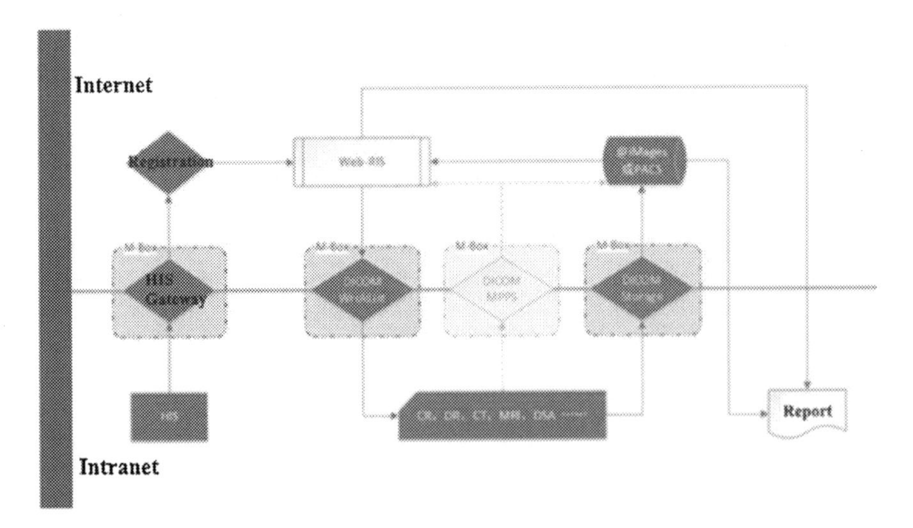

Fig. 9 External process of medical image cloud

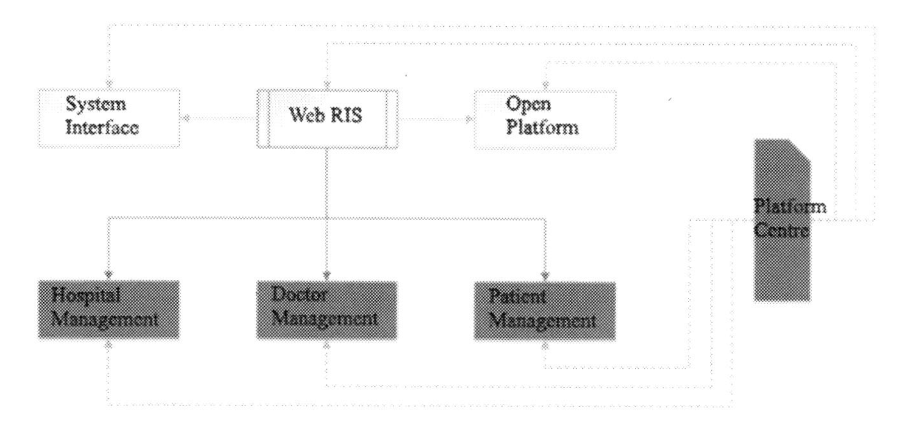

Fig. 10 Internal process of medical image cloud

6.3 *Operational Services Enabled on MIC*

The medial image cloud platform also supports other services related to operations such as image statistics, image management, user account and organisation account management, FEP monitoring and early warning in operation.

No.	Processes	Process descriptions
1	Event warning	Automatic warning on FEP error and offline, cloud storage close to limits, account membership expiry
2	Image statistics	Real-time statistics on upload images by equipment, date/month for operational monitoring
3	Image management	Managing the availability and correctness of the images on cloud
4	Accounts management	Management organisation's account registration and allocate doctor's personal account for access
5	FEP monitoring	Real-time comprehensive monitoring of all FEPs' status (e.g. CPU, memory, HD I/O, network) for smooth business operation

6.4 *Comparison in Operational Costs Between MIC and Traditional PACS*

The comparison between medical image cloud solution and traditional PACS system in operational costs are as follows. Clearly cloud-based solution is very cost-effective especially for those secondary and primary level hospitals.

Item	Medical image cloud	Traditional PACS
Initial investment (Software/hardware)	0	Millions RMB
Implementation	Extremely simple (one M-Box, one network cable)	Complicated (servers, software system configurations)
Deployment time	Very fast (from hours to days)	Long (normally 6 months+)
Storage cost	Clear and explicit accounting (e.g. DR, CT by case and type)	Hundreds of thousands RMB
System maintenance cost	0	10–15% of initial cost
Shared computing room cost	0	High (increasing yearly)

6.5 Basis for Medical Image Big Data

By getting more and more volume and types of data on the cloud, the medical image cloud contributes to a base for medical Big Data in the future. In the overall Big Data analysis process, medical image data mining plays an important role, which is considered an advanced feature and function of medical image cloud.

(1) Medical image data mining approaches

Medical image data mining mainly works in two models: function-driven model and information-driven model [1].

Function-driven model is to use different functional modules for specific requirements, normally involves image acquisition (extracting image data from the image database), image pre-processing (image feature extraction and storage), search engine (using image features for inquiry), and knowledge discovery (using image data analysis algorithms to find the related data, characteristics and relationships).

Information-driven model works on contents of the images. It starts from meaningful segmentation of images based on original characteristics using data mining algorithms and domain knowledge, then carries out higher-level analysis, and derives more accurate and understandable semantics [29]. Normally the model works at four different levels accordingly from pixels, objects and semantics to the highest knowledge level.

In the context of medical image cloud, it is more effective to use the information driven model by making use of annotated/embedded information in DICOM image data and related EMR information.

(2) Medical imaging big data task force

Medical imaging big data is the most challenging subdomain in interdisciplinary medical big data research and development [5]. Requirements and solutions may vary depending on disease contexts. It is so complicated that neither doctors nor IT experts could work out a successful solution alone. It requires close cooperation between clinical experts (domain knowledge) and IT experts (computing technology). An experimental task force for medical image big data is now initiated between hospitals and companies specialised in medical imaging.

The operation model of the multi-discipline task force works like this: "medical experts describe the requirements → engineering specialist provide technical solutions → Medical experts verifies results" in order to solve the dilemma. Led by famous doctors in top teaching hospital, medical experts collate medical records and related information especially medical image data disease by disease. IT experts then start to build models on the pre-organised data for machine learning and cross referencing. With powerful computation capacity on the cloud, intermediate results could be shown to medical experts for evaluation or approval, and to make adjustment to algorithms and even original data/information sets if necessary. By experimenting on certain diseases first, and extend to other diseases later, gradually build an efficient medical big data research framework, and eventually to be applied in clinical practices.

7 Case Study: Cloud Teleconsultation in Real Practice

7.1 *Processes of Cloud Teleconsultation*

In order to demonstrate how mobile healthcare works on cloud in real practice, a scenario of teleconsultation is illustrated as an example, it happens quite frequently when junior doctors face difficult and complex cases and ask for senior doctor's help. Part of the tele-consultation practice process is illustrated as Fig. 11.

It is a relatively simple process. The requester initiates the teleconsultation, and sends the invitation to one or multiple recipients in the same hospital or other collaborative hospitals, and wait for the advice and report back from the teleconsultation in the end. The requester could join the discussion over the phone or on the cloud if needed. A corresponding detailed process flow of the requestor in real practice is shown as Fig. 12.

On the teleconsultation receiver side, the cloud will send out a notification message automatically when the request is initiated. When the consultant receives a mobile message, he/she could then log on to the website, and follow the instructions on the website or mobile phone, view the medical image on the cloud and fill in the necessary form for advice and comments for the requester. The corresponding processes are shown as Fig. 13.

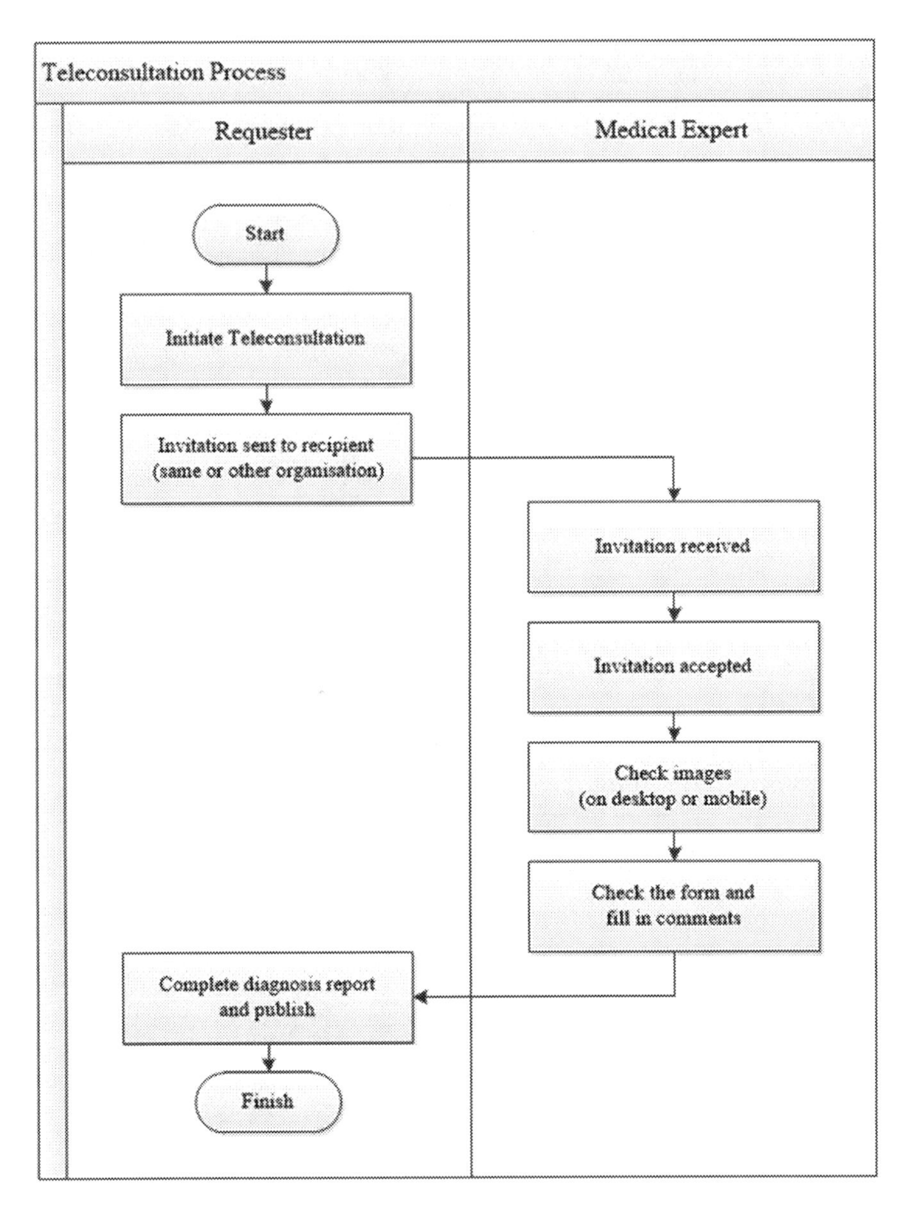

Fig. 11 Example: process of teleconsultation on cloud

During the cloud image viewing process, it could be opened from cloud via desktop application as shown in Fig. 14, or via mobile applications as shown in Fig. 15 (note: images below are for illustration purpose, not necessarily correspond to each other).

(Step 1). invitation: choose the patient record and click "initiate teleconsultation":

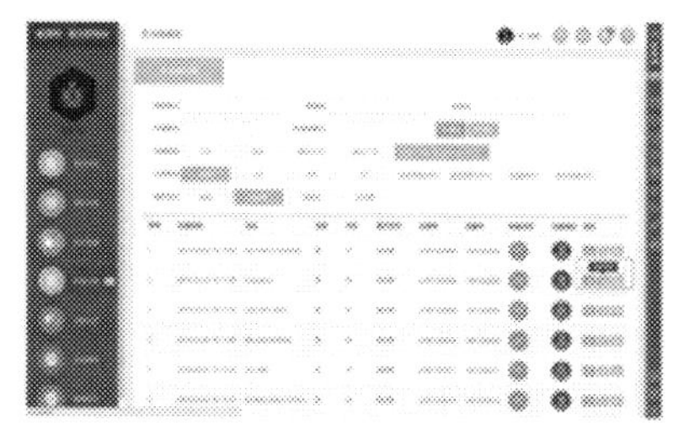

(Step 2). Choose "recipient in the same organisation" or "recipient in other organisation":

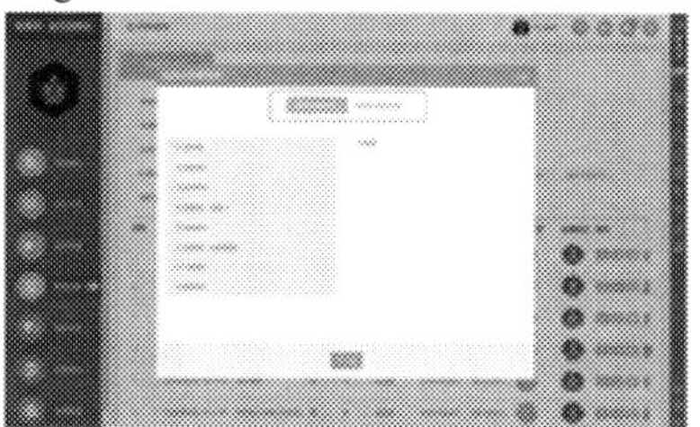

(Step 3). Select doctor (same organisation/ other organisation), click "next":

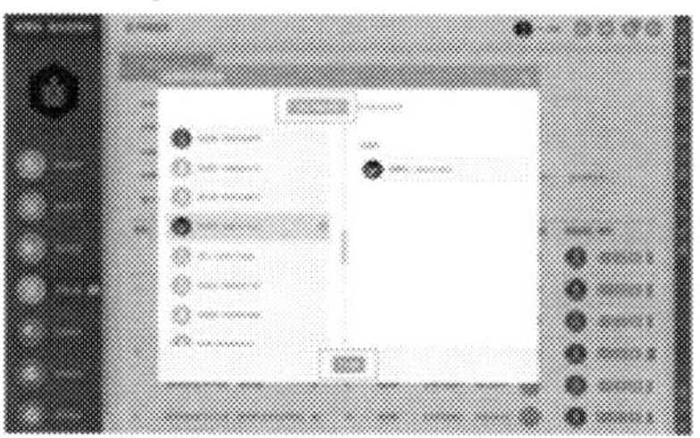

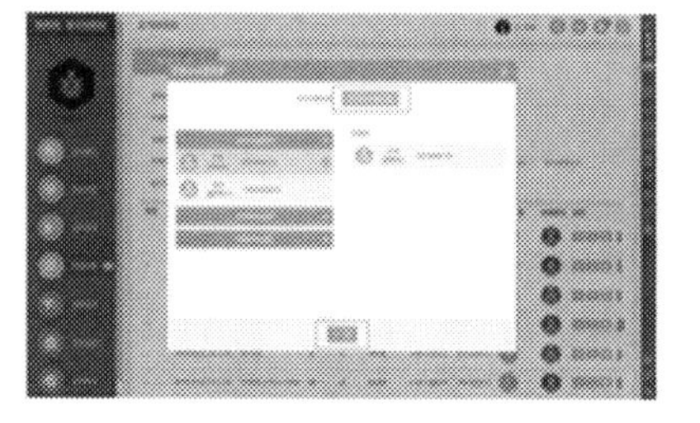

(Step 4). Set time, fill in the notes for consultation, click "finish".

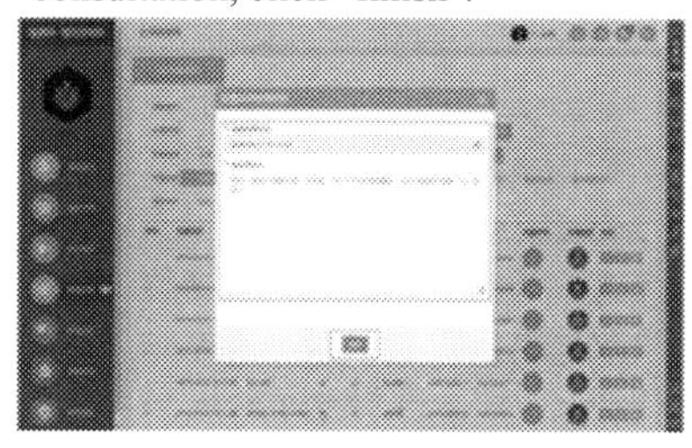

(Step 5) After the teleconsultation, complete the diagnosis report and publish the report.

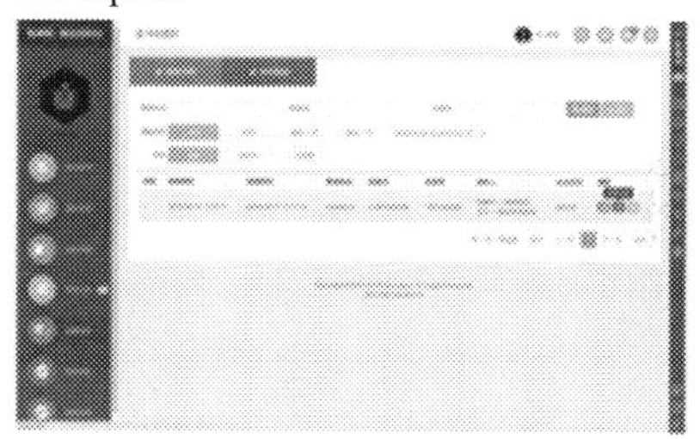

Fig. 12 Requestor process illustration

7.2 Recommended System Specification for MIC

In terms of recommended system specification in implementation, the system actually requires no special configuration apart from a high-speed (20 Mbps plus) network connection between the front-end gateway FEP (provided by the manufacturer) sitting between the medical imaging device and the Internet all computation is done on the cloud. The only thing requires for the desktop client side is an up-to-date browser (e.g. Chrome) on a typical mainstream office desktop computer (e.g. Intel i3 with 2 GB RAM). The mobile client runs very smoothly on any

(Step 1) On the top right corner of the interface, click "My mailbox" to view and select the consultation request.

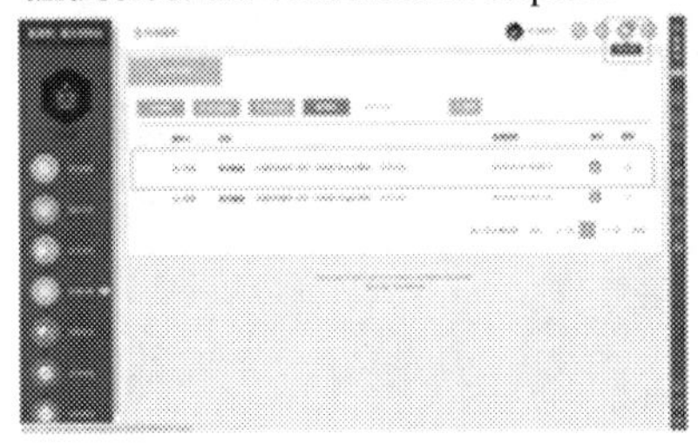

(Step 2). Check the teleconsultation details.

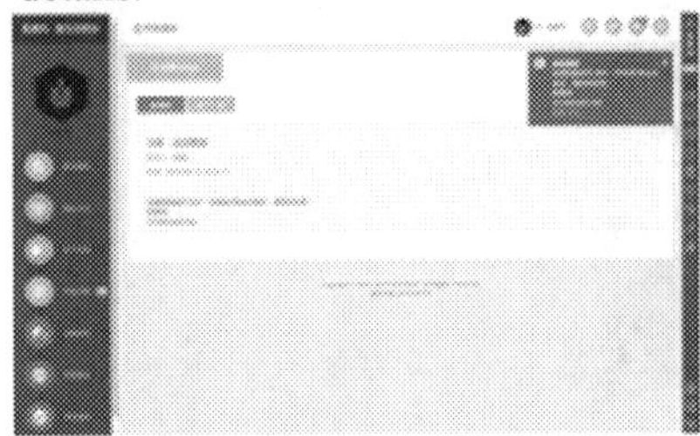

(Step 3) Accepts the consultation request.

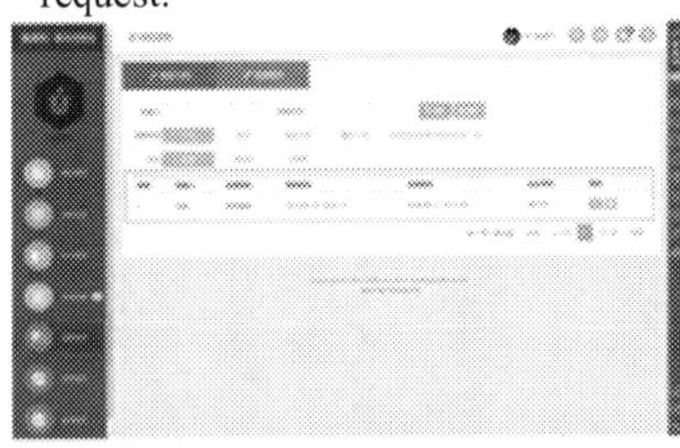

(Step 4) Choose "continue" or "check image".

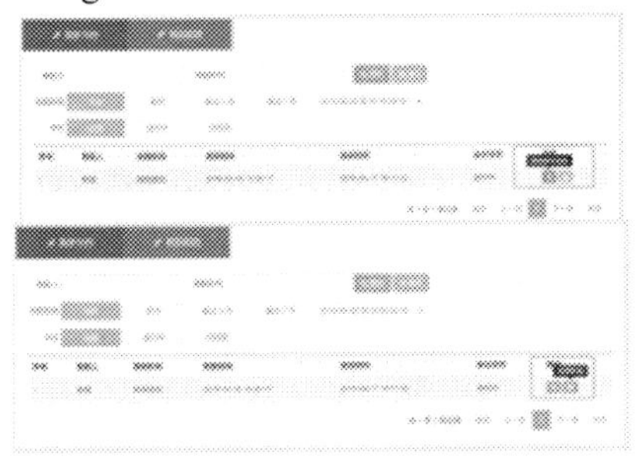

(5) check the consultation information and fill in the comments, then publish.

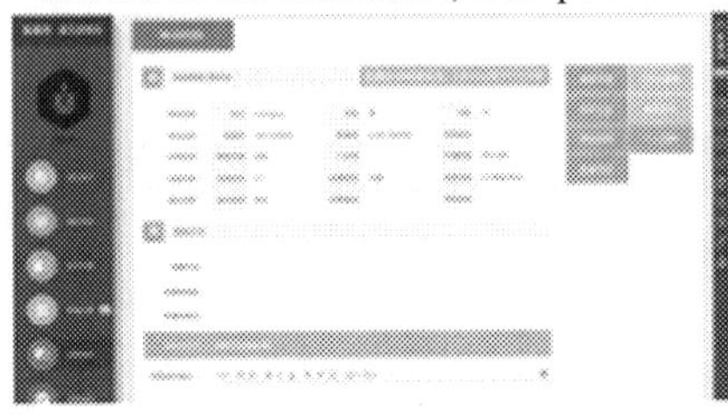

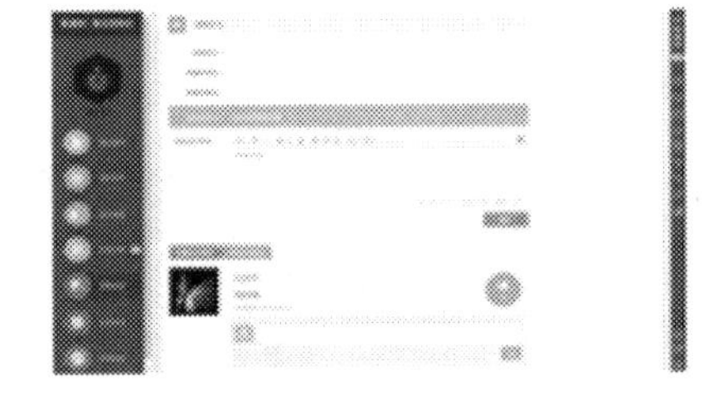

Fig. 13 Receiver process illustrations

mainstream Android and iOS smart phones with 2 GB RAM, preferably with 4 screen for better viewing result.

7.3 Photos of Teleconsultations on MIC and More

It would be interesting to see some photos of teleconsultation and other applications on medical image cloud in real practices (Figs. 16, 17 and 18).

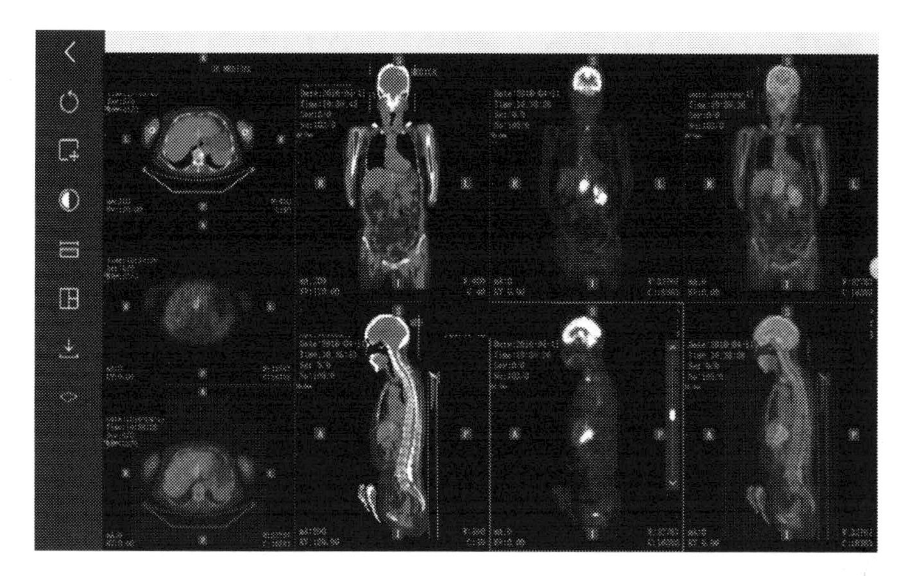

Fig. 14 Cloud RIS desktop application screenshot

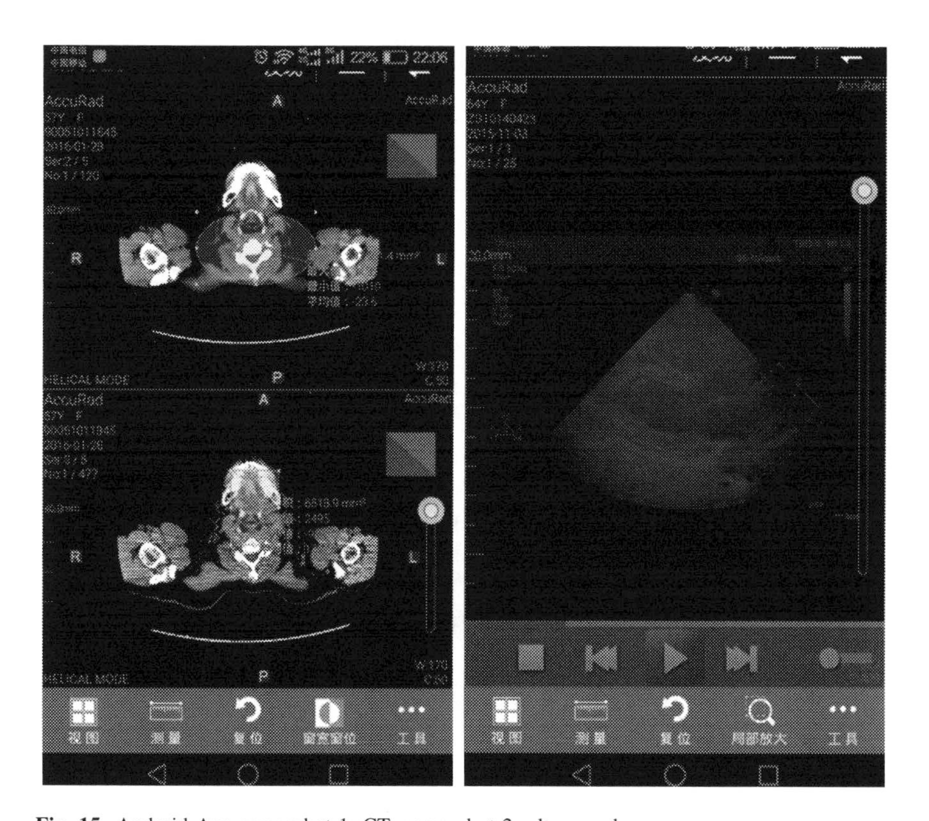

Fig. 15 Android App screenshot 1: CT, screenshot 2: ultrasound

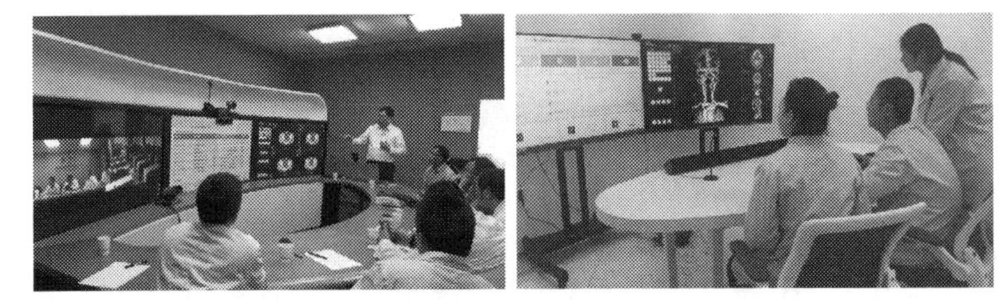

Fig. 16 Two different teleconsultation rooms with big screen TVs connected to the cloud

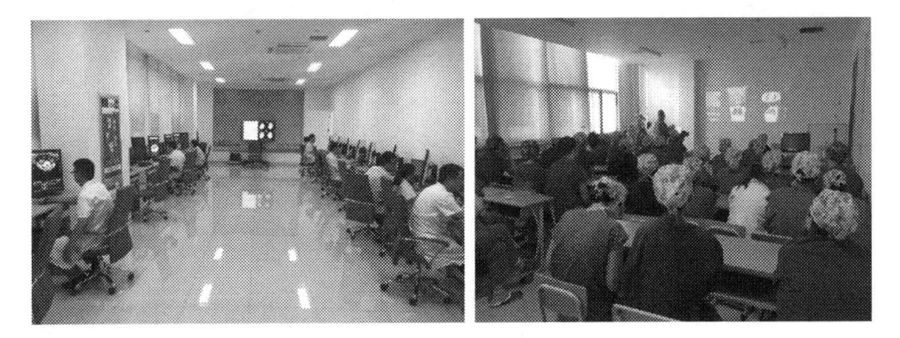

Fig. 17 *Left* A regional medical imaging centre in China; *Right* using medical image cloud for education

These photos present a recent successful case just launched in China. Under the support from local Health and Family Planning Commission, a regional medical image cloud is now online, which covers over 8 million residents across 2 city districts and 9 counties, connects 1 referral hospital, 20 secondary county hospitals, and 107 primary level health centres. This project is highly approved and appraised by local government that it is nominated as one of the model projects of "top 10

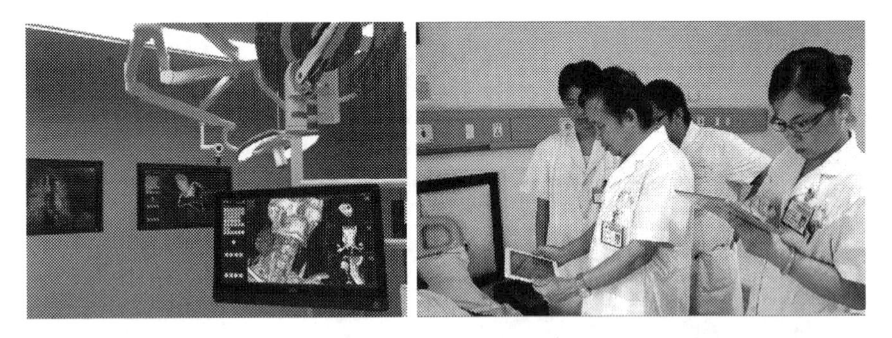

Fig. 18 *Left* cloud imaging in operating room; *Right* using tablet in department rounding

practical projects for the people in 2016 in the region". This example shows that medical image cloud is also feasible, practical at the small regional levels organised by regional hospitals, and it is replicable to other regions in different part of China.

8 Conclusions and Future Work

To address the most challenging issue of mobile imaging service in mobile healthcare and to form a solid base for future medical Big Data processing in healthcare, this chapter systematically presents an innovative medical image cloud solution. This chapter not only describes how a medical image cloud is implemented, but also shows how technology solutions like medical image cloud could contribute to a regional hierarchical medical system construction in China by connecting medical experts and patients safely and seamlessly on the cloud across the traditional hospital barrier. With dedicated system architectural design and enabled collaborative processes such as teleconsultation, the medical image cloud enables easy installation and configuration of a cloud-based PACS, universal access of different types of medical image data on various terminal including desktops, tablets and smart phones. From the management and operational perspective, the medical image cloud assures mobile healthcare quality, reduces care costs for both government and patients, provides reliable, secure, and convenient access to medical images for doctors and patients, and literally creates a win-win ecosystem in modern healthcare system in China.

Current hardware products and software architecture in the presented medical image cloud system are mature and stable for large scale deployment in China. A promising direction for future development would be medical image Big Data analysis. This has been a world-class challenging issue in healthcare information technology industry. Based on the powerful computing capacity and constant-growing medical image data and related medical information on cloud, medical experts could now work closely with computing scientists towards a promising breakthrough in Medial Image Big Data will be expected in the near future.

References

1. Antonie, M. L., Zaïane, O. R., & Coman, A. (2001). Application of Data Mining Techniques for Medical Image Classification. *International Workshop on Multimedia Data Mining, Mdm/kdd'2001, August, 2001, San Francisco, CA, USA*.
2. Breant, C. M., Taira, R. K., Tashima, G. H., & Huang, H. K. (1992). Issues and solutions for interfacing a PACS database with an RIS. *Medical Imaging VI* (pp. 255–263). International Society for Optics and Photonics.

3. Chen, F. X., Mao, Y., & Wang, J. H. (2012). Two-way referral of patients with infectious diseases between community health care organizations and specialized hospitals in beijing. *Chinese General Practice, 15*, 775–777.
4. Cox, R. D., Henri, C. J., Rubin, R. K., & Bret, P. M. (1998). DICOM-compliant PACS with CD-based image archival. *Medical Imaging*. International Society for Optics and Photonics.
5. Dilsizian, S. E., & Siegel, E. L. (2014). Artificial intelligence in medicine and cardiac imaging: harnessing big data and advanced computing to provide personalized medical diagnosis and treatment. *Current Cardiology Reports, 16*(1), 1–8.
6. Fang, P. Q., Zou, X. X., & Sun, Y. (2014). Key points of the hierarchical medical system research in china. *Chinese Hospital Management*.
7. Garlan, D., Monroe, R. T., & Wile, D. (2000). *Acme: architectural description of component-based systems*. Cambridge University Press.
8. Gilmour, Campbell, Loane, Esmail, Griffiths, & Roland, et al. (1998). Comparison of teleconsultations and face-to-face consultations: preliminary results of a United Kingdom multicentre teledermatology study. *British Journal of Dermatology, 139*(1), 81–7.
9. Hany, T. F., Steinert, H. C., Goerres, G. W., Buck, A., & von Schulthess, G. K. (2002). Pet diagnostic accuracy: improvement with in-line pet-ct system: initial results. *Radiology, 225* (2), 575–81.
10. Hays, R. (2001). Rural initiatives at the James cook university school of medicine: a vertically integrated regional/rural/remote medical education provider. *Australian Journal of Rural Health, 9 suppl 1*(9 Suppl 1), 2–5.
11. Istepanian, R., Laxminarayan, S., & Pattichis, C. S. (2006). M-health: emerging mobile health systems. 237–246.
12. Karlsson, G., Hedman, K., & Fridlund, B. (2011). Views on patient safety by operations managers in somatic hospital care: a qualitative analysis. *Open Journal of Nursing, 01*(33), 5125–5131.
13. Kong, X., Feng, M., & Wang, R. (2015). The current status and challenges of establishment and utilization of medical big data in china. *European Geriatric Medicine, 6*(6), 515–517.
14. Levine, B. A., Cleary, K. R., Norton, G. S., Cramer, T. J., & Mun, S. K. (1997). Challenges encountered while implementing a multivendor teleradiology network using DICOM 3.0. *Medical Imaging* (pp. 237–246). International Society for Optics and Photonics.
15. Liu, J., & Dai, R. (2013). The inquiry into telecom enterprises' cloud computing strategy: A case study of China telecom. *IEEE International Conference on Digital Ecosystems and Technologies*. IEEE.
16. Mahoney, C. D., Berard-Collins, C. M., Coleman, R., Amaral, J. F., & Cotter, C. M. (2007). Effects of an integrated clinical information system on medication safety in a multi-hospital setting. *American journal of health-system pharmacy: AJHP: official journal of the American Society of Health-System Pharmacists, 64*(18), 209–215.
17. Martinez, A. W., Phillips, S. T., Carrilho, E., Sindi, H., & Whitesides, G. M. (2008). Simple telemedicine for developing regions: camera phones and paper-based microfluidic devices for real-time, off-site diagnosis. *Analytical Chemistry, 80*(10), 3699–707.
18. Mates, J., Branstetter, B. F., Morgan, M. B., Lionetti, D. M., & Chang, P. J. (2007). 'wet reads' in the age of pacs: technical and workflow considerations for a preliminary report system. *Journal of Digital Imaging, 20*(3), 296–306.
19. Mauro, A. D., Greco, M., & Grimaldi, M. (2016). A formal definition of big data based on its essential features. Library Review, 65(3), 122–135.
20. Mell, P. M., & Grance, T. (2011). SP 800–145. The NIST Definition of Cloud Computing. National Institute of Standards & Technology.
21. MIIT Report on the Quality of Telecommunications Services (No. 1 of 2016), Ministry of Industry and Information Technology of China, Retrieved 1 October 2016, from http://www.miit.gov.cn/.
22. Neame, R. L. (2014). Privacy protection for personal health information and shared care records. *Journal of Innovations in Health Informatics, 21*(2), 84–91.

23. Pasha, M. F., Supramaniam, S., Liang, K. K., Amran, M. A., Chandra, B. A., & Rajeswari, M. (2012). An android-based mobile medical image viewer and collaborative annotation: development issues and challenges. *International Journal of Digital Content Technology & Its Applications, 6*(1).
24. Peck, D. (2010). *Digital Imaging and Communications in Medicine (DICOM): A Practical Introduction and Survival Guide. Biomedical Image Processing*. Springer Berlin Heidelberg.
25. Robinson, M., & Cottrell, D. (2005). Health professionals in multi-disciplinary and multi-agency teams: changing professional practice. *Journal of Interprofessional Care, 19*(6), 547–60.
26. Rodríguez, N. J., Borges, J. A., Crespo, G., Pérez, C., Martinez, C., & Colónrivera, C. R., et al. (2009). Users Can Do Better with PDAs Than Paper: A Usability Study of PDA-Based vs. Paper-Based Nursing Documentation Systems. *Universal Access in Human-Computer Interaction. Applications and Services, International Conference, Uahci 2009, Held As* (Vol. 5616, pp. 395–403).
27. WeChat – Free messaging and calling app, Retrieved 1 October 2016, from https://www.wechat.com/en/.
28. Yizhen.cn, Retrieved 1 October 2016, from http://www.yizhen.cn.
29. Zhang, J., Hsu, W., & Lee, M. L. (2003). *An Information-driven Framework for Image Mining. Database and Expert Systems Applications*. Springer Berlin Heidelberg.

Large-Scale Innovations and Approaches for Community Healthcare Support in Developing Nations

Shah Jahan Miah

Abstract Over the past two decades, many large-scale innovations have been designed for the individuals' information support in improving public healthcare. Studies show rapidly growing interests on cloud computing and telecommunication-based technologies such as mobile-based innovations that are mainly evident in form of improving the social healthcare support systems for community, organisations and individuals. Approaches for various innovations to healthcare support delivery enable people to build on their strengths and to improve the independence and overall wellbeing in the community. The objective of such innovations for community healthcare has been well-established in developed nations, but still emergent to achieve various goals for many developing nations. A lot of application aspects are therefore under-researched to achieve the outcomes such as for encouraging healthy lifestyle choices [4, 8], for individual's wellness monitoring [31], and in providing general-healthcare information and advice for self-management [21]. This chapter describes issues of the innovative large-scale technological developments for the community healthcare and well-being in context of developing nations, from an angle of service receivers' perspective. The discussion in the chapter will also capture on various useful large-scale technologies and their effective provisions. In relation to the software-as-service and other forms of cloud technologies as well as the mobile health infrastructure are discussed as they would be useful for the benefit of healthcare service receivers, and through them how individuals can be able to achieve services in the community for enhanced self-management-oriented healthcare.

S.J. Miah (✉)
College of Business, Victoria University, Footscray Park Campus, Melbourne, Australia
e-mail: shah.miah@vu.edu.au

© Springer International Publishing AG 2017

S.U. Khan et al. (eds.), *Handbook of Large-Scale Distributed Computing in Smart Healthcare*, Scalable Computing and Communications,
DOI 10.1007/978-3-319-58280-1_13

1 Introduction

Large-scale computing technologies become essential in improving healthcare systems, especially both to improve processes for efficient care facility and to address organisational and managerial changes in industries. Approaches for various innovations to healthcare support delivery enable people to build on their strengths and to improve the independence and overall wellbeing in the community. Implications of large-scale computing provisions, such as cloud computing and relevant telecommunication service options such as e-health and m-health (mobile health) for improving healthcare delivery, demonstrate potential to significantly improve the accessibility and quality of public or community health and their well-being. The service related to public health includes advisory, emergency and any form of consultation support, treatment and enhanced patient diagnosis through the provisions of m-health and cloud computing are well-established in developed nations [11, 27] but still emergent to fully adopt the applications in many developing nations.

The limitations of medical resources and skilled healthcare professionals are common in rural areas of developing nations. Specifically, resources and healthcare expertise on various support care are inadequate in most of the district towns of developing countries. Network of transportation are also not robust in rural and remote areas; however, wireless and cable based infrastructure and Internet facilities are quite rapidly growing (3G mobility), in rural areas of developing countries [32]. It is due to new research on sustainable and demand-driven technological provisions development. There are scopes to develop sustainable large-scale technological solutions for healthcare industry to maintain and improve information dissemination in relation to various supports such as diagnosis, clinical consultations and for business operations in rural areas.

Cloud computing can be seen as large-scale computing resources as the technological provisions are demand-driven, end-user enabled, resource pooling based and easy to access and manage [3]. For instance, [3] propose a cloud computing based solution for diagnosing neurological diseases in developing countries. The solution uses patient's voice sample for diagnosing the diseases via mobile application. The system uses an artificial neural network classifier for the diagnosis. Rural patients can communicate to healthcare professionals if they use Internet to access the cloud-based solution through their mobile or other form of computing tool. The cloud-based solution also ensures large-scale infrastructure as a service, large-scale platform as a service (PaaS), and user demand oriented large-scale software as a service [3]. Such huge hierarchical view can exemplify the development and use of sustainable public healthcare in order to meet its diverse demands across the huge population.

A large-scale technology in from of telecommunication infrastructure base, m-health provides health service through mobile communication on medical issues and diagnosis of both—well-known and complex diseases, by electronically connected to healthcare professionals who are geographically dispersed. The growth of m-health adaptations in forms of telemedicine, mobile applications, telehealth, and telematics are widely accepted provisions for their service delivery capability and they successfully address issues to bridge social and economic gaps between rural and urban communities [24]. Such m-health infrastructure improves access and provides options for various health services to enhance wellbeing and quality of life of underserved people who are living in the rural, regional and remote locations. For the huge population, m-health innovations have been gained numerous attentions to both—researchers and service industries, because of its basis is on telecommunication infrastructure. Since telemedicine has become a prosperous evidence to be an useful approach for information exchange and transferring, mobile phone convert as an ubiquitous electronic tool for rather than communication and shopping [16].

Having mentioned about the provisions of the large-scale computing technologies for improving rural healthcare, it is imperative task for exploring aspects that are under-researched but hold promises to achieve potential improvements for the rural communities, such as, for encouraging healthy lifestyle choices [4, 8], for individual's wellness monitoring [31], and in providing healthcare information and advice for self-management [21]. The aim of the chapter is to describe issues of the innovative large-scale technological developments for the rural community healthcare and well-being in the developing nations. The discussion in the chapter will also capture on various useful large-scale technological innovations and their effective provisions for improving public healthcare delivery.

The chapter is organised through five sections as follows. The Sect. 2 presents background of relevant large-scale technologies for various healthcare service innovations. The section after that provides two vital but common general solution frameworks for enabling healthcare services to rural community. The next section presents the issues of the service provisions followed by a discussion and further research directions drawn from the study.

2 Large Scale Innovations

The innovations around the large-scale technologies have demonstrated its positive impacts on the structural transformation in organisations, specially for achieving various business, economic and social objectives. Tegenu [26] described that

> Large scale technologies are the means for the reallocation of resources between and across sectors, particularly in a country such as Ethiopia where there is high population growth and pressure. I am of the opinion that incremental approach to technological change in a model designed for small scale production does not help us to cope up with the demand and speed of growing population of the country (pp. 1).

In healthcare sector, digital healthcare became a rapidly-growing discipline that deals with various ICT based innovations for addressing health service problems and challenges encountered by healthcare professionals, patients and relevant administrative managements. The healthcare is a multi-disciplinary platform in which different sectors are interconnected to serve the healthcare operations and functions, therefore complex and large computing technologies for improving the functions and operations are essential for providing benefits to relevant people and management in organisations [30].

In an editorial note titled *"What is e-Health: the death of telemedicine"*, Mea [15] described telemedicine, as a type of healthcare systems, that is related to medical professionals, while e-health is driven by non-professionals, namely patients (or, in the e-health jargon, consumers) that hold potentials to drive innovative services of healthcare delivery, typically for general parients' empowerment through their freedom of access to relevant information and knowledge. Although the central focuses of the large-scale innovations are considered as drivers of three main aspects in organisations: for large-scale change management, for large-scale integration in service management and for large-scale process maximisations, latest innovations lead the development and innovation for improving public focused process and practices, through which empowerment of users is vital for designing technological solutions.

The ultra large scale technologies are not new aspect in healthcare domain for meeting various stakeholders' service demands. The large-scale technologies are mainly used for addressing integration issues and often with conflicting purposes where interchangeable needs are necessary. The concept was first introduced by Northrop et al. [19] as a problem concept for solving issues in the United States Department of Defence. The technology represents complex IT systems that involved many stakeholders from multiple organizations, in heterogeneous forms that signify complex dependencies and growing properties. Northrop et al. [19] also reported on key characteristics of the ultra large scale technologies that can be viewed as aspects for innovations. The aspects of innovations development are given below:

- Technological provisions for managing decentralized data and their operational control.
- Technological features for continuously addressing conflicts and incomprehensible requirements.
- Technological improvement for evolving operational capabilities.
- Technological improvement for continuously meeting user's demand for encountering failure and exception.
- Technological features that are required for acquisition of new knowledge, policy and control methods for re-adjustments.

The country wide national healthcare system can have lots of benefits from the concept of an ultra large scale system. National healthcare builds on projects that demands not just from the cutting-edge innovative technological development, but involved latest software, system engineering and operations managements of information processing systems. Although Sullivan [25] explained the ultra large scale system as a "Cyber-Social Systems Approach" for meeting the demand of cyber-infrastructure requirements for healthcare system, all most none of the studies previously, so far, discussed the ultra large scale digital technologies for the advancement of the public access, their empowerment and appropriate service delivery options for their self-management.

3 Common General Framework of Large Scale Innovations

Various public-focused healthcare innovations have been introduced over the past few years for the developing nations. Such large-scale innovations are mainly for the purpose of countrywide healthcare service delivery. Two vital technologies are used as the basis: cloud computing and telecommunication based such as mobile-based service allows options both—healthcare professionals for maintaining and monitoring heath records, collaborate with healthcare professionals, analyse patient health record (PHR) as well as for patients for their freedom of information access.

3.1 Cloud Based Innovations

Relatively new information technologies based research movement such as cloud computing provides a strong infrastructure and offer a true enabler for e-health services over the Internet. Cloud computing is a large-scale ICT service model where computing services (both hardware and software) are delivered on-demand to customers over a network in a self-service fashion, independent of device and location [14]. Cloud computing adopts a service oriented architecture that enables functionalities in form of an integrated e-health system in order to offer various inter-operable software services [12]. Such services exchange and share healthcare data among patients, healthcare workers/professionals, facilitators, nurses, and doctors in order to improve the overall quality of healthcare diagnosis and consultation offered to people. The adoption of cloud computing for e-health introduces many opportunities to innovate healthcare service delivery in various ways, especially for developing nations. However, existing e-health solutions utilized in developing nations has been incomplete, under quality remarks, inefficient and in most of the cases, requires extensive internal and external resources and considerations to be operationalised [6, 9].

As mentioned earlier the end user or internal system can be a part of cloud based platform that services can be as Infrastructure as a Service, Software as a Service, and Platform as a Service in order to ensure appropriate and effective storage, processing, and controlling services for supporting applications without physical computing hardware or devices. This clearly represents an option with none or minimal technological intervention needing at user-end and enable less chances of service interruption or access restrictions, as long as the Internet connection is provided. Two vital examples of cloud computing based innovations for the benefits of public healthcare are given in the section below, for better understanding on the growing demand of the field.

Framework 1

Hossain and Muhammad [11] reported an innovative country-wide approach of cloud-based system in which a platform for collaborative services were offered among service or care-givers and healthcare professionals. In the large-scale system, cloud computing provisions mainly facilitated an environment for effective collaboration by considering a voice pathology assessment scenario, in which all stakeholders such as healthcare professionals, care-givers and patients in the communities can collaborate to assess voice pathology, using an *extensible messaging and presence protocol* and the sensing capability of the smart phones's audio components [11]. This collaboration was mainly aimed for delivering quality patient care.

Figure 1 illustrates the overall framework which is developed based on the model of Hossain and Muhammad [11]. In the framework, a patient can give his or her voice through a smartphone, which is used as a media sensor then the media content server (a component of the cloud-based framework) receives and transmits it to the other node, cloud manager. The could manager then sends the voice data to a collaborative service manager for uploading the information to the website for the use of a family doctor. The collaborative service manager are key part of the framework dedicated to the extraction of features from the patient's voice, to modelling pathological samples or/and to classifying the samples.

After analysing the doctor prepares a report or feedback for sending it to collaborative service manager. If the family doctor needs to check the report by an external doctor, the report can be accessed by the doctor and they can analyse the report prior to process in the collaborative service manager for storage. The patient can get the feedback from the doctor from the CM. One of the main problems of this collaboration between the patients and the doctors is to maintain the quality of the voice during transmission, because pathological voice is already noisy [11]. Central focuses are to empower patient community by giving them option to actively collaborate and participate for their own potential health monitoring, quality care, and decision.

Framework 2

Miah et al. [16] introduced a consultancy system utilizing cloud computing that enabled healthcare professionals and field workers to identify and treat non-communicable diseases in rural and remote communities. The framework is called as "On-Cloud Healthcare Clinic". Figure 2 illustrates below an overall architecture of the solution.

According to Miah et al. [16], the idea of designing the cloud-computing tool is mainly the intermediary tier through which patients were introduced and linked up

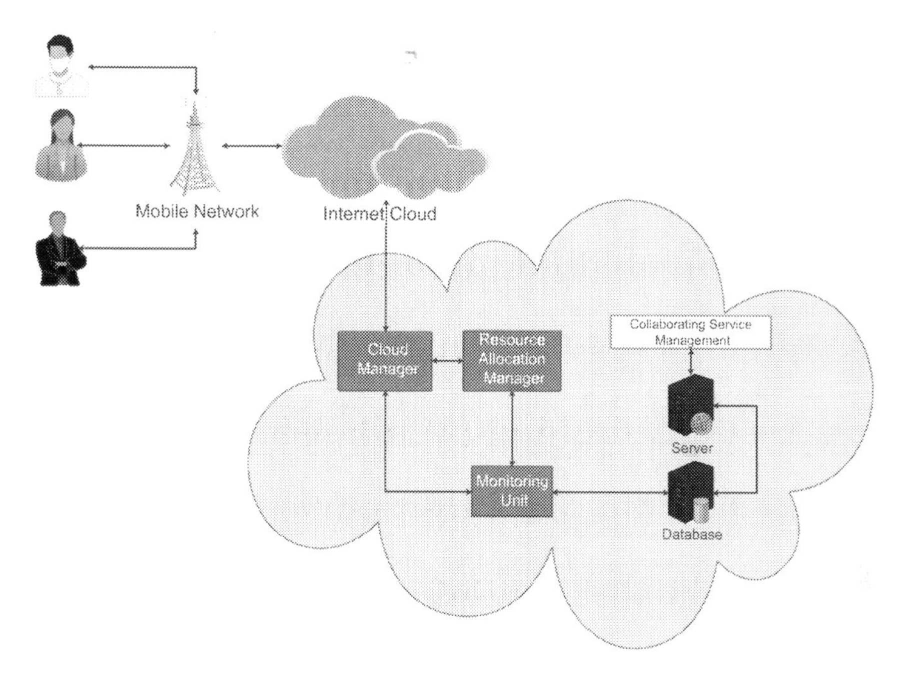

Fig. 1 Solution framework of the cloud based collaborative environment for patients

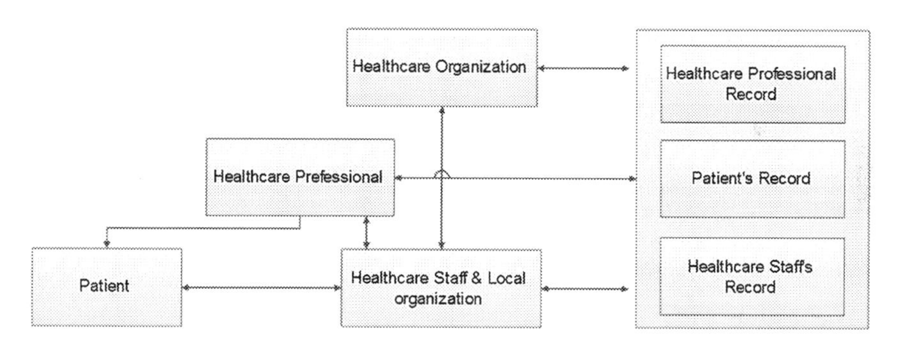

Fig. 2 Solution framework of On-Cloud Healthcare Clinic

with the doctors. Such cloud-based approach could be local hospitals or in a form of healthcare centres. Access to the cloud based service was managed through local or assisted IT services. The solution structure allowed front-end applications at end users' level that can be seen as an extension to this, addressing the problem on intermediary assistance, and shifting the burden of data inputs to the patient. This option also enables monitoring and assessment role at intermediate level. For various diseases management, such solution can work with body sensors, wearable monitors and other specialised devices potentially to generate accurate data as required in real time, and without necessitating physical travel.

The cloud computing solution provides storage support for patient initials records, patient medical history, and diseases conditions with treatments details for mobile healthcare professionals. Access controls via login forms, and registration processes for new patients have been designed for web access using technologies such as MySQL and PHP in the server side. Appointments are managed through the features of the system that were populated from the database of existing medical records, input—verified by healthcare workers. Using open or cloud-based software means, the solution is not locked into proprietary data forms or devices and liable to commercial pricing concepts.

In the cloud-based system, healthcare professionals also are to be registered with their expertise and availability details. Load balancing allocations can be naturally handled in the cloud, so the system was entirely scalable, and because it is located on cloud, appears unified to the people in the community for their information aids. Person specific details and medical conditions are formulated in terms of medical "rules of thumb" that begin to specify diagnosis and other information control and delivery to specific actions [16].

The cloud-based approach allows storage of detailed record of workflow, tests or medicines required, time spent and the like, making both individual and collective pricing and informing future resourcing and provisioning decisions. There is no overhead for such record keeping, as it is all mediated within the flow of the system. Healthcare professionals can do evaluation through patient details and concerns, perform an initial diagnosis, so that they can convey additional advice through the system, in case any further diagnostic tests are required or emergency is considered. That does mean that healthcare professionals and patient can meet up online as required through an intermediary platform [16].

Medicine prescriptions or lifestyle adjustment guidance can be provided and followed up on over time, especially in the case of diabetes treatment, as a case. In the same way, details of healthcare professionals and healthcare workers can be populated for the coverage of areas. They are also in terms of providing necessary support during and after healthcare professionals' specific patient consultation process. Comprehensive reporting for the patients the system provides options for healthcare professionals but any complete online-based healthcare system would need to be monitored for patient data security and privacy details [16].

3.2 M-health Innovations

M-health aims to provide health professionals, patients, clinicians and other relevant users with information support services to manage, disseminate, collect, administer, control and monitor healthcare information and improve health service delivery and quality of care support. The service eliminates geographical and temporal constraints while enhancing the coverage, quality, cost savings and other user provisions of healthcare [7, 18, 28]. Moreover, the m-health innovations allow acquisition, monitoring, forecasting, sharing and control of various health conditions. Such provision is designed for healthcare personnel and patients with various needs to make decisions regarding treatments and care support, and administration requirements for developing anytime-anywhere service support. Illustrative examples include: m-health systems for remote patient monitoring [5], disease prevention and wellbeing [29], knowledge exchange [22] and medication management [13].

Many current m-health innovations are, however, designed that encompass steps or iterations for identifying and analysing requirements, designing or implementing a system solution and testing the system within the problem domain. For instance, Radzuweit and Lechner [23] utilised prototyping for designing a consultation service that supported effective interaction between individuals and health professionals. Oluwafemi and Olanrewaju [20] proposed a patient communication solution through messaging but, although the study used phases such as design, development and evaluation, the authors did not evaluate the solution with the target user patient group. In the following sections two vital frameworks are introduced for better understanding on the growing demand of the field. Milošević et al. [17] used a basic software engineering methodology for designing an m-health application for community well-being by monitoring individuals' health conditions such as physical activity, weight and heart activity. The methodology consisted of common phases such as problem definition, (mobile) architecture design and implementation. Many of the m-health innovations designs, however, did not develop the large-scale capacity and evaluate the solution capacity directly or indirectly with the target user groups.

Framework 1

Wayne and Ritvo [31] designed a health coach intervention for patients with diabetes in the community that promoted adoption and maintenance of health behaviours. The solution framework was so-called "Connected Health and Wellness Platform Health Coach app" offers advisory support for helping people to attain personal goals through their intrinsic health-oriented motivations. The smartphone-based application framework supported multi-channel communications between stakeholders such as patients in the community and health (professionals) coaches and supportive family members. The solution framework in a form of prototype version established positive gains in terms of medication adherence and improved psychological functioning, as the people's positive illness-coping strategies [31].

According to Wayne and Ritvo [31], the solution framework was collaboratively developed by application designers and researchers to support participants in electronically tracking health behavioural matters. These matters are mainly exercise, diet, stress reduction practices and self-monitoring health data such as—blood glucose, blood pressure, mood, pain, and level of energy. In the solution framework, security provisions were vital for the service provider-patients interactions through the two-way communication channel in which certificate-based authentication and individual's password were encrypted with entered data recalled by the patients and healthcare professionals or service providers. Figure 3 illustrates an example of mobile healthcare support system for rural communities.

Framework 2

Thomas and Wing [27] introduced an innovative m-health approach so-called "Health-E-Call" and the main objectives of the innovative smartphone application was to determine whether key components of behavioural weight loss treatments such as self-monitoring, feedback, and skills training could be accomplished and potentially enhanced. The idea was to reducing the need for intensive care for person specific treatment. Main aim of the solution is to enhance patient's self-monitoring, given the importance of this skill for successful weight loss. Use of an electronic handheld device already popularised not only for self-monitoring improved adherence to the self-monitoring procedures, but also to improve accuracy of self-monitoring. Figure 4 illustrates an example GUI of this type of mobile-based applications. The vital outcome measures in the system were weight loss and devotion to the self-monitoring procedure and transparent reporting for self-satisfaction by patients [27].

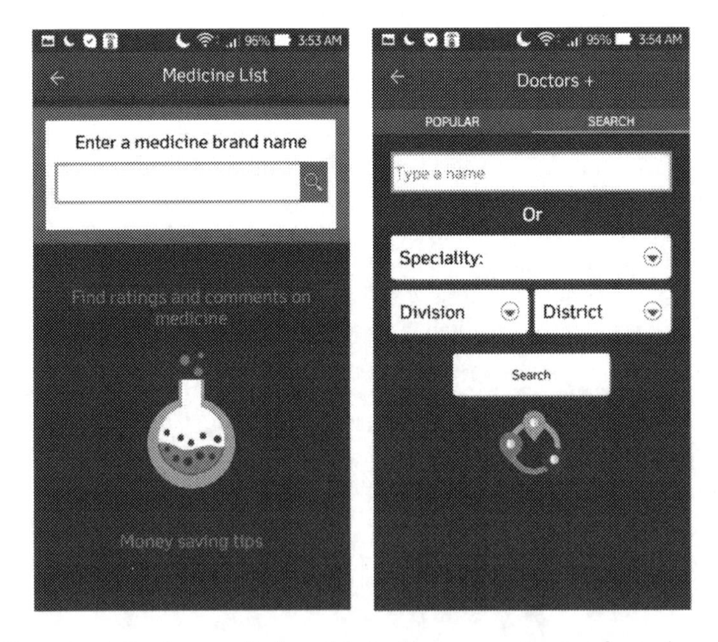

Fig. 3 Example solution framework of a mobile healthcare support system for rural communities

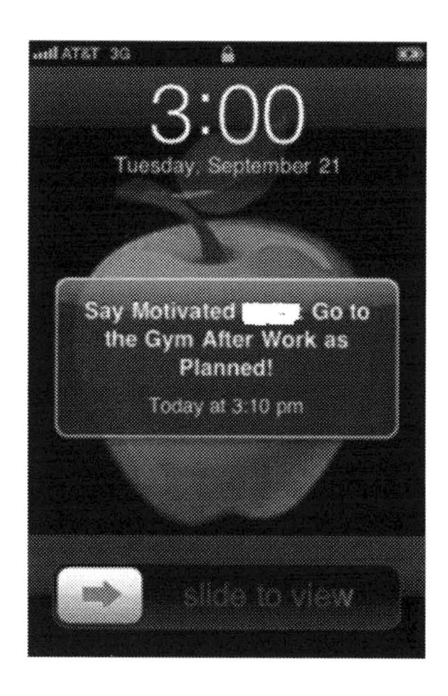

Fig. 4 Example GUI of a mobile-based approach (adopted from [27])

4 Potential Aspects of General Large-Scale Framework

In this section potential aspects in which various applications are designed are described. For both technological innovations top ten aspects are only given as case demonstration. The findings are collected through a literature review study to investigate relevant literature in both fields. Following Figs. 5 and 6 represent various aspects of existing application design through the innovations of cloud computing and m-health technologies.

The importance of utilizing cloud computing for providing health analysis, diagnosis and consultancy made strong argument for it to be adopted for rural and remote communities where a trained professionals or nurses would be able to record and enabled the entry of data on cloud based e-health systems using preferably mobile computing devices. With the extensive usage of mobile computing and telecommunication infrastructure, such a system solution would be feasible to quick design and implement for meeting any healthcare information service demands. The mobile platform allowed for direct healthcare professional patient discussion for effective medical diagnosis, monitoring, consultations and follow-up.

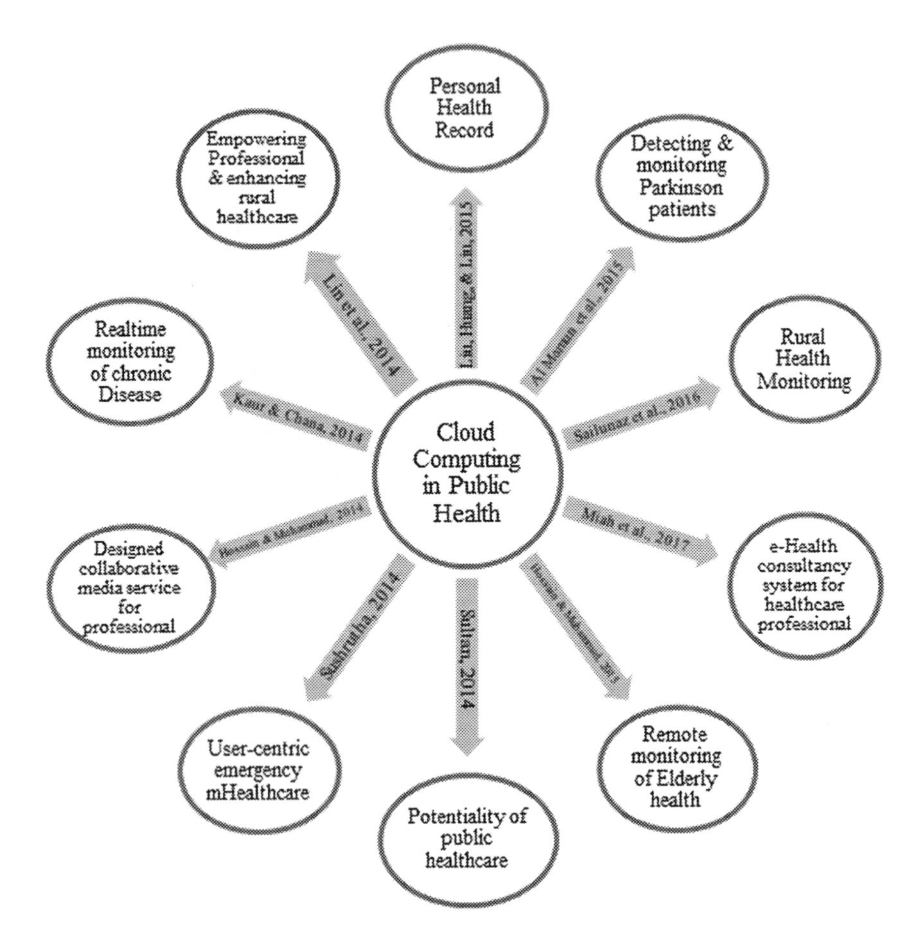

Fig. 5 Various aspects of cloud computing based application innovations

5 Discussion

In this book chapter, large-scale innovations and approaches for community healthcare support have been discussed. The aim was to focus the emergent technological perspectives in healthcare for developing countries. We focused on two divergent of large-scale technologies related innovations with their applications. These are cloud computing and telecommunication infrastructure for m-health that were described with its provisions and benefits for improving healthcare support and service delivery for citizen/patients in developing countries. The discussion also highlighted existing aspects of both cloud and telecommunication based interventions that could be of paramount for underdeveloped nations particularly when they aim to adapt large-scale computing resources through the implementation of cloud computing and m-health systems/services. Based on the theoretical

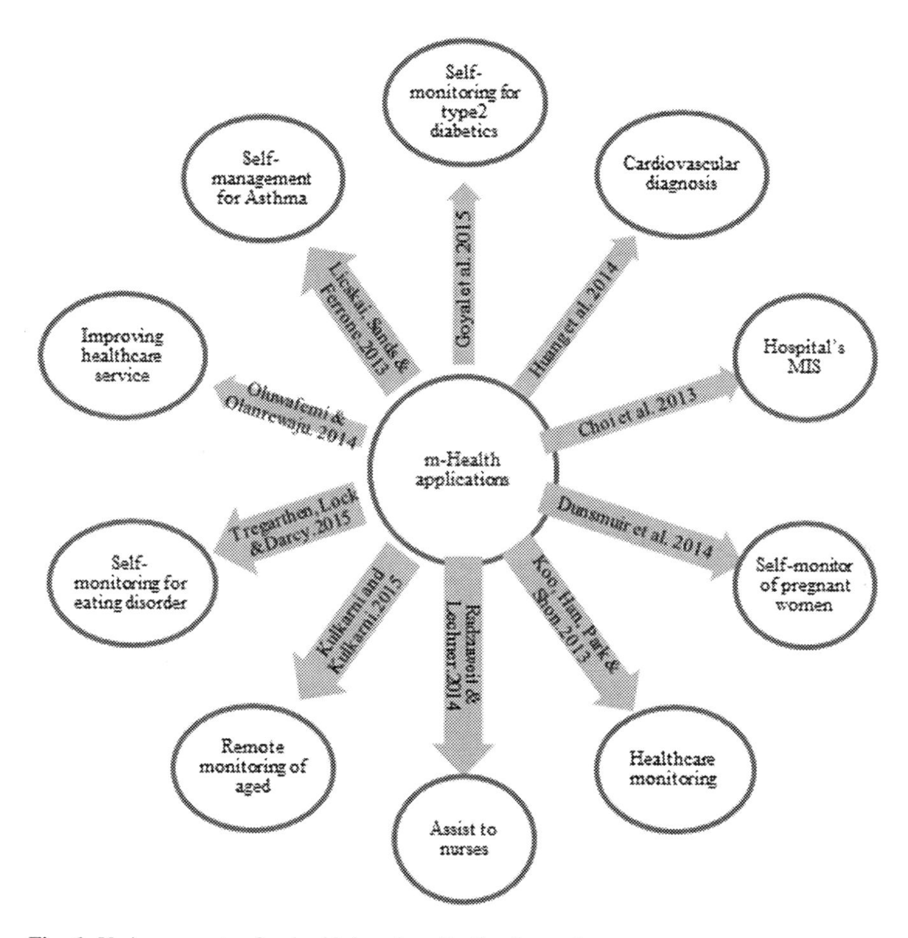

Fig. 6 Various aspects of m-health based application innovations

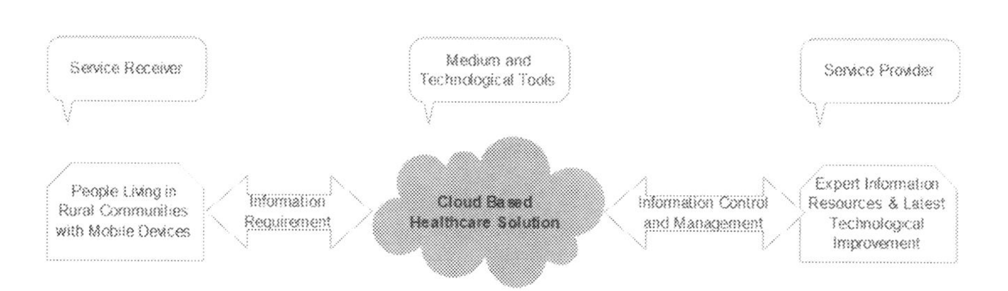

Fig. 7 Conceptual framework of a large-scale healthcare service

analysis, a conceptual framework was proposed that combines both cloud and mobile computing provisions as a platform of large-scale healthcare service. Figure 7 illustrates the diagram of the combined solution platform.

In developing countries, the public healthcare situation is considerably overlooked over the past years. The situation has changed a lot in the current era. Government, NGOs and private organisations are concerned to put forward their effort and financial budgets to improve the situations. Relevant researchers are keen to investigate the practical issue for meeting the complex healthcare demand of rural communities. South-Asian developing countries have large remote populations, but lack of balanced medical and healthcare expertise. For example, Bangladesh has only one healthcare professional for every 1700 patients, against a Millennium Development Goal of at least 2.5 healthcare professionals per 1000 people [32]. The healthcare sectors in Bangladesh are undeveloped due to inappropriate use of ICT for the need of the remote communities [16]. The majority of the population in Bangladesh live in remote areas without access to modern healthcare facilities and specialized hospitals [2, 10, 16].

The government authorities in developing countries have been considered the public healthcare a priority agenda due to the growing interests of the international donner and aids agencies such as United Nations and World Bank. Without large-scale technologies it would be nearly impossible to deliver a satisfactory and effective level of health care for the public demand of medical support. One of the reasons of that is, the healthcare and its underlying issues are include from large and widely spread population. Most of the nations at their developing stage or still lack of medical infrastructure due to many issues such as organisational heritages and bureaucracy in civil services, and limited financing for improving healthcare sector [1]. In some cases, there is a recognised shortage of well-trained healthcare professionals and nurses but they do not have required skills and motivation to work on a large-scale technological platform for providing support services to rural and regional people. In some other cases, telecommunication infrastructures and support services are quite advanced, with extensive and rapidly growing coverage. They just need to commence new projects on large-scale systems development. Developing large-scale system solutions utilizing these infrastructures such as cloud computing therefore suggests functional methods to deliver healthcare services to meet the demand of individuals in rural areas.

6 Conclusion and Future Aspects for Research

The chapter discussed both the issues and potential solutions for more sustainable healthcare service delivery. In this chapter, we reinforced on the requirements of developing large-scale technologies for the communities in developing nations. We reinforced the requirement of a comprehensive approach using cloud-based and telecommunication based technologies for various aspects such as community care, treatment support, patient self-management support, medical consultation support etc. we also discussed various examples in Sect. 4 for both technological divergence. We focused on the public care aspect, but professionals at specific problem domain may have their own opinions about a variety of different system that may be used involving different management concerns that were not covered in the chapter. We may only covered the technological aspects on limited organizations that may not have appropriate reflections in terms of resource allocations and infrastructure required associated to particular service management. Although the cloud-based solution can support flexibility and easier access to real-time data and mobile infrastructure can support every-where any-where access and presence, both technological provisions involve common issues of security and privacy of information and integrity of data or information resources including access control policy and other legislative and management concerns.

Although individual or end user computing techniques have grown to a sophisticated level, the large-scale technologies and their relevant services through the use of cloud-based and mobile computing are still in the emergent stage. Many relevant tools and technologies are still being developed. The topic area introduced in the chapter on public healthcare aspects of developing nations is just based on existing studies and concepts. There is a need for considerable research on developing new knowledge and technological innovations in this field to address the complex practical demand in public healthcare. The author attempts to bring an overview of the relevant technological developments and introduce the application area of large-scale techniques to enhance readers' knowledge in the field.

References

1. Afsana, K., Grant, J., and Evans, J. (2014). Crisis of health workforce in Bangladesh: a non-government organization's experience in deploying community health workers in primary health care, Perspectives in Public Health, 34 (5), 253–254.
2. Akter, S., Rahman, MM., Abe, SK., and Sultana, P. (2014). Prevalence of diabetes and prediabetes and their risk factors among Bangladeshi adults: a nationwide survey, Bulleting of the World Health Organization, 92 (3), 204–213.
3. Al Mamun, K.A., Alhussein, M., Sailunaz, K. and Islam, M.S. (2016). Cloud based framework for Parkinson's disease diagnosis and monitoring system for remote healthcare applications, Future Generation Computer Systems 66, 36–47.
4. Alshurafa N, Xu W, Liu JJ, Huang M, Mortazavi B, Roberts CK, et al. (2014), Designing a robust activity recognition framework for health and exergaming using wearable sensors. IEEE J Biomed Health Inform Sep;18(5):1636–1646.
5. Baig, M. M., GholamHosseini, H., & Connolly, M. J. (2015). Mobile healthcare applications: system design review, critical issues and challenges, Australasian Physical & Engineering Sciences in Medicine, 38(1), 23–38.
6. Barjis, J., Kolfschoten, G., Maritz, J., (2013). A sustainable and affordable support system for rural healthcare delivery. Decis. Support Syst. 56, 223–233.
7. Duarte, J.L., Crawford, J.T., Stern, C., Haidt, J., Jussim, L. and Tetlock, P.E. (2015). Political diversity will improve social psychological science, Behavioral and Brain Sciences, Cambridge University Press 2015, 1–58.
8. Fatima I, Fahim M, Lee Y, Lee S. (2013), A unified framework for activity recognition-based behavior analysis and action prediction in smart homes. Sensors (Basel) 13(2):2682–2699.
9. Hage, E., Roo, J.P., van Offenbeek, M., Boonstra, A., (2013). Implementation factors and their effect on e-health service adoption in rural communities: a systematic literature review. BMC Health Serv. Res. 13 (19), 1–16.

10. Hasan, J., (2012). Effective telemedicine project in Bangladesh: Special focus on diabetes health care delivery in a tertiary care in Bangladesh. Telematics and Inform. 29, 211–218.
11. Hossain, M. S. and Muhammad, G. (2014). Cloud-Based Collaborative Media Service Framework for HealthCare, Hindawi Publishing Corporation, International Journal of Distributed Sensor Networks, Volume 2014, Article ID 858712, pages 1–11, doi:10.1155/2014/858712.
12. Hu, Y., Bai, G., (2014). A systematic literature review of cloud computing in e-health. Health Inf. Int. J. 3 (4), 11–20.
13. Lee, J.-A., Nguyen, A. L., Berg, J., Amin, A., Bachman, M., Guo, Y., & Evangelista, L. 2014. Attitudes and preferences on the use of mobile health technology and health games for self-management: interviews with older adults on anticoagulation therapy, JMIR mHealth and uHealth, 2(3). e32.
14. Marston, S., Li, Z., Bandyopadhyay, S., Zhang, J., Ghalsasi, A., (2011). Cloud computing—the business perspective. Decis. Support Syst. 51 (1), 176–189.
15. Mea, V.D. (2001). What is e-Health (2): The death of telemedicine?, J Med Internet Res, 3(2): e22, doi:10.2196/jmir.3.2.e22.
16. Miah, S. J., Hasan, J., & Gammack, J. G. (2017). On-Cloud Healthcare Clinic: An e-health consultancy approach for remote communities in a developing country. Telematics and Informatics, 34(1), 311–322.
17. Milošević, M., Shrove, M. T., & Jovanov, E. (2011). Applications of Smartphone for Ubiquitous Health Monitoring and Wellbeing Management, Journal of Information Technology and Applications, 1, 7–15.
18. Nhavoto, J. A., & Grönlund, Å. (2014). Mobile technologies and geographic information systems to improve health care systems: a literature review, JMIR mHealth and uHealth, 2(2), e21.
19. Northrop, L. (2006). Ultra-Large-Scale Systems: The Software Challenge of the Future, Software Engineering Institute, Carnegie Mellon, URL: http://www.sei.cmu.edu/library/assets/uls_book20062.pdf.
20. Oluwafemi, A. J., & Olanrewaju, K. M. (2014). Mobile-Health Application Software Design and Development, International Journal of Computer Science and Information Security, 12(7), 59.
21. Pitt M, Monks T, Allen M. (2015) Systems modelling for improving healthcare. In: Richards D, Hallberg I, editors. Complex Interventions in Health: An Overview of Research Methods. Abingdon: Routledge, 312–25.
22. Pulijala, Y., Ma, M. and Ayoub, A. (2015). Design and Development of Sur-Face: An Interactive Mobile App for Educating Patients Regarding Corrective Surgery of Facial Deformities, JCSG 2015, LNCS 9090, 26–35, 2015.
23. Radzuweit, M., & Lechner, U. (2014). Introducing tablet computers into medical practice: design of mobile apps for consultation services. Health and Technology, 4(1), 31–41.
24. Ruxwana, N.L., Herselman, M.E., Conradie, D.P., (2010). ICT applications as e-health solutions in rural healthcare in the Eastern Cape Province of South Africa Health. Inf. Manage. J. 39 (1), 17–30.
25. Sullivan, K. (2011). A Cyber-Social Systems Approach to the Engineering of Ultra-Large-Scale National Health Information Systems, Institute of Medicine, University of Virginia, URL: http://www.nationalacademies.org/hmd/~/media/56E105203D1046C7B519EEB328840E0A.ashx.
26. Tegenu, T. (2011). Large-scale Technology is at Heart of Economic Structural Transformation in Ethiopia, Economic Structural Transformation in. Ethiopia, URL: https://www.diva-portal.org/smash/get/diva2:938615/FULLTEXT01.pdf.
27. Thomas, J.G. and Wing, R.R. (2013). Health-E-Call, a Smartphone-Assisted Behavioral Obesity Treatment: Pilot Study, JMIR Mhealth Uhealth,1(1):e3, doi:10.2196/mhealth.2164.
28. Varshney, U. (2014). A model for improving quality of decisions in mobile health, Decision Support Systems, 62, 66–77.
29. Walton, R., & DeRenzi, B. (2009). Value-sensitive design and health care in Africa, IEEE Transactions on Professional Communication, 52(4), 346–358.

30. Warwick (2013). Digital Healthcare Master's Programme for 2013, Institute of Digital Healthcare, Retrieved from: http://www2.warwick.ac.uk/fac/sci/wmg/idh/study/mastersprogramme, accessed on 23 January, 2017.
31. Wayne, N. and Ritvo, P. (2014). Smartphone-Enabled Health Coach Intervention for People With Diabetes From a Modest Socioeconomic Strata Community: Single-Arm Longitudinal Feasibility Study, J Med Internet Res, 16(6): e149.
32. World Bank (2014, 2015) Health Nutrition and Population Statistics report http://databank.worldbank.org/data/reports.aspx?source=health-nutrition-andpopulation-statistics.

Part IV
Wearable Computing for Smart Healthcare

Wearable Computers for Sign Language Recognition

Jian Wu and Roozbeh Jafari

Abstract A Sign Language Recognition (SLR) system translates signs performed by deaf individuals into text/speech in real time. Low cost sensor modalities, inertial measurement unit (IMU) and surface electromyography (sEMG), are both useful to detect hand/arm gestures. They are capable of capturing signs and are complementary to each other for recognizing signs. In this book chapter, we propose a wearable system for recognizing American Sign Language (ASL) in real-time, fusing information from an inertial sensor and sEMG sensors. The best subset of features from a wide range of well-studied features is selected using an information gain based feature selection approach. Four popular classification algorithms are evaluated for 80 commonly used ASL signs on four subjects. With the selected feature subset and a support vector machine classifier, our system achieves 96.16 and 85.24% average accuracies for intra-subject and intra-subject cross session evaluation respectively. The significance of adding sEMG for American Sign Language recognition is explored and the best channel of sEMG is highlighted.

Keywords American sign language recognition · IMU sensor · Surface EMG · Feature selection · Sensor fusion

J. Wu (✉)
Department of Computer Science and Engineering, Texas A&M University, College Station, USA
e-mail: jian.wu@tamu.edu

R. Jafari
Departments of Biomedical Engineering, Computer Science and Engineering, and Electrical and Computer Engineering, Center of Remote Health Technologies and Systems, Texas A&M University, College Station, USA
e-mail: rjafari@tamu.edu

© Springer International Publishing AG 2017

S.U. Khan et al. (eds.), *Handbook of Large-Scale Distributed Computing in Smart Healthcare*, Scalable Computing and Communications,
DOI 10.1007/978-3-319-58280-1_14

1 Introduction

According to World Health Organization (WHO), over 5% of the world's population—360 million people—has disabling hearing loss (328 million adults and 32 million children) by March, 2015. Disabling hearing loss refers to hearing loss greater than 40 decibels (dB) in the better hearing ear in adults and a hearing loss greater than 30 dB in the better hearing ear in children. The majority of people with disabling hearing loss live in low- and middle-income countries. Hearing loss may result from genetic causes, complications at birth, certain infectious diseases, chronic ear infections, the use of particular drugs, exposure to excessive noise and ageing. 50% of hearing loss can be prevented by taking medicines, surgery and the use of hearing aids and other devices. However, there are still a large number of people who have profound hearing loss which is also defined as deafness. They often use sign language for communication.

A sign language is a language which uses manual communication to convey meaning, as opposed to acoustically conveyed sound patterns. It is a natural language widely used by deaf people to communicate with each other [1]. However, there are communication barriers between hearing people and deaf individuals either because signers may not be able to speak and hear or because hearing individuals may not be able to sign. This communication gap can cause a negative impact on lives and relationships of deaf people. Two traditional ways of communication between deaf persons and hearing individuals who do not know sign language exist: through interpreters or text writing. The interpreters are very expensive for daily conversations and their involvement will result in a loss of privacy and independence of deaf persons. The text writing is not an efficient way to communicate because writing is too slow compared to either spoken/sign language and the facial expressions during performing sign language or speaking will be lost. Thus, a low-cost, more efficient way of enabling communication between hearing people and deaf people is needed.

A sign language recognition (SLR) system is a useful tool to enable communication between deaf people and hearing people who do not know sign language by translating sign language into speech or text [2, 3]. Figure 1 shows a typical

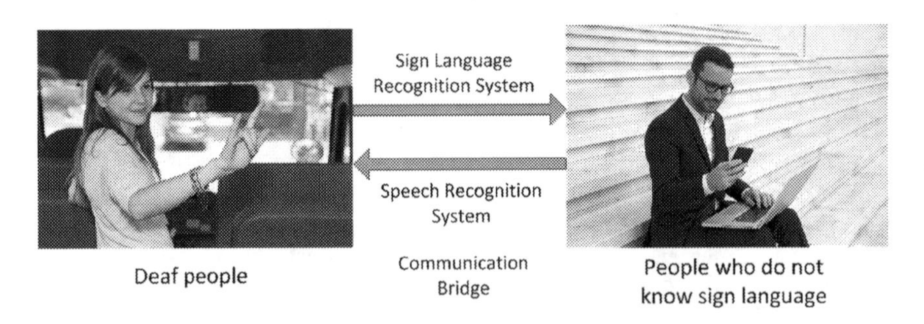

Fig. 1 Typical application of sign language recognition system

application of sign language recognition system. The SLR system worn by deaf people facilitates the translation of the signs to text or speech and transfer it to the smart phones of the people who can hear and speak. The spoken language of individuals who do not know sign language is translated into sign language images/videos by speech recognition systems. The speech recognition systems is not considered in this book chapter. The real-time translation of sign language enable deaf individual to communicate in a more convenient and natural way.

Similar to spoken languages, different countries have different sign languages. About 300 sign languages are currently being used all over the world. Due to the differences, the SLR should be trained and customized for every individual sign language. In our work, we have considered ASL. ASL dictionary includes thousands of signs, but most of them are not commonly used. In this chapter, 80 most commonly used signs are selected from 100 basic ASL signs [4, 5]. A sign is made up by five parts: hand shape, hand orientation, hand location, hand and arm movement and facial expression. Facial expression is more complicated and is not considered in this chapter.

Vision-based and glove-based SLR systems are well-studied systems which capture signs using cameras and sensory glove devices, respectively [6–10]. However, each of these two modalities has their own limitations. Vision-based systems suffer from occlusion due to light-of-sight factor. Moreover, cameras are mounted fixed in the environment and thus they can only be used in a limited range of vision. They are also considered to somewhat invasive to user's privacy. The glove-based systems are usually expensive which limits their usage in daily life.

Wearable inertial measurement unit (IMU) based gesture recognition systems attract much research attention due to their low cost, low power consumption and ubiquitous sensing ability [11, 12]. An IMU consists of a 3-axis accelerometer and a 3-axis gyroscope. The accelerometer measures 3-axis acceleration caused by motion and gravity while the gyroscope measures 3-axis angular velocity. A surface electromyography (sEMG) sensor is able to capture muscle electrical activities and can be used to distinguish different gestures since different gestures have different muscle activity patterns [13, 14]. For sign language recognition systems, the wrist worn IMU sensor is good at capturing hand orientations and hand and arm movements while sEMG does well in distinguishing different hand shapes and finger movements when the sensors are placed on the forearm. Thus, they are complementary to each other capturing different information of a sign and the fusion of them will improve the system performance [15]. Fortunately, the IoT platforms offer information from various sensor modalities and thus the performance of SLR would be enhanced by data fusion. However, additional sensor modalities will generate highly complex, multi-dimensional and larger volumes of data which introduce additional challenges. Challenges to address include increase in power consumption of wearable computers which will impact the battery life negatively and reducing the impact of modalities that appear to be too noisy and will degrade the performance of the classifiers.

In this book chapter, we propose a real-time wearable system for recognizing ASL by fusing inertial and sEMG sensors. Although such a system has been studied for Chinese Sign Language [16], to the best of the authors' knowledge this is the first time such a system is studied for the ASL. In this chapter, we first propose an adaptive auto-segmentation algorithm that determines the period during which the sign is performed. A wide range of well-established features are studied and the best subset of features are selected using an information gain based feature selection scheme. The feature selection determines the smallest feature subset which still provides good performance. It reduces the possibility of over-fitting and the smaller feature size is more suitable for wearable systems. Four commonly used classification algorithms are evaluated for intra- and inter-subject testing and the significance of adding sEMG for SLR is explored. When the best classifier is determined, the power consumption and the scalability of the classifiers are also considered.

The remainder of this book chapter is organized as follows. The related work is discussed in Sect. 2. Our lab customized sEMG data acquisition and IMU hardware platforms are introduced in Sect. 3. The details of our system are explained in Sect. 4, followed by the experimental setup in Sect. 5. The experimental results are explained in Sect. 6 and limitations are discussed in Sect. 7. At last, the chapter is concluded in Sect. 8.

2 Related Work

SLR systems are broadly studied in the field of computer vision with camera as a sensing modality. Two vision-based real-time ASL recognition systems are studied for sentence level continuous American Sign Language using Hidden Markov Model (HMM) [6]. The first system is evaluated for 40 signs and achieves 92% accuracy with camera mounted on the desk. The second system is also evaluated for 40 signs and achieves 98% accuracy with camera mounted on a cap worn by the user. A framework for recognizing the simultaneous aspects of ASL is proposed and it aims at solving the scalability issues of HMM [7]. The signs are broken down into phonemes and are modeled with parallel HMM. It reduces HMM state space dramatically as the number of signs increases. Another vision-based SLR system is studied for a medium vocabulary Chinese Sign Language [17]. It has two modules and the first module consists of three parts: robust hand detection, background subtraction and pupil detection. The second module is a tiered-mixture density HMM. With the aid of a colored glove, this system achieves 92.5% accuracy for 439 Chinese Sign Language words. In another work, three novel vision based features are learned for ASL recognition [18]. The relationship between these features and the four components of ASL is discussed. It yields 10.99% error rate on a published dataset. A Chinese Sign Language recognition system is proposed to address the issue of complex background in the environment [19]. The system is able to update the skin color model under various lighting conditions. A hierarchical classifier is used which integrates Linear Discriminant Analysis (LDA), Support Vector Machine (SVM) and Principle Component Analysis (PCA).

Glove-based SLR systems recognize signs using multiple sensors on the glove. They are usually able to capture finger movements precisely. A glove-based Australian SLR system is proposed using some simple features and achieves 80% accuracy for 95 AUSLAN signs [20]. Another glove-based system is studied using artificial neural network classifier and it offers 90% accuracy for 50 ASL signs [9]. A flex sensor based glove is introduced recently that can be used to recognize 26 alphabets [21].

Similar to glove-based systems, the low cost wearable accelerometer and sEMG based SLR systems do not require cameras to be mounted at a certain location while they cost less than glove-based systems. Therefore, this kind of wearable SLR system is gaining more popularity. The importance of accelerometer and sEMG for recognizing gestures is studied [22]. The results show accelerometer and sEMG do well in capturing different information of a gesture and the fusion of them improve the system performance. In another work, 5–10% performance improvement is achieved after fusing these two modalities [23]. The sample entropy based feature set is proven to be effective for both accelerometer and sEMG and the system achieves 93% accuracy for 60 Greek Sign Language signs using this feature set [24]. A Chinese SLR framework is proposed fusing data from an accelerometer and 4-channel sEMG sensors [16]. It automatically determine the beginning and ending of a sign based on sEMG signal strength. Multi-stage classifications are applied to achieve an accuracy of 96.8% for 120 Chinese signs with sensors deployed on two hands. At the first stage, LDA is used for both accelerometer and sEMG to detect hand shape and hand orientation, respectively. In the meantime, a multi-stream HMM is applied for sEMG and accelerometer features. At the second stage, the decisions achieved from the first stage are fused with a Gaussian mixture model. Despite the good performance, multiple stages and multiple classifiers are not favorable for real-time wearable computers based applications. Recently, the same group proposes a component-based vocabulary-extensible sign language recognition system [25]. In this work, the sign is considered to be a combination of five common sign components, including hand shape, axis, orientation, rotation, and trajectory. There are two parts of this system. The first part is to obtain the component-based form of sign gestures and establish the code table of target sign gesture set using data from a reference subject. In the second part, which is designed for new users, component classifier are trained using a training set suggested by the reference subject and the classification of unknown gestures is performed with a code matching method. Another system is proposed to detect seven German sign words with 99.82% accuracy achieved using an accelerometer and one channel sEMG [26]. However, this work is not extensively evaluated for a large number of signs and does not include auto-segmentation which makes it difficult to operate in real time. The major differences between our work and the previous works are as follows: (1) An adaptive auto-segmentation is proposed to extract periods during which signs are performed using sEMG. (2) The best feature subset is selected from a broad range of features using information gain criterion and the selected features from different modalities (e.g. accelerometer, gyroscope and 4-channel sEMG) are discussed. (3) Gyroscope is incorporated and the significance of adding sEMG is analyzed. (4) Although such a system has been studied for Chinese Sign Language [16], our work is the first study for American Sign Language recognition fusing these two modalities.

3 Hardware Description

A. *IMU Sensor*

Figure 2 shows the 9-axis motion sensor customized in our lab. The InvenSense MPU9150, a combination of 3-axis accelerometer, 3-axis gyroscope and 3-axis magnetometer, severs as the IMU sensor. A Texas Instruments (TI) 32-bit microcontroller SoC, CC2538, is used to control the whole system. The board also includes a microSD storage unit and a dual mode Bluetooth module BC127 from BlueCreation. The system can be used for real-time data streaming or can store data for later analysis. It also has an 802.15.4 wireless module which can offer low power proximity measurement or ZigBee communication. In this book chapter, the sampling rates for accelerometer and gyroscope are chosen to be 100 Hz which is sufficient for the sign language recognition system [27].

B. *sEMG Acquisition System*

sEMG measures the electrical activity generated by skeletal muscle. Figure 3 shows a customized 16-channel Bluetooth-enabled physiological signal acquisition system. It can be used for ECG, sEMG and EEG data acquisition. The system is used as a four channel sEMG acquisition system in this study. A TI low power analog front end, the ADS1299, is used to capture four channel sEMG signals and a TI

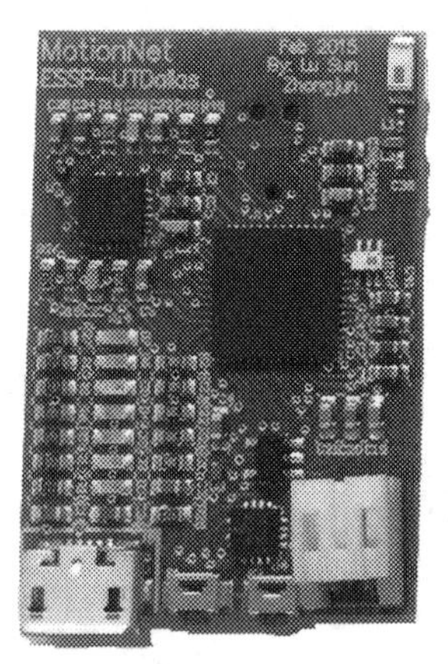

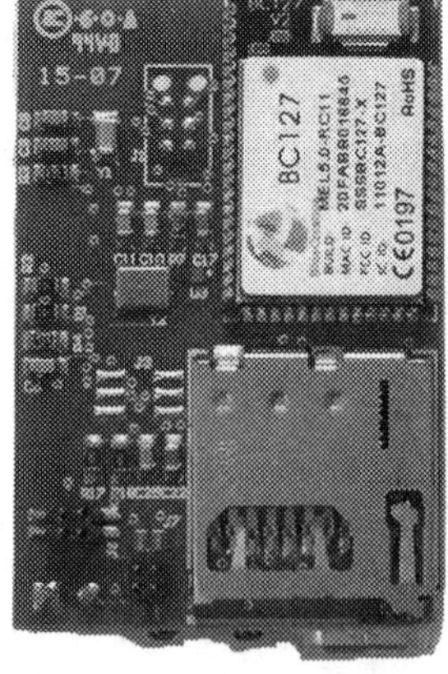

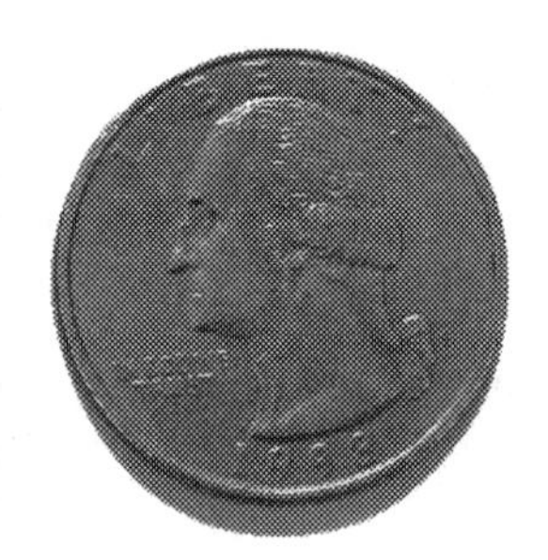

Fig. 2 Motion sensor board

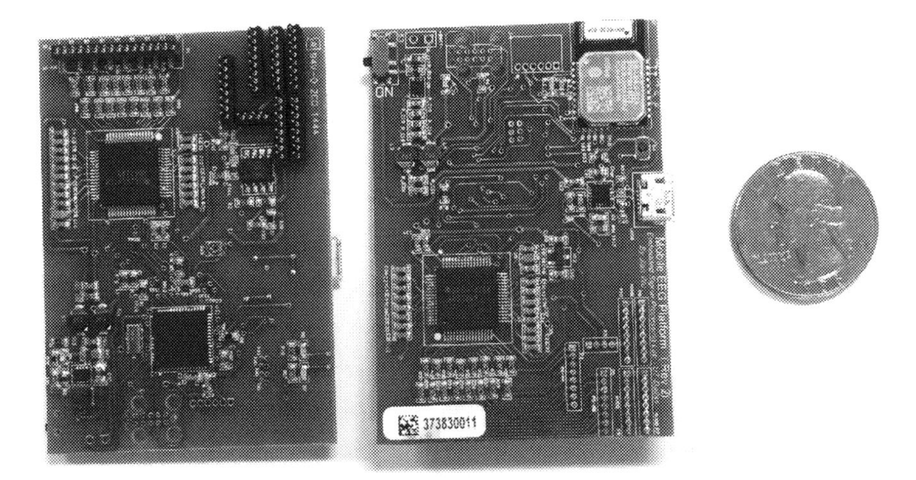

Fig. 3 8-channel sEMG acquisition system

MSP430 microcontroller is responsible for forwarding data to a PC via Bluetooth. A resolution of 0.4 μV is achieved setting a gain of 1 on the ADS1299. Covidien Kendall disposable surface EMG patches are attached to skin and the same electrodes are used as introduced in our previous work [28].

Generally, sEMG signals are in the frequency range of 0–500 Hz depending on the space between electrodes and muscle type [29]. To meet the Nyquist criterion, the sampling rate is chosen as 1 KHz, which is usually used in surface EMG based pattern recognition tasks [30].

4 Proposed SLR System

The block diagram of our proposed multi-modal ASL recognition system is shown in Fig. 4. Two phases are included: training phase and testing phase. In the training phase, the signals from 3-D accelerometer (ACC), 3-D gyroscope (GYRO) and four channel sEMG are preprocessed for noise rejection and synchronization purposes. The sEMG based auto-segmentation technique obtains the beginning and ending of a sign for both IMU and sEMG. As the segmentation is done, a broad set of well-established features are extracted for both IMU and sEMG signals. All extracted features are then put into one feature vector. The best feature subset is obtained using an information gain (IG) based feature selection scheme. Four different classifiers are evaluated (i.e. decision tree, support vector machine, NaïveBayes and nearest neighbor) on the selected feature subset and the best one is selected. In the testing phase, the same techniques are repeated for preprocessing and segmentation. The selected features are extracted and recognition of the sign is achieved by the chosen classifier.

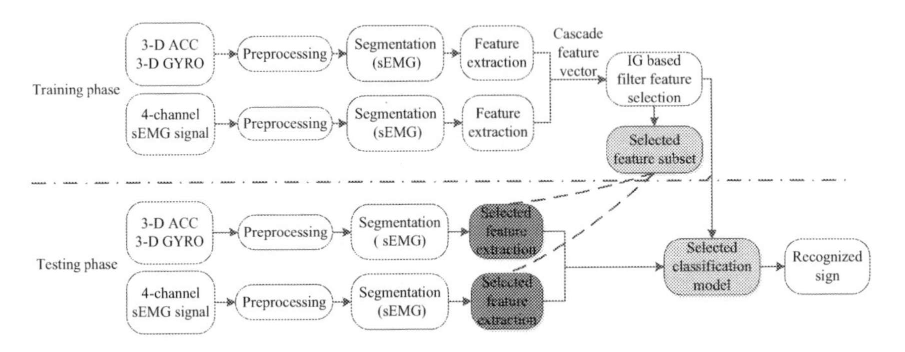

Fig. 4 Diagram of proposed system

A. *Preprocessing*

The synchronization between IMU and sEMG data is important for fusion. In our system, IMU data samples and sEMG data samples are sent to a PC via Bluetooth and time-stamped with the PC clock. The synchronization is done by aligning samples with the same PC clock. Bluetooth causes a transmission delay (5–20 ms) for both IMU and sEMG data and this small synchronization error is negligible for the purposes of our system. To remove low frequency noise in sEMG, a 5 Hz IIR high pass filter is used since the frequency components of sEMG beyond the range of 5–450 Hz are negligible [31]. The raw data is used for accelerometer and gyroscope.

B. *Segmentation*

Automatic segmentation is crucial for real-time applications. It extracts the period during which each sign word is performed such that the features can be extracted on the correct segment before classification is done. For certain parts of some signs, only finger movements are observed and no obvious motion signal can be detected from the wrist. Thus, sEMG signals are used for our automatic segmentation technique since sEMG signals can capture larger number of movements.

To explain our segmentation technique, we first define the average energy E of four sEMG channels in an n sample window in Eq. (1). $S_c(i)$ denotes ith sample of cth channel of sEMG. m is total number of channels which equals four in our case. A non-overlapping sliding window is used to calculate E in every window. The length of the window is set to 128 ms, which covers 128 samples with the 1000 Hz sampling frequency. If E in five continuous windows are all larger than a threshold T, the first sample of the first window will be taken as the beginning of a gesture. If E in four continuous windows are all smaller than the threshold, the last sample in the last window is considered to be the ending of this gesture.

$$E = \frac{1}{n}\sum_{i=1}^{n}\sum_{c=1}^{m} s_c^2(i) \tag{1}$$

Different people have different muscular strengths which will result in different E. A simple threshold may not be suitable for all subjects. An adaptive estimation technique is proposed to adjust the threshold according to different subjects and different noise levels on-line. The proposed approach is explained in two steps. In the first step, the average energy E is calculated for five continuous windows. If all five E is smaller than $a * T$, it is assumed no muscle activity is detected and the threshold is updated with $b * T$ in the second step. a is called the converge parameter and this reduces the threshold T when quiet periods are detected. b is the diverge parameter which enlarges the threshold T as the noise level increases. The values of a, b and T are set to be 0.5, 4 and 0.01 for the system empirically. 0.01 is much bigger than E for all subjects and the user is requested to have a 2–3 s quiet period at the beginning of system operation to have the system converge to a suitable threshold.

C. *Feature Extraction*

A broad range of features have been proposed and studied for both sEMG and IMU sensors for recognizing activities or gestures. In this chapter, these well-studied features are investigated [32–36]. Tables 1 and 2 list features and their dimensions from sEMG and IMU, respectively. The sEMG features are extracted for all four channel signals and the total dimension is 76. The IMU sensor features are extracted for 3-axis accelerometer, 3-axis gyroscope and the magnitude of accelerometer and

Table 1 sEMG features

Feature name (dimension)	Feature name (dimension)
Mean absolute value (1)	Variance (1)
Four order reflection coefficients (4)	Willison amplitude in 5 amplitude ranges (5)
Histogram (1)	Modified median frequency (1)
Root mean square (1)	Modified mean frequency (1)
Four order AR coefficients (4)	

Table 2 IMU sensor features

Feature name (dimension)	Feature name (dimension)
Mean (1)	Variance (1)
Standard deviation (1)	Integration (1)
Root mean square (1)	Zero cross rate (1)
Mean cross rate (1)	Skewness (1)
Kurtosis (1)	First three orders of 256-point FFT coefficients (3)
Entropy (1)	Signal magnitude area (1)
AR coefficients (10)	

gyroscope. The number of total IMU features is 192. The sEMG and IMU features are cascaded into a 268 dimension feature space.

D. *Feature Selection*

For classification, it is important to select the most useful features. There are usually two approaches to select the most useful features. The first approach is to define most useful and relevant features from a domain expert. For those experts who are familiar with their field, they usually know what the useful features are for certain tasks. The second approach is to select a certain subset features from an extensive number of features. Since even a domain expert may not be aware of all best features, thus the second approach is preferred. In this chapter, we use the second approach to select a subset of features from a wide range of features. It reduces over fitting problems and information redundancy in the feature set. It is also helpful if a small feature set is required by certain applications with limited computational power.

There are three different feature selection methods which are filter methods, wrapper methods, and embedded methods [37]. Wrapper methods generate scores for each feature subset based on a specific predictive model. Then, cross validation is done for each feature subset. Based on the prediction performance, each subset is assigned a score and the best subset is chosen. Filter methods use general measurement metrics of a dataset to score a feature subset instead of using the error rate of a predictive model. Some common measures are mutual information and inter/intra class distance. The embedded methods perform the feature subset selection in conjunction with the model construction. In our work, an information gain filter method is used in conjunction with a ranking algorithm to rank all the features. The best n features form the best feature subset which is evaluated with different classifiers. The choice of n is discussed in Sect. 5. Compared to wrapper methods, the features selected by filter methods will operate for any classifier instead of working only with a specific classifier.

E. *Classification*

Four commonly used classification algorithms are investigated in this chapter: decision tree (DT) [38], support vector machine (LibSVM) [39], nearest neighbor (NN) and NaiveBayes. The implementations of these classifiers are achieved by Weka, a popular open source machine learning tool [40]. LibSVM uses radial basis function (RBF) kernel and uses a grid search algorithm to determine the best kernel parameters. The default parameters are applied for other classifiers. In machine learning, it is usually hard to determine which classifier is more suitable for a specific application and thus it is worth testing several algorithms before we choose one.

5 Experimental Setup

A. *Sensor Placement*

The signs can involve one hand or two hands. In our work, we only look at the right hand movements for both one-hand or two-hand signs. If they system is deployed on two hands, it will increase the recognition accuracy. Figure 5 shows the sensor placement on right forearm of the user. Four major muscle groups are chosen to place four channel sEMG electrodes: (1) extensor digitorum, (2) flexor carpi radialis longus, (3) extensor carpi radialis longus and (4) extensor carpi ulnaris. The IMU sensor is worn on the wrist where a smart watch is usually placed. To improve signal-to-noise ratio of sEMG readings, a bi-polar configuration is applied for each channel and the space between two electrodes for each channel is set to 15 mm [41]. The electrode placements are also annotated in the figure.

B. *Data Collection*

In this chapter, we selected 80 most commonly used ASL signs in daily conversations. The data is collected from four subjects (three male subjects and one female subject). The subjects performed the signs for the first time and did not know the ASL prior to the experimentation. For each subject, the data collection includes three sessions which were performed on three different days. During each session, all signs were performed 25 times. The dataset has 24,000 instances in total.

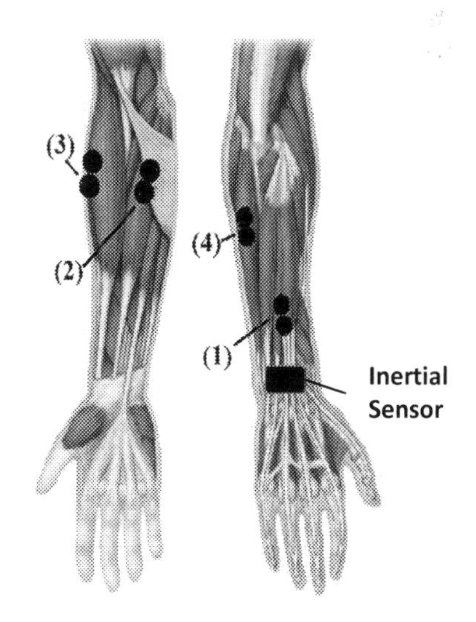

Fig. 5 Placement of sEMG electrodes

C. *Experiments*

To evaluate our system, four experiments are carried out: intra-subject testing, all cross validation, inter-subject testing and intra-subject cross session testing. In intra-subject testing, the data from the same subject from all sessions are combined and for each subject, a ten-fold cross validation is conducted. Ten-fold validation means that the data is split into 10 parts randomly and the model is trained with 9 parts and is tested on the 10th part. This process is carried out 10 times and the average performance outcome is considered the cross validation result. In all cross validation, all the data from different subjects from different days are combined. The ten-fold cross validation is performed similarly. In the inter-subject testing, the model is trained with data from three subjects and is tested on the fourth subject. This process is repeated four times. The feature selection for the first three experiments is performed during all cross validation since it has all the data and it will offer better generalization for classification models. The fourth experiment is called intra-subject cross session testing. The feature selection and model training are done with two sessions of data from the same subject and tested on the third session. This process is repeated three times for each subject and the average is taken over. The experiment indicates how well the model will perform with new data and a new subject.

6 Experimental Results

A. *Auto-segmentation*

In this chapter, no gold standard (e.g. video record) is included to determine the accuracy of our auto-segmentation technique. However, we approximately evaluate our auto-segmentation performance by looking at the difference in the number of signs each subject performed and the number of signs our system recognized. We define an error rate as in (2):

$$ER = \frac{|detected\ nums - performed\ nums|}{perfomed\ nums} \tag{2}$$

detected nums and *performed nums* are the numbers of signs our algorithm detected and numbers of signs the user actually performed, respectively. Our approach achieves 1.3% error rate which means our auto-segmentation algorithm performs well. The intra-subject classification results in Sect. 5. C also indicate suitable performance of the segmentation.

B. *Feature Selection*

All features are ranked with information gain criterion and the features with highest scores are chosen to form the best feature subset. To decide the size of best feature set, all cross validation is performed on four different classifiers as feature subset size increases from 10 to 268.

Figure 6 shows the accuracies of four classifier as the selected feature size increases. All classifier accuracies increase as the feature size increases. However, when the feature size is larger than 120 for the LibSVM and nearest neighbor, the accuracies decrease due to the over-fitting. This proves the feature selection is necessary. Table 3 shows the data points for four classifiers when they achieve the best accuracy.

It is shown in Fig. 6, when feature subset size becomes 40, LibSVM already offers 96.16% accuracy. The feature size is determined to be 40 in order to save computational cost for wearable systems. Among the 40 features, the numbers of features selected from different sensors are shown in Table 4. More than half of the features are selected from accelerometer which means accelerometer plays the principal role in recognizing signs. Accelerometers measure both gravity and acceleration due to the motion. Gravity is the major part of accelerometer measurements and captures the hand orientation information. It indicates hand orientation plays a more important role when recognizing different signs. 10 gyroscope

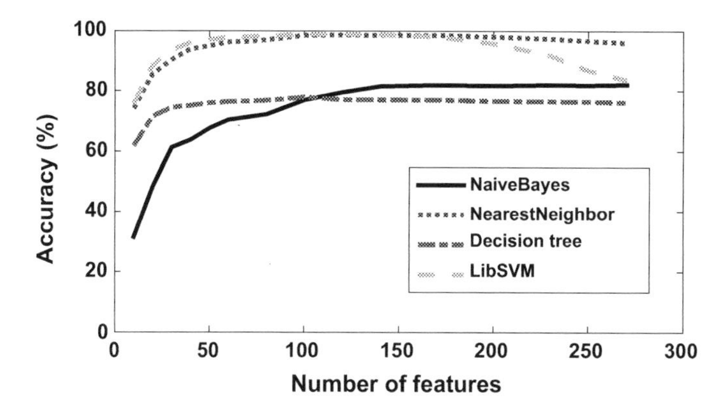

Fig. 6 Results of feature selection

Table 3 Optimal data point of feature selection

Classifier	Optimal point (feature number, accuracy) (%)
NaiveBayes	(270, 82.13)
Neareast neighbor	(120, 98.73)
Decision tree	(100, 78.00)
LibSVM	(120, 98.96)

Table 4 Number of features selected from different sensors

Sensor	Number of feature selected	Sensor	Number of feature selected
Accelerometer	21	sEMG2	2
Gyroscope	10	sEMG3	0
sEMG1	4	sEMG4	3

features are chosen which indicates the hand and arm rotation is also important. It is necessary to include sEMG sensors since nine features are selected from sEMG.

To have a better understanding of the importance of each individual feature, the rankings of 40 features are listed in Table 5. In the table, Acc_x, Acc_y and Acc_z represent accelerometer readings along *x-axis*, *y-axis* and *z-axis*, respectively. Similarly, Gyro_x, Gyro_y and Gyro_z are gyroscope readings along *x-axis*, *y-axis* and *z-axis*, respectively. From the table, the accelerometer contributes to the most highly ranked features which means the most significant modality of our system is the accelerometer. The gyroscope features are not as highly ranked as the accelerometer, but they have higher rankings than sEMG features. From the table, sEMG contribute least among all three. Among accelerometer and gyroscope features, the most important ones include mean, integration, standard deviation, RMS and variance. Mean absolute value, variance and RMS are valuable features for sEMG signal. One interesting observation of sEMG features is that four selected features from channel one have higher ranks than the others from channel two and channel four. Channel one is placed near the wrist where a smart watch is usually worn. In reality, if only one electrode is allowed, channel one could selected and it can be integrated into a smart watch without introducing a new device.

C. *Classification Results*

Table 6 shows the classification results of intra-subject testing on four subjects. In this experiment, each classifier is trained and tested with data from the same subject. We can see that nearest neighbor and LibSVM achieve high accuracies while decision tree classifier obtains the lowest accuracy. Nearest neighbor classifier is a lazy learning classifier and it does not require a trained model. In the testing phase, it compares the testing instance with all instances in the training set and assigns it a same class label as the most similar instance in the training set. It will require a large computation power as the number of training samples increase and thus is not suitable for our wearable SLR system. LibSVM trains a model based on training data. As the size of training set increases, it only increase the training time without affecting the time needs in testing phase. This is crucial for real time wearable computer based applications. Therefore, LibSVM is selected for our system. The results achieved for 80 signs are consistent with the results obtained for 40 signs in our prior investigation [42]. It indicates our technique scales well for intra-subject testing.

Table 7 shows classification results of all cross validation. For all classifiers, the classification results with sEMG and without sEMG are given. The performance with sEMG is when the performance achieved using all 40 selected features while

Table 5 Fourty selected features

Rank#	Feature name	Rank#	Feature name	Rank#	Feature name	Rank#	Feature name
1	Mean of Acc_y	11	RMS of Gyro_x	21	RMS of sEMG1	31	Signal magnitude area of Acc_x
2	Mean of Acc_z	12	RMS of amplitude of accelerometer	22	Zero cross rate of Acc_y	32	Variance of sEMG4
3	RMS of Acc_x	13	Mean of amplitude of accelerometer	23	Variance of Gyro_z	33	Entropy of Gyro_x
4	RMS of Acc_z	14	Mean of Acc_x	24	Standard deviation Of Gyro_z	34	RMS of sEMG4
5	RMS of Acc_y	15	Signal magnitude area of Acc_x	25	Variance of Acc_y	35	Signal magnitude area of Gyro_x
6	Integration of Acc_y	16	Standard deviation of Acc_z	26	Standard deviation of Acc_y	36	Zero cross rate of Acc_z
7	Integration of Acc_x	17	Variance of Acc_z	27	Modified mean frequency of sEMG1	37	Mean absolute value of sEMG4
8	Integration of Acc_z	18	Standard deviation of Gyro_z	28	Mean absolute value of sEMG1	38	Signal magnitude area of Gyro_z
9	Entropy of Acc_x	19	Variance of Gyro_x	29	First auto-regression coefficient of Acc_x	39	RMS of sEMG2
10	RMS of Gyro_z	20	Variance of sEMG1	30	Mean absolute value of sEMG2	40	Mean of amplitude of gyroscope

performance without sEMG is when the performance obtained using 31 features selected from accelerometer and gyroscope. The performance improvements by adding sEMG are also listed in the table. Among four classifiers, LibSVM achieves the best performance in accuracy, precision, recall and F-score while NaiveBayes gives the worst performance. The accuracy, precision, recall and F-score are very close to each other for all classifiers which indicates all classifiers achieve balanced performance on our dataset. With 40 features, LibSVM achieves 96.16% accuracy. It is consistent with the results (95.16%) we obtained for 40 sign words with 30 features in our prior study [42]. This proves the scalability of approach for all cross validation test.

Table 6 Results of intra-subject validation

	NaiveBayes (%)	DT (%)	NN (%)	LibSVM (%)
Subject 1	88.81	83.89	96.6	98.22
Subject 2	97.01	91.54	99.16	99.48
Subject 3	92.74	81.97	92.89	96.61
Subject 4	91.15	77.98	95.77	97.23
Average	93.68	83.85	96.11	97.89

Table 7 Results of all-cross validation

	NaiveBayes (%)	DT (%)	NN (%)	LibSVM (%)
Accuracy with sEMG	63.87	76.18	94.02	96.16
Accuracy without sEMG	48.75	68.93	87.62	92.29
Improvement	15.12	7.25	6.4	3.84
Precision with sEMG	66.9	76.3	94.0	96.7
Precision without sEMG	51.8	69.0	87.7	92.3
Improvement	15.1	7.3	6.3	4.4
Recall with sEMG	63.9	76.2	94.0	96.7
Recall without sEMG	48.8	68.9	87.7	92.3
Improvement	15.1	7.3	6.3	4.4
F-score with sEMG	63.6	76.2	94.0	96.7
F-score without sEMG	47.6	68.9	87.6	92.3
Improvement	16.0	7.3	6.4	4.4

The improvement after adding the sEMG modality is most significant for NaiveBayes classifier. It achieves about 15% improvement for all four classification performance metrics. However, for our chosen classifier LibSVM, the accuracy improvement is about 4% while the error rate is reduced by 50%. It indicates the sEMG is necessary and significant. The significance of sEMG is further analyzed in next section.

Figure 7 shows the average accuracy of inter-subject testing for both 80 sign words and 40 sign words. The figure shows none of four classifier achieves good performance. LibSVM is still the best classifier. There are three reasons for such low accuracies. First, different people perform the same signs in different ways. Second, all subjects in our experiment are first time ASL learners and never had experience with ASL before. Even though they follow the instructions, the gestures for the same signs are different from each other. Third, different subjects have very different muscular strength and thus leading to different sEMG features for same signs. From the comparison between accuracy of 40 signs and 80 signs, our technique offers low accuracy for all classifiers consistently. The low performance suggests our system is not suitable for inter-subject applications and it is recommended that our system should be trained on each individual to provide good performance.

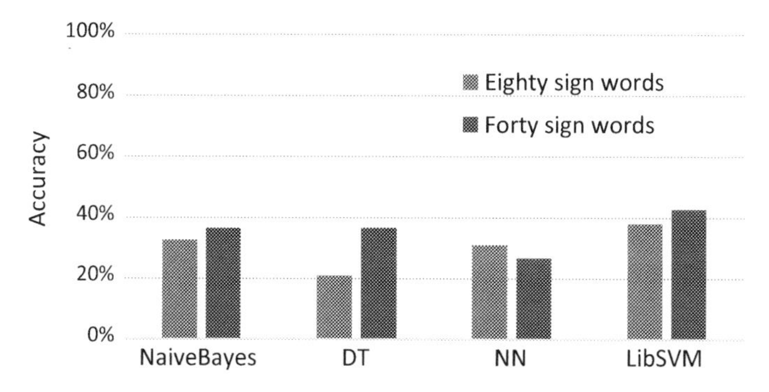

Fig. 7 Results of inter-subject testing

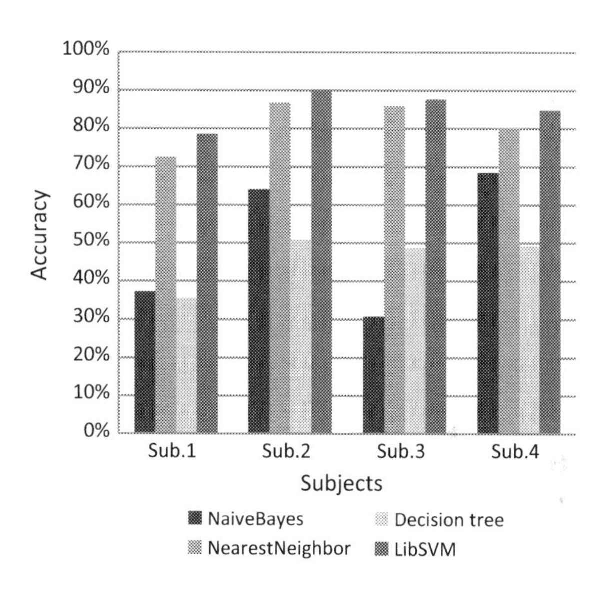

Fig. 8 Results of intra-subject cross session testing

The first three experiments show our system achieves suitable performance if the system is trained and tested for the same subject and the system obtains less ideal performance for inter-subject testing. We further investigate how well the system will generalize for new data collected in future for the same subject. Figure 8 shows the results of the intra-subject cross session testing in which the feature selection is performed and the classifier is trained with two days data from the same each subject and is tested on data of the third day for the same subject. This process is repeated three times for the same subject and the accuracy measures are averaged. We can see that both NaiveBayes and decision tree yield poor accuracies while LibSVM offers best accuracy. Table 8 shows the average accuracy of different classification algorithms between four subjects. LibSVM achieves 85.24% which is less suitable than the 96.16% of intra-subject testing. Two reasons may explain this performance decrease. The first reason is that the user may have placed the sensors

Table 8 Results of intra-subject cross session testing

Classifier	Accuracy (%)	Classifier	Accuracy (%)
NaiveBayes	50.11	NN	81.37
DT	46.01	LibSVM	85.24

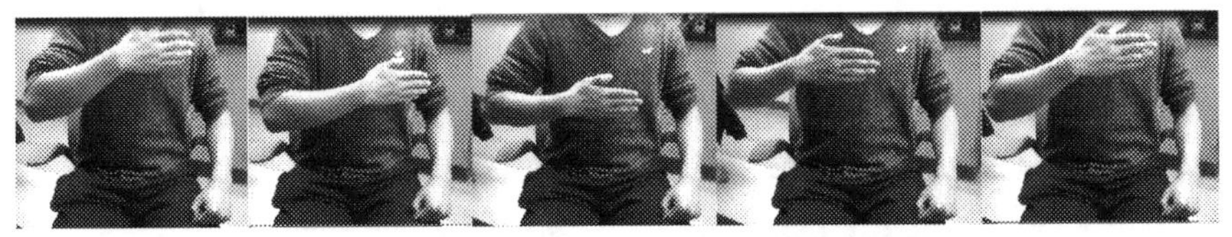

(a). Sequence of postures when performing 'Please'.

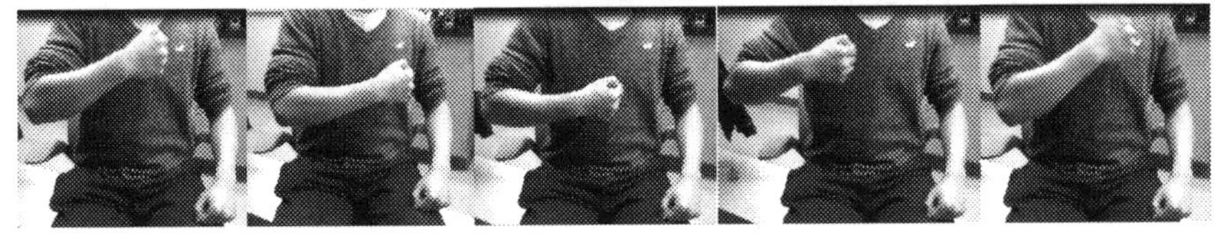

(b). Sequence of postures when performing 'Sorry'.

Fig. 9 Sequence of postures when performing 'Please' and 'Sorry'

at slightly different locations for the sEMG and IMU sensors, and with a slightly different orientation for the IMU sensor. The second reason is that all four subjects are first time learner who have not developed consistent patterns for signs. They may have performed the same signs somewhat differently on different days.

D. *Significance of sEMG*

From the analysis of inter-subject testing in previous section, the error rates for the accuracy, precision, recall and F-score are reduced by about 50%. In this section, we analyze the importance of sEMG in details. From the previous discussion, accelerometer and gyroscope are more important than sEMG. However, in ASL, there are some signs that have similar arm/hand movement and different hand shape and finger configurations (e.g. fist and palm). For these signs, they will have similar accelerometer and gyroscope readings and the IMU is not able to distinguish these signs. The sEMG is able to capture the difference of these signs since they will have different muscle activities. Figure 9 shows an example of sequences of postures when the user is performing two signs 'Please' and 'Sorry'. We can see from the figures, the arm has the same movement which is drawing a circle in front of chest. The inertial sensor will offer same readings for these two different signs. However, the hand is closed (i.e. fist) when performing 'Sorry' while it is open (i.e. palm) when performing 'Please'. This difference can be captured by sEMG and thus they will be distinguishable if sEMG is included.

In order to show how sEMG will enhance recognition performance of each individual sign, the improvement on the true positive (TP) rate of each individual sign is investigated. TP rate is rate of true positive and true positives are number of instances which are correctly classified as a given class. Figure 10 shows the TP rate improvement for 80 signs and the improvement is sorted in descend order. From the figure, we can see that for most of signs (last 29–80), the rate of improvement is within the range of [−5, 5]%. However, for the signs from 1 to 11, the improvement is bigger than 10% which is very helpful for recognizing these signs. In Table 9, 10 signs are listed with the highest TP rate improvement. We can see that 'Sorry' and 'Please' are both improved significantly since they are confused with each other. In reality, it is important to eliminate the confusion between signs which have similar motion profile but different sEMG characteristics. Therefore, the sEMG is significant for our system.

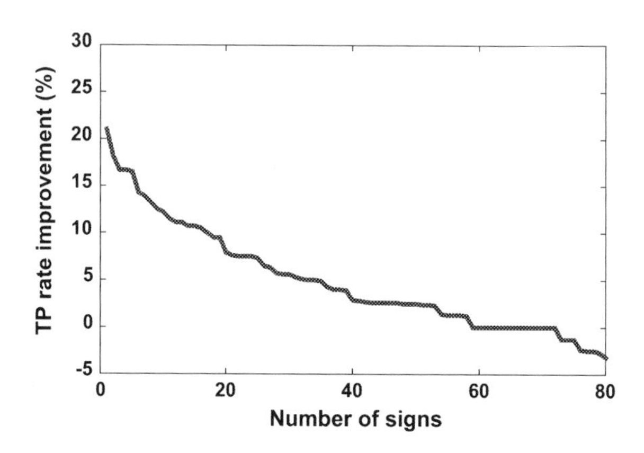

Fig. 10 TP rate improvement of all signs

Table 9 10 signs with most TP rate improvement

Sign ID	Sign	Improvement (%)
29	Thank	21
19	My	18.2
9	Have	16.7
24	Please	16.7
37	Work	16.5
57	Tall	14.3
67	Girl	13.9
26	Sorry	13.8
76	Doctor	12.5
66	Boy	12.5

7 Limitations and Discussion

The wearable inertial sensor and sEMG sensors based sign language recognition/gesture recognition systems have become more and more popular in recent years because of low-cost, privacy non-intrusive and ubiquitous sensing ability compared with vision-based approaches. They may not be as accurate as vision-based approaches. A vision-based approach achieves 92.5% accuracy for 439 frequently used Chinese Sign Language words [17]. Although we have not tested for such a large number of signs, it may be challenging with wearable inertial and sEMG systems to recognize such a big number of signs. Another disadvantage with wearable inertial sensor and sEMG based sign language recognition system is that the facial expression is not captured.

In our study, we observe that the accelerometer is the most significant modality for detecting signs. When designing such systems, if fusion of multiple modalities is not possible, the suggested choice order of these three are: accelerometer, gyroscope and sEMG. The significance of sEMG is to distinguish sets of signs which are similar in motion and this is crucial for sign language recognition. For some gesture recognition tasks, if gesture number is not big and there are no gestures which are very similar in motion, one inertial sensor may be sufficient for the task to reduce the system cost.

Our system offers high accuracy for both 40 signs and 80 signs for intra-subject testing and all cross validation. This shows our system is scalable for American Sign Language recognition if the system is trained and tested on the same subjects. However, very low accuracy is achieved for inter-subject testing which indicates our system is not very suitable for use on individuals if the system is not trained for them. We have talked to several experts of American Sign Language and they think it is reasonable to train for each individuals since even for expert, they will perform quite differently from each other for the same signs based on their preference and habits. This is the major limitation of sign language recognition systems. Our system is studied and designed to recognize individual signs assuming a pause exists between two sign words. However, in daily conversation, a whole sentence may be performed continuously without an obvious pause between each words. To recognize continuous sentence, a different segmentation technique or other possibility models should be considered.

Machine learning is a powerful tool for different applications and is gaining a lot of popularity in recent years in wearable computer based applications. However, it is important to use it in a correct way. For different applications, different features and different classifiers may have significantly different performance. It is suggested to try different approaches to determine the best one. The other point is that the classifier parameters should be carefully tuned. In our approach, if we do not choose the correct parameters for LibSVM, only 68% accuracy can be achieved.

As IoT emerges, the information from different sensing modalities could be explored. When designing applications, data from different sources should be considered and verified if they are complementary and the fusion of the modalities could potentially enhance the application performance.

8 Conclusion

A wearable real-time American Sign Language recognition system is proposed in this book chapter. This is a first study of American Sign Language recognition system fusing IMU sensor and sEMG signals which are complementary to each other. Our system design is an example of fusing different sensor modalities and addressing computation cost challenge of wearable computer based SLR due to the high-dimensional data. Feature selection is performed to select the best subset of features from a large number of well-established features and four popular classification algorithms are investigated for our system design. The system is evaluated with 80 commonly used ASL signs in daily conversation and an average accuracy of 96.16% is achieved with 40 selected features. The significance of sEMG to American Sign Language recognition task is explored.

Acknowledgements This work was supported in part by the National Science Foundation, under grants CNS-1150079 and ECCS-1509063. Any opinions, findings, conclusions, or recommendations expressed in this material are those of the authors and do not necessarily reflect the views of the funding organizations.

References

1. W. C. Stokoe, "Sign language structure: An outline of the visual communication systems of the American deaf," *Journal of deaf studies and deaf education*, vol. 10, no. 1, pp. 3–37, 2005.
2. D. Barberis, N. Garazzino, P. Prinetto, G. Tiotto, A. Savino, U. Shoaib, and N. Ahmad, "Language resources for computer assisted translation from italian to italian sign language of deaf people," in *Proceedings of Accessibility Reaching Everywhere AEGIS Workshop and International Conference, Brussels, Belgium (November 2011)*, 2011.
3. A. B. Grieve-Smith, "Signsynth: A sign language synthesis application using web3d and PERL," in *Gesture and Sign Language in Human-Computer Interaction*, pp. 134–145, Springer, 2002.
4. B. Vicars, "Basic ASL: First 100 signs."
5. E. Costello, *American sign language dictionary*. Random House Reference &, 2008.
6. T. Starner, J. Weaver, and A. Pentland, "Real-time american sign language recognition using desk and wearable computer based video," *Pattern Analysis and Machine Intelligence, IEEE Transactions on*, vol. 20, no. 12, pp. 1371–1375, 1998.
7. C. Vogler and D. Metaxas, "A framework for recognizing the simultaneous aspects of American sign language," *Computer Vision and Image Understanding*, vol. 81, no. 3, pp. 358–384, 2001.

8. T. E. Starner, "Visual recognition of American sign language using Hidden Markov models.," tech. rep., DTIC Document, 1995.
9. C. Oz and M. C. Leu, "American sign language word recognition with a sensory glove using artificial neural networks," *Engineering Applications of Artificial Intelligence*, vol. 24, no. 7, pp. 1204–1213, 2011.
10. E. Malaia, J. Borneman, and R. B. Wilbur, "Analysis of ASL motion capture data towards identification of verb type," in *Proceedings of the 2008 Conference on Semantics in Text Processing*, pp. 155–164, Association for Computational Linguistics, 2008.
11. A. Y. Benbasat and J. A. Paradiso, "An inertial measurement framework for gesture recognition and applications," in *Gesture and Sign Language in Human-Computer Interaction*, pp. 9–20, Springer, 2002.
12. O. Amft, H. Junker, and G. Troster, "Detection of eating and drinking arm gestures using inertial body-worn sensors," in *Wearable Computers, 2005. Proceedings. Ninth IEEE International Symposium on*, pp. 160–163, IEEE, 2005.
13. A. B. Ajiboye and R. F. Weir, "A heuristic fuzzy logic approach to EMG pattern recognition for multifunctional prosthesis control," *Neural Systems and Rehabilitation Engineering, IEEE Transactions on*, vol. 13, no. 3, pp. 280–291, 2005.
14. J.-U. Chu, I. Moon, and M.-S. Mun, "A real-time EMG pattern recognition based on linear-nonlinear feature projection for multifunction myoelectric hand," in *Rehabilitation Robotics, 2005. ICORR 2005. 9th International Conference on*, pp. 295–298, IEEE, 2005.
15. Y. Li, X. Chen, X. Zhang, K. Wang, and J. Yang, "Interpreting sign components from accelerometer and sEMG data for automatic sign language recognition," in *Engineering in Medicine and Biology Society, EMBC, 2011 Annual International Conference of the IEEE*, pp. 3358–3361, IEEE, 2011.
16. Y. Li, X. Chen, X. Zhang, K. Wang, and Z. J. Wang, "A sign-component-based framework for chinese sign language recognition using accelerometer and sEMG data," *Biomedical Engineering, IEEE Transactions on*, vol. 59, no. 10, pp. 2695–2704, 2012.
17. L.-G. Zhang, Y. Chen, G. Fang, X. Chen, and W. Gao, "A vision-based sign language recognition system using tied-mixture density hmm," in *Proceedings of the 6th international conference on Multimodal interfaces*, pp. 198–204, ACM, 2004.
18. M. M. Zaki and S. I. Shaheen, "Sign language recognition using a combination of new vision based features," *Pattern Recognition Letters*, vol. 32, no. 4, pp. 572–577, 2011.
19. T.-Y. Pan, L.-Y. Lo, C.-W. Yeh, J.-W. Li, H.-T. Liu, and M.-C. Hu, "Real-time sign language recognition in complex background scene based on a hierarchical clustering classification method," in *Multimedia Big Data (BigMM), 2016 IEEE Second International Conference on*, pp. 64–67, IEEE, 2016.
20. M. W. Kadous *et al.*, "Machine recognition of AUSLAN signs using powergloves: Towards large-Lexicon recognition of sign language," in *Proceedings of the Workshop on the Integration of Gesture in Language and Speech*, pp. 165–174, Citeseer, 1996.
21. M. G. Kumar, M. K. Gurjar, and M. S. B. Singh, "American sign language translating glove using flex sensor," *Imperial Journal of Interdisciplinary Research*, vol. 2, no. 6, 2016.
22. D. Sherrill, P. Bonato, and C. De Luca, "A neural network approach to monitor motor activities," in *Engineering in Medicine and Biology, 2002. 24th Annual Conference and the Annual Fall Meeting of the Biomedical Engineering Society EMBS/BMES Conference, 2002. Proceedings of the Second Joint*, vol. 1, pp. 52–53, IEEE, 2002.
23. X. Chen, X. Zhang, Z.-Y. Zhao, J.-H. Yang, V. Lantz, and K.-Q. Wang, "Hand gesture recognition research based on surface EMG sensors and 2D-accelerometers," in *Wearable Computers, 2007 11th IEEE International Symposium on*, pp. 11–14, IEEE, 2007.
24. V. E. Kosmidou and L. J. Hadjileontiadis, "Sign language recognition using intrinsic-mode sample entropy on sEMG and accelerometer data," *Biomedical Engineering, IEEE Transactions on*, vol. 56, no. 12, pp. 2879–2890, 2009.
25. S. Wei, X. Chen, X. Yang, S. Cao, and X. Zhang, "A component-based vocabulary-extensible sign language gesture recognition framework," *Sensors*, vol. 16, no. 4, p. 556, 2016.

26. J. Kim, J. Wagner, M. Rehm, and E. André, "Bi-channel sensor fusion for automatic sign language recognition," in *Automatic Face & Gesture Recognition, 2008. FG'08. 8th IEEE International Conference on*, pp. 1–6, IEEE, 2008.
27. J.-S. Wang and F.-C. Chuang, "An accelerometer-based digital pen with a trajectory recognition algorithm for handwritten digit and gesture recognition," *Industrial Electronics, IEEE Transactions on*, vol. 59, no. 7, pp. 2998–3007, 2012.
28. V. Nathan, J. Wu, C. Zong, Y. Zou, O. Dehzangi, M. Reagor, and R. Jafari, "A 16-channel bluetooth enabled wearable EEG platform with dry-contact electrodes for brain computer interface," in *Proceedings of the 4th Conference on Wireless Health*, p. 17, ACM, 2013.
29. C. J. De Luca, L. Donald Gilmore, M. Kuznetsov, and S. H. Roy, "Filtering the surface emg signal: Movement artifact and baseline noise contamination," *Journal of biomechanics*, vol. 43, no. 8, pp. 1573–1579, 2010.
30. I. Mesa, A. Rubio, I. Tubia, J. De No, and J. Diaz, "Channel and feature selection for a surface electromyographic pattern recognition task," *Expert Systems with Applications*, vol. 41, no. 11, pp. 5190–5200, 2014.
31. R. Merletti and P. Di Torino, "Standards for reporting EMG data," *J Electromyogr Kinesiol*, vol. 9, no. 1, pp. 3–4, 1999.
32. A. Phinyomark, C. Limsakul, and P. Phukpattaranont, "A novel feature extraction for robust EMG pattern recognition," *arXiv preprint* arXiv:0912.3973, 2009.
33. M. Zhang and A. A. Sawchuk, "Human daily activity recognition with sparse representation using wearable sensors," *Biomedical and Health Informatics, IEEE Journal of*, vol. 17, no. 3, pp. 553–560, 2013.
34. S. H. Khan and M. Sohail, "Activity monitoring of workers using single wearable inertial sensor."
35. O. Paiss and G. F. Inbar, "Autoregressive modeling of surface EMG and its spectrum with application to fatigue," *Biomedical Engineering, IEEE Transactions on*, no. 10, pp. 761–770, 1987.
36. A. M. Khan, Y.-K. Lee, S. Y. Lee, and T.-S. Kim, "A triaxial accelerometer-based physical-activity recognition via augmented-signal features and a hierarchical recognizer," *Information Technology in Biomedicine, IEEE Transactions on*, vol. 14, no. 5, pp. 1166–1172, 2010.
37. I. Guyon and A. Elisseeff, "An introduction to variable and feature selection," *The Journal of Machine Learning Research*, vol. 3, pp. 1157–1182, 2003.
38. J. R. Quinlan, *C4. 5: programs for machine learning*. Elsevier, 2014.
39. C.-C. Chang and C.-J. Lin, "LIBSVM: A library for support vector machines," *ACM Transactions on Intelligent Systems and Technology*, vol. 2, pp. 27:1–27:27, 2011. Software available at http://www.csie.ntu.edu.tw/~cjlin/libsvm.
40. M. Hall, E. Frank, G. Holmes, B. Pfahringer, P. Reutemann, and I. H. Witten, "The weka data mining software: an update," *ACM SIGKDD explorations newsletter*, vol. 11, no. 1, pp. 10–18, 2009.
41. M. Z. Jamal, "Signal acquisition using surface EMG and circuit design considerations for robotic prosthesis," 2012.
42. J. Wu, Z. Tian, L. Sun, L. Estevez, and R. Jafari, "Real-time american sign language recognition using wrist-worn motion and surface EMG sensors," in *Wearable and Implantable Body Sensor Networks (BSN), 2015 IEEE 12th International Conference on*, pp. 1–6, IEEE, 2015.

Real-Time, Personalized Anomaly Detection in Streaming Data for Wearable Healthcare Devices

Bharadwaj Veeravalli, Chacko John Deepu and DuyHoa Ngo

Abstract Ubiquitous deployment of low cost wearable healthcare devices and proactive monitoring of vital physiological data, are widely seen as a solution for the high costs and risks associated with personal healthcare. The healthcare data generated from these sensors cannot be manually analyzed for anomalies by clinicians due to its scale and therefore automated techniques has to be developed. Present approaches in literature depends on accurate detection of features from the acquired signal which is not always realistic due to noisy nature of the ambulatory physiological data obtained from the sensors. In addition, present anomaly detection approaches require manual training of the system for each patient, due to inherent variations in the morphology of physiological signal for each user. In this chapter, we will first introduce the system architecture for wearable health-care monitoring systems and present discussions on various components involved. Then we discuss on the complexities involved in realizing these methods and highlight key features. We then present our experiences in extracting the ECG segments in real-time and detecting any anomalies in the streams. Particularly, we apply real-time signal processing methods and heuristics to estimate the boundary limits of individual beats from the streaming ECG data. We discuss the importance of designing methods, which are blind to inherent variations among multiple patients and less dependent on the accuracy of the feature extraction. The proposed methods are tested on public database from physionet (QTDB) to validate the quality of results. We highlight and discuss all the significant results and conclude the chapter by proposing some open-ended research questions to be addressed in the near future.

B. Veeravalli · C.J. Deepu (✉) · D. Ngo
Department of Electrical & Computer Engineering,
National University of Singapore (NUS), 4 Engineering Drive 3,
117583 Singapore, Singapore
e-mail: deepu.john@ieee.org

B. Veeravalli
e-mail: elebv@nus.edu.sg

D. Ngo
e-mail: elendh@nus.edu.sg

© Springer International Publishing AG 2017

S.U. Khan et al. (eds.), *Handbook of Large-Scale Distributed Computing in Smart Healthcare*, Scalable Computing and Communications,
DOI 10.1007/978-3-319-58280-1_15

1 Introduction

Healthcare expenditure has been steadily increasing worldwide over the past several decades. This increase is primarily attributed to (1) a fast aging population and declining birth rates, (2) chronic conditions which need sustained medical care, and (3) focus on treatment of diseases rather than pro-actively preventing it. Cardiovascular diseases (CVDs) is one of the major contributors for this spending and is one of the leading causes for death [1]. It is noted that even with the large spending on CVDs, 47% of all CVD related deaths happen outside of the hospital premises [2]. All of these triggered a renewed interest in developing wearable healthcare systems which can proactively monitor the user's health to reduce the risks and costs associated with personal healthcare. Thanks to ultra-low power circuit design and device integration, several miniature wearable sensors which can continuously acquire user's physiological signals like Electrocardiogram (ECG), Bio impedance has been developed [3–8].

The top level architecture of a wearable healthcare monitoring setup is illustrated in Fig. 1. The physiological signals like ECG, from the subject is continuously acquired using wearable sensors and is streamed in real-time to a gateway device. Typically, low power radios like Bluetooth *Smart* are used in the wearable sensor for data transfer. The gateway can be a dedicated hardware device or simply a smartphone app, which collects data from all connected sensors and transfers it to a cloud server. The data collected in the cloud server is constantly examined for signal patterns that matches potentially anomalous conditions. Also various predictive algorithms that can identify different types of arrhythmias can be deployed. A client interface web application can be used to visualize real-time data streaming from the sensor.

Electrocardiogram (ECG) signal, which represents the electrical activity of heart, is one of the most commonly measured physiological signal for monitoring patients. For healthy subjects, ECG rhythm variations are minimal. Also morphology and timing intervals of various ECG wave segments will be within defined limits. The variations in morphology, wave timing intervals and rhythm can potentially an indicator of various ailments that is associated with the human heart.

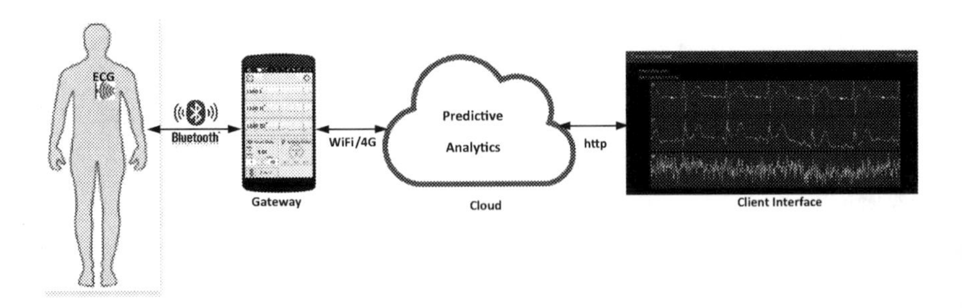

Fig. 1 System architecture for wearable healthcare monitoring system

ECG can be measured in different lead configurations, i.e. from a single lead up to 12 leads. Typical lead configurations are (1) Single lead, (2) 3 Leads which are typically the limb leads, (3) 6 leads—which includes the limb leads and augmented leads, and (4) 12 leads, which include the limb leads, augmented leads and the 6 precordial leads.

Different cardiac arrhythmias can be detected by identifying the changes in rhythm, morphology and timing interval of various segments across all or some of the 12 leads of ECG Signal. Many of these arrhythmias are 'asymptomatic' and doesn't cause any noticeable discomfort or uneasiness to the subject in the initial stages. However, if not treated in-time these can trigger other complex and fatal conditions. For e.g., Atrial fibrillation an often unnoticed arrhythmia is one of the leading causes for stroke related fatalities [9]. An early detection of the onset of these conditions are necessary for responding with treatment options and making proactive changes in lifestyle. Since many of cardiac arrhythmias are paroxysmal in nature, regular hospital visits won't help to identify these ailments [10]. Therefore, continuous monitoring of ECG is essential to improve the diagnostic yield. Automated methods for detection of anomalies in ECG signals are needed to continuously analyse the vast amount of data collected.

2 Related Works

There are several approaches proposed in literature for automatic detection of cardiac conditions. Majority of them focuses on automatic detection of arrhythmias from single or multi lead ECG signals [11–13]. However, till date none of these techniques can classify arrhythmias with a high level of accuracy. Often the algorithms are tuned for lower level false negatives at the expense of higher false positives. Therefore, participation of clinicians is still essential and often they are desensitized to the automatic alerts due to large false positives.

Cardiac arrhythmia classification is a pattern recognition task which can be done using **syntactic** or **machine learning** methods. In syntactic methods the features of ECG signal are carefully extracted using signal processing and feature extraction methods and after which rules are applied to the extracted features to detect arrhythmias [14, 15]. For example, a PR interval longer than 0.2 s is potentially caused by a first degree heart block; a QRS duration greater than 0.12 s could be the result of a ventricular premature complex [16]. Obviously, the accuracy of this method extremely depends on the precision of the features extraction. Due to the ambulatory nature of wearable sensors, the signals acquired by the sensors are often noisy and hence would require complex signal processing approaches (wavelet transforms [17], empirical mode decomposition [18] etc.) for accurate feature extraction.

Machine learning based methods uses a combination of signal features and morphology as feature vectors [19, 20]. Learning methods such as decision tree [11], SVM [12], ANN [13], etc., train the model using existing training data, annotated by clinicians. The trained classifier can be then used to classify/identify the real time streaming ECG signals into various arrhythmias. However, the accuracy of those methods heavily depends on the selected learning schemes and the distribution of training data. The classification accuracy can be improved by ensemble learning [21, 22], but it has very high computational complexity. Another major issue with this approach is that the training data set are often very limited and has large variation between patients, therefore the classifiers which performs well on one data set performs poorly with other data sets [23].

Our approach differentiates with the above methods, in terms of the required ECG signal analysis, to detect the abnormality in ECG pattern. In our technique, we treat the problem similar to that of anomaly detection problem in a time series data [24, 25], where precise characteristics of the ECG signal is not necessary to be extracted. Instead, such methods compare signal patterns within a stream to detect the anomalies. Most of these methods do not need or need very little of existing data for configuration of system parameters.

A popular approach in time series data mining is to approximate the streaming binary data into a sequence of text data. Some approximation methods such as Symbolic Aggregate Approximation (SAX) [26, 27], Piecewise Linear, and Piecewise Constant models (PAA) [28] have been widely studied in time series mining, but might not be useful in ECG data. Our observation is that even for the same type of ECG heart cycle, the wave timing intervals and morphology varies among different people. Therefore, those approximations may cause high inaccuracy.

Some approaches that are closely related to our approach are [29, 30]. We segment the streaming ECG data and apply DTW algorithm to compare ECG segments. In [29], author still use some existing data for pre-training system, whereas, in [30], authors require accurate detection of ECG wave onsets, offsets and peak of P, QRS and T wave. In contrary, our approach neither requires precise detection of P, QRS, T waves, nor require any training data for configuring the system.

3 Requirements for Data Analysis Algorithms

To be used for analysing the huge volume of streaming ECG data from wearable devices, the algorithms should possess the following desirable characteristics.

Single lead based anomaly detection: Although ECG signal can be measured using up to 12 leads, in the case of wearable devices typically only single lead or three lead ECG signal is acquired [3]. This is because wearable devices are made to be minimally obtrusive with small form factors and therefore has minimal number of leads acquired. For single lead devices typically only lead II signal is acquired. Many of the existing arrhythmia classification algorithms requires the multiple ECG leads, i.e. signal from limb leads as well as precordial leads. This is because arrhythmias can be reflected in multiple ECG leads. Since wearable devices can pick up only one or a few leads, the algorithm used should be able to work with a single lead. It is understood that an accurate identification of a specific arrhythmia may not be possible from a single lead ECG signal. However, in the context of wearable devices, detection of an anomaly is good enough to alert the user for a more thorough analysis at a hospital.

Minimal training or calibration requirements: The algorithm should be able to detect the anomalous patterns in the streaming ECG with no or minimal pre training and calibration. For optimal performance in learning based algorithms, significant amount of training with pre marked ECG signals are required for each patient. However, this is not practical for real life use cases. The algorithms should be self-adaptive and no calibration/modifications should be made for individual subjects.

Low computational complexity and high accuracy: The techniques used for wearable health monitoring should have a high detection accuracy and lower computational complexity. Often these two requirements contradict each other and therefore a balanced tradeoff is desirable. Usage of syntactic or machine learning methods, which require ECG delineation, wave morphology identification etc. will increase overall computational complexity due to the complex signal processing methods involved.

Real-time detection: The algorithms used should be able to detect the anomalies in the incoming streaming data in a real time fashion. The user/clinicians should be alerted as and when an event occurs. The storage requirements for past data should be minimal to limit overall complexity. Some of the existing feature detection algorithms need to analyze the entire dataset at once to decide on the computational thresholds which is not practical for real time usage.

The above requirements necessitate simple RR interval based algorithms for arrhythmia detection, like the one mentioned in [31]. However, RR interval based algorithms are not able detect abnormalities causing variations in the morphology of the ECG signal. Therefore, in this paper we propose a novel method for ECG anomaly detection, which has low computational complexity and yet has high detection accuracy. The proposed method doesn't individually identify each arrhythmia; however, it can classify a cardiac beat as normal versus abnormal based on the RR interval and the signal morphology. For a wearable health monitoring system, such a classification is a more appropriate choice, considering the limitations mentioned above. The proposed technique can be used individually for ECG anomaly detection or in conjunction other arrhythmia detection approaches for improving its accuracy. The main contributions of this work are:

1. A technique for real-time detection and adaptive segmentation of each cardiac beat.
2. A method to compute similarity between two adaptive beat segments of different length.
3. A technique to automatically detect the normal beat for individual patients in the monitoring process.
4. A fast and effective incremental algorithm to identify abnormal heart beat in the real-time mode.

We evaluated the proposed method using publicly available QT database from physionet library. The QT Database includes ECGs that represent various heart beat morphologies, in order to challenge detection algorithms with real-world variability. The experimental result shows that the proposed approach is suitable to be used in wearable healthcare monitoring applications.

4 Proposed Methodology

4.1 Overview

The overview of the proposed ECG monitoring technique is shown in the Fig. 2 [32]. The data streamed from wearable ECG device is processed using a real-time signal processing block which will extract the R-peak locations from the ECG signal. Typically, the ECG Lead II signal from the wearable device is used for processing since the morphologies of the normal and abnormal beats can be clearly and easily distinguished compared to other ECG leads [33]. Once the R-peak is extracted, the beat segment surrounding the R-peak is identified and fed into the anomaly detection block. The *current beat segment* to be monitored is adaptively detected, so as to make sure to include the P-wave and T-wave from each individual beat from the ECG Signal. The variations in morphology of these wave segments may indicate various anomalies. The timing of the onset and offset of T-wave and P-wave varies among different subjects as well as within the ECG of the same subject. Hence the wave onsets and offsets has to be detected in real-time to make sure T-wave and P-wave is included in the extracted *current beat segment*. However, the exact detection of the wave onsets and offsets is a complex signal processing task [34, 35]. Therefore, to reduce the computational complexity, we used a heuristic to approximate a left and right signal boundary which will include the all ECG waves (P-QRS-T) in its entirety. The next sections will describe details about R-peak detection and how the *current beat segment* is extracted for anomaly detection.

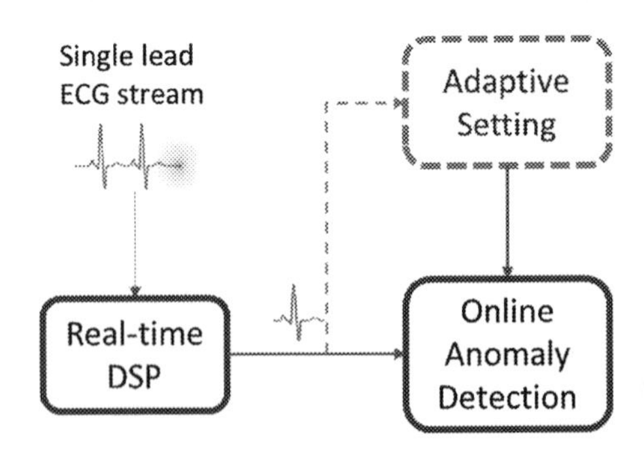

Fig. 2 Overview of the proposed methodology [32]

Once an adaptive beat segment, which captures the P-QRS-T waves from every beat in the ECG signal is extracted, a quantitative measurement of similarity of the adaptive *current beat segment* with a *normal beat segment* is to be calculated. Based on the similarity measure, the current beat can be classified into a normal or anomalous beat. Since the length of the extracted adaptive beat segments are not always constant, typical similarity measures like Euclidean distances, Cosine distances, Correlation measures is not suitable for computation of the similarity between 2 different beat segments. Therefore, in this work, we propose to use a time series based similarity measure called discrete time warping, which quickly computes the similarity between beat segments.

Identification of anomalous beat segments from a stream of incoming data is a time series data analysis task, which is usually complex due to the high dimensional features of the data objects. Typically, dimensionality reduction is required in such cases to reduce the computational complexity. However, in the proposed scheme we converted a multivariate stream of beat segments into a uni-variate stream of numbers by calculating the similarity measure between the *current beat segment* and the *normal beat segment* and thus limits the computational complexity. The *normal beat segment* is identified individually for each subject to represent the normal status of the heart rhythm during the time of monitoring. However, the *normal beat segment* isn't necessarily a clinically normal beat as found in a normal sinus rhythm. For e.g., in patients with chronic arrhythmia conditions like left bundle branch block, the occurrence of a beat segment with arrhythmia is very frequent compared to the normal sinus rhythm and hence occurrence of normal sinus rhythm is to be considered abnormal. Therefore, the identification of *normal beat segment* must be patient adaptive. An initialization routine, which is one-time process is used for identifying *normal beat segment* template for each patient. Once the *normal beat segment* template is selected as a reference, the incoming data, which is a stream of *current beat segments* are transformed into a stream of numerical values, where each of them is the measure of similarity between the current and the normal beat segments. Finally, the online Anomaly detection technique, described in Sect. 4.5 will detect if the *current beat segment* is an outlier among the streaming data, to classify it is as a regular or anomalous beat.

4.2 Real-Time Signal Processing for Extracting Current Beat Segment

The signal processing block extracts individual non overlapping beat segments from the incoming ECG data stream in a real-time fashion. The R-peaks from the ECG stream is detected in real-time using an adaptive linear predictor based QRS detection technique (Fig. 3) [36]. The linear predictor effectively estimates the low frequency components of the ECG signal, including the P, T waves and slow

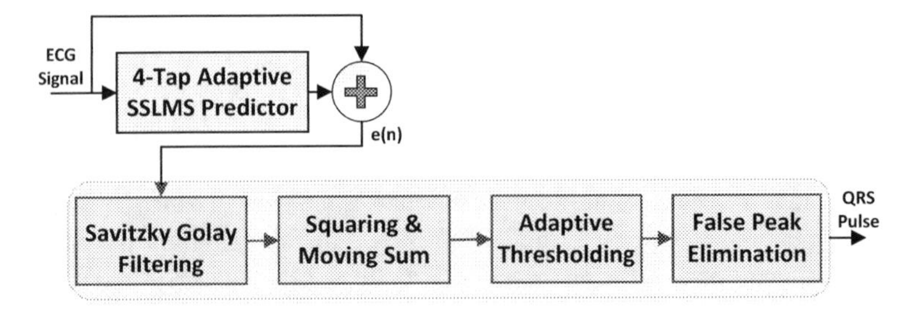

Fig. 3 Block diagram for the R-peak extraction block

varying baseline noises. The prediction error computed therefore contains the high frequency noise components and the QRS segment only. The prediction error is passed through a Savitzky-Golay (SG) [37] filter which will filter out all the high frequency impulse noises, while preserving high order moments which corresponds to the QRS Peaks. The SG filtered signal is further de-noised using a squaring and moving average filter to smoothen and amplify the QRS peaks. Further, an adaptive threshold is used to detect the R-peaks from the smoothened signal. The adaptive threshold used for detection is computed as 25% of average of the past 4 detected peaks. The overall algorithm is simple with low computational complexity and is implemented in real-time and operates on the streaming input on a sample by sample basis. The detection accuracy of the QRS detection scheme was measured using MIT-BIH Arrhythmia database and found to be very high with a sensitivity of 99.64% and positive predictivity of 99.81%. More detail about the implementation and evaluation results can be found at [36].

Ideally the *current beat segment* should start from the onset of P-wave and end at the offset of T-wave. However, detection of the wave onset and offset involves using complex signal processing methods. Therefore, to reduce the complexity of the *current beat segment* extraction we used a heuristic to estimate the maximum left and right boundaries within which the onset and offset of the waves are contained (Fig. 4). Once an R-peak (red circle), the beat segment of the previous R-peak will be extracted as shown in Fig. 4. The boundary estimation is inspired from [38, 39] and is determined as follows.

$$P_{window} = QR_{max} + 0.2 \times RR_{prev} + 0.1$$

$$T_{window} = 1.5 \times QTc_{max} \times \sqrt{RR_{prev}} - QR_{max}$$

Here, $QTc_{max} = 0.42$ corresponds to the maximum value for the QT coefficient in Bazet's formula; and $QR_{max} = 0.08$ is a half of the maximum of QRS duration [33].

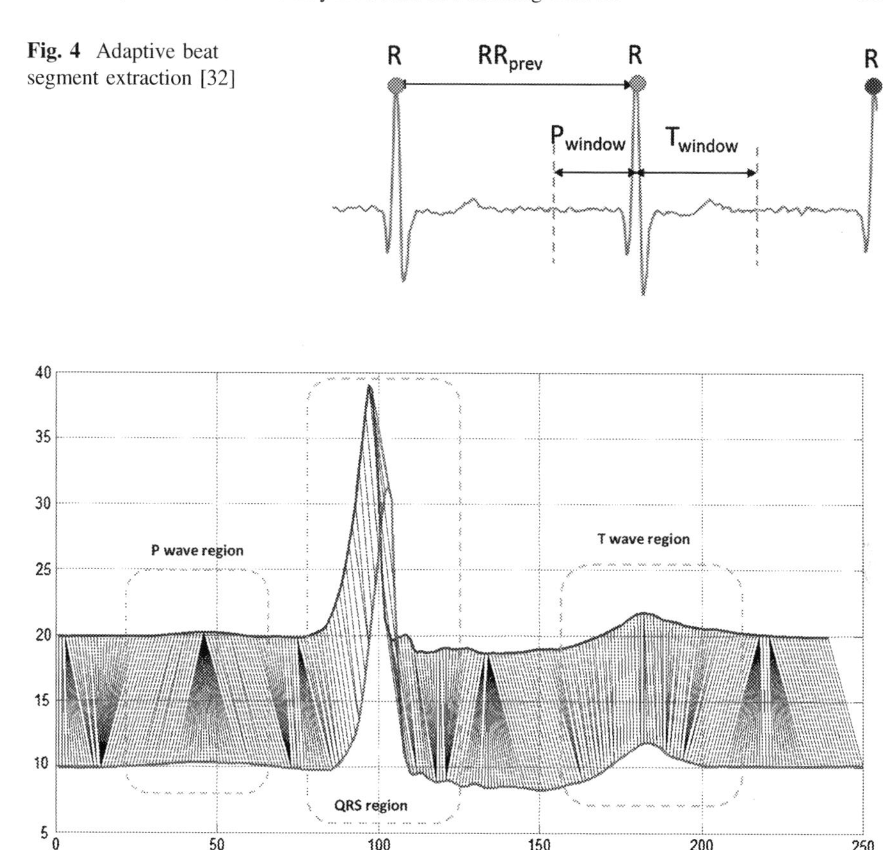

Fig. 4 Adaptive beat segment extraction [32]

Fig. 5 Dynamic time warping (DTW) distance [32]

4.3 Similarity Measure for Beat Segment Comparison

To compare the similarity between beat segments, we propose a modified dynamic time warping (DTW) based similarity measure. DTW is a common algorithm used in time series analysis for measuring similarity between two temporal sequences [40]. It calculates an optimal match between two given sequences (e.g. time series) with certain restrictions. DTW can compare 2 beat segments of different lengths while aligning waveforms and peaks that are significantly similar as shown in Fig. 5. The two ends of the sequences are also involved in the alignment. The computational complexity of DTW operation is minimal and suitable for real-time applications as well.

For each of the extracted *current beat segment*, the beat segment is split into 2 segments w.r.t R-peak, i.e. RP which has length P_{window} and contains left P region, and RT, which has length T_{window} and contains right T region. To compare the corresponding sequences from the two beat segments, we have implemented a fast

DTW algorithm [41] with warping window constraint [42].The measure of similarity between two beat segments s and t is calculated as below.

$$DtwDist(s,t) = DTW(RP_s, RP_t, w) + DTW(RT_s, RT_t, w)$$

Here, the value of warping window is chosen that the P wave and T wave do not overlap the R wave during the DTW alignment. In our experiments, we set $w = 0.1 \times$ Fs where Fs is sampling frequency of the ECG record.

Ideally, a similarity measure should not only be identifying similar beat types but also distinguish them with the other types based on their morphologies. For example, in Fig. 6, the similarity measure has to detect beat 2 and beat 6 are highly similar because they belong to the same type, i.e., normal beat (N). Whereas, they are highly different with beat 344 (V—premature ventricular contraction) and beat 341 (F—fusion of ventricular and normal beat). Using the proposed DTW based similarity measure, the distance between beat 6, beat 344 and beat 341 in comparison with beat 2 are 5.9984e-04, 0.5851 and 0.2281 respectively. It is obvious that our proposed DTW measure finds the two beats number 2 and 6 are highly similar, but clearly different with beats number 344 and 341.

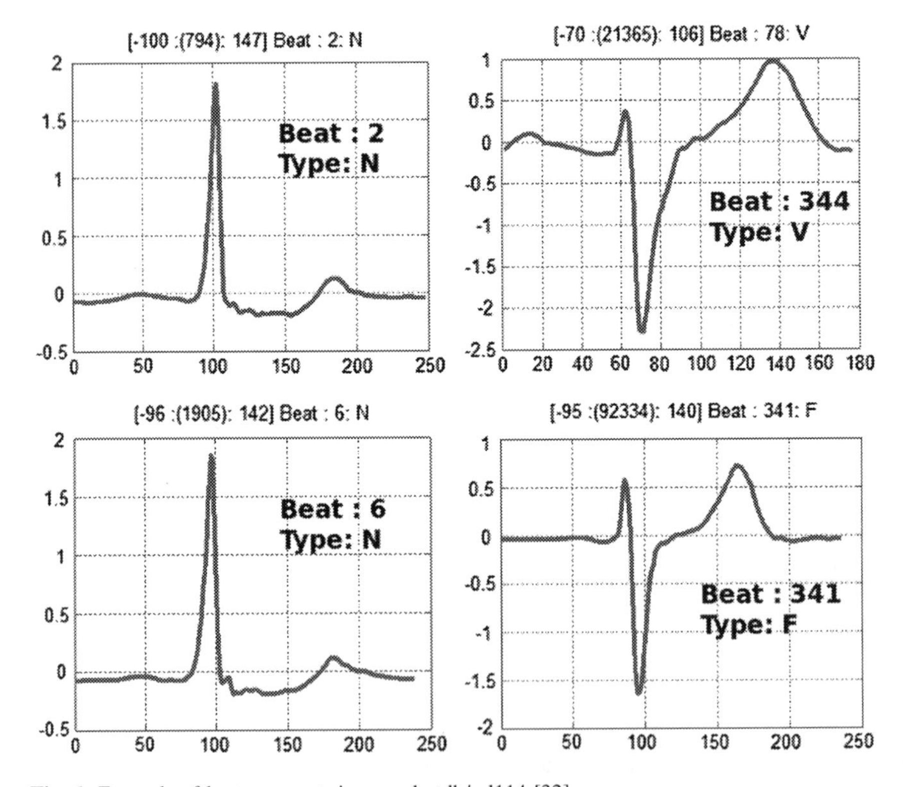

Fig. 6 Example of beat segments in record qtdb/sel114 [32]

4.4 *Extracting* Normal Beat Segment

A *normal beat segment,* which corresponds to the normal status of patient's ECG has to be extracted as a reference for performing anomaly detection. The *normal beat segment* template should be automatically extracted from the individual's ECG stream instead of statistical datasets, as it will vary among different patients. Due to its quasi-periodic property, most anomalous beat patterns are repeated with irregular periodicity. Moreover, a normal beat pattern appears much more frequently than an anomalous beat pattern. Therefore, without the prior knowledge of the data, our heuristic assigns a normal beat status to the one which occurs most frequently from the stream, since abnormalities occur intermittently. This idea is widely adopted in the unsupervised anomaly and outlier detection methods [25, 43] for the real cases.

Algorithm 1: Selection of a normal beat segment

Input: $Seg_{[1:N]}$: list of extracted beat segments
K : number of partitioned clusters
Output: I_{norm} : index of the selected normal beat

// build a feature matrix
1. $V = \{V_{i,j} = DtwDist(Seg_i, Seg_j) \mid i,j \in [1:N]\}$;

// partition by K-mean algorithm
2. $\{Clus\}_{[1:K]} \leftarrow Kmeans(V, K)$;

//get the largest cluster
3. $MaxClus \leftarrow findMaxSize(\{Clus\}_{[1:K]})$;

// internal, external average distances
4. $ID \leftarrow [\, ID_i = avg_{j \in MaxClus} V(i,j) \mid i \in MaxClus]$;
5. $ED \leftarrow [\, ED_i = avg_{j \notin MaxClus} V(i,j) \mid i \in MaxClus]$;

// select an index for normal beat
6. $A \leftarrow [a_i = (ED_i - ID_i) \mid i \in MaxClus]$;
7. $I_{norm} \leftarrow k \mid a_k = \max(A)$;

By adopting this heuristic, clustering analysis techniques have been applied in order to determine the normal beat status. In particular, the beat segments from the first 30 s ECG stream are collected and analyzed by K-means clustering algorithm [44]. The procedure in detail is shown in Algorithm 1. Assume that $Seg_{[1:N]}$ is a list of beat segments extracted from the first 30 s and are statically stored in the main (executable) memory. The K-means clustering algorithm will partition those segments into K clusters. In our approach, we select K = 2 corresponding to normal and abnormal beats. In order to provide input to the K-means algorithm (See line 1), the feature matrix *V* is built by pairwise similarity using *DtwDist* (ref. Sect. 4.3) between segments. In the matrix *V*, each row is a representative feature vector of the corresponding beat segment. After performing partitioning by K-means algorithm on matrix *V*, in line 2, each cluster $Clus_i$ contains a list of indices of beat segments and, in line 3, the largest size cluster *MaxClus* is selected. For each item *i* in the *MaxClus*, we compute the internal (ID_i) and external (ED_i) average distances from the corresponding beat segment to all other beat segments in the same cluster (line 4) and to all beat segments outside (line 5). The normal beat will be the one that has low internal average distance and high external average distance. Therefore, in lines 6 and 7, we select the index of a normal beat segment by finding the maximum difference between the two average distances, i.e., $a_i = ED_i - ID_i$ over all items inside the *MaxClus* cluster. Thereafter only the normal beat segment is stored in the memory and other segments are erased for saving memory space.

4.5 Online Anomaly Detection

Once a *normal beat segment* is identified from patient's incoming ECG data stream, the algorithm starts comparing it with *current beat segments* extracted in real-time to detect the anomalies. Figure 7 shows an example of comparison from Physionet QTDB record sel114, when lead MLII is used. The y-axis shows the value of similarity measure computed in real-time against the *normal beat segment* which was identified to be beat 2 (type N).

It can be observed from the Fig. 7, that the numerical values corresponding to the normal beats (type N) are much smaller than the ones corresponding to other beats (type V and F). A threshold method potentially can distinguish the normal beats and abnormal ones. However, finding an appropriate threshold value is a challenge because the range of values are unknown. Moreover, a fixed threshold value may work for one patient but fails for the others.

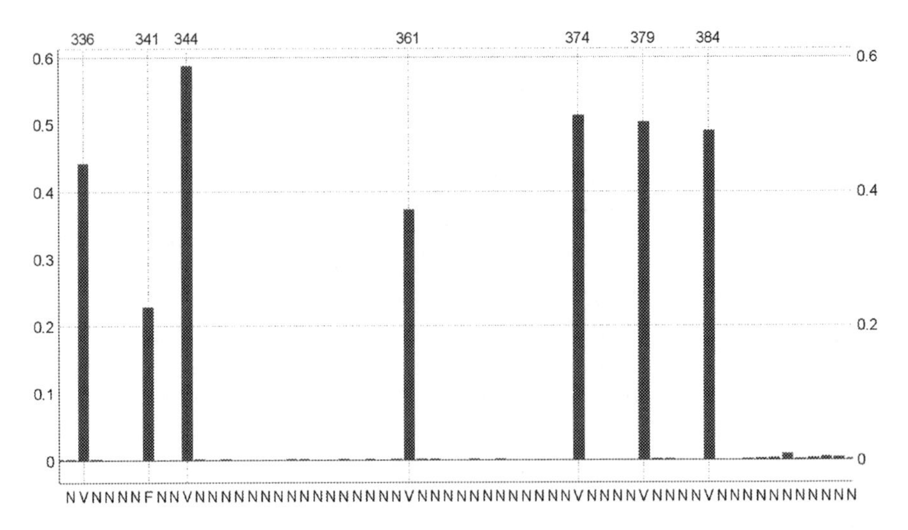

Fig. 7 Transform ECG stream to numerical stream [32]

Actually, the anomaly detection here is indeed a detection of outliers from the uni-variate data set, which can be solved by various methods [43]. Among uni-variate outlier detection methods, Hampel identifier is often found to be practically very robust and effective. Additionally, in term of dynamic data, a dynamic Hampel filter obtained by applying the Hampel identifier on moving windows has been proposed to effectively work with streaming data in different real cases [45]. Based on those advantages, a modification of the dynamic Hampel filter has been implemented in our approach.

Algorithm 2: Real-time anomaly detection

```
Input: X: streaming of numerical values,
       W: haft-width of moving window,
       θ: threshold value for anomaly detection
Output: AnomalyInds: indexes of the detected anomaly

  1.  AnomalyInds ← 0;
// stat. info of anomaly
  2.  N ←0; S ←0; D ←0; lastOutlier ←0;
// index of the incoming value
  3.  i ← 1;
  4.  while true do
// suspected index & sliding window
  5.      I ← i - W; IW ← [I - W: I + W];
// median absolute deviation (MAD)
  6.      X_median ←median (X_k | k ∈ IW);
  7.      DX_median ← 1. 4826 x median (abs(Xk - X_median));
// Hampel condition
  8.      rule1 ←abs(X(I) - X_median) ≥ θ x DX_median;
// 3σ condition
  9.      rule2 ←X(I) ≥ lowerBound(N, S, D, 3);
// anomaly detection
  10.     if rule1 or rule2 then
  11.         AnomalyInds ←AnomalyInds U I;
// update stat. infor.
  12.         N ← N + 1; S ← S + X(I); D ← D + X(I)^2;
  13.         if not rule2 then
  14.             X(I) ← X_median;
  15.             lastOutlier ← X(I);
  16.         else if not rule1 then
  17.             X(I) ←lastOutlier;
  18.         end
  19.     end
  20. end
```

Algorithm 2 summarizes the idea of dynamic Hampel filter as described in [45]. Indeed, for each incoming value X_i from the stream data X, a sliding window X [i −2 W:i] will be inspected for detecting outlier at center value $X(I)| \; I = i - W$ (line 5). On this window, the Hampel breakpoints, i.e., median absolute deviation (MAD), are calculated at lines 6 and 7. Those values are used in the Hampel condition (line 8) to check if the center $X(I)$ is an outlier. If it is as an outlier, value at index *I* will be marked (line 10) and the outlier value *X*(*I*) is removed by assigning a current median value of the window X_{median} (line 14).

Due to the locality property of the dynamic Hampel filter, the filter output can be incorrect when the outliers are continuous and lasting longer than the width of the moving window. For example, assume that the window data showing in ***Window 1*** in the Fig. 8 are [0.2, 0.6, 0.4, 8.2, 8.0, 8.4, 8.6] with the half-width of moving window W = 3, threshold θ = 1 and the inspected value *X*(*I*) = 8.2 at the center. According to median absolute deviation (MAD) computation, we have X_{median} = 8.0, DX_{median} = 0.8896, $X(I) - X_{median}$ = 0.2. Obviously, even with small θ, the Hampel rule fails. Thus, the center point (red circle) is not detected as an outlier and its value is kept the same. Consequently, in the ***Window 2***, outlier will not be detected neither. In order to overcome this problem, we amend a global rule as a compensation to the Hampel local identifier rule. The statistical information pertaining to the previous detected outliers will be used to identify the new incoming outlier. Particularly, at line 9, function *lowerBound* determines the lower bound value of the 3σ limits computed from overall detected outliers. The mean value μ and standard deviation σ can be easily computed through: *N*—number of data items, *S*—sum of all values and *D* sum of square values.

$$\mu = \frac{S}{N}; \ \sigma = \sqrt{\frac{D - \frac{s^2}{N}}{N-1}}$$

$$lowerBound(N, S, D, 3) = \mu - 3\text{x}\sigma$$

The second rule will check if the suspected value *X*(*I*) is higher the lower bound value. If the *X*(*I*) is detected as an outlier, the statistical information is updated (line 12) and *X*(*I*) is replaced by the last updated outlier value (line 17).

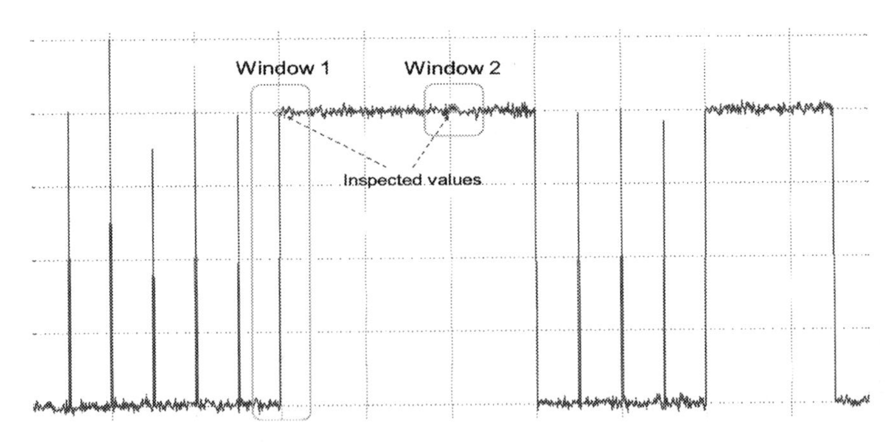

Fig. 8 Weakness of moving Hampel identifier over long continuous outliers [32]

5 Evaluation

The complexity and accuracy of the proposed technique is evaluated in this section. As mentioned in the requirement section, the proposed method can be used for anomaly detection in a single lead ECG signal acquired from wearable sensors. The algorithm doesn't need long training to start functioning as opposed to typical machine learning based approaches. The proposed technique comprises several incremental algorithms that can be used in real-time. In particular, the signal processing algorithm given in Sect. 4.2 handles sample-by-sample in order to detect the R-peak of the heartbeat. Consequently, beat segments can be extracted online from the streaming ECG data. Thereafter each incoming beat segment is transformed into a numerical value, which is then used in the modified Hampel filter to detect anomaly in the current moving window in Sect. 4.5. On the other hand, the identification of *normal beat segment* in Sect. 4.4 is done offline with static data for just first 30 s. It run only once during initialization, and thus it does not impact the real-time monitoring process. In the rest of this section, the computational complexity, memory usage and accuracy performance will be studied.

5.1 Complexity Analysis

The computational complexity and memory usage will be considered for (i) signal processing block for extracting *current beat segment,* (ii) morphology-based similarity measure, (iii) identification of *normal beat segment*, and (iv) online anomaly detection.

In the signal processing block for R-peak detection and *current beat segment* extraction, different filters are used for processing and de-noising the data stream. Assume that the length of filter coefficients is k, then the complexity of convolution operations performing inside filters for each incoming sample data is $O(k)$. The convolution requires an array buffer with size k numeric values. On the other hand, to extract a beat segment, we need a buffer storing 03 consecutive detected R-peaks. This buffer size is around $\frac{3 \times Fs \times 60}{HR} = 750$, where Fs = 250 Hz is sampling frequency of the ECG record; HR $\approx$ 60 bpm is a heart rate value. Therefore, it requires around 1.5 K (bytes) of memory for buffering 750 numeric 2-byes values. For computing similarity between beat segments, the time complexity of the fast DTW algorithm [41] x is $O(N)$, where N is the length of beat segment (around Fs = 250 samples). Additionally, the memory space used to store input and warp path is $2 \times N \approx 500$ 2-byes numeric values ($\approx$1 K bytes). The adaptive setting component requires memory allocation for storing ECG data in the first 30 s (around 30 beat segments), which is around $250 \times 30 = 7500$ samples. It also needs to store the feature matrix of size $30 \times 30 = 900$ cells. The total buffering memory is $(7500 + 900) \times 2 \approx 16$ K. The computational complexity of the K-means algorithm for one dimensional data is $O(IKN)$, where, K is number of clusters, N is number of data items and I is a fixed number of iterations. However, this component runs only one time, so with small N $\approx$ 30, this process can be done fast. Finally, for the online anomaly detection, the algorithm incrementally works with a small moving window of data, i.e., an array of numerical values with length $N = 2\ W$, where W $=$ 5 is set in our approach. Finding median for moving window is done by rolling median filter [46] which yields a linear-time algorithm.

As per the above discussion, the computational and space complexity of our approach is relatively minimal and therefore is suitable for deploying in cloud servers for monitoring several patients at once.

5.2 Accuracy Evaluation

To analyze the accuracy of the proposed technique, we used the physionet QT database (QTDB) [47]. QTDB consists of 15 min ECG records acquired from 105 patients, which were specifically chosen from existing databases, to represent a wide variety of QRS and ST-T morphologies, with reference annotations for arrhythmias. In the MIT-BIH Arrhythmia (15 records) and MIT-BIH Supraventricular Arrhythmia (13 records) groups in QTDB, abnormal heart beats appear in various types with high frequency. The MIT-BIH Normal Sinus Rhythm group (10 records) in QTDB does not contain any abnormality; and in the MIT-BIH Long-Term ECG group (4 records), abnormalities are sparse and intermittent. The MIT-BIH ST Change (6 records) and European ST-T (33 records) groups mainly focus on harmful ventricular arrhythmias. Since in our approach, individual arrhythmias are not identified, the default physionet annotations are converted into AAMI recommended categories as showing in Table 1.

The statistical values, i.e., true positive (TP), false positive (FP), true negative (TN) and false negative (FN) are as defined in Table 2. Here, the detected normal and abnormal beats are identified by our anomaly detection algorithm. Whereas, the annotated normal beats are determined from the gold standard annotation of the ECG record. Once an annotation is determined as a normal beat, the other beat annotation will be assumed as abnormal.

Technically, anomaly detection performance is measured using the standard metrics, i.e., Sensitivity (Se), Specificity (Sp) and Accuracy (Acc) as follows:

Table 1 AAMI recommended beat categories

AAMI categories	Physionet heart beat annotations
N (normal)	N, L, R, e, j
Y (ventricular)	Y, E
S (supraventricular)	A, a, J, S
F (fusion)	F
Q (unclassified)	f, /, Q

Table 2 Definition of statistical values

	Annotated abnormal	Annotated normal
Detected abnormal	TP	FP
Detected normal	FN	TN

Table 3 Detection on arrhythmia group

Sel	Se	Sp	Acc	Sel	Se	Sp	Acc
100	1.0	1.0	1.0	**102**	1.0	1.0	1.0
103	1.0	1.0	1.0	**104**	0.998	0.997	0.999
114	1.0	0.997	0.998	**116**	1.0	0.988	0.989
117	1.0	1.0	1.0	**123**	1.0	1.0	1.0
213	0.972	0.987	0.984	**221**	1.0	1.0	1.0
223	0.973	0.997	0.992	**230**	1.0	0.997	0.997
231	1.0	0.989	0.989	**232**	1.0	0.997	0.997
233	0.990	0.992	0.992				

$$Se(\%) = \frac{TP}{TP + FN} \quad Sp = \frac{TN}{TN + FP} \quad Acc = \frac{TP + TN}{TN + TP + FN + FP}$$

Qualitatively, Sensitivity and Specificity corresponds to the performance of the technique in picking up actual anomalies and skipping the normal beats respectively. Accuracy refers to the detection performance in terms for both normal and abnormal beats.

Table 3 shows the experimental results for each record in the *Arrhythmia* group. The average of Sensitivity, Specificity and Accuracy overall records are 0.995, 0.996 and 0.996 respectively. There are several types of arrhythmia in the ECG signal of these records and the normal beat status is different in different records. For e.g., in record sel100, the normal beat status is a sinus normal heart beat (physionet—N) but in the record sell02 and record se1232, the normal beats status is paced beat (physionet—/) and atrial premature beat (physionet—A). Due to the adaptive *normal beat segment* identification method, the normal beat status is selected accurately for each record, resulting in good detection performance. Record sel213 which contains 1308 normal beats (N) and 332 abnormal beats (V and F) performed the worst, with 9 F beats are un-identified and 17 beats are incorrectly marked as anomalous beat. By manually checking form the signal visualization, we realized that those mis-identified F beats are quite similar to the normal beats because by the definition, it is a fusion of ventricular and normal beat. On the other hand, some of the wrongly detected beats are indeed atrial premature type (physionet—A). This is not a dangerous arrhythmia (that is why it still belongs to AAMI category N), however, it causes the shorter RR-interval, thus makes the morphology of the current beat segment different from the selected normal beat status and this behavior happens the same for the record se1223. The other records do not suffer from this issue, consequently, they obtain high (≈1.0) sensitivity.

The detection performance from the *Supraventricular* group is given in Table 4. The records in this group includes ECG with supraventricular premature or ectopic beats (S type). Although most of S beats are successfully detected, due to the wide variety S-type morphologies involved, a few are not detected and shows up as low sensitivity and specificity for some records. The average of Sensitivity, Specificity and Accuracy are still acceptable at 0.839, 0.981 and 0.979 respectively.

The performance results from the *Normal Sinus Rhythm* and *Long-Term* groups are given in Tables 5 and 6. The proposed method performs well for both these groups. For the *Normal Sinus Rhythm* group, there isn't any anomalous beat in the record and the technique achieves 100% accuracy. For the *Long-Term* group, most abnormalities are V or F types, which are highly different with normal beat N in term of morphology. An average Sensitivity, Specificity and Accuracy of 0.994, 0.999 and 0.999 is achieved respectively for this group.

The performance results of *MIT-BIH ST-change* and *European ST-T* groups are shown in Tables 7 and 8 respectively. The average Sensitivity, Specificity and Accuracy for all records of the both groups are 0.996, 0.997 and 0.997 respectively. Generally, the sensitivity values in most records are 1.0, i.e. all anomalous beats are successfully detected. On the record sele0606, among 6 beats V, the first beat is

Table 4 Detection on supraventricular group

Sel	Se	Sp	Acc	Sel	Se	Sp	Acc
803	1.0	0.997	0.997	**808**	0.75	0.975	0.974
811	1.0	0.987	0.987	**820**	1.0	0.980	0.980
821	0.987	0.964	0.968	**840**	1.0	0.960	0.960
847	0.909	0.986	0.984	**853**	0.75	0.987	0.986
871	0.714	0.941	0.938	**872**	0.783	1.0	0.992
873	0.375	0.998	0.987	**883**	0.773	0.993	0.987
891	0.996	0.987	0.989	–	–	–	–

Table 5 Detection on normal sinus rhythm group

Sel	Se	Sp	Acc	Sel	Se	Sp	Acc
16265	1.0	1.0	1.0	**16272**	1.0	1.0	1.0
16273	1.0	1.0	1.0	**16420**	1.0	1.0	1.0
16483	1.0	1.0	1.0	**16539**	1.0	1.0	1.0
16773	1.0	1.0	1.0	**16786**	1.0	1.0	1.0
16795	1.0	1.0	1.0	**17453**	1.0	1.0	1.0

Table 6 Detection on long-term group

Sel	Se	Sp	Acc	Sel	Se	Sp	Acc
14046	1.0	0.998	0.998	**14157**	1.0	1.0	1.0
14172	1.0	0.998	0.998	**15814**	1.0	1.0	1.0

Table 7 Detection on ST-change group

Sel	Se	Sp	Acc	Sel	Se	Sp	Acc
301	1.0	0.995	0.995	**302**	1.0	0.995	0.995
306	1.0	1.0	1.0	**307**	1.0	1.0	1.0
308	1.0	0.998	0.998	**310**	1.0	0.994	0.994

Table 8 Detection on European ST-T group

Sel	Se	Sp	Acc	Sel	Se	Sp	Acc
e0104	1.0	1.0	1.0	**e0106**	1.0	1.0	1.0
e0107	1.0	0.996	0.996	**e0110**	1.0	0.973	0.973
e0111	1.0	1.0	1.0	**e0112**	1.0	1.0	1.0
e0114	1.0	1.0	1.0	**e0116**	1.0	0.998	0.998
e0121	1.0	1.0	1.0	**e0122**	1.0	0.999	0.999
e0124	1.0	1.0	1.0	**e0126**	1.0	1.0	1.0
e0129	1.0	1.0	1.0	**e0133**	1.0	1.0	1.0
e0136	1.0	1.0	1.0	**e0166**	1.0	0.992	0.992
e0170	1.0	1.0	1.0	**e0203**	1.0	1.0	1.0
e0210	1.0	1.0	1.0	**e0211**	1.0	1.0	1.0
e0303	1.0	1.0	1.0	**e0405**	1.0	1.0	1.0
e0406	1.0	0.997	0.997	**e0409**	1.0	0.993	0.993
e0411	1.0	0.999	0.999	**e0509**	1.0	1.0	1.0
e0603	1.0	1.0	1.0	**e0604**	1.0	1.0	1.0
e0606	0.833	1.0	0.999	**e0607**	1.0	1.0	1.0
e0609	1.0	0.999	0.999	**e0612**	1.0	0.994	0.994
e0704	1.0	0.995	0.995	–	–	–	–

quite similar to the normal beat thus the algorithm fails to identify it. The specificity values are not high as the sensitivity values in some records, since normal beats N have been incorrectly detected as abnormalities. Checking the waveforms in simulation, we realize that in those beats, despite the fact that the ST segment and T wave are significantly different, are still identified as normal beats in the annotations. A typical example is shown in the Fig. 9, in which, both of the beats number 1 and 783 have beat type N. However, we can see that they are very different in term of both P wave (marked by red ovals), ST segment and T wave regions (marked by yellow ovals). This behavior can happen because the high changing range of ST segment deviation and T wave morphology in different normal heart beats [33].

The average values for Sensitivity, Specificity and Accuracy on the whole 105 ECG records in QTDB are 0.971, 0.995 and 0.994 respectively. These high performance results prove the reliability of the proposed approach. Indeed, almost all of the anomalous beats (i.e., V, F and Q categories) are absolutely detected. This success will limit the life threatening risks caused by heart diseases. On the other

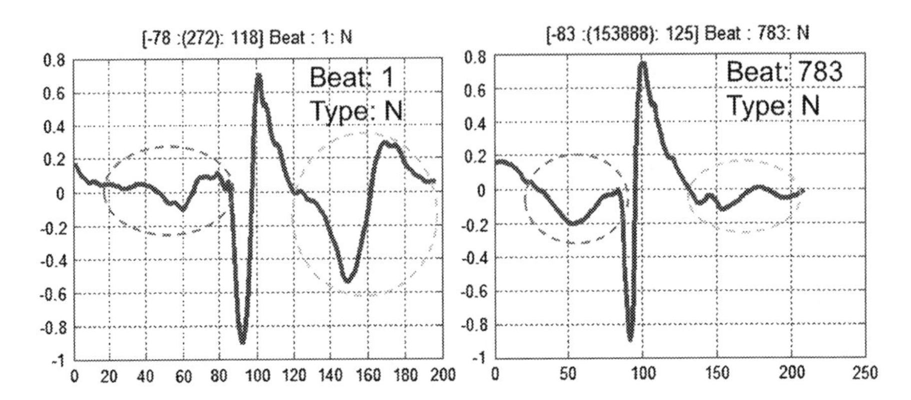

Fig. 9 Differences between beats of the same type [32]

hand, detection of the abnormal heart beats belonging to the S categories is less accurate due to their high similarity to the normal heart beats. However, most of the supra-ventricular (S)\ beats are not dangerous that unable or wrong detection few of them does not cause a serious problem.

6 Conclusions

In this paper, we have proposed a novel ECG anomaly detection technique to be implemented in cloud systems for wearable healthcare monitoring. A low complexity technique with high accuracy, which can work on single lead ECG data and doesn't require personalized calibration for individual users is the fundamental requirement for practical, large scale wearable cardiac monitoring deployments. The proposed technique which works by comparing the beat segments against a normal beat, succeeds in fulfilling all the necessary prerequisites for large scale monitoring. The complexity of the proposed technique is kept under control by using simple SG filtering for signal processing and Discrete time warping for measuring the similarity between two multi-dimensional beat vectors. The ECG stream is converted into a stream of numerical values, which is then monitored by an online anomaly detection method to classify incoming beats to be a normal or abnormal types. To avoid calibration of the technique for individual users, we automatically identified the *normal beat segment* using K-means clustering technique. The performance of the proposed method has been evaluated on publicly available QTDB which consists of a wide variety of ECG Signal morphologies and found to be very high with an average sensitivity and specificity of 0.971 and 0.995 respectively. We demonstrated that complexity of the technique is very modest and therefore the proposed method can be easily deployed in HPC platforms for monitoring of large scale wearable healthcare data.

7 Future Works

The technique proposed in this paper can be improved by using more accurate extraction of the *current beat segment* from the streaming ECG signal. In this paper we used heuristics to estimate the maximum possible limits which would include the P wave in the right side of the R-peak and T wave in the left side of R-peak. However, this can potentially reduce the accuracy of the beat segment limits extracted for comparing the similarity. If we can use a low complexity method, to extract the onset and offset of P wave and T wave respectively, then the beat segments extracted are more accurate representation of the signal segment that needs to be compared. We propose to use a wavelet based ECG delineator for this purpose. The added complexity can be mitigated by using the wavelet delineator for R-peak extraction along with P, T wave onset/offset extraction and replacing the current linear predictor based R-peak extractor. We propose the usage of Haar based ECG delineator which proven to have lower complexity [48].

The proposed technique currently can be augmented by a ECG classifier so that the exact arrhythmia can be detected. A plethora of methods currently exists for ECG classification, with lower detection accuracies. The proposed method when used in combination with existing classification methods can help to (1) improve the detection/classification accuracy, and (2) distribute the processing load of anomaly detection and classification on different elements in the wearable healthcare system.

Acknowledgements The authors would like to thank the funding support from National Research Foundation (NRF), under the project entitled, "*Self-powered body sensor network for disease management and prevention oriented healthcare*", (NRF) CRP-8-2011-01 grant.

References

1. "World Health Statistics 2013," *World Health Organisation.*
2. "Heart Disease Facts," *Centres Dis. Control Prev.*, no. http://www.cdc.gov/heartdisease/facts.htm, 2015.
3. C. J. Deepu, X. Zhang, W.-S. Liew, D. L. T. Wong, and Y. Lian, "Live demonstration: An ECG-on-Chip for wearable wireless sensors," in *2014 IEEE Asia Pacific Conference on Circuits and Systems (APCCAS)*, 2014, vol. 4, pp. 177–178.
4. C. J. Deepu, X. Zhang, W.-S. Liew, D. L. T. Wong, and Y. Lian, "An ECG-on-Chip With 535 nW/Channel Integrated Lossless Data Compressor for Wireless Sensors," *IEEE J. Solid-State Circuits*, vol. 49, no. 11, pp. 2435–2448, 2014.
5. C. J. Deepu, X. Xu, X. Zou, L. Yao, and Y. Lian, "An ECG-on-Chip for Wearable Cardiac Monitoring Devices," *2010 Fifth IEEE Int. Symp. Electron. Des. Test Appl.*, pp. 225–228, 2010.
6. D. R. Zhang, C. J. Deepu, X. Y. Xu, and Y. Lian, "A wireless ecg plaster for real-time cardiac health monitoring in body sensor networks," in *2011 IEEE Biomedical Circuits and Systems Conference (BioCAS)*, 2011, pp. 205–208.

7. C. J. Deepu, Z. Xiaoyang, C. Heng, and L. Yong, "A 3-lead ECG-on-Chip with QRS Detection & Lossless Compression for Wireless Sensors," *IEEE Transactions on Circuits and Systems II: Express Briefs*, vol. PP, no. 99. p. 1, 2016.
8. C. J. Deepu, C. H. Heng, and Y. Lian, "A Hybrid Data Compression Scheme for Power Reduction in Wireless Sensors for IoT," *IEEE Transactions on Biomedical Circuits and Systems*, vol. PP, no. 99. pp. 1–10, 2016.
9. P. A. Wolf, R. D. Abbott, and W. B. Kannel, "Atrial fibrillation as an independent risk factor for stroke: the Framingham Study," *Stroke,* vol. 22, no. 8, pp. 983–988, Aug. 1991.
10. R. L. Page, W. E. Wilkinson, W. K. Clair, E. A. McCarthy, and E. L. Pritchett, "Asymptomatic arrhythmias in patients with symptomatic paroxysmal atrial fibrillation and paroxysmal supraventricular tachycardia," *Circulation*, vol. 89, no. 1, p. 224 LP-227, Jan. 1994.
11. A. M. Bensaid, N. Bouhouch, R. Bouhouch, R. Fellat, and R. Amri, "Classification of ECG patterns using fuzzy rules derived from ID3-induced decision trees," *Fuzzy Information Processing Society - NAFIPS, 1998 Conference of the North American*. pp. 34–38, 1998.
12. A. Kampouraki, G. Manis, and C. Nikou, "Heartbeat Time Series Classification With Support Vector Machines," *IEEE Transactions on Information Technology in Biomedicine*, vol. 13, no. 4. pp. 512–518, 2009.
13. T.-F. Yang, B. Devine, and P. W. Macfarlane, "Artificial neural networks for the diagnosis of atrial fibrillation," *Med. Biol. Eng. Comput.*, vol. 32, no. 6, pp. 615–619, 1994.
14. P. W. Macfarlane, B. Devine, and E. Clark, "The university of glasgow (Uni-G) ECG analysis program," *Computers in Cardiology, 2005*. pp. 451–454, 2005.
15. D. Ngo and B. Veeravalli, "Applied semantic technologies in ECG interpretation and cardiovascular diagnosis," *Bioinformatics and Biomedicine (BIBM), 2014 IEEE International Conference on*. pp. 17–24, 2014.
16. A. R. Houghton and D. Gray, *Making Sense of ECG*. 2007.
17. J. P. Martinez, R. Almeida, S. Olmos, a P. Rocha, and P. Laguna, "A wavelet-based ECG delineator: evaluation on standard databases," *Biomed. Eng. IEEE Trans.*, vol. 51, no. 4, pp. 570–581, 2004.
18. B. Weng, M. Blanco-Velasco, and K. E. Barner, "ECG Denoising Based on the Empirical Mode Decomposition," in *2006 International Conference of the IEEE Engineering in Medicine and Biology Society*, 2006, pp. 1–4.
19. P. de Chazal, M. O'Dwyer, and R. B. Reilly, "Automatic classification of heartbeats using ECG morphology and heartbeat interval features," *IEEE Transactions on Biomedical Engineering*, vol. 51, no. 7. pp. 1196–1206, 2004.
20. J. Rodríguez, A. Goñi, and A. Illarramendi, "Real-time classification of ECGs on a PDA," *IEEE Trans. Inf. Technol. Biomed.*, vol. 9, no. 1, pp. 23–34, 2005.
21. M. Javadi, R. Ebrahimpour, A. Sajedin, S. Faridi, and S. Zakernejad, "Improving ECG Classification Accuracy Using an Ensemble of Neural Network Modules," *PLoS One*, vol. 6, no. 10, p. e24386, Oct. 2011.
22. J. Macek, "Incremental learning of ensemble classifiers on ECG data," *18th IEEE Symposium on Computer-Based Medical Systems (CBMS'05)*. pp. 315–320, 2005.
23. Y. H. Hu, S. Palreddy, and W. J. Tompkins, "A patient-adaptable ECG beat classifier using a mixture of experts approach," *IEEE Transactions on Biomedical Engineering*, vol. 44, no. 9. pp. 891–900, 1997.
24. C.. Aggarwal, *Outlier Analysis*. Springer Publishing Company, 2013.
25. V. Chandola, A. Banerjee, and V. Kumar, "Anomaly Detection: A Survey," *ACM Comput. Surv.*, vol. 41, no. 3, p. 15:1–15:58, Jul. 2009.
26. J. Lin, E. Keogh, L. Wei, and S. Lonardi, "Experiencing SAX: a novel symbolic representation of time series," *Data Min. Knowl. Discov.*, vol. 15, no. 2, pp. 107–144, 2007.
27. J. Lin, E. Keogh, S. Lonardi, and B. Chiu, "A Symbolic Representation of Time Series, with Implications for Streaming Algorithms," in *Proceedings of the 8th ACM SIGMOD Workshop on Research Issues in Data Mining and Knowledge Discovery*, 2003, pp. 2–11.

28. K. Chakrabarti, E. Keogh, S. Mehrotra, and M. Pazzani, "Locally Adaptive Dimensionality Reduction for Indexing Large Time Series Databases," *ACM Trans. Database Syst.*, vol. 27, no. 2, pp. 188–228, Jun. 2002.
29. M. C. Chuah and F. Fu, "ECG Anomaly Detection via Time Series Analysis," in *Frontiers of High Performance Computing and Networking ISPA 2007 Workshops: ISPA 2007 International Workshops SSDSN, UPWN, WISH, SGC, ParDMCom, HiPCoMB, and IST-AWSN Niagara Falls, Canada, August 28-September 1, 2007 Proceedings*, P. Thulasiraman, X. He, T. L. Xu, M. K. Denko, R. K. Thulasiram, and L. T. Yang, Eds. Berlin, Heidelberg: Springer Berlin Heidelberg, 2007, pp. 123–135.
30. H. Sivaraks and C. A. Ratanamahatana, "Robust and Accurate Anomaly Detection in ECG Artifacts Using Time Series Motif Discovery," *Computational and Mathematical Methods in Medicine*, vol. 2015. 2015.
31. M. G. Tsipouras, D. I. Fotiadis, and D. Sideris, "Arrhythmia classification using the RR-interval duration signal," *Comput. Cardiol.*, pp. 485–488, 2002.
32. D. Ngo and B. Veeravalli, "Design of a real-time morphology-based anomaly detection method from ECG streams," *Bioinformatics and Biomedicine (BIBM), 2015 IEEE International Conference on*. pp. 829–836, 2015.
33. G. Tomas B and H. Neil E, *12-Lead ECG The Art of Interpretation.* Jonesand Bartlett Publishers, 2001.
34. N. Boichat, N. Khaled, F. Rinconz, and D. Atienza, "Wavelet-based ECG delineation on a wearable embedded sensor platform," in *Proceedings - 2009 6th International Workshop on Wearable and Implantable Body Sensor Networks, BSN 2009*, 2009, pp. 256–261.
35. J. P. Martinez, R. Almeida, S. Olmos, A. P. Rocha, and P. Laguna, "A wavelet-based ECG delineator: evaluation on standard databases," *IEEE Transactions on Biomedical Engineering*, vol. 51, no. 4. pp. 570–581, 2004.
36. C. J. Deepu and Y. Lian, "A Joint QRS Detection and Data Compression Scheme for Wearable Sensors," *IEEE Trans. Biomed. Eng.*, vol. 62, no. 1, pp. 165–175, 2015.
37. R. W. Schafer, "What Is a Savitzky-Golay Filter?," *Signal Processing Magazine, IEEE*, vol. 28, no. 4. pp. 111–117, 2011.
38. N. Boichat, N. Khaled, F. Rinconz, and D. Atienza, "Wavelet-based ECG delineation on a wearable embedded sensor platform," *Proc. - 2009 6th Int. Work. Wearable Implant. Body Sens. Networks, BSN 2009*, pp. 256–261, 2009.
39. L. Johannesen, U. Grove, J. Sorensen, M. Schmidt, J.-P. Couderc, and C. Graff, "A wavelet-based algorithm for delineation and classification of wave patterns in continuous Holter ECG recordings," *2010 Comput. Cardiol.*, pp. 979–982, 2010.
40. "Dynamic Time Warping," in *Information Retrieval for Music and Motion*, Berlin, Heidelberg: Springer Berlin Heidelberg, 2007, pp. 69–84.
41. S. Salvador and P. Chan, "Toward Accurate Dynamic Time Warping in Linear Time and Space," *Intell. Data Anal.*, vol. 11, no. 5, pp. 561–580, Oct. 2007.
42. H. Sakoe and S. Chiba, "A dynamic programming approach to continuous speech recognition," 1971, pp. 65–69.
43. V. J. Hodge and J. Austin, "A Survey of Outlier Detection Methodologies," *Artif. Intell. Rev.*, vol. 22, no. 2, pp. 85–126, 2004.
44. J. A. Hartigan, *Clustering Algorithms*, 99th ed. New York, NY, USA: John Wiley & amp; Sons, Inc., 1975.
45. R. K. Pearson, "Outliers in process modeling and identification," *IEEE Transactions on Control Systems Technology*, vol. 10, no. 1. pp. 55–63, 2002.
46. J. T. Astola and T. G. Campbell, "On computation of the running median," *IEEE Transactions on Acoustics, Speech, and Signal Processing*, vol. 37, no. 4. pp. 572–574, 1989.

47. P. Laguna, R. G. Mark, A. Goldberg, and G. B. Moody, "A database for evaluation of algorithms for measurement of QT and other waveform intervals in the ECG," *Comput. Cardiol. 1997*, vol. 24, pp. 673–676, 1997.
48. E. B. Mazomenos, D. Biswas, A. Acharyya, T. Chen, K. Maharatna, J. Rosengarten, J. Morgan, and N. Curzen, "A low-complexity ECG feature extraction algorithm for mobile healthcare applications.," *IEEE J. Biomed. Heal. informatics*, vol. 17, no. 2, pp. 459–69, Mar. 2013.

Activity Recognition Based on Pattern Recognition of Myoelectric Signals for Rehabilitation

Oluwarotimi Williams Samuel, Peng Fang, Shixiong Chen, Yanjuan Geng and Guanglin Li

Abstract Limb-amputation, stroke, trauma, and some other congenital anomalies not only decrease patients' quality of life but also cause severe psychological burdens to them. Several advanced rehabilitation technologies have been developed to help patients with limb disabilities restore their lost motor functions. As a kind of neural signal, surface electromyogram (sEMG) recorded on limb muscles usually contain rich information associated with limb motions. By decoding the sEMG with pattern recognition techniques, the motion intents can be effectively identified and used for the control of rehabilitation devices. In this chapter, the control of upper-limb prostheses and rehabilitation robots based on the pattern recognition of sEMG signals was detailedly introduced and discussed. In addition, the clinical feasibility of sEMG-based pattern recognition technique towards an improved function restoration for upper-limb amputees and stroke survivors is also described.

O.W. Samuel · P. Fang · S. Chen · Y. Geng · G. Li
Chinese Academy of Sciences (CAS), Key Laboratory of Human-Machine Intelligence-Synergy Systems, Shenzhen Institutes of Advanced Technology (SIAT), Shenzhen 518055, China
e-mail: samuel@siat.ac.cn

P. Fang
e-mail: peng.fang@siat.ac.cn

S. Chen
e-mail: sx.chen@siat.ac.cn

Y. Geng
e-mail: yj.geng@siat.ac.cn

O.W. Samuel · P. Fang · S. Chen · Y. Geng · G. Li
The Institute of Biomedical and Health Engineering, SIAT, Shenzhen 518055, China

O.W. Samuel · P. Fang · S. Chen · G. Li
Shenzhen College of Advanced Technology, University of Chinese Academy of Sciences, Shenzhen 518055, China

G. Li (✉)
1068 Xueyuan Avenue, University Town, Nanshan, Shenzhen 518055, China
e-mail: gl.li@siat.ac.cn

© Springer International Publishing AG 2017

S.U. Khan et al. (eds.), *Handbook of Large-Scale Distributed Computing in Smart Healthcare*, Scalable Computing and Communications,
DOI 10.1007/978-3-319-58280-1_16

Keywords Myoelectric signal • Pattern recognition • Limb motion • Upper-limb amputee • Stroke survivor • Prosthesis • Rehabilitation robot • Distributed computing

1 Introduction

Individuals with upper-limb disabilities from amputations or strokes are often found all around the world. For instance, over 1 million persons in the USA were reported to be leaving with limb amputations, and about 10% of them suffer from different forms of upper-limb amputations [39]. Report from a previous study indicated that approximately 15 million people suffer from stroke-related diseases yearly in the world, among which one third are permanently disabled [48]. Meanwhile, stroke was reported as the principal cause of adult disability with an annual incidence of about 152,000 patients in the UK [34]. Hence, both limb amputation and stroke would lead to a decreased quality of life, because such patients have lost their upper-limb motion functions [1], and as well an important communication tool needed in daily life.

Over the years, different types of prostheses have been developed to restore the limb functions of amputees. As categorized in Table 1, there are different levels of upper-limb amputations. Usually, prostheses are specifically designed for each individual by considering the length of residual limb, limb activity level, limb prognosis, employment status, as well as the individual's specific needs for assistance. In addition, developing prostheses for individuals with high-level amputations such as FQ or SD would require more efforts than that for those with low-level amputations like PH or FA (Fig. 1).

The body-powered prostheses were firstly introduced as an alternative to lost limbs to aid amputees in performing some simple tasks [35]. However, the body-powered prostheses could only provide support for motions with single degree of freedom (DOF) and are counter-intuitive. In addition, they require a significant amount of energy to perform a simple motion, which would cause strong burdens to amputees and impede their use for a long period of time. Later, motorized prostheses that are controlled based on the amplitude and rate of change of surface electromyogram (sEMG) signals were invented [30]. This type of

Table 1 Levels of upper-limb amputation

S/N	Amputation categorization	
1	Forequarter (FQ)	Transhumeral (AE)
2	Shoulder disarticulation (SD)	
3	Elbow disarticulation (ED)	
4	Wrist disarticulation (WD)	Transradial (BE)
5	Partial hand (PH)	
6	Finger amputation (FA)	

[a]AE and BE represent *above elbow* and *below elbow*, respectively

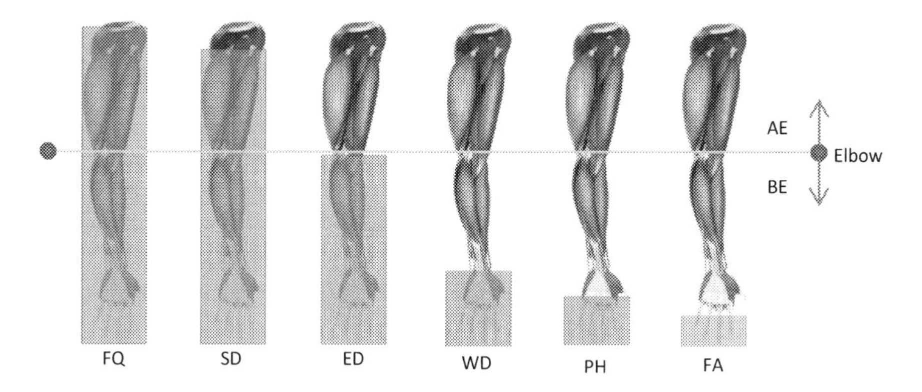

Fig. 1 Illustration of upper-limb amputation of different levels

Table 2 Levels of impairment by stroke

S/N	Stroke severity	Score
1	No stroke symptoms	0
2	Minor stroke	1–4
3	Moderate stroke	5–15
4	Moderate to severe stroke	16–20
5	Severe stroke	21–42

prostheses could decrease the body burden for amputees to a certain extent, but still provide a control of single DOF due to insufficient residual muscles for signal generation. Although the concept of mode switching among different joints has been proposed to realize the control of additional DOFs [14], but the switching itself would lead to a cognitive burden to the users and reduce the control performance of the prosthetic systems.

Besides prosthetic limbs, a number of therapeutic rehabilitation robots have been developed to facilitate the recovery of motor disorders for stroke survivors. The different levels of impairment caused by strokes have been objectively quantified by the National Institutes of Health Stroke Scale (NIHSS), as presented in Table 2 [46].

In like manner with the amputation levels described above, stroke patients with high-level severity would need to recover from a number of motor function disorders while those with low-level severity only require less motor function restoration.

Generally, the end-effectors and exoskeletons are two types of robots that have proven to be effective compliments to the conventional physiotherapy approach for limb motor function restoration in stroke patients [7]. Robot-aided rehabilitation devices such as the MIT-MANUS robot [11, 23] and the MINE robot [32, 33] among other mechatronic robots have been developed. These devices often assist patients to perform exercises which involve repetitive movement of their paretic limbs in a passive or active manner [9, 24, 25]. Examples of the rehabilitation devices that could help restore the limb functions for stroke survivors are shown in Fig. 2.

Generally, most functional tasks are accomplished through a complex temporal and spatial coordination of multiple muscles. It is therefore difficult to realize a control of multiple DOFs via the one-to-one mapping principle adopted by the above described mechatronic robot-aided rehabilitation devices. In addition, such mechatronic devices cannot support volitional control which would be very important for the motor function recovery.

Pattern recognition (PR) technique was proposed several years ago as a potential method for the control of rehabilitation devices such as the prostheses [18, 22]. A number of recent studies [1, 6, 17, 27, 31, 41, 48] suggested that PR of myoelectric signals might potentially facilitate the development of an efficient rehabilitation device that could help restore upper-limb function for amputees and stroke survivors. The remaining part of the chapter is structured as follow: in Sect. 2, a detailed description of pattern recognition technique for upper-limb motion intents decoding, Sect. 3 discusses the potential of large-scale distributed processing as applied to myoelectric signals, Sect. 4 discusses the clinical feasibility of myoelectric pattern-recognition, while Sect. 5 concludes the chapters.

2 Pattern-Recognition Technique for Rehabilitation

In the control of rehabilitation devices like the prostheses and assistive robot, the PR technique is considered as a promising alternative to the conventional amplitude-based method. The PR-based control is grounded on the assumption that the patterns of sEMG signals regarding the intended limb motions are consistent

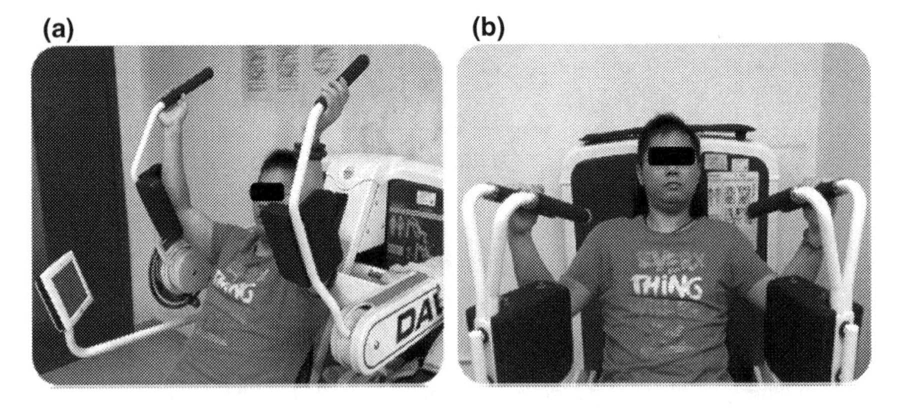

Fig. 2 Therapeutic devices for the restoration of upper-limb and backside functions. **a** David F400 Pullover for the restoration of latissius dorsi, teres major, and trapezius muscle. **b** David F450 Rowing Torso/Pec Deck for the restoration of targeted muscles (pectoralis major, pectoralis minor, serratus anterior, and deltoideus posterior)

and repeatable over time. Also, each limb motion is characterized by a series of consistent muscle activations that can be described by a set of features, and the features should be reproducible across trials for the same limb motion and discriminative between different ones [15]. The PR technique primarily provides a more intuitive mapping of physiologically appropriate muscle contractions to the corresponding prosthetic movements. Also, it requires less specific electrode placement compared to the conventional myoelectric control methods. The PR technique easily adapts to changing conditions, and thus users could wear the prosthesis and calibrate the arm to recognize the current location of multiple myoelectric signals [45].

The development of rehabilitation devices based on PR technique to restore limb functions of patients could be generally divided into two stages. Firstly, the limb motion intents of the patients are decoded from a set of acquired myoelectric signals. In the second stage, the output of the first stage (the decoded limb motion intents) is used as a command to control a motorized assistive device such as prosthesis, an exoskeleton, or other forms of rehabilitation robots. The next section in this chapter shall focus more on the first stage which involves the decoding of various upper-limb motions from a set of acquired myoelectric signals based on PR method. This stage fundamentally consist of recording myoelectric signals from the disabled limb, preprocessing the myoelectric signal, segmentation of the preprocessed signals, extraction of features from the segmented data, and decoding of the limb motion intents. These processes are described sequentially as follows. Additionally, the PR-based control strategies for rehabilitation devices are introduced.

2.1 *Myoelectric Signal Acquisition*

Myoelectric signals are recorded during muscle contractions either invasively with needles or wires inserted into muscles or non-invasively with electrodes placed on the skin surface overlying the muscles. The intramuscular recordings have the ability to maintain robust electrode contact with the muscle and could acquire signals from deep muscles with little or no crosstalk. For several years, the intramuscular recordings have not been clinically feasible because it requires the use of percutaneous wire/needle electrodes for signal transmission [44]. On the other hand, the non-invasive method has been widely adopted in both research and clinical applications due to their relative ease of acquisition. The non-invasive collection of myoelectric signals often requires the placement of a certain number of electrodes on the skin surface as shown in Fig. 3a, b. It is important to note that before electrode placement, the skin needs to be properly cleaned with alcohol swabs to guarantee good electrode-skin contact, which would minimize the impedance and improve the signal quality [16, 20]. The sEMG electrodes are usually placed at some selected positions experientially. Muscle crosstalk, an important factor that

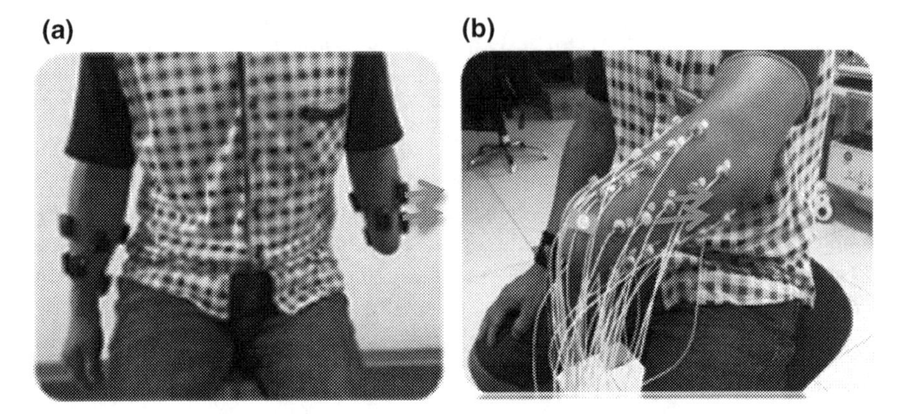

Fig. 3 sEMG electrode placement on patient's residual limb, **a** Wireless sEMG electrodes, **b** Wired sEMG electrodes

affects the quality of sEMG recordings, could be minimized by choosing an appropriate electrode conductive area as well as the inter-electrode distance during electrode placement. Decreasing the size of conductive area on the skin leads to a reduction in effective sEMG measurement, and decreasing the inter-electrode distance usually shifts the sEMG bandwidth to higher frequencies [26].

After a successful electrode placement, participants are often instructed based on the experimental design to elicit a number of upper-limb motions for a specific period of time based on either an audio or video prompt. Then, sEMG signals from muscle contractions corresponding to the intended limb motions are recorded by the electrodes and stored for further analysis in offline scenarios.

2.2 *Myoelectric Signal Preprocessing*

The recorded sEMG signals are usually sampled at a frequency range of between 1000 and 2500 Hz depending on the objective of the experiment. Power line interference should be firstly attenuated from the sEMG recordings by using a 50–60 Hz notch filter. In addition, a band-pass filter with certain range of cutoff frequency is adopted to improve the signal quality. The low frequency cutoff of the band-pass filter is designed to eliminate baseline drift that is sometimes associated with movement, perspiration, as well as any direct current offset, and typical values of the low frequency cutoff range between 5 and 20 Hz. The high frequency cutoff of the band-pass filter basically removes high frequency noise and prevents aliasing in the sampled sEMG signals. This frequency should be quite high so that rapid on-off bursts of the sEMG signals could still be clearly identified. In practice, values for the high frequency cutoff usually range between 200 and 1000 Hz.

2.3 Data Segmentation

The preprocessed signals are segmented into a series of analysis windows with a window length raging between 150 and 250 ms [15, 31, 41, 43] and an increment of about 100–150 ms. and usually with an overlap of about 50–100 ms [28, 29] (Fig. 4). The fundamental trade-off in selecting the window length is that longer windows will improve the stability of features by reducing the variance and increasing the classification performance, but may result in a longer delay in the motion classification decision [42].

The concept of overlapping the analysis window is often adopted to maximally utilize the continuous stream of data that could produce an acceptable decision stream as fast as possible with regards to the available computing capacity [43]. For overlapping analysis windows, the operational delay in real-time control due to data buffering would simply be the duration of the overlapping window instead of the window length [30]. Therefore, an operational delay (T) between 50 and 100 ms in real-time use may be considered.

2.4 Feature Extraction

After segmenting the preprocessed sEMG data into a series of analysis windows, a set of features characterized by rich neural information that could aid the decoding

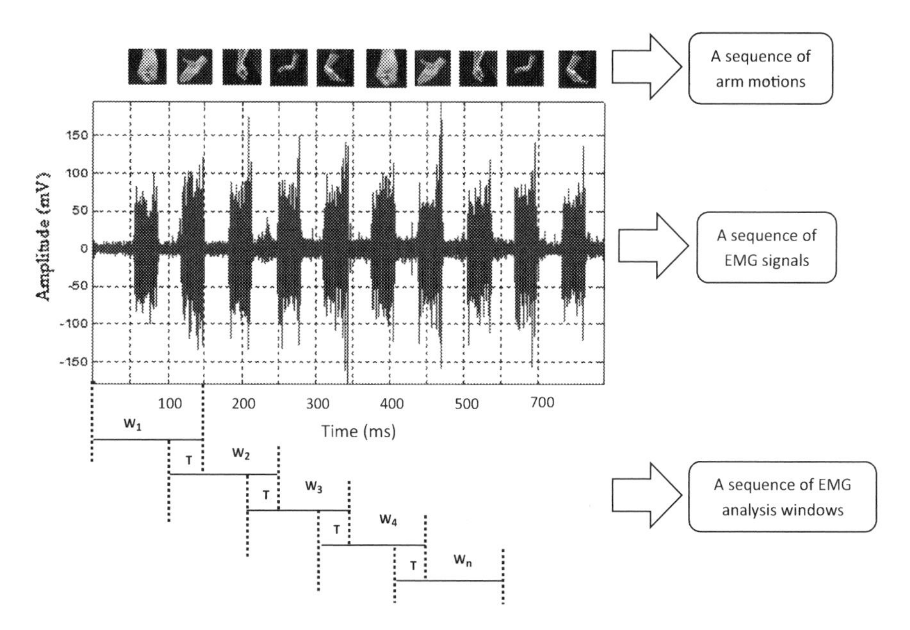

Fig. 4 Segmentation of sEMG data based on the "sliding windows" technique. $\mathbf{W_1}$ to $\mathbf{W_n}$ represent the analysis windows and **T** is the delay between any two consecutive windows

of different upper limb motion intents are often extracted from each analysis window. A proper extraction of signal features from the preprocessed sEMG data would eventually lead to a high performance in terms of motion classification. In several previous studies, features from time, frequency, and time-frequency domains have been proposed for limb motion classification [38]. Four time-domain features shown in Table 3 were widely adopted in myoelectric signal classification because of their relative ease of computation and good performance. Then, the desired feature sets are extracted and projected into a matrix of feature vector that contains the coefficients of the features.

2.5 *Motion Recognition*

The classification of limb motion intents of patients from extracted feature sets constitutes an integral part of myoelectric PR based method since the classifier's output directly serve as the control commands for rehabilitation devices. Due to the nature of myoelectric signals, it is sometimes reasonable to expect a large variation in the value of a particular feature between individuals. Instances of this kind could be observed in situations where the muscle structure is disrupted as a result of

Table 3 Conventionally used time-domain features

S/N	Commonly used time domain features	Description
1	$\mathrm{MAV} = \frac{1}{k}\sum_{n=1}^{k} \lvert x_n \rvert$	**Mean Absolute Value** is an average of the absolute value of the EMG signal amplitude per time
2	$\mathrm{WL} = \sum_{n=1}^{k-1} \lvert (x_{n+1} - x_n) \rvert$	**Waveform Length** (WL) gives a measure of the complexity of the EMG signal in each analysis window
3	$\mathrm{NZC} = \sum_{n=1}^{k-1} [\mathrm{sgn}(x_n * x_{n+1}) \cap (x_n - x_{n+1}) \geq \mathrm{Thres}]$	**Number of Zero Crossings** (ZC) is the number of times that the signal (x_n) crosses the zero point within an analysis window and it has been reported to have association with the frequency of the signal
4	$\mathrm{SSC} = \sum_{n=2}^{k-1} [f(x_n - x_{n-1}) * (x_n - x_{n+1})]$	**Slope Sign Changes** (SSC) is related to the signal frequency and is defined as the number of times that the slope of the EMG waveform changes sign within an analysis window

amputation or congenital defect [22]. Also, factors such as electrode shift, variation in muscle contraction level, change in limb position, and body-weight fluctuation may lead to changes in the feature values over time. Considering all these factors, choosing an efficient classifier becomes necessary to ensure accurate and consistent classification performance. In line with this, several machine learning and statistical classifiers have been examined with respect to their classification performance in the identification of different upper-limb motions. For instance, classifiers based on Bayesian Statistical Method [21], Adaptive Neural Networks [22], Fuzzy Logic [3], Support Vector Machine [38], and Linear Discriminant Analysis [19, 28, 31] have been investigated. Among those classifiers, the Liner Discriminant Analysis classifier has been considered as the most prominent candidate because it was reported to be relatively less complex in terms of implementation but still with good performance compared to some existing complex classification scheme [19].

The decided classifier is built and trained with a portion of the extracted feature sets. Subsequently, the trained classifier is tested with the remaining portion of the feature vector to determine the classification performance in identifying the different limb motion intents. The control performance of a myoelectric PR-based method is assessed in both real-time and off-line scenarios by using a number of standard metrics. Evaluation metrics such as classification accuracy across different limb motions, motion completion rate, motion completion time, and motion selection time are some common metrics.

2.6 Device Control

Currently, there are two types of PR control methods for prostheses and robots namely the "sequential PR" and "simultaneous PR" method. Figure 5 shows the two methods together with the conventional one, which depends on signal amplitude and rate of change. Take a 2-DOF upper-limb prosthesis as example, which contains four active motions of hand-open (HO), hand-close (HC), elbow-flexion (EF), and elbow-extension (EE). The conventional control scheme (A) requires two different decision nodes, and each consisting of two channels to determine a motion output based on the amplitude of recorded sEMG signals. In the "sequential PR" control method (B), sEMG recordings from more than two channels often serve as a single input that is used to determine any of the four discrete motion classes or no movement. Meanwhile, the "simultaneous PR" control method (C) also receives its input from more than two sEMG channels and outputs any of the four discrete motions or no movement. In addition, the simultaneous PR method could provide output for any combination of elbow and hand movements [47].

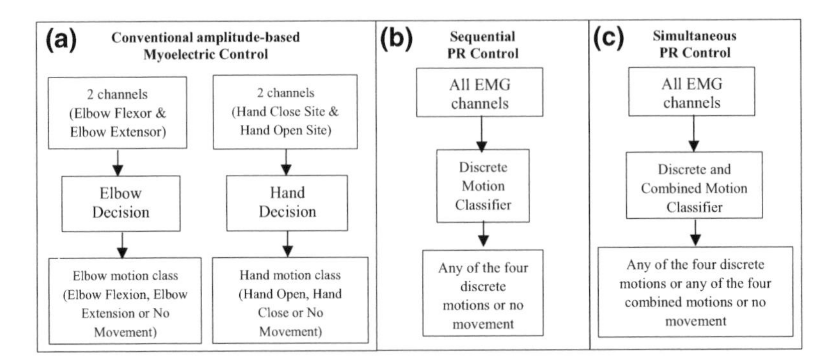

Fig. 5 A block diagram of different myoelectric control strategies

3 Clinical Feasibility of Pattern Recognition Technique for Rehabilitation

The myoelectric PR approach for prosthesis and assistive robot control was hypothesized several decades ago as a prospective method that would revolutionize the rehabilitation industry due to the advantages it has over the conventional control methods. Though lots of research efforts have been made to advance this control technique, however, the clinical performance of the current myoelectric PR-based prostheses for upper-limb amputees is not yet satisfactory. The limited translation of advances in academic researches relating to upper-limb prosthetic devices into commercially available products for amputees can be attributed to a number of factors which are described as follows.

In laboratory researches, only a limited number of conditions could be considered when carrying out an experiment. Under this limited condition, relatively stable and good performances are usually achieved relating to the controllability of myoelectric PR-based prostheses. Meanwhile, in clinical applications, some other conditions which were not considered in the laboratory are often encountered and thereby compromises most of the results reported in the laboratory. This in turn affects the performance of the assistive devices as well as their acceptance for clinical use. It is worthy to note that rehabilitation devices such as the upper-limb prostheses would generally need to undergo extensive evaluation in accordance with strict medical device requirements. And in most cases, a sizable number of upper-limb amputees are usually not easily accessible to extensively test the functionality of the developed assistive devices. Also, the development of upper-limb prosthetic devices would require lots of funding and such devices may be quite expensive for patients with average to low income in the developed countries. In addition, considering the fact that the market for upper-limb prostheses is small compared to that of the lower-limb prostheses, not many investors would be interested in funding projects relating to the development of upper-limb prostheses. At the long run, the issue of inadequate funding would result in less innovative ideas since the numbers of researchers working on such project are limited by fund. In a way, this has been slowing down the clinical realization of upper-limb prostheses. Another important issue that may be limiting the clinical viability of upper-limb PR-based prostheses is the lack of intelligent feedback mechanism that could provide users with the ability to intuitively operate the device. With proper feedback mechanism, it is believed that a reliable control could be achieved with ease. Also, such closed loop would enable proper integration of the whole device consisting of the socket, the prosthetic device, and other components.

One way to guarantee the clinical feasibility of myoelectric PR-based prostheses for upper-limb amputees would be to carefully consider the above discussed challenges with the aim of resolving them. In addition, the introduction of an iterative user-centered design approach would be instrumental to establishing a close relationship among the necessary stakeholders (researchers, clinical experts, professionals, and end-users). Furthermore, integrating some adaptation features into the prosthesis would make users feel that the device is part of their body. Though achieving this may be challenging, but we believe it would improve users' confidence and level of reliance on the devices. It is also important to note that for PR technique to be a success in rehabilitation robots for stroke survivors, the above highlighted issues limiting the clinical success of myoelectric prostheses would need to be properly addressed.

It also is important to note that apart from the rehabilitation of amputees and stroke survivors, upper limb EMG signals have found more applications such as post-surgery evaluation where there is articular instability and/or damage to ligaments [4], sports and occupational medicine to determine the existence or absence fatigue and analyze its development over time [5, 36], quantitative analysis of neuromuscular disorder [37], and personal entertainment.

4 Large-Scale Distributed Computing in EMG Pattern Recognition

Distributed systems consist of a group of networked computers, which have been designed to achieve the same goal with respect to a task. Basically, the processing of the whole task is shared among the computers on the network in order obtain timely results [12]. Typically in such systems, the processors have associated memories and they run concurrently in parallel. For instance, a schematic view of a typical distributed system is shown in Fig. 6a, where the system is represented by a network topology in which each node is a computer and each line connecting the nodes is a communication link. Meanwhile, Fig. 6b shows the same distributed system in more detail: each computer has its own local memory, and information can be exchanged only by passing messages from one node to another by using the available communication links.

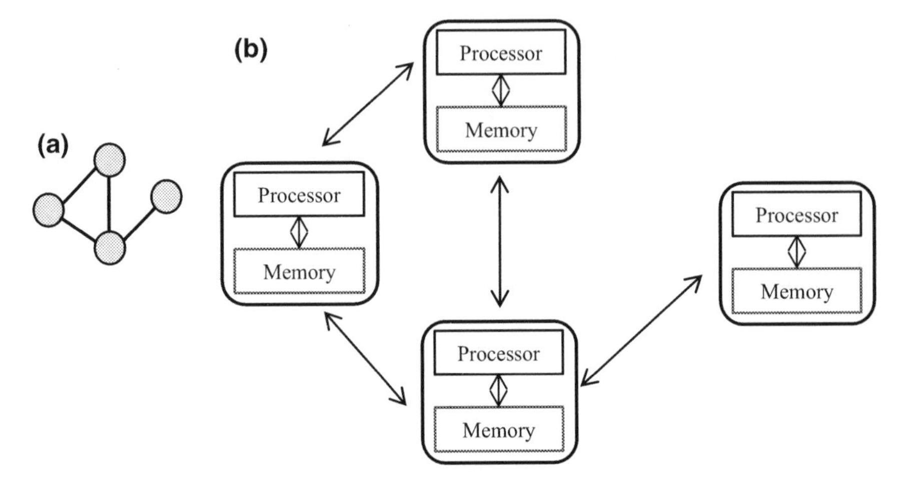

Fig. 6 An illustration of a typical distributed computing system; **a** a schematic view, **b** a detail view

A common characteristic of distributed systems is that they can support efficient processing of data (especially large-scale dataset) within short space of time. And such platforms are usually readily accessible at a relatively low cost and this makes them indispensable in the modern day society. Some recent studies indicated that distributed computing offers new possibilities that can improve healthcare services and benefit biomedical research [2, 13, 40]. Machine learning assisted decision support systems are often designed for centralized systems that require a relatively small amount of data. In Big data systems, such designs may not be efficient and redesigning another platform for such systems are often challenging due to computational cost and network bandwidth requirements especially when there is need to integrate some learning algorithms into the system. However, with technologies like the Hadoop and MapReduce [10], efficient distributed systems could be incorporate learning algorithms could be developed. The benefits of such distributed systems in healthcare include higher performance at a lower cost, higher reliability, and more scalability [8].

Considering the fact that microcontrollers embedded in upper-limb prostheses or rehabilitation robots are often limited by their memory size and processing power, the overall performance of such devices would be affected in some ways by these factors, especially when a high-density EMG electrode array and a high sampling rate are required in some applications. With such limited hardware capability, integrating additional features into the prostheses or assistive robots that could make them more attractive to users may be challenging. For individuals who mostly carry out their daily life activities within a confined space (especially the elderly), upper-limb prostheses could be designed for them in a way that the processing and memory requirements would be distributed remotely to a computing platform for smooth operation. For instance, the sensors on a prosthesis or even rehabilitation robot could be configured to acquire and transmit myoelectric signals from muscle contractions wirelessly to a server installed within the confined space. Subsequently, the data will be processed on the server and the output would be communicated back to the prosthetic or rehabilitation device. Such distributed computing approach may enable the integration of additional features into a prosthesis or rehabilitation robot easily and also enhance the performance of the whole device. This idea is relatively new and we believe that it may be beneficial to future designs of upper-limb prosthesis as well as other rehabilitation devices.

5 Conclusion

The field of rehabilitation robotics has been a major research focus in recent years due to the roles played by such assistive technologies in ensuring that the functions of certain body parts are restored. In line with this, a number of prosthesis and robot aided rehabilitation devices have been developed over the years. Therefore, this chapter presents motion recognition method for the control of upper-limb prosthetic and robotic devices with emphasis on myoelectric pattern recognition technique. The fundamental procedures for the decoding of upper-limb motion intents of amputees and stroke survivors from myoelectric signals have been described with emphasis on the commonly adopted practices in research and clinical applications. In addition, the potential of distributed computing concept in healthcare especially its prospects in the development of robust upper-limb rehabilitation device has been discussed. Finally, several factors currently challenging the clinical success of myoelectric PR-based rehabilitation devices for patients, and some possible solutions have been presented.

Acknowledgements The work was supported in part by the National Key Basic Research Program of China (2013CB329505), the National Natural Science Foundation of China under Grants (#61135004, #91420301, #61203209, #61403367), the National High Technology Research and Development Program of China (#2105AA042303), the Natural Science Foundation for Distinguished Young Scholars of Guangdong Province, China (2014A030306029), the Special Support Program for Eminent Professionals of Guangdong Province, China (2015TQ01C399), and the Shenzhen Peacock Plan Grant (#KQCX2015033117354152, #JCYJ20150401145529005). Lastly, I (O.W. Samuel) sincerely appreciate the support of CAS-TWAS President's Fellowship in the pursuit of a Ph.D. degree at the University of Chinese Academy of Sciences, Beijing, China.

References

1. Adewuyi A.A., Hargrove L.J., & Kuiken, T.A. (2016). An analysis of intrinsic and extrinsic hand muscle EMG for improved pattern recognition control. IEEE Transactions on Neural Systems and Rehabilitation Engineering, 24(4), 485–494.
2. Ahuja, S.P., Mani, S., & Zambrano, J. (2012). A survey of the state of cloud computing in healthcare. Network and Communication Technologies, 1(2), 12–19.

3. Ajiboye, A.B. & Weir, RF. (2005). A heuristic fuzzy logic approach to EMG pattern recognition for multifunctional prosthesis control. IEEE Transactions on Neural Systems and Rehabilitation Engineering, 13, 280–291.
4. Benoit, D.L., Lamontagne, M., Cerulli, G., Liti, A. (2003). The clinical significance of electromyography normalisation techniques in subjects with anterior cruciate ligament injury during treadmill walking. Gait Posture, 18, 56–63.
5. Bonato, P., Roy, S.H., Knaflitz, M., De Luca, C.J. (2001). Time-frequency parameters of the surface myoelectric signal for assessing muscle fatigue during cyclic dynamic contractions. IEEE Transactions on Biomedical Engineering, 48, 745–53.
6. Cesqui, B., Tropea, P., Micera, S., & Krebs, H.I. (2013). EMG-based pattern recognition approach in post stroke robot-aided rehabilitation: A feasibility study. Journal of NeuroEngineering and Rehabilitation 2013, 10:75.
7. Chang, W.H. & Kim, Y.H. (2013). Robot-assisted Therapy in Stroke Rehabilitation. Journal of Stroke, 15(3), 174–181.
8. Che N., Janusz W. (2013). Learning from Large-scale distributed health data: An approximate logistic regression approach. Proceedings of the 30th International Conference on Machine Learning, Atlanta, Georgia, USA, JMLR: W&CP volume 28.
9. Cozens, J.A. (1999). Robotic assistance of an active upper limb exercise in neurologically impaired patients. IEEE Transactions on Neural Systems and Rehabilitation Engineering, 7(2) 254–256.
10. Dean, J. and Ghemawat, S. (2008). Mapreduce: simplified data processing on large clusters. Communications of the ACM, 51(1):107–113.
11. Dipietro, L.H. et al. (2007). Changing motor synergies in chronic stroke. J. Neurophysiol., 98 (2), 757–768.
12. Distributed computing: (2016) https://en.wikipedia.org/wiki/Distributed_computing#cite_note-18 Date Last Accessed: 2016-10-31.
13. Eugster, M.J.A., Schmid, M., Binder, H., & Schmidberger, M., (2013). Grid and cloud computing methods in biomedical research. Methods of Information in Medicine, 1, 62–64.
14. Fang, P., Geng, Y., Wei, Z., Zhou, P., Tian, L., & Li, G. (2015). New control strategies for multifunctional prostheses that combine electromyographic and speech signals. IEEE Intelligent Systems, 30(4), 47–53.
15. Farina, D. et al. (2014). The extraction of neural information from surface EMG for the control of upper-limb prostheses: Emerging avenue and challenges. IEEE Transactions on Neural Systems and Rehabilitation Engineering, 22(4), 797–809.
16. Freriks, B., Hermans, H.J., Disselhorst-King, C., & Rau, G. (1999). European Recommendations for surface electromyography. Results of the SENIAM Project, B.V., ISBN: 90-75452-14-4.
17. Geng, Y., Zhang, L., Tang, D., Zhang, X., & Li, G. (2013). Pattern recognition based forearm motion classification for patients with chronic hemiparesis, 35th Annual International Conference of the IEEE EMBS Osaka, Japan, 3–7 July, 2013.
18. Hargrove, L.J., Lock, B.A., & Simon, A.M. (2013). Pattern recognition control outperforms conventional myoelectric control in upper limb patients with targeted muscle reinnervation. 35th Annual International Conference of the IEEE EMBS Osaka, Japan, 3–7 July, 1599–1602.
19. Hargrove, L., Englehart, K., & Hudgins, B. (2007). A comparison of surface and intramuscular myoelectric signal classification, IEEE Transactions on Biomedical Engineering, 54, 847–853.
20. Hewson, D.J., Hogrel, J.Y., Langeron, Y., & Ducêne, J. (2003). Evolution in impedance at the electrode–skin interface of two types of surface EMG electrodes during long-term recordings. Journal of Electromyography and Kinesiology, 13, 273–279.
21. Huang, Y.H., Englehart, K., Hudgins, B., & Chan, AD. (2005). A Gaussian mixture model based classification scheme for myoelectric control of powered upper limb prostheses. IEEE Transactions on Biomedical Engineering, 52, 1801–1811.

22. Hudgins, B., Parker, P., & Scott, R.N. (1993). A new strategy for multifunction myoelectric control. IEEE Transactions on Biomedical Engineering, 40(1), 82–94.
23. Krebs, H.I. et al. (2007). Robot-aided neurorehabilitation: A robot for wrist rehabilitation. IEEE Transactions on Neural Systems and Rehabilitation Engineering, 15(3), 327–335.
24. Levy, C.E., Nichols, D.S., Schmalbrock, P.M., Keller, P., & Chakeres, D.W. (2001). Functional MRI evidence of cortical reorganization in upper-limb stroke hemiplegia treated with constraint-induced movement therapy. Am. J. Phys. Med. Rehabil., 80(1), 4–12.
25. Liepert, J. et al. (2000). Treatment-induced cortical reorganization after stroke in humans. Stroke, 31(6), 1210–1216.
26. Lindstrom, L.H. & Magnusson, R.I. (1977). Interpretation of myoelectric power spectra: a model and its applications. Proceedings of the IEEE 65: 653–662.
27. Liu, J. & Zhou, P. (2013). A novel myoelectric pattern recognition strategy for hand function restoration after incomplete cervical spinal cord injury. IEEE Transactions on Neural Systems and Rehabilitation Engineering, 21(1), 96–103.
28. Li, G., Schultz, A.E, & Kuiken, T.A. (2010). Quantifying pattern recognition-based myoelectric control of multifunctional transradial prostheses. IEEE Transactions on Neural Systems and Rehabilitation Engineering, 18(2), 185–192.
29. Li, G., Li, Y., Yu, L., & Geng, Y. (2011). Conditioning and sampling issues of EMG signals in motion recognition of multifunctional myoelectric prostheses. Annals of Biomedical Engineering 39(6), 1779–1787.
30. Li, G. (2011). Electromyography pattern-recognition-based control of powered multifunctional upper-limb prostheses. Advances in Applied Electromyography, Prof. Joseph Mizrahi (Ed.), ISBN: 978-953-307-382-8, Chap. 6: 99–117.
31. Li, X., Chen, S., Zhang, H., Samuel O.W., Wang, H., Fang, P., Zhang, X., & Li, G. (2016) Towards reducing the impacts of unwanted movements on identification of motion intentions. Journal of Electromyography and Kinesiology, 28, 90–98.
32. Lum, P.S., Burgar, C.G., Kenney, D.E., & Van der Loos, H.F. (1999). Quantification of force abnormalities during passive and active-assisted upper-limb reaching movements in post-stroke hemiparesis. IEEE Transactions on Biomedical Engineering, 46(6), 652–662.
33. Lum, P.S., Burgar, C.G., & Shor, P.C. (2004). Evidence for improved muscle activation patterns after retraining of reaching movements with the MIME robotic system in subjects with post-stroke hemiparesis. IEEE Transactions on Neural Systems and Rehabilitation Engineering, 12(2), 186–194.
34. Kutlu, M. et al. (2016). Upper-limb stroke rehabilitation using electrode-array based functional electrical stimulation with sensing and control innovations. Medical Engineering & Physics, 38, 366–379.
35. Muilenburg, A.L. & LeBlanc, M.A. (1999). Body-powered upper-limb components. D. J. Atkins et al. (eds.) Comprehensive Management of the Upper-Limb Amputee, Springer-Verlag, New York Inc.
36. Nordander, C. et al. (2000). Muscular rest and gap frequency as EMG measures of physical exposure: The impact of work tasks and individual related factors. Ergonomics, 43, 1904–19.
37. Núria, M. et al. (2010). Surface electromyography applications in the sport, Apunts Med Esport., 45(165), 121–130.
38. Oskoei, M.A. and Hu, H. (2008). Support vector machine-based classification scheme for myoelectric control applied to upper limb. IEEE Transactions on Biomedical Engineering, 55 (8), 1956–1965.
39. Patricia, F.A. et al. (1999). Current Estimates from the National Health Interview Survey, 1996. Vital and Health Statistics 10:200.
40. Rosenthal, A. et al. (2010). Cloud computing: A new business paradigm for biomedical information sharing. Journal of Biomedical Informatics, 43, 342–353.
41. Samuel, O.W., Li, X., Fang, P., & Li, G., (2016). Examining the effect of subjects' mobility on upper-limb motion identification based on EMG-pattern recognition. IEEE Asia-Pacific Conference on Intelligent Robot Systems, July 20–24, Tokyo, Japan, 139–141.

42. Scheme, E. & Englehart, K. (2011). Electromyogram pattern recognition for control of powered upper-limb prostheses: state of the art and challenges for clinical use. Journal of Rehabilitation Research & Development, 48, 643–660.
43. Smith, L.H., Hargrove, L.J., Lock, B.A., & Kuiken, T.A. (2011). Determining the optimal window length for pattern recognition-based myoelectric control: balancing the competing effects of classification error and controller delay. IEEE Transactions on Neural Systems and Rehabilitation Engineering, 19(2), 186–192.
44. Smith, L.H. & Hargrove, L.J. (2013). Comparison of surface and intramuscular EMG pattern recognition for simultaneous wrist/hand motion classification. 35th Annual International Conference of the IEEE EMBS, Osaka, Japan, 3–7 July.
45. Soulis, J., (2016) Utilizing pattern recognition to improve myoelectric control: A case study. http://www.oandp.org/AcademyTODAY/2015Jul/5.asp Date Last Accessed: 2016-08-15.
46. Ver Hage. The NIH stroke scale: a window into neurological status. Nurse.Com Nursing Spectrum (Greater Chicago) [serial online]. September 12, 2011; 24(15):44–49.
47. Young, A.J., Smith, L.H., Rouse, E.J., & Hargrove, L.J. (2014). A comparison of the real-time controllability of pattern recognition to conventional myoelectric control for discrete and simultaneous movements. Journal of NeuroEngineering and Rehabilitation, 11:5.
48. Zhang, X. & Zhou, P. (2012). High-density myoelectric pattern recognition toward improved stroke rehabilitation, IEEE Transactions on Biomedical Engineering, 59(6), 1649–1657.

Infrequent Non-speech Gestural Activity Recognition Using Smart Jewelry: Challenges and Opportunities for Large-Scale Adaptation

Mohammad Arif Ul Alam, Nirmalya Roy, Aryya Gangopadhyay and Elizabeth Galik

Abstract Wearable Body Area Network (BAN) based activity recognition is one of the fastest growing research areas in activity recognition and context reasoning. However, wearable physical sensor based Infrequent Non-Speech Gestural Activity (IGA) recognition is not well studied problem because IGAs are not directly observable from BAN sensor devices. Due to the recent proliferation of smart jewelries capable of monitoring locomotive and physiological signals from certain specific human body positions which are currently hitherto impossible to measure by traditional fitness and smart wristwatch devices opens up unprecedented research and development opportunities in anatomical gestural activity recognition. Inspired by this, we propose a new wearable smart earring based framework which is capable of differentiating IGAs in a daily environment with a single integrated accelerometer sensor. The natural gestures associated with the first portion of the human alimentary canal, i.e., human mouth can broadly be categorized in two types; frequent (talking, silence etc.) or infrequent (coughing, deglutition, yawning) gestures. Infrequent Gestural Activities (IGAs) help create an abrupt but distinct change in accelerometer sensor signal streams of an earring pertaining to specific activities. Mining and classifying the abrupt changes in sensor signal streams require high sampling frequency which in turn depletes the limited battery life of any smart ornaments. Extending the battery life of smartened designer jewelry requires probing those devices less which in turn prohibits of achieving high precision and recall for non-frequent gestural activity discovery and recognition. In this book chapter, we propose a novel data segmentation technique that harnesses the power of change-point detection algorithm to detect and quantify any abrupt changes in sensor data streams of smart earrings. This

---

M.A.U. Alam (✉) · N. Roy · A. Gangopadhyay · E. Galik
University of Maryland Baltimore County, Baltimore, MD, USA
e-mail: alam4@umbc.edu

N. Roy
e-mail: nroy@umbc.edu

A. Gangopadhyay
e-mail: gangopad@umbc.edu

E. Galik
e-mail: galik@son.umaryland.edu

© Springer International Publishing AG 2017

S.U. Khan et al. (eds.), *Handbook of Large-Scale Distributed Computing in Smart Healthcare*, Scalable Computing and Communications,
DOI 10.1007/978-3-319-58280-1_17

helps to distinguish between frequent and infrequent gestural acclivities at a high precision with a low sampling frequency, energy, and computational overhead. Experimental evaluation on one real-time and two publicly available benchmark datasets attests the scalability and adaptation of our techniques for both IGAs and postural activities in large-scale participatory sensing health applications.

Keywords Infrequent gesture · Activity recognition · Smart segmentation

1 Introduction

Modeling fine-grained physiological symptoms and chronic psychological conditions of older adults have significant impacts on smart connected elderly healthcare. The fine-grained insights about the human health and wellness can be obtained from the physiological and psychological data processing if they are combined with Activities of Daily Living. Human contexts refer to a variety of dynamically changing states, relevant to either activities, biomedical states, or behavioral conditions. Such contexts enable critical capabilities, such as alerting a first responder on an abnormal behavioral incident or recommending avoidance of a potential health risk behavior by analyzing health data related to continuous deglutition or coughing after every day eating [1]. Cognitive dissonance and psychological disorders often evolve from abnormal physical behaviors. For example, while suffering with different kinds of physiological health issues, patient may show irregular gestures such as frequent coughing, yawning, breathing irregularities etc. Therefore mental and physical health of older adults are correlated and if harnessed appropriately may provide meaningful microscopic physiological and psychological contexts. For example, a person feeling a headache from anxiety or anger might shout loudly or show irregular interpersonal traits. Thus the mental hygiene or physical wellness of a particular person can be inferred by monitoring the IGAs which reflect the emotional or behavioral state of the individual. In this chapter, we explore the recognition of non-speech infrequent gestural activities (henceforth defined as IGAs) which provide significant insights about the long-term well-being of the older adults.

With the technological advancements and emergence of sophisticated microelectronic technologies, the modern age has seen the advent of smaller devices. These advancements have also enabled the development of intelligent and miniaturized biomedical sensors. Very small biomedical sensors can be either worn or implanted inside the body to collect a variety of physical information and services. The multimodal networking ability between these body node mounted devices and integration with existing device infrastructure can convey health-related information between the user's contexts and the caregivers. On the other hand, the employment of wireless networks is becoming more and more extensive with the increase in the number of devices being able to communicate wirelessly. With such an advent, studies ensued whether electronic devices could be operated on and near the human body. It was during this time that the idea of Body Area Network or BAN was invented.

In this chapter, we propose a new wearable smart Body Area Network (BAN) device (say earring) based framework which is capable of differentiating infrequent movements of the wearable sensor attached body parts in a daily environment with a single integrated accelerometer sensor. The framework is inspired by the change-point detection based segmentation and feature extraction that can effectively perform higher in terms of accuracy in very low sampling frequency confirming lower battery power consumption in the daily environment. We built a customized accelerometer sensor integrated wearable jewelry (earring) and implement our proposed framework to distinguish non-speech infrequent gestural activities (IGAs) to prove the efficacy of our framework.

2 Design Considerations and Contributions

Most of the prior works focused on speech based acoustic signal processing to detect human speech and non-speech gestures [2–5]. While acoustic signal can help determine the speech and non-speech human gestures but undermine significantly the computational cost and life longevity of wearable devices. Recording, pre-processing, ambient noise reduction, segmentation, features extraction and classification processes cause huge computational overhead which rapidly drains out the battery power of source devices. However, continuous sensing of acoustic signals causes privacy violations.

More specifically, any ubiquitous wearable device must facilitate the following **critical requirements**:

- **Long Battery Life**: Earring has become very common for men and women to have both ears pierced, and is becoming more acceptable for teenagers as well. The advantage of smart earring based physical/gestural activity recognition is its ubiquitous usage of all time even during sleep. However, the most advantageous fact also creates the most disadvantageous charge. Since users keep it worn for a long time, it is obvious that they are reluctant of changing batteries frequently. Moreover, if the batteries must be replaced often (every day or every week), not only will the primary benefit (freedom from wiring constraints and costs) of wireless networks be lost, but also many remote sensing applications may become impractical. Therefore, long battery life is essential in earring sensor networks.
- **Small Form Factor**: Devices used as wearable data collector must be small enough to be embedded in their operating environment. This requirement affects the choice of batteries which possibly could be very small in size with very low powers.
- **Lower Sampling Rate**: In our framework, sensor data is captured in the earring but transmitted, stored and processed by a remote node before it is transmitted to the central base station. The entire data streaming, transmission, storage and local processing are exhilarated with low sampling rate. However, low sampling rate costs the accuracy of the recognition process which also needs to be handled.

In this chapter, we first describe the anatomy of non-speech infrequent gestural activities that includes IGAs selection, analyzing non-speech gesture patterns and critical requirements for BAN based IGAs recognition framework design considerations. Next, we describe a retrospective change-point detection framework that helps represent the instant transition of gestural signals as an abrupt change and continuous perturbation as a specific pattern. We use this framework (i) to detect appropriate position of wearable jewelry and (ii) data segmentation technique for gestural activity recognition confirming highest detection accuracy with lowest sampling frequency.

The structure of our entire chapter is as follows. We start with the relevant works. Next, we describe our proposed change-point scoring method and its application on device position setup and dynamic segmentation. We highlight the anatomy of non-speech gestural activities which includes gestural activities selection process, device position setup details and gestural activity patterns analysis. Next, we describe our experimental methodology that comprises of device customization, data collection, feature extraction, feature selection and description of performance metrics. We describe our evaluation method that consists of segmentation, device position setup and classification performance analysis, baseline classification algorithm development and comparisons of performances. To attest the scalability and adaptation of our techniques for other activity and large-scale participatory sensing health applications, we evaluate our framework on two wearable sensor-based daily activity benchmark datasets.

3 Related Works

This chapter builds on previous works on wearable sensor-based context recognition techniques that offer better healthcare and physical well-being. Here we compare and contrast our contributions with the most relevant existing literature.

3.1 Acoustic Signal Processing

Most of the oral gestural activities i.e. non-speech infrequent gestural activity involve vision feed (sequence of images) analysis for tracking facial expressions or body postures. Previous works for detecting oral gestures were based on only one criterion such as vocal features, body postures, facial expressions or physiological changes [6–12]. Some researchers used microphones [13], weight detection panels [14], cameras [15], and water usage detectors [13] to detect gestural activities. [5] proposed a mobile sensing system that leveraged microphone sensor to detect non-speech oral gestural activities. DeepEar has been proposed a mobile audio sensing framework built from coupled Deep Neural Networks (DNNs) that simultaneously perform common audio sensing tasks and distinguish speech and non-speech human sounds in the mobile environment [2]. However, audio sensing based speech or non-speech human gesture recognition costs higher battery power consumption for a mobile device.

3.2 Accelerometer Sensor Signal Processing

Among the various wearable devices, the most popular wearable for activity detection purposes is the accelerometer [16, 17]. Besides being inexpensive, accelerometers tend to be small and lightweight, and so are fairly unobtrusive and user-friendly [18]. RisQ presents a single wrist worn 9-axis inertial measurement unit (IMU) based smoking gesture detection [19] along with a static point detection based segmentation technique to improve detection accuracy in lower sampling rate. However, accelerometers or IMU based non-speech gesture recognition techniques rely on hand mounted sensor system [19, 20] which is extremely inconvenient if the non-speech human gestures are infrequent or not relevant to hand (for example, deglutition, yawning, chewing etc.). Accelerometers gather data at a high frequency, and as such may be used to collect a sizeable amount of data in a relatively short amount of time. To differentiate between different variants of vocal sounds *Mel-Frequency Cepstral Coefficient (MFCC)* has been applied achieving 66% average accuracy in detecting human emotions [3]. [4] added acceleration of pitch with MFCCs in forming cintinuous feature streams.

3.3 Multi-modal Sensor Signal Processing

Researchers have proposed multimodal signal processing approaches where multiple sensors have been considered simultaneously [16, 21–24]. While Coulson et al. [25] and Gunes et al. [26] proposed the bi-modal approach to capture human gestures using both facial expressions and body postures Ginerva et al. [27] used facial expressions, vocal features, body movements and gestures fused altogether. Silve et al. [28] proposed a rule based classification technique on audio-visual data. Whether or not an accelerometer yields data that is discriminative for a set of activity types depends partially on where the accelerometer is worn on a subject's body [29]. For example, an accelerometer worn on the ankle will be more discriminative for the activity of cycling than it would be if it was worn on the hip, and different types of arm movements will likely be discriminated only by an accelerometer worn on the arm. For this reason, some researchers have considered to use multiple accelerometer systems to capture movement information from different parts of the body [30]. This approach can be cumbersome for the wearer, so a single accelerometer is preferred when it is reasonable to assume that it will be discriminative for the relevant set of activities. However, wireless sensor network based activity recognition imposes several other issues like performance expectancy in terms of hardware cost and processing delay, human training effort expectancy, social influence, facilitating condition and privacy issues [31, 32]. In the past few years researchers have begun to recognize the need to test on realistic free-living data [33, 34]. The time required to detect that a change in activity has occurred was considered in [35], but in the context of the very different problem of video activity recognition. We consider the feasibility of performing accelerometer based IGA recognition in real time by using both accuracy and detection time as performance metrics.

3.4 Reduced Sampling Rate for Activity Recognition

Reducing sampling rates to save energy is also a well investigated research problem. Some prior researchers have proven that it is not necessary for sensors be at full sampling rate to achieve higher accuracy [36]. Krause et al. [37] addresses the tradeoffs between accuracy and energy consumption which reports that for both time and frequency domain features there are some knee exists for sampling rate and accuracy. Below the knee, there is a significant accuracy degradation. It suggests using the sampling rate at the knee to save energy while enjoying a relatively high accuracy. In addition, Chu [38] achieves significant accuracy of mobile sensor data classification based on Krause et al. proposed energy latency accuracy tradeoffs. However, we proposed a novel approach of segmentation by accumulating change-point scoring based feature extraction method that significantly enhances IGAs recognition performances in lower sampling rate which confirms energy savings as well as computational cost.

4 Application of Change-Point Detection Algorithm

Change point detection refers to detect the instances or the point of occurances when the probability distribution of a continuous (time-series) process. While the traditional statistical features fail to expedite the abrupt changes in infrequent oral gestural signals (infrequency of signal refers abruptness in nature), we propose to use change-point scoring to capture the signal divergence. We design a change-point scoring method taking relative Pearson divergence as a divergence measure estimated by a method of direct density-ratio estimation method [39]. We first describe the mathematical background of change-point scoring for single dimensional time series sample and extend to multi-dimensional abrupt change-point score estimation relevant to three axis-accelerometer sensor signal values.

4.1 Change-Point Scoring Method

Let us consider $x(t)$ as a 1-dimensional time series with one sub-sequence sample at time t where $x(t)$ =[x-axis reading, t]. Then, the sub-sequence of the time series at t time with length k will be,

$$X(t) = [x(t)^T, x(t+1)^T, \ldots, x(t+k-1)^T]^T \in \mathbf{R}^{\mathbf{k}} \tag{1}$$

Here, $x(t)^T$ = transpose of $x(t)$.

Let us consider $\mathbf{X(t)}$ be a set of n retrospective sub-sequence samples starting at time t. Then, $\mathbf{X(t)}$ will be

$$\mathbf{X(t)} = X(t), X(t+1), \ldots, X(t+n-1) \in \mathbf{R}^{k \times n} \tag{2}$$

Now, consider $x(t)$ be a d-dimensional time series (3 dimensional accelerometer values say x, y and z axis values) with n sub-sequence sample where $x(t) = \begin{pmatrix} x\ t \\ y\ t \\ z\ t \end{pmatrix}$ Then, the sub-sequence of time series at time t be:

$$\mathbf{X(t)} = X(t), X(t+1), \ldots, X(t+n-1) \in \mathbf{R}^{dk \times n} \tag{3}$$

Here, $\mathbf{X(t)}$ forms a Hankel matrix [40]. We considered $k = 10$, $n = 50$ and $d = 3$ which was proved to be optimal in our case. We estimate the dissimilarity measure between two consecutive segments $\mathbf{X(t)}$ and $\mathbf{X(t+n)}$, and use it as the plausibility of change-points i.e., the higher the dissimilarity measure, the more likely the point is an abrupt change-point as shown in Fig. 1.

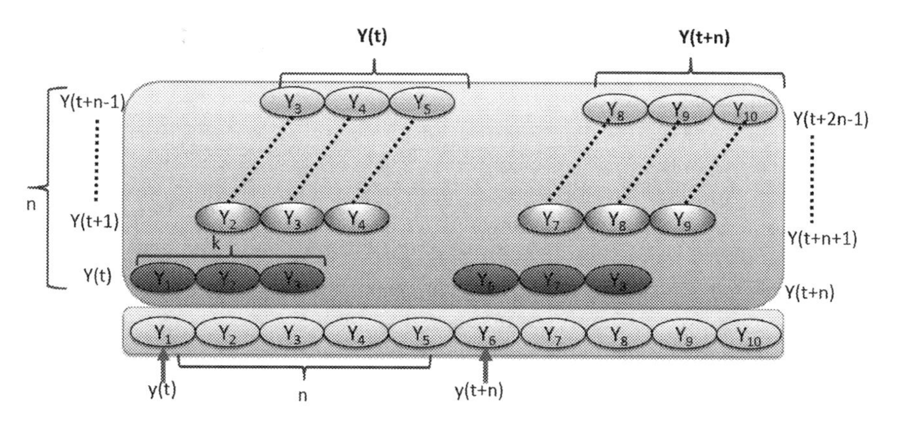

Fig. 1 One-dimensional time-series data for Pearson divergence estimation based Change-point detection.

4.2 Optimal Device Position Detection

While change-point score measures the abrupt changes over time-series data stream, we argue that, it also can be used in determining the informativeness of the data. In general, to find the informativeness of any data stream, researchers collect entire dataset with maximum fine-grained granularity with several cross-validated fine-grained labelings. Then, use different classifiers to find the best dataset to be the best position of the device. We argue that, we can detect the best position setup of the device only taking the advantage divergence measure achieved of the transition points from the change-point scoring method. Our proposed position setup method is stated as following steps:

1. We first define and label the transition points of activities i.e., a small segment of data streams where two consecutive activities are present while transiting from one activity to another. In our scenario, we defined five gestural activities to be distinguished (silence, talking, coughing, yawning and deglutition) which generated 28 $(5 \times 2 + 4 \times 2 + 3 \times 2 + 2 \times 2)$ bilateral transition points. For example, silence to talk, talk to silence, silence to cough, cough to silence, silence to yawn, yawn to silence etc.
2. We take the change-point scores of each segment that signify the divergence measures of the transition point. If the divergence is more significant (higher value), then the data stream contains higher informativeness of that position of the device.

4.3 Change-Point Detection Based Segmentation

For this approach, we split data stream (x, y and z axis of accelerometer data) into non-overlapping segments using a statistical field of change-point detection. Change-point detection in general is used to analyze time series data from dynamic systems, including failure detection [41], quick detection of attacks on computer networks [42], monitoring of heartbeat fluctuations during sleep [43]. Very few of prior works applied change-point detection in segmentation but most of these were related to vocal or non-vocal sound segmentation [44, 45]. We are the first of a kind to apply change-point detection in segmenting accelerometer data stream. We identify the best change-point score threshold to segment time series data, apply supervised classification techniques and show how we can get more fine-grained performance in classifying infrequent gestural activities.

To explain how Change-point scores are used for segmentation, we have to consider each tick of a time series as some sort of probability distribution, but that the distribution may suddenly change as time passes. The goal of change-point detection is to predict when these changes have occurred, a significant score is generated for each time tick (described in the previous section). If the score is above a given threshold a change is predicted to have occurred between that tick and its immediate

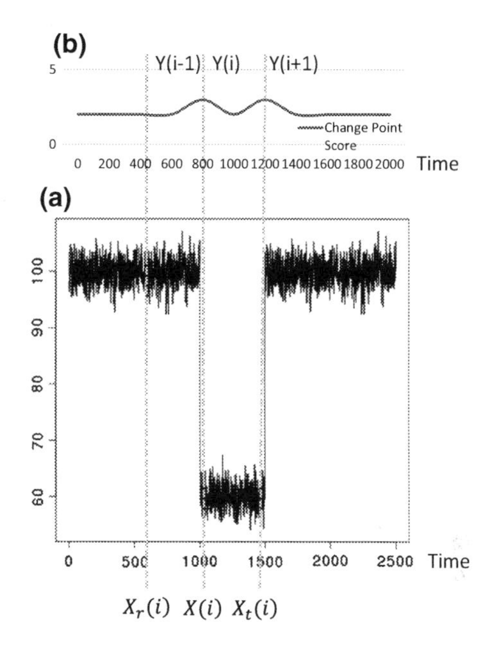

Fig. 2 Change-point detection based segmentation

predecessor. This change-point is considered as a partition between two consecutive segments. We then extract the features of each segment throughout the data stream for next level of classification. Figure 2a illustrates the data stream where $X_r(i)$ and $X_t(i)$ represent two consecutive sub-sequence of data stream associated with the ith tick. Figure 2b represents the change-point score based segmentation. Here, change-point score $S(i)$ goes below the minimum threshold resulting an end of previous segment $Y(i-1)$ as well as a start of next segment $Y(i)$.

5 Anatomy of Non-speech Gestural Activities

The goal of this chapter is that we can detect IGAs from an earring placed on ear location using only integrated accelerometer with lower battery power consumption. Towards this broader goal, we analyze the anatomy of infrequent non-speech gestures and recognizing their patterns in terms of acceleration in details. We start with infrequent gestural activities selection which carries significance in determining behavioral and physical health status. Next, we test using our proposed change-point score based informativeness heuristic to setup possible position of the accelerometer. Then, we analyze the gestural activity patterns in terms of acceleration for the selected position towards recognizing through machine learning algorithm.

5.1 Selection of Gestural Activities

The major goal of this study is to provide both behavioral and physical health status in terms of non-speech gestures. Towards this broader perspective, we choose 5 important non-speech gestural activities which are closely relevant to proactive healthcare and abnormal physical behaviors: (i) silence, (ii) talking, (iii) coughing, (iv) yawning and (v) deglutition. 'Silence' is the most common form of human non-speech gesture which defines a state when the person does no significant sound through her mouth and stays the mouth close to normal position. The silence movement does not change the jaw and ear positions of the face. However, it also can be considered as a separator from one IGAs to another due to its universal presence in-between all IGAs natural performance. 'Talking' is the speaking state of human gesture which has been considered in this study to distinguish it from other IGAs. 'Coughing' is a sudden and often repetitively occurring reflex which helps to clear the large breathing passages from secretions, irritants, foreign particles and microbes. 'Deglutition' or 'Swallowing' is the process in the human or animal body that makes something pass from the mouth, to the pharynx, and into the esophagus, while shutting the epiglottis. 'Yawning' is a reflex consisting of the simultaneous inhalation of air and the stretching of the eardrums, followed by an exhalation of breath. 'Yawning' most often occurs in adults immediately before and after sleep, during tedious activities and as a result of its contagious quality. It is commonly associated with sleepiness, tiredness, stress or even boredom and hunger, though studies show it may be linked to the cooling of the brain [46]. The above activities can be related to each other based on their nature. For example, 'Coughing' can be followed by 'Deglutition', 'Silence' or 'Talking' which represent a different form of pattern and may consist of clinical significance in nature of 'coughing' detection. However, 'Coughing' followed by 'Yawning' could be an indication of sleep disturbance caused by couching. However, our baseline framework has an opportunity to add more activities too.

5.2 Device Position Setup

To investigate the appropriate device position, we engaged 10 users and collected data in a controlled lab environment. This experiment consisted of two parameters: (i) change of body positions (pant pocket, chest pocket, neck and ear) and (ii) change of gestural activities (silence, talking, coughing, yawning and deglutition). We recorded accelerometer signal streams on five gestural activities, label the transition points and took the average accelerometer magnitudes and average change-point scores of accelerometer magnitude to compute the average acceleration changes on each transition point segment. Then, we compute and compared average change-point scores, average magnitudes of the captured accelerometer data and machine learning classification method of the features with respect to different body positions for different gestures. Figure 3 shows a comparison of average magnitude and

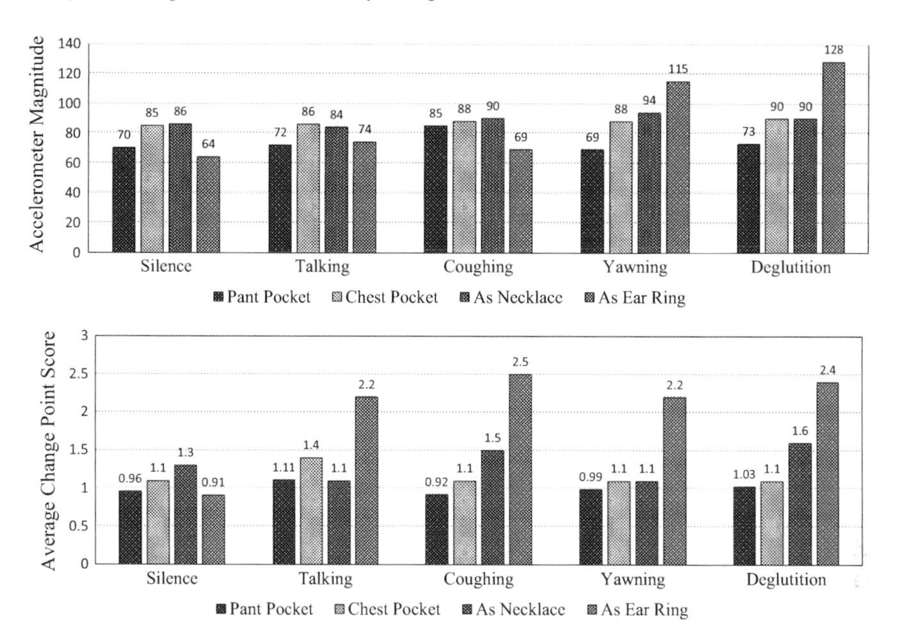

Fig. 3 Comparing different body positions (pant pocket, chest pocket, neck, ear) to capture different types of gestural motion

change-point detection scores of each activity in different position. We can clearly see that consideration of average change-point scores gives us ear position as most values for each gestural activities except silience which coincides with the real-life scenario. The breathing motion only affects chest and neck creating abrupt changes in acceleration than at pant pocket or ear. This continuous changes in acceleration due to the inherent breathing activity poses challenges to detect our finer IGAs based on chest or neck mounted accelerometer. Through the device position experiment (as shown in Fig. 3), we establish that the position ear is always less affected by any external noise sources providing more information about the relevant gestural activities in presence of regular ADLs.

5.3 Analysis of Oral Gestural Activity Patterns

The continuous and instantaneous periodicity of oral gestural activities and their impacts on human motion pose significant challenges on dintinguishing them from each other successfully. Different gestural activities have different motion characteristics and intensity that posit valuable movement information to differentiate them. Every infrequent oral gestural activity (e.g., yawning, coughing, talking etc.) occurs when a sequence of events is stimulated by the presence of sputum or foreign particles in the main, central airways of a person [47]. For example, normal coughing can

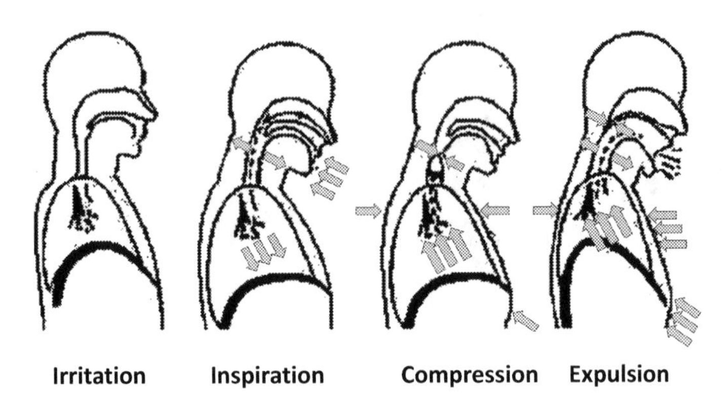

Fig. 4 Usual coughing consists of four events: **a** irritation, **b** inspiration, **c** compression and **d** expulsion

be referred as the sequence of irritation, inspiration, compression and expulsion [47]. Irritation is an abnormal stimulus which provokes sensory fibers to send impulses to the brain's medullary cough center. In inspiration phase, the glottis becomes wide open due to reflex muscle contraction. Each phase of coughing causes a unique pattern of movement associated with the human body (as shown in Fig. 4). In Fig. 4, we see sudden upward and downward movements during different coughing phases of movements. To capture these slightest movements and acceleration changes of the user, we place an accelerometer as a smart jewelry earring.

From the above discussion, we can firmly say that different micro events that construct human gestures can be defined with a sequence of micro events. However, the duration, occurrence sequence and acceleration features in terms of body movements of those micro events vary from one gesture to another. For example, single cough consists of four events: irritation, inspiration, compression, and expulsion but normal yawning consists of only irritation, inspiration and expulsion having different duration [47]. On the otherhand, dry coughing caused by tuberculosis, consecutive coughing can be occurred which may cause intense pain in the throat creating several extra compression events. Thus it is extremely challenging to recognize IGAs using a unified model. While using smart earring to capture the acceleration of the different types of coughing, the x and z axis accelerometer sensor data are always steady, but y axis acceleration increases when the transition from irritation to inspiration occurs. On the other hand the acceleration decreases when the transition from compression to expulsion occurs (see Fig. 5). In Fig. 6, if we consider raw acceleration signals, different gestural activities have almost similar movement patterns that makes it is impossible to classify. To distinguish these similar statistical features we propose to use change-point scoring method on each statistical feature. Figure 6 shows the change-point scores of magnitudes applied on each statistical feature which visualize the unique pattern of each IGA.

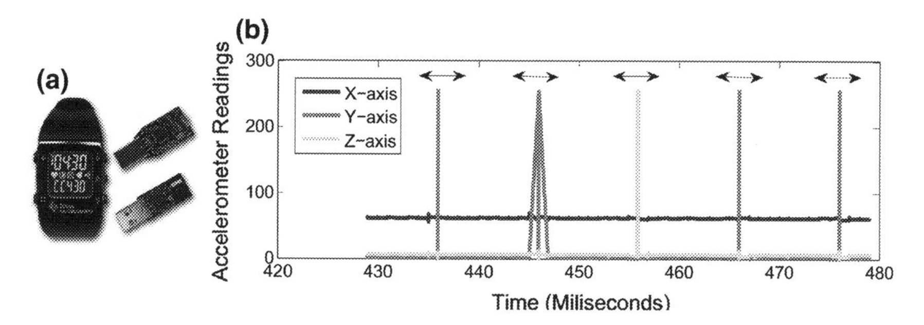

Fig. 5 **a** Chronos. Wrist Watch, CC1111 USB RF access point, eZ430 USB programming and debugging interface **b** Coughing data from Chronos used as earring

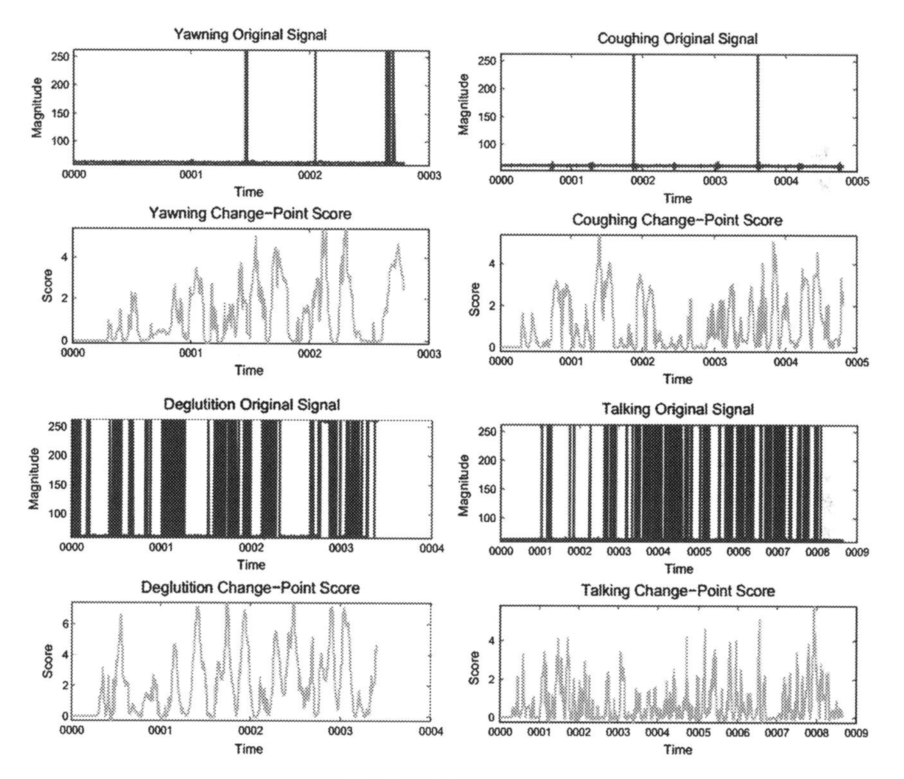

Fig. 6 Acceleration (magnitude $= \sqrt{x^2 + y^2 + z^2}$) and corresponding Change-Point Score of talking, coughing, yawning and deglutition

6 Experimental Methodology

Detection of abrupt changes based on change-point scores can be classified into two categories:

- Real-time detection: It targets applications that require immediate responses such as intrusion detection, robot control etc.
- Retrospective detection: It targets more robust results in detecting abrupt signal changes although detection may require longer reaction periods.

In this paper, we incorporate retrospective change-point detection based method along with a unique segmentation algorithmic approach to distinguish different IGAs with more fine-grained granularity.

6.1 Device Setup and Customization

We choose Texas Instruments Chronos development [48] device which was found to fit our needs and used for the development. 'Chronos' an MSP430-compatible system-on-chip with an integrated wireless modem is usually being used as a smart watch. We customized the basic communication firmware establishing communications between computer and the integrated modem through wireless "access point". The accelerometer integrated with the Chronos device is a Bosch BMA250 [49] which offers a bandwidth of up to 1000 Hz. Though the pre-programmed device provides an evaluation firmware that demonstrates the features of the device it does not provide an option to save the data received to disk or in the computer. We develop interfacing software, communications between the Texas Instruments host-side software and the virtual COM port parser. The software was written in C# and the data was saved to computer hard drive in a CSV format (Fig. 7).

6.2 Data Collection

We recruited 20 student volunteers (5 female and 15 male) with different heights (mean 170.3 cm with standard deviation 5.83 cm), weights (mean 176.3 pounds with standard deviation 15.3) and ages (19–30 years old with mean 25.3 and standard deviation 2.6) to collect five different IGAs as mentioned before in two postural positions (i.e., standing and sitting). The participants were asked to wear our customized earring device on their ear and to perform 5 different gestural activities (IGAs are listed in Table 1). While most of the previous works considered talking and silence activities as noise [5, 50], in our system we consider them one of the gestural activities that also should be distinguished from each other as well. In total, each of our

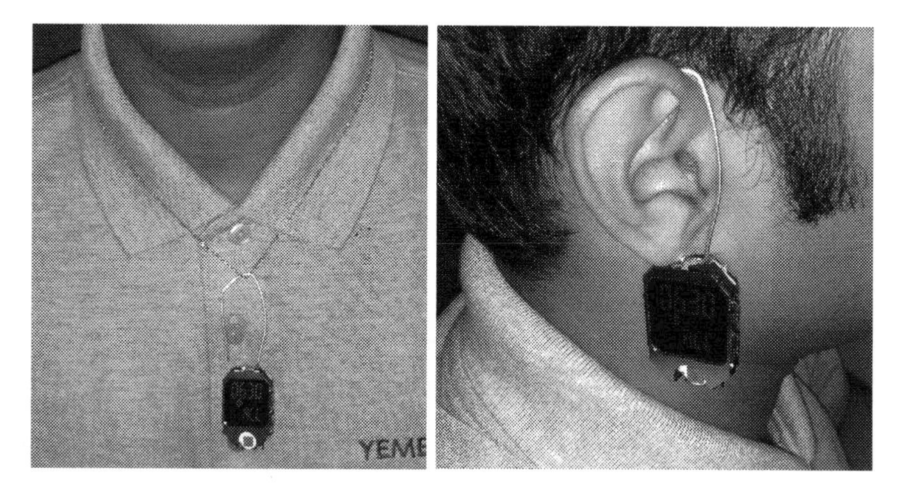

Fig. 7 Chronos in different position

Table 1 Gestural activities with distribution details

Index	Gestures	Details	# Samples	Time distribution (min)
1	Silence	No gestural activities		181.6
2	Coughing	Natural two consecutive coughing (single, consecutive two and three)	263 (186, 49 and 28)	12.6 (7.7, 3.2 and 1.7 respectively)
3	Yawning	Natural yawning	285	19.3
4	Deglutition	Natural water deglutition	281	31.15
5	Talking	Normal talking	220	55.3
		Total		300

participants performed a session of data collection of 15 min with proper instructions and sequences. Table 1 shows the detailed description of our captured IGAs and gestural activities.

6.2.1 Description of Data Collection Session

We build a video manual instructing how the participants require to perform the IGAs. The manual starts with an instruction about the entire experiment, the goals of the experiment, final outcomes and a consent form. Then, the participants are asked to read several segments of paragraphs in natural talking voice chosen from recent articles published in New York Times newspaper displayed on the screen. Then, the video displays an instruction requesting to cough for 1–3 consecutive times as natural as possible. Similarly, the participants are asked through the video instruction to perform all of the IGAs and silence activities in two different positions, (i) sitting and (ii) standing. A glass of water is kept in front of the participants to help perform 'deglutition'. However, the participants are allowed to do any of the 5 activities at any time in the middle of the session. A webcam camera enabled with an audio recording has been configured with time to record entire session. The nature of 'coughing' is designed very carefully in three coughing forms (single, two consecutive and three consecutive) as rest of the activities (i.e., 'silence','talking', 'yawning' and 'deglutition') do not have diversity like 'coughing' in natural scenario.

Two trained graduate student annotators are recruited to properly annotate the ground truth of the entire session and another one graduate student is recruited to validate the annotation. To help them annotate the ground truth, a continuous graph of acceleration magnitude (similar to Fig. 6 spectrogram) has been displayed along with the video. Table 1 shows the details of our dataset, class distribution and subclass of coughing (single, consecutive two and consecutive three coughing samples) distribution with sample sizes.

We plot corresponding spectrograms of our collected gestural activities in Fig. 6. In the spectrograms visualization, 'Silence' is not shown separately due to its presence in between of every two consecutive gestural events. While the distinct spectral pattern is not clearly visible in the original graph of raw accelerometer spectrum, change-point scoring for all of the gestural activities makes it more clear.

6.3 Feature Extraction

We split each time series data stream into a set of non-overlapping windows of feature vectors. We used 18 statistical features that have uni-axial and bi-axial statistical properties. The uni-axial statistics were applied to data from each axis separately and the bi-axial statistic was applied to data from each of the $C_2^3 = 3$ possible pairs of axes for a total of $18 \times 3 + 3 = 57$ features [51]. We briefly describe our feature sets below.

The sum and the sample mean act such properties that as more intense activities will tend to involve higher rates of acceleration during movement. We also used the 10th, 25th, 50th, 75th, and 90th percentiles of the data, as well as signal power and log energy as supplemental measures of overall activity intensity. The standard deviation, coefficient of variation, amplitude, zero crossings count and the interquartile range are useful for discriminating between activities with a consistent level of intensity and activities. Lag-one-autocorrelation, skewness, kurtosis, and peak intensity are useful for discriminating between activities that tend to be similar in their overall intensity and variation in intensity. The correlation coefficient feature, which discriminates between activities where acceleration values in one axis are predictive of acceleration values in another axis, versus activities where that is not the case. We also applied change-point scoring [39] on each axis value and extracted above mentioned 57 statistical features on these. We used efficient feature selection algorithm to find out the best features out of 114 (57 + 57) features separately.

6.4 Feature Selection

Our above mentioned feature extraction method generates 114 statistical features. We use the correlation feature selection (CFS) algorithm to select the subset of features to improve the computational efficiency of our method [52].

6.5 Performance Metrics

To measure the performance of our classification algorithms we used two performance metrics, accuracy and detection time. Accuracy is computed by counting the number of correctly predicted ticks for each true window separately, summing the counts, and dividing by the total number of ticks. From Fig. 8, the accuracy of the prediction is given as follows:

$$Accuracy = \frac{CPT(A_1) + CPT(B) + CPT(C) + CPT(A_2)}{(Total\ number\ of\ ticks)} = \frac{3+3+0+4}{20} = 50\% \tag{4}$$

where $CPT(.)$ is the number of correctly predicted ticks in an interval, and A_1 and A_2 are the true class "A" windows.

Detection time is computed by counting how many ticks are required for a prediction algorithm to start correctly predicting the class, after a true window begins. From Fig. 8 the true window begins at tick 1 (class A), the algorithm predicts A immediately, so the detection time for that window is 0. Over the second true window beginning at tick 4 (class B), the algorithm does not start predicting B until tick

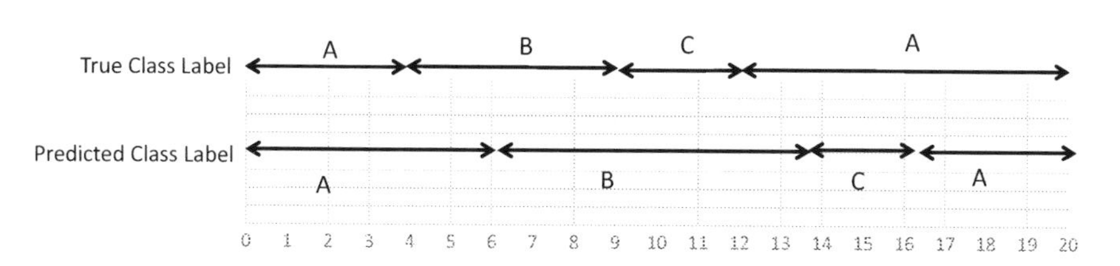

Fig. 8 Time series example with 20 ticks from a dataset of three classes A, B and C with true labels and predicted labels

6 so the detection time for that window is $6 - 4 = 2$ and so on. Thus the average detection time over the time series segment is:

$$\frac{(0 + 2 + 3 + 4)\ ticks}{4\ windows} = \frac{9}{4}\ ticks\ per\ window$$

7 Evaluation

Activity recognition using accelerometer data is a rapidly emerging field with many real-world applications. We apply accelerometer data based activity recognition for infrequent gestural behavior analysis and detection. Though much of the prior works in this area have assumed that the accelerometer data has already been segmented into pure activities, in reality, activity recognition would need to be applied to "free-living" data, which is collected over a continuous time period and would consist of a mixture of activities. We applied our proposed novel change-point segmentation based method and compare their performances with traditional fixed segment based HMM method as follows.

7.1 Change-Point Scoring Based Segmentation

In this approach, we used [39] written Matlab implementation of relative density ratio based change-point scoring algorithm [53] (explained in Sect. 5). Once change-point detection scores were generated, we tested a number of threshold values that determined which scores were high enough to be considered a predicted change-point. Threshold values were chosen by considering the false positive rates of change prediction for the change-point detection algorithms. A smaller false positive rate corresponded to a higher and more conservative threshold, which split the time series into fewer segments. A larger false positive rate corresponded to a lower threshold, which split the time series into more segments. After segmenting the data, we extracted features (114 features), applied feature selection and finally classify using mostly explored classifiers for IGAs recognition. Towards the classification, we split data stream into three equal parts: training, validation and testing.

7.2 Baseline Classification Method

In this method, we partitioned each time series into small non-overlapping windows, where each window corresponded to a discrete time index in the HMM (explained in Sect. 6). Then we applied feature extraction on each window. We build and tunes classification models (SVM, C4.5 and Neural Networks) to select observation state.

We split data into 4 equal parts: training base classifier, validation, training (HMM), and testing. Here we formulated the problem of making predictions on the testing set in terms of an HMM by treating the second training set as a training HMM. In our dataset we let X be the ground truth activity classes of the windows, and O be the predicted activity classes of the windows. We used the procedure above to calculate $\hat{T}$ and $\hat{S}$, and assumed that these estimates held for the testing set as well as the second training set. We then used the tuned base classifier to predict on the testing set, giving us O. Finally, we used O, $\hat{T}$ and $\hat{S}$ to run the Viterbi algorithm on the testing set and predict the ground truth activity classes X.

7.3 *Performance Analysis*

We tested our approaches with five base classifiers: decision tree, support vector machines, neural networks, naive Bayes and Bayesian network. We used WEKA API in java platform for our experiments. For decision tree, we chose C4.5 (J48 in WEKA API) with a confidence factor of 0.25. J48 implementation of WEKA API provides auto pruning for tuning the classifier which helped avoid the usage of validation dataset. We used [54] implementation of support vector machine called sequential minimal optimization (SMO). For neural network, we used the iteration number of 1000 with 100 hidden layers. We implemented Hidden Markov Model (HMM) in java platform using HMMWeka [55] package. The details of results of our two approaches are described as follows.

7.3.1 Change-Point Scoring Segmentation Method

In this approach, we followed two different strategies. First, we have extracted 57 pre-defined features using the raw sensor data stream (x, y and z axis values) and used CFS algorithm to choose 13 best features for target classifiers. In Fig. 9a and b, we illustrated details of performance metrics (accuracy and detection time) of our chosen 5 different classifiers with increasing of change-point score threshold for segmentation. Second, we have extracted 57 features using the change-point score of the data stream and used CFS algorithm to choose 11 best features for final classification. Figure 9c and d presented details performance metrics of our base classifiers with increasing of change-point score. Figure 9 clearly shows that change-point score threshold 3 gives the best performance of each base classifier. We also can say that though Naive Bayes classifier performs better in terms of detection time, Decision Tree algorithm outperforms another classification algorithms as it provides the most accurate classification and close to best detection time.

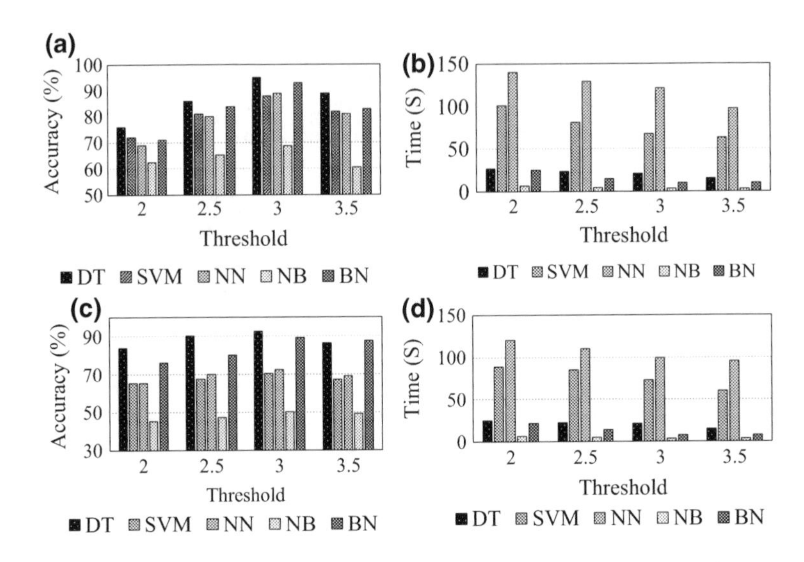

Fig. 9 Comparisons of different base classifiers with the increasing of change-point score segmentation threshold with features from raw sensor **a** accuracy versus threshold **b** detectiontime versus threshold and features from change-point scores of time series data stream **c** accuracy versus threshold **d** detection time versus threshold

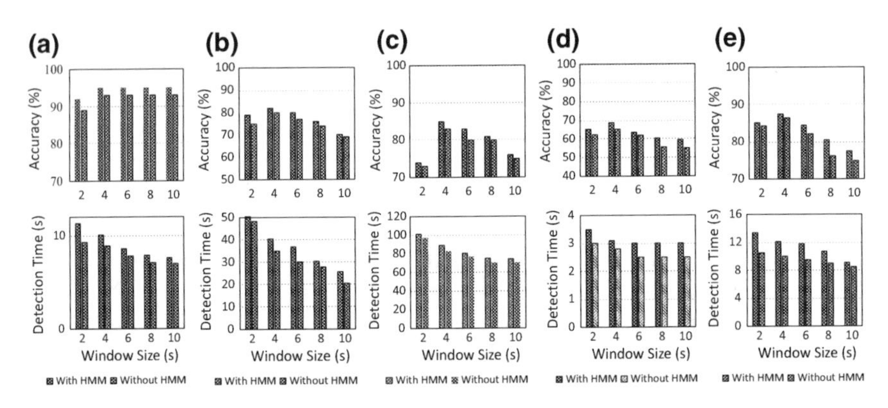

Fig. 10 Comparisons of HMM performance (accuracy on the top and detection time on the bottom) with the increasing of window sizes based on different base classifiers **a** Decision Tree **b** Support Vector Machine **c** Neural Network **d** Naive Bayes **e** Bayesian Networks

7.3.2 HMM Based Method

In this approach, we split each time series into windows of fixed length corresponding to discrete time 'ticks' in an HMM, and results for windows of length 2; 4; 6; 8; 10 s are shown in Fig. 10. We can see the window size of 4 s always gives better classification accuracy as Decision Tree outperforms other base classifiers. It also depicts that in every case, incorporating HMM increases the accuracy measure for all base classifier. Meanwhile, the increment of window size is inversely proportional to the detection time.

7.3.3 Comparison

From the above results, we can see, for change-point scoring based segmentation method, the best performance can be achieved if we use raw sensor data stream for feature extraction and change-point score threshold of 3 for segmentation with Decision Tree classification algorithm. On the other hand, for HMM based classification method, we can achieve best performance if we use raw sensor data stream and 4 s window size of segmentation with Decision Tree classification algorithm as base classifier. For the first method, we achieved maximum accuracy of $\approx$95% with 21.1 s of detection time on average. On the other hand, for HMM-based method, we achieved maximum accuracy of $\approx$96% with 10.5 s of detection time on an average. Tables 2 and 3 show the true positive rate (TP rate), false positive rate (FP rate), recall, precision and F-measure from the 10-fold cross validation experiment of both baseline and our method. Though, our first method shows significant accuracy, the second approach slightly outperformed in terms of both accuracy and detection time. HMM-based approach does not include the computation of a change-point detection

Table 2 The TP rate, FP rate, Precision, Recall and F-measure for each class from the LOPO experiment using C4.5 as classifier and change-point score as frame-level features

Accuracy	TP rate (%)	FP rate (%)	Precision (%)	Recall (%)	F-measure (%)
Silence	95.7	5.8	96.4	95.7	96.0
Coughing	86.0	00.3	84.0	86.0	85.0
Yawning	90.5	0.1	93.8	90.5	92.1
Deglutition	88.5	1.9	85.8	88.5	87.1
Talking	96.5	1.2	95.9	96.5	96.2
Weighted Avg.	95.1	4.1	95.3	95.1	95.1

Table 3 The TP rate, FP rate, Precision, Recall and F-measure for each class from the HMM Experiment

Accuracy	TP rate (%)	FP rate (%)	Precision (%)	Recall (%)	F-measure (%)
Silence	97.8	7.5	96.4	97.5	97.1
Coughing	88.4	00.7	90.1	88.4	89.2
Yawning	81.5	0.3	89.5	87.3	88.4
Deglutition	87.3	0.5	89.5	87.3	85.8
Talking	92.4	1.3	93.0	92.4	92.7
Weighted Avg.	95.8	5.7	96.1	96.3	96.0

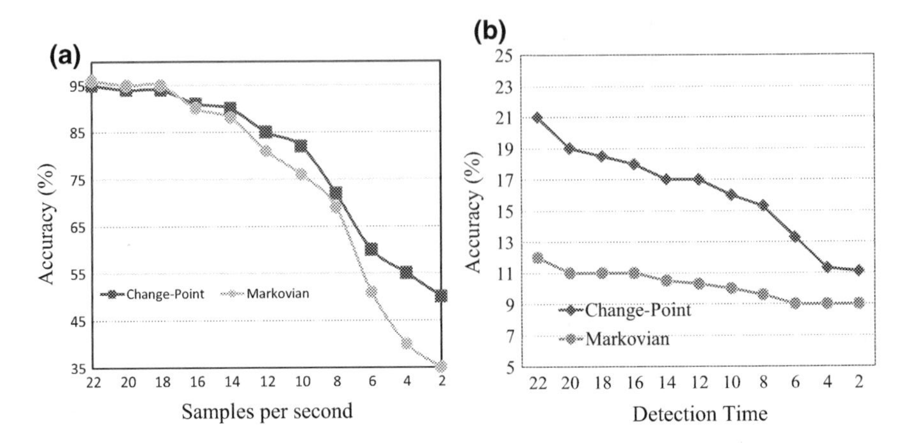

Fig. 11 Comparisons of HMM and change-point based classification performances with the decreasing of sampling rate in terms of **a** accuracy and **b** detection time

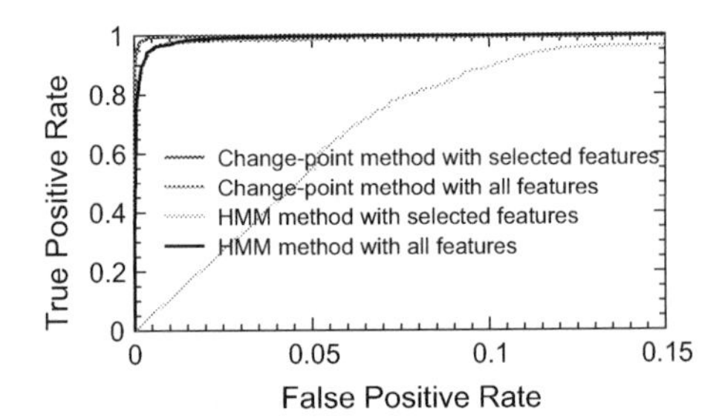

Fig. 12 ROC curve true positive versus false positive rate

score, but does include a final step the computation (via the Viterbi algorithm) of the set of hidden states in an HMM that are most likely to correspond with classifier predictions on the windows in the test data. The Viterbi algorithm is an offline algorithm that considers all of the windows in the time series rather than just the latest window, but it nonetheless runs quickly.

From the above results, it is really difficult to disseminate that HMM-based model outperforms change-point detection based model as the outperformance is not significant ($\approx 1\%$). To expurgating the comparison more clearly, we reduce our sampling rate from 22 to 2 samples per second and analyze the accuracy and detection time for both of our approaches illustrated in Fig. 11. From Fig. 11, we can depict that for low sampling rate, change-point score based classification outperforms HMM-based approach. Figure 12 shows the ROC curve for both of our method that clearly depicts that change-point based method outperforms HMM-based method significantly. However, Fig. 12 also depicts that how correlation feature selection can improve the classification accuracies for both change-point and HMM-based method. Table 4 clearly depicts that our model outperforms other existing solutions in classifying different types of IGAs.

Table 4 Comparison with prior works' classification recalls measure

Methods	Hayley Hung [50] 2013	BodyBeat [5] 2014 (%)	1st approach (%)	2nd approach (%)
Silence	N/A	74.38	95.9	97.6
Coughing	N/A	80.0	82.7	88.4
Yawning	24%	75.0	80.2	81.5
Deglutition	21%	72.09	81.1	87.3
Talking	82.0%	81.06	89.0	92.4
Weighted Avg.	N/A	71.2	95.3	96.7

7.4 Performance on Benchmark Datasets

It has become really hard to come up with a firm conclusion that our proposed change-point detection based segmentation outperforms existing HMM-based method significantly in lower sampling rate from the above analysis. To strengthen our method's outperformance precisely, we choose two benchmark datasets with high sampling rate, HHAR [56] and REALDISP [57], to evaluate our novel change-point detection based segmentation method in terms of sampling rate.

HHAR dataset consist of 6 postural activities (biking, sitting, standing, walking, stair up and stair down), accelerometer and gyroscope sensors integrated 12 wearable devices (4 smartwatches, 8 smartphones) with 9 users. We choose only one Samsung Galaxy S3 smartphone integrated accelerometer sensor streams (sampling frequency 100 Hz) placed in the right pocket of each user for detecting 6 postural activities performances to evaluate the efficiency of our approach. On the other hand, REALDISP dataset consists of 33 activities, multi sensors (accelerometer, gyroscope and magnetometer) integrated wearable devices in 9 difference nodes of the body with 17 users. We choose right thigh worn wearable sensor device integrated accelerometer signal streams (sampling frequency 50 Hz) and 6 activities (walking, jogging, running, jump up, jump sideways, and cycling) dataset to evaluate our approach's efficiency.

For change-point detection based approach, we apply change-point scores and find the segments, apply accelerometer feature extraction and feature selection to extract 12 best features then finally apply decision tree algorithm to evaluate results. For fixed length segmentation technique, we first set the segment window to 4 s, apply accelerometer feature extraction and feature selection to extract 12 best features and apply HMM method (explained before) for classifying activities (Fig. 13).

In REALDISP dataset, classification accuracies with change-point based decision tree method shows 86.9% (FP rate 11.5%) while fixed length segmentation based HMM algorithm shows 82.3% (FP rate 13.3%). On the other hand, on HHAR dataset, our change-point segmentation based decision tree algorithm shows 93.4% (FP rate 3.5%) accuracy while HMM-based classification accuracy stagnates at 87.3% (FP rate 9.3%). We downsample the sensor signal by a fixed factor to test the algorithms

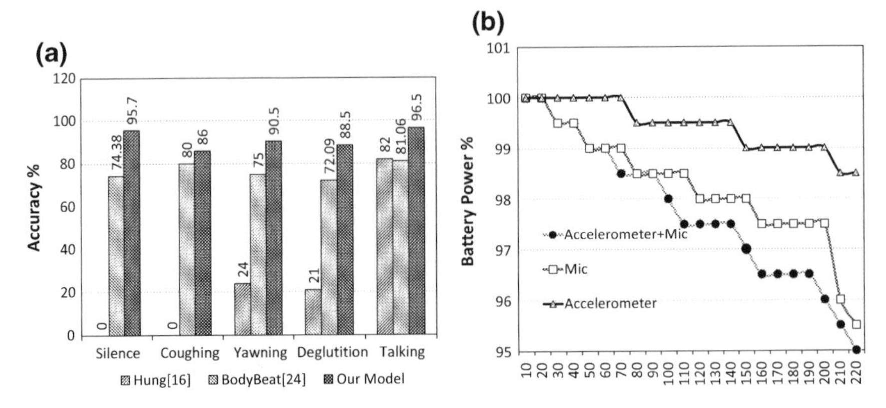

Fig. 13 **a** Comparison of Results with prior works **b** Comparison of battery power drop of sensors

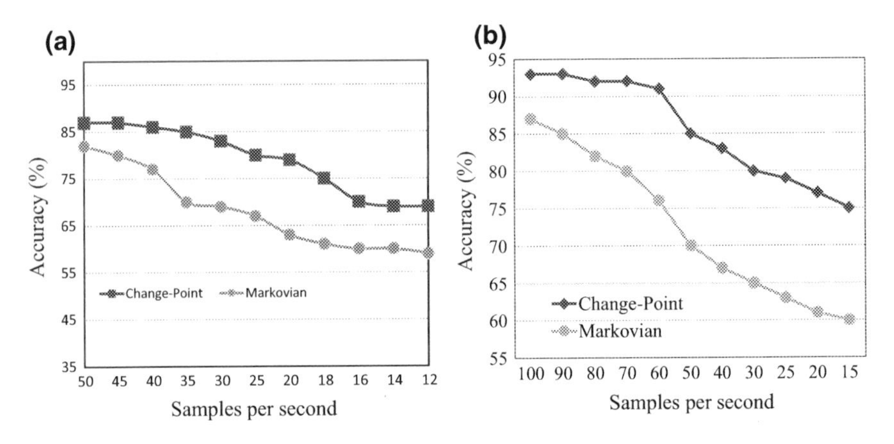

Fig. 14 Comparisons of change-point segmentation method based decision tree algorithm and fixed length segmentation based HMM algorithm accuracies on **a** REALDISP and **b** HHAR datasets

performances in lower sampling frequency. Figure 14 shows the comparisons of the accuracies for both of our method and HMM method on two benchmark datasets which clearly depicts that in lower sampling rate, our method outperforms traditional fixed length based HMM method significantly.

8 Discussion

The body motion and social behavior of the people are highly correlated [58–60]. It has also been proven that, social psychology has strong correlation with both the speech and body gestures among the speaker and listener [59, 60]. In lower sampling

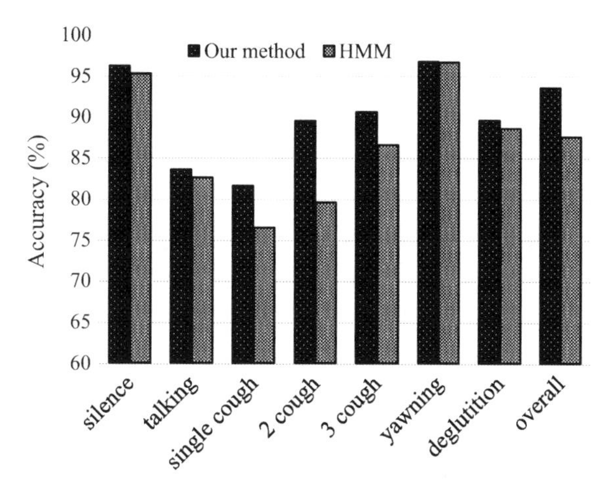

Fig. 15 Accuracy comparison for 7-class problem based on our proposed method and fixed length HMM method

rate, the traditional accelerometer feature-based activity recognition fails to achieve higher accuracy for infrequent gesture recognition because each infrequent gestural activity executes completely different pattern with different episode duration. Fixed length segmentation fails to find fine-grained classification accuracy which necessitates to apply different segmentation for different activity classification. In this chapter, we show that CPS approach outperforms the fixed length based traditional activity recognition methods in terms of accuracy and close enough in terms of the detection time toward classification of IGAs. GeSmart also attests significant energy savings sustaining the detection accuracy compared to the existing methods (Fig. 13). We do more microscopic analysis of 'coughing' activity recognition performance to evaluate our proposed change-point segmentation based method and fixed length segmentation based HMM method. If we consider, three 'coughing' states (single, two and three consecutive coughing) as three classes, then our total classification problem consists of 7 classes ('silence','talking','single coughing', 'consecutive two coughing', 'consecutive three coughing', 'yawning' and 'deglution'). Figure 15 shows the classification accuracies for 7 class problem of the two approaches which clearly depicts that the detection accuracy of 'consecutive three coughing' is much higher for both of the method followed by 'consecutive two coughing' and 'single coughing' IGAs. However, it also can be seen that our method outperforms for both overall and individual coughing IGAs classification accuracies. To test our feature selection performance, we train

Privacy and energy efficiency: Collecting data from microphone or camera involves serious privacy concern that doing so without proper consent of the users is unethical and often illegal. Hence, most of the people especially the elderly people, are reluctant of wearing some devices which capture audio or video of ADLs. Our system values user's privacy by applying a highly privacy concerned sensor accelerometer. However, only using accelerometer itself reduces significant amount of energy consumptions. For example, as shown in Fig. 13b, a simple measure of battery power drainage of different sensors in Google Nexus 4 smartphone shows that accelerometer sensor helps improve the battery life of smartphone 2.3 and 3.3 times respectively compared to an audio and audio cum accelerometer sensor based activity recognition approach.

9 Conclusion and Future Work

Behavioral health safety assurance of older adults has become increasingly important as the number of older adults living worldwide and average life expectancy of them increases. In this chapter, we presented an energy efficient infrequent IGAs recognition model to predict the chronic behavioral conditions. We explored one online (CPS), one offline (HMM) method and a smart segmentation method towards classification of IGAs in different human postures. Change-point detection is a field of statistics popular in control theory and other similar applications. This method takes as input an initial time series and partitions it into smaller pieces using change-point detection. While, regular activity recognition can be exploited easily using fixed length window based traditional activity recognition algorithm, infrequent gestural level activity recognition fails with it in terms of lower sampling rate which is usual case for available cheap devices. We are the first of a kind used Change-point scoring based segmentation to provide more fine-grained classification accuracy for IGAs detection than existing works.

The objective of this work is to make an energy efficient, computationally fast and accurate classification of activities which are subjected to be abrupt changes (infrequent non-speech gestures like coughing, deglution and yawning) and distinguish them from other frequent gestures (such as talking and silence). For any sensor device, sensing with low sampling rate is one of the primary ways of reducing computational cost and energy consumption. However, low sampling rate costs the accuracy which can be reduced using proper segmentation rather than using fixed length segmentation. We propose a new segmentation technique (change-point detection based) and compare its performance with the most popular fixed length segmentation based technique (HMM).

Our device is customized in the lab and not commercially marketable. The device needs more miniaturization and light weight conversion to use it as an ubiquitous wearable earring for older adults. Our initial goal of this study is to find out the opportunity to detect IGAs using only a single accelerometer integrated earring with very lower sampling rate thus the data length and transmission consume less power. That is why, we customize a device that facilitates a controllable sampling rate. In our future goal, we will build a complete, light weight, energy efficient, micro accelerometer sensor integrated earring that can come up with all commercial requirements.

Acknowledgements The work is supported in part by the National Science Foundation (NSF) under grants CNS-1344990, CNS-1544687, and IIP-1559752; the ONR under grant N00014-15-1-2229; Constellation: Energy to Educate; and the University of Maryland Baltimore-University of Maryland Baltimore County (UMB-UMBC) Research and Innovation Partnership grant.

References

1. Mohammad Arif Ul Alam, Nirmalya Roy, Michelle Petruska, Andrea Zemp, Smart-Energy Group Anomaly Based Behavioral Abnormality Detection, IEEE Wireless Health Conference 2016, WH
2. Nicholas D. Lane, Petko Georgiev, Lorena Qendro: DeepEar: robust smartphone audio sensing in unconstrained acoustic environments using deep learning. UbiComp 2015: 283–294
3. F. S. Wei, L. C. D. Silva, Speech based emotion classification, International Conference on Electrical Electronic Technology, 2001, 1, 297–301
4. Oh-Wook Kwon, Kwokleung Chan, Jiucang Hao, Te-Won Lee, Emotion Recognition by Speech Signals, In proceeding of: 8th European Conference on Speech Communication and Technology, EUROSPEECH, 2003, 125–128
5. T. Rahman, A. Adams, E. Carroll, B. Zhou, H. Peng, Mi Zhang, T. Choudhury, BodyBeat: A Mobile System for Sensing Non-Speech Body Sounds, International Conference on Mobile Systems, Applications and Services (MobiSys), 2014
6. R. Cowie, E Douglas-Cowie, Automatic statistical analysis of the signal and prosodic signs of emotion in speech, Fourth International Conference on Spoken Language, 1996. ICSLP 96. Proceedings, 1996, 3, 1989–1992
7. Xia Mao, Bing Zhang, Yi Luo, Multi-level Speech Emotion Recognition Based on HMM and ANN, WRI World Congress on Computer Science and Information Engineering, 2009, 7, 225–229
8. Xin Min Cheng, Pei Ying Cheng,Li Zhao, A Study on Emotional Feature Analysis and Recognition in Speech Signal, Proceedings of the International Conference on Measuring Technology and Mechatronics Automation (ICMTMA), 2009, 1, 418–420
9. K. H. Kim, S. W. Bang, S. R. Kim, Emotion recognition system using short-term monitoring of physiological signals, Medical and Biological Engineering and Computing, 2004, 42, 419–427
10. R. W. Picard , E. Vyzas , J. Healey, Toward machine emotional intelligence: analysis of affective physiological state, IEEE Transactions on Pattern Analysis and Machine Intelligence, 2001, 23, 1175–1191
11. I.A. Essa, A.P. Pentland, Coding, analysis, interpretation, and recognition of facial expressions, IEEE Transactions on Pattern Analysis and Machine Intelligence, 1997, 19, 757–763
12. Ying-Li Tian, T. Kanade, J.F. Cohn, Recognizing action units for facial expression analysis, IEEE Transactions on Pattern Analysis and Machine Intelligence, 2001, 23, 97–115
13. J. Fogarty, C. Au, and S.E. Hudson. Sensing from the basement: a feasibility study of unobtrusive and low-cost home activity recognition. In Proceedings of the 19th annual ACM symposium on User interface software and technology, UIST '06, pages 91–100, New York, NY, USA, 2006. ACM
14. J. Rowan and E.D. Mynatt. Digital family portrait field trial: Support for aging in place. In Proceedings of the SIGCHI Conference on Human Factors in Computing Systems, CHI '05, pages 521–530, New York, NY, USA, 2005. ACM
15. T.V. Duong, H.H. Bui, D.Q. Phung, and S. Venkatesh. Activity recognition and abnormality detection with the switching hidden semi-markov model. In IEEE Computer Society Conference on Computer Vision and Pattern Recognition, pages 838–845, June 2005
16. Mohammad Arif Ul Alam, Nirmalya Roy, GeSmart: A Gestural Activity Recognition Model for Predicting Behavioral Health, International Conference on Smart Computing, SmartComp 2014, Hong Kong

17. Mohammad Arif Ul Alam, Nirmalya Roy, Aryya Gangopadhyay, Elizabeth Galik, A Smart Segmentation Technique Towards Improved Infrequent Non-Speech Gestural Activity Recognition Model, Pervasive and Mobile Computing (PMC) Special Issue on Gerontechnology
18. Drew Williams, Mohammad Arif Ul Alam, Sheikh Iqbal Ahamed, William Chu, Considerations in Designing Human-Computer Interfaces for Elderly People, International Conference on Quality Software, 2013, QSIC/SQHE
19. A. Parate, M. Chiu, C. Chadowitz, D. Ganesan, E. Kalogerakis: RisQ: recognizing smoking gestures with inertial sensors on a wristband. MobiSys 2014
20. Sougata Sen, Vigneshwaran Subbaraju, Archan Misra, Rajesh Krishna Balan, Youngki Lee: The case for smartwatch-based diet monitoring. PerCom Workshops, WristSense, 2015
21. Mohammad Arif Ul Alam, Nilavra Pathak, Nirmalya Roy, Mobeacon: An iBeacon-Assisted smart-phone-Based Real Time Activity Recognition Framework, 12th International Conference on Mobile and Ubiquitous Systems: Computing, Networking and Services, Mobiquitous 2015
22. Mohammad Arif Ul Alam, Nirmalya Roy, Sarah Holmes, Aryya Gangopadhyay, Elizabeth Galik, Automated Functional and Behavioral Health Assessment of Older Adults with Dementia, IEEE Conference on Connected Health: Applications, Systems and Engineering Technologies, CHASE 2016
23. Mohammad Arif Ul Alam, Nirmalya Roy, Archan Misra, Joseph Taylor, CACE: Exploiting Behavioral Interactions for Improved Activity Recognition in Multi-Inhabitant Smart Homes, 36th International Conference on Distributed Computing Systems, ICDCS 2016
24. Mohammad Arif Ul Alam, Nilavra Pathak, Nirmalya Roy, Mobeacon: An iBeacon-Assisted smart-phone-Based Real Time Activity Recognition Framework, 12th International Conference on Mobile and Ubiquitous Systems: Computing, Networking and Services, EAI Endorsed Transactions on Ubiquitous Environments, January, 2016
25. M. Coulson, Attributing emotion to static body postures: recognition accuracy, confusions, and viewpoint dependence, Journal of Nonverbal Behavior, 1992, 28, 2, 117–139
26. H. Gunes, M. Piccardi, Bi-modal emotion recognition from expressive face and body gestures, Journal of Network and Computer Applications, 2007, 30, 4, 1334–1345
27. Ginevra Castellano, Loic Kessous, George Caridakis, Multimodal emotion recognition from expressive faces, body gestures and speech, Artificial Intelligence and Innovations 2007: from Theory to Applications IFIP The International Federation for Information Processing, 2007, 247, 375–388
28. L.C De Silva, Pei Chi Ng, Bimodal emotion recognition, Fourth IEEE International Conference on Automatic Face and Gesture Recognition, 2000. Proceedings, 2000, 332–335
29. Mohammad Arif Ul Alam, Weiqiang Wang, Sheikh Iqbal Ahamed, William Chu, Elderly Safety: A Smartphone Based Real Time Approach, International Conference On Smart homes and health Telematics, ICOST, 2013
30. L. Bao and S.S. Intille. Activity recognition from user-annotated acceleration data. pages 1–17. Springer, 2004
31. Alaiad, A. Zhou, L. Patient Behavioural Intention toward Adopting Healthcare Robots. The 19th Americas Conference on Information Systems (AMCIS), Chicago, USA, 2013
32. Alaiad, A., & Zhou, L. (2015, January). Patients' Behavioral Intentions toward Using WSN Based Smart Home Healthcare Systems: An Empirical Investigation. In System Sciences (HICSS), 2015 48th Hawaii International Conference on (pp. 824–833). IEEE. doi:10.1109/HICSS.2015.104
33. T. Gu, Z. Wu, X. Tao, H.K. Pung, and J. Lu. Epsicar: An emerging patterns based approach to sequential, interleaved and concurrent activity recognition. In Pervasive Computing and Communications, IEEE International Conference on, 2009
34. J.R. Kwapitz, G.M. Weiss, and S. Moore. Activity recognition using cell phone accelerometers. SIGKDD, 12(2):74–82, 2010
35. K. Grauman. Efficient activity detection with max-subgraph search. In Proceedings of the 2012 IEEE Conference on Computer Vision and Pattern Recognition (CVPR), CVPR '12, IEEE Computer Society, 2012

36. Patrick S. Hamilton and E.P. Limited. Open Source ECG Analysis Software Documentation. 2002
37. Andreas Krause, Matthias Ihmig, and et al. Trading off prediction accuracy and power consumption for context-aware wearable computing, ISWC 2005
38. David Chu, Nicholas D.Lane, and et al. Balancing energy, latency and accuracy for mobile sensor data classification. In Proc. of Sensys 2011
39. Song Liu, Makoto Yamada, Nigel Collier, Masashi Sugiyama, Change-point detection in time-series data by relative density-ratio estimation, Neural Networks. 2013; 72–83
40. Y. Kawahara, T. Yairi, and K. Machida. Change-point detection in time-series data based on subspace identification. In Proceedings of the 7th IEEE International Conference on Data Mining, pages 559–564, 2007
41. S.J. Bae, B.M. Mun, and K.Y. Kim. Change-point detection in failure intensity: A case study with repairable artillery systems. Computers and Industrial Engineering, 64:11–18, January 2013
42. A.G. Tartakovsky, B.L. Rozovskii, R.B. Blazek, and H. Kim. A novel approach to detection of intrusions in computer networks via adaptive sequential and batch sequential change-point detection methods. IEEE Transactions on Signal Processing, 54:3372–3382, September 2006
43. M. Staudacher, S. Telserb, A. Amannc, H. Hinterhuberb, and M. Ritsch-Marte. A new method for change-point detection developed for on-line analysis of the heart beat variability during sleep. Statistical Mechanics and its Applications, 349:582–596, April 2005
44. Ni-Chun Wang and Hudson, R.E. and Lee Ngee Tan and Taylor, C.E. and Alwan, A. and Rung Yao, Change point detection methodology used for segmenting bird songs, Signal and Information Processing (ChinaSIP), 2013 IEEE China Summit International Conference on, 2013
45. Zhang, Chi and Hansen, John HL, Effective segmentation based on vocal effort change point detection, Speech Analysis and Processing for Knowledge Discovery, 2008
46. James. R. Anderson, Pauline Meno, Psychological Influences on Yawning in Children, Current psychology letters, 2003
47. McGarvey LP, Patterns of cough in the clinic, Pulm Pharmacol Ther. 2011 Jun;24(3):300-3
48. Chronos: http://processors.wiki.ti.com/index.php/EZ430-Chronos
49. Bosch: http://www.bosch-sensortec.com/de/homepage/products_3/3_axis_sensors/acceleration_sensors/bma250_1/bma250
50. Hayley Hung, Gwenn Englebienn, Jeroen Kools, Classifying social actions with a single accelerometer, UbiComp '13 Proceedings of the 2013 ACM international joint conference on Pervasive and ubiquitous computing, 2013, 207–210
51. Michael Mason, Physical activity recognition of free-living data using change-point detection algorithms and hidden Markov models, Masters Thesis, Oregon State University, 2013
52. Hall, M. A. Correlation-based Feature Selection for Machine Learning. PhD Thesis (April 1999)
53. Source code: http://www.makotoyamada-ml.com/RuLSIF.html
54. J. Platt: Fast Training of Support Vector Machines using Sequential Minimal Optimization. In B. Schoelkopf and C. Burges and A. Smola, editors, Advances in Kernel Methods—Support Vector Learning, 1998
55. HMMWeka, Marco Gillies, http://doc.gold.ac.uk/~mas02mg/software/hmmweka/
56. Allan Stisen, Henrik Blunck, Sourav Bhattacharya, Thor Siiger Prentow, Mikkel Baun Kjrgaard, Anind Dey, Tobias Sonne, and Mads Moller Jensen, Smart Devices are Different: Assessing and Mitigating Mobile Sensing Heterogeneities for Activity Recognition, SenSys 2015
57. O. Banos, M. A. Toth, M. Damas, H. Pomares, I. Rojas,Dealing with the effects of sensor displacement in wearable activity recognition. Sensors vol. 14, no. 6, 2014
58. T. L. Chartrand and J. A. Bargh, The chameleon effect: the perception-behavior link and social interaction, Journal of Personality and Social Psychology, 1999, 76, 6, 893–910
59. A. Kendon, Conducting Interaction: Patterns of Behavior in Focused Encounters, Cambridge University Press, 1990
60. D. McNeill, Language and Gesture, Cambridge University Press New York, 2000

Smartphone Based Real-Time Health Monitoring and Intervention

Daniel Aranki, Gregorij Kurillo and Ruzena Bajcsy

Abstract Smartphones are often dubbed as "a doctor in your pocket" as they have in recent years become one of the most notable platforms for health management and monitoring. In this chapter we discuss the potentials for real-time health monitoring of chronic health conditions and data-driven intervention that aim to improve patient care at a lower cost. We outline several challenges that developers, patients, and providers face with respect to this new technology. We then review several commercial platforms for health monitoring and discuss their pros and cons. Furthermore, we present Berkeley Telemonitoring Framework, a recently developed Andorid-based open source solution for development of health-monitoring applications with security and privacy in mind. In particular, our framework offers an easy-to-use API for building client apps, deploying data-hosting servers, fault-tolerant data retrieval and storage, access to event-based Bluetooth and BLE stacks with standards for personal health devices, access to phone sensors, implementation of several vital signs estimators, gait analysis, etc. We demonstrate the use of the framework on an example fitness application MarathonCoach. We further discuss several challenges facing real-time telemonitoring. In particular, we focus on privacy and propose a novel information-theoretic framework called Private Disclosure of Information (PDI). The PDI framework formalizes a scheme for encoding the collected health data in a manner that minimizes the ability of an adversary from gaining knowledge about the patient's diagnosis (or other information private by implication) through statistical inference, while allowing the authorized provider to use this information with no loss in utility.

D. Aranki (✉) · G. Kurillo · R. Bajcsy
University of California, Berkeley, USA
e-mail: daranki@cs.berkeley.edu

© Springer International Publishing AG 2017

S.U. Khan et al. (eds.), *Handbook of Large-Scale Distributed Computing in Smart Healthcare*, Scalable Computing and Communications,
DOI 10.1007/978-3-319-58280-1_18

1 Introduction

The current prevalent healthcare model is reactive in nature. That is, in most cases, an individual seeks medical care or advice *after* a deterioration of her or his health status is perceived. In general, the current healthcare model does not encourage people to invest into their health until notable symptoms that indicate serious conditions occur. There are some exceptions to this rule. For instance, women are encouraged to get checked regularly for breast cancer, even before any signs of deterioration are present. As such, a healthcare model where health changes can be detected in advance and intervened upon is desired. We will call this model *the proactive healthcare model* in the remainder of this chapter. Other names for this model exist in the literature, including *predictive healthcare* and *preventive healthcare*. The potential benefits of the proactive healthcare model include: (i) improvement in individuals' well-being; (ii) reduction in healthcare costs; (iii) reduction in readmission rates in chronic health conditions; and ultimately (iv) reduction in all-cause mortality.

For example, the cost of healthcare in the United States of America reached $3.0 trillion in 2014 ($9,523 per person), a 5.3% increase following the growth of 2.9% in 2013. The spending for hospital care increased 4.1% to $971.8 billion in 2014 compared to the 3.5% growth in 2013. The spending on physician and clinical services followed a similar trend by increasing 4.6% in 2014 to reach $603.7 billion from a 2.5% growth in 2013. In contrast, the acceleration in spending on prescription drugs was significantly higher in 2014 at 12.2% to reach $297.7 billion compared to the 2.4% growth in 2013 [21]. A more proactive healthcare model may help reduce these costs for individuals, healthcare institutions, the government, and insurance companies.

To reduce the rising cost of healthcare in the United States, the US legislation under President Barack Obama passed Patient Protection and Affordable Care Act (PPACA) in March 2010. One of the main mechanisms to achieve this goal was to reduce readmission rates in chronic health conditions [60, 65]. Chronic health conditions are particularly prevalent in older population which is by and large covered by the Medicare program. The Medicare program, which in 2015 covered 46 million people age 65 and older and 9 million younger people (with disabilities), is funded by taxpayers. Fig. 1 depicts the 12-month moving average of 30-day all-condition hospital readmission rates for discharges occurring in each month in Medicare. Although there is an improvement in the all-condition 30-day readmission rates following the enactment of PPACA in 2010, the full potential of improvement however is yet to be attained. For example, 26.9% of patients with congestive heart failure (CHF) in Medicare were readmitted within 30 days of discharge between October 1, 2003 and December 31, 2003 24.6% of patients with psychosis in Medicare, 22.6% of patients with chronic obstructive pulmonary disease (COPD) in Medicare and 20.1% of patients with pneumonia in Medicare were readmitted within 30 days of discharge in the same period [51]. In another study, it was reported that 50% of patients with CHF were readmitted within 6 months of discharge [43].

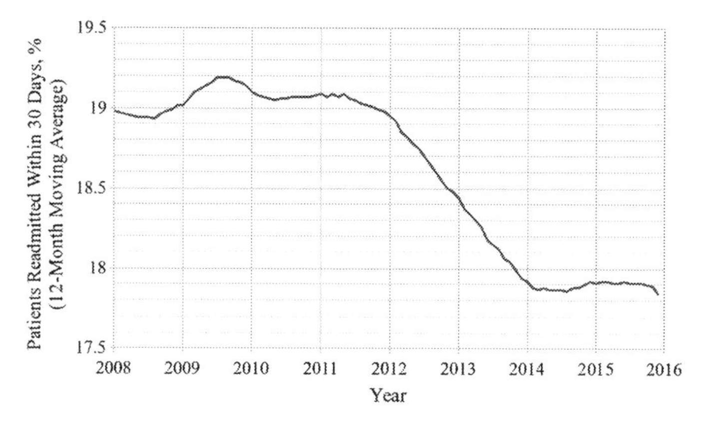

Fig. 1 Medicare 30-Day, all-condition hospital readmission rate. Data were provided by the Centers for Medicare and Medicaid Services. The plotted series reflects a 12-month moving average of the hospital readmission rates reported for discharges occurring in each month [60]

In current medical practice, patients typically visit their physician only a few times a year. This provides a limited number of data points that may not be sufficient to forecast the patient's health prognosis. In order to implement a more proactive healthcare model, more data points are needed, however with the increasing amount of information, the doctors cannot review all the data manually to provide appropriate feedback to each patient. Instead, predictive models have to be utilized to provide the decision-making support [10]. Furthermore, the data collection does not necessarily have to happen only in the clinical environment, but can be instead, with the support from technology, accomplished from home by patient self-reporting or in a more continuous manner via the real-time telemonitoring. In the last decade, smartphones have become one of the most notable platforms for health management and monitoring, giving rise to the term mHealth for services accessed through mobile technologies. In the context of healthcare, smartphones can be used not only to seek medical information online almost anytime and anywhere, but also to keep track of one's health status through various apps. However, due to the complexity of health regulations and various technical obstacles, the use of smartphones for health management has been to date primarily limited to various fitness and wellness purposes. Many clinical and technology researchers have on the other hand explored the use of smartphones in various health-related applications, including monitoring of chronic health conditions, such as CHF, diabetes, hypertension, depression and others (e.g., [62, 67]). Although such studies demonstrated the utility of mHealth technologies for telemonitoring, they were typically only observational and limited to short-term experiments in the laboratory controlled environments.

The smartphone however has the potential to not only facilitate the data collection but also to provide intervention for the proactive healthcare model. Unfortunately, continuous health monitoring comes with several challenges that need to be addressed in order to maximize the potential benefits of this approach. For example, predictive models that utilize the collected health data and the population data to assess risks of clinical deterioration first need to be developed before they can provide reliable information to patients. Predictive models for healthcare are challenging to develop and to validate clinically. For starters, the development of these predictive models requires collection of preliminary patient data, which may pose a challenge to technology researchers and data scientists who have no direct access to patients. Second, the development of the models requires expertise in medical sciences and practice; in addition to expertise in data science (for example, statistical machine learning). This usually requires collaboration between researchers from both disciplines which may pose an extra challenge in the process. Third, the clinical validation of such predictive models is a long and costly process, requiring long-term monitoring of both healthy subjects and patients with specific health conditions in order to collect sufficient data. Take, for example, the Framingham Heart Study, a study that aims to unveil facts about the epidemiology of cardiovascular diseases, which has been ongoing since 1948 [29].

Subsequently, the involvement of healthcare professionals and researchers in the development of medical apps in general, and health monitoring apps specifically, is necessary and currently lacking [48]. There are several barriers that hinder such involvement from reaching its maximum potential; most notably, the complexity of designing such apps in a technologically robust way, ensuring reliability of collected data, ensuring data security and privacy, and designing apps in a way that keep the patients engaged over time. In this chapter, we will discuss these challenges in detail and argue for the need of a more systematic approach. We will introduce a number of attempts to address them through generalized frameworks for mobile health monitoring in research and commercial space and discuss the features and potential drawbacks of these platforms. Furthermore, we will examine some of the remaining challenges and propose directions of addressing them.

Almost by definition, mobile health monitoring is a distributed paradigm. That is, the health data authored by patients are collected and partially processed at distributed nodes and submitted to distributed servers (often referred to as "the cloud"). This provides the opportunity to apply and recycle many of the techniques that are well-studied in the field of distributed computing. It is also of importance to note that incorporating distributed systems design principles when designing health monitoring systems is a requirement, if health monitoring is to be scaled beyond a small number of patients. On the other hand, the distributed nature of health monitoring systems also provides some challenges. For instance, in parallel to the technological challenges in mHealth, privacy is an important issue that needs to be addressed by design. At the same time, distributed computing could potentially help in certain privacy challenges arising in mobile health monitoring. For example, allowing medical apps to compute certain functions on the cloud allows patients to protect their privacy in case their data are needed to assess the health status of an individual patient (for example, if population data are used in the process). This goal can be achieved because the health status factor can now be calculated on trusted nodes without disclosing any particular patient data to the client app running on the smartphone. Unfortunately, a survey of the literature reveals a lack of studies on the security and privacy aspects of health apps, which have received considerable attention in the literature on more traditional eHealth technologies, such as electronic health records and databases [48]. Therefore, at the end of this chapter we provide a view of privacy from a perspective relevant to mobile health monitoring.

In the reminder of this chapter, we first review the literature for related studies in the field of telemonitoring (Sect. 2). We then survey existing solutions to smartphone-based health and fitness monitoring (Sect. 3). Finally, we introduce and describe the Private Disclosure of Information (PDI) framework, which is applicable to patient privacy in telemonitoring scenarios (Sect. 4).

2 Potential, Feasibility and Related Work

In this section we briefly review three topics that closely relate to continuous smartphone based health monitoring addressed in this chapter: (a) clinical telemonitoring, (b) use of smartphone apps in mHealth, (c) measurement of physical activity, and (d) privacy. These related works provide the background information and motivation for some of the solutions that are discussed in subsequent sections.

2.1 Telemonitoring

We first review several examples of telemonitoring for proactive healthcare which gave rise to the idea of continuous real-time monitoring with smartphone. We particularly focus on the chronic heart failure (CHF) as one of the notable examples where telemonitoring and timely intervention based on collected data could reduce the re-hospitalization rates and overall cost of care. For brevity, we summarize results from several systematic reviews while interested readers are encouraged to refer to the cited papers—and the references therein—for more information.

Telemonitoring of CHF has been the focus of several studies even before the conception of mHealth. Chaudhry et al. [22] conducted a telemonitoring randomized clinical trial, where telemonitoring was accomplished by means of telephone-based interactive voice-response system that collected daily information about symptoms and weight of patients with CHF (826 patients in the telemonitoring group and 827 in the standard care group). The collected data were subsequently reviewed by the patients' clinicians. The study reported no significant difference in hospital readmissions or mortality within 180 days from the enrollment between the two groups.

In [26], Clark et al. reviewed 14 randomized controlled trials (4,262 patients in total) of telemonitoring and/or structured telephone support for patients with CHF. Among the reviewed trials, only one study collected some form of daily physical activity information, which was self-reported to a nurse via telephone. Only five of the studies collected vital signs (e.g., weight, blood pressure, heart rate and/or periodic electrocardiogram) on a daily basis; four of which also collected information about related symptoms (e.g., fatigue). The authors reported average reduction of hospital readmissions by 21% (95% confidence interval 11–31%) and average reduction in all-cause mortality by 20% (8–31%).

The review by Giamouzis et al. reported results of 12 studies on telemonitoring of patients with CHF in [44], two of which were also included in the review by Clark et al. [26]. Although some of the studies collected self-reported data about physical activity, none of the trials captured any quantitative information, such as energy expenditure (EE), that could provide a more objective estimate of patients' physical activity levels [44].

Inglis [49] reviewed a set of 30 studies on telemonitoring and structured telephone support with medical intervention mechanisms for patients with CHF. Only one study provided subjects with activity monitors; however, the data were used for self-monitoring only and were not transmitted to the medical staff [42]. One structured telephone support study inquired daily about patients' physical activity (the study was also included in the review by Clark et al. in [26]). However, none of the reviewed studies performed continuous activity monitoring. From the above literature review it is clear that there is a need to implement more continuous monitoring that could alert physicians when changes in physical activity or relevant vital signs occur. In Sect. 2.3, we review and discuss various methods of obtaining continuous measures of physical activity that can be applicable for mHealth purposes.

2.2 mHealth and Smartphones

In this section we briefly review the smartphone app development related to mobile health (mHealth). We summarize the results of a comprehensive survey article by Hussain et al. who reviewed 133 articles on mHealth from MEDLINE, Web of Science, ScienceDirect, and IEEE Xplore [48]. The aim was to examine the trends of using smartphone apps for medical purposes (from the beginning of 2010). In their report they found that the majority of existing research literature (68/133) either concerns specific medical apps or provides an overview of apps dedicated to specific clinical specialty, disease area, or usage as a clinical tool. These areas include anesthesia, surgery (including plastic surgery), oncology, internal medicine, palliative medicine, ophthalmology, dentistry, pharmacy, psychiatry, pediatrics, infectious diseases, public health, women's health, dermatology, family medicine, endocrinology, cardiopulmonary resuscitation (CPR), asthma, cardiology, rehabilitation, and sports medicine. Another group of articles (43/133) reported on the usability and design aspects of the apps, such as evaluating existing apps or exploring desired features of mHealth systems. They further found that only a few researchers (17/133) reported on the experience in developing new medical apps. The rest of the articles (5/133) were dedicated to general frameworks that would address several aspects of medical app development and their operation. The review by Hussain et al. emphasizes (i) that medical apps development is not standarized, resulting in a relatively small number of researchers developing medical apps; and (ii) that there is a need for clinical validation of medical apps. We believe that standardization of mHealth is crucial in order to facilitate progress in the field addressing both of these shortcomings. In the rest of this chapter, we discuss several frameworks which attempt some degree of standardization for the development and operation of mHealth systems and outline the outstanding challenges in the field.

2.3 *Measurement of Physical Activity*

Regular physical activity is one of the most important factors in the primary and secondary prevention of several chronic diseases (e.g., cardiovascular disease, diabetes, cancer, hypertension, obesity, depression, and osteoporosis) and premature death [73]. Although many of the previous works used telephone support to monitor patients' activity, such service requires substantial involvement of the staff and may as such be cost-prohibitive to track larger number of patients. In addition, self-reporting through telephone creates additional burden to the patients and does not provide objective way to quantify the activity levels and vital signs in order to make reliable predictions needed for an automated alert system. In this context, an expert report by Dhurandhar et al. argues that self-reported physical activity EE data are too inaccurate to be used in scientific research [32].

Objective measurement of physical activity could thus facilitate relevant information on the patient's health status for prediction and intervention that would encourage individuals to initiate the change and sustain a positive health behavior over a longer time period, as it has been demonstrated in various wellness applications [53]. Physical activity can be in general quantified by estimating EE. Some research efforts are aimed at incorporating activity monitoring capabilities in daily-life consumer products such as the design of smart clothes and smart gloves [12, 54]. In the consumer market, several off-the-shelf products for EE data collection are currently available. Some examples include Nike+ FuelBand[1]; Fitbit's Activity Wristbands and Trackers,[2] and others. Several research studies that examined the accuracy of such monitoring showed that many of these devices are accurate in counting steps but inaccurate in EE estimation [30, 61]. In another study, researchers found smartphone applications to be more accurate in counting steps than some of the wearable devices [20]. This emphasizes the need to take into account the model of the sensor accuracy and the measurement distribution when developing predictive healthcare models.

Many wearable devices require (or benefit from) a smartphone (or other internet-connected device) and would as such require patients to carry with them an additional device at all times while having to keep track of the battery charge and connectivity. With smartphones becoming ubiquitous, we believe that the smartphone alone is currently the most convenient device for continuous EE estimation as opposed to a

[1] http://www.nike.com/us/en_us/c/nike-plus.

[2] http://www.fitbit.com/.

dedicated wristband, hip clip, heart rate monitor or other discrete tracking device [64]. One of the limiting factors in adopting wearable devices for health monitoring is the battery life [2]. Majority of the wearables work in conjunction with a smartphone and thus require charging two or more devices. Using the smartphone alone for the activity monitoring reduces the burden of keeping track of battery levels across devices, which is especially important for less tech-savvy users. Smartphones have thus the necessary sensory (e.g., accelerometer) and computing capabilities to accomplish this task. Accelerometers have been used for activity monitoring and recognition in many previous studies (for example, [33, 61]). These studies have shown that accelerometers can be used reliably to estimate EE [61]. In a study on CHF, Aranki et al. included continuous estimation of EE using the algorithm developed by Chen and Sun [24] and validated by Donaire-Gonzalez et al. [33]. The algorithm solely relies on the built-in triaxial accelerometer sensor available on the phone [10].

2.4 Privacy

Attention to privacy has been rising in the healthcare domain with the spread of electronic health-records usage and the growing data sharing between medical institutions. It has been reported that consumers are expressing increasing concerns regarding their health privacy [15, 46, 48]. Most of the research in privacy from the health community focuses on medical data publishing and is therefore database centric. For a survey of results in this domain, we refer the reader to [45].

In more general-purpose scenarios, the privacy of statistical databases and data publishing has been extensively studied. Denning et al. presented some of the early privacy threats related to inference in statistical databases and reviewed controls that are based on the lattice model [31]. Duncan et al. studied methods for limiting disclosure and linkage risks in data publishing [34, 35]. Sandhu provided a tutorial on lattice-based access controls for information flow security and privacy [69]. Later, Farkas et al. provided a survey of more results in the field of access controls to the inference problem in database security [40]. For rigorous surveys in the fields of data publishing privacy and statistical databases privacy, we refer the reader to [1, 41].

Two semantic models of database privacy of growing interest in the privacy literature are k-anonymity [71] and differential privacy [36, 37]. In k-anonymity, given a set of quasi-identifiers that can be used to re-identify subjects, a table is called k-anonymous if every combination of quasi-identifiers in the table appears in at least k records. If a table is k-anonymous, assuming each individual has a single record in the table, then the probability of linking a record to an individual is at most $1/k$. Other extensions and refinements of k-anonymity have been proposed including l-diversity [56], t-closeness [55] and others.

In differential privacy, the requirement is that the output of a statistical query should not be too sensitive to any single record in the database. Formally, given a statistical query M, then M is ϵ-differentially private if $\mathbb{P}\left(M\left(D_1\right) \in S\right) \leq e^{\epsilon} \times$

$\mathbb{P}\left(M\left(D_2\right) \in S\right)$ for any two realizations D_1 and D_2 of the database such that $|D_1 \Delta D_2| = 1$ and all $S \subset Range(M)$, where $D_1 \Delta D_2$ is the symmetric difference between D_1 and D_2 [36, 37]. Cormode showed that sensitive attribute inference can be done on databases that are differentially private and l-diverse with similar accuracy [27].

As can be seen from the review above, most of the research in data-privacy is focused on privacy-preserving data publishing and privacy-preserving statistical databases. In contrast, in Sect. 4 we will focus on preventing adverserial statistical inference of a piece of private information based on the disclosed messages in an individual's information exchange scenario during communication applicable to health telemonitoring systems.

3 Solutions

3.1 Apple Health, ResearchKit, and CareKit

Recognizing the need for smartphones to include a central data collection point for health related data, Apple in September of 2014 released Health app with an accompanying *HealthKit* Application Program Interface (API). The framework addressed the fragmentation and lack of interoperability of third-party health apps and connected health devices. Health app thus provides users with controls to grant other applications access to health and fitness data. Furthermore, it includes a dashboard with an overview that displays the data, such as heart rate, calories burned, weight, blood pressure, measured blood sugar, etc. An example screenshot is depicted in Fig. 2a.

With the release of Apple Watch in March 2015, Apple introduced *ResearchKit*, an open-source software framework designed to collect data for health and medical research. ResearchKit enables researchers to develop mobile applications that can accumulate various types of data from surveys and patient-reported vital signs, access data from Apple Health (given user permission), track movements from the phone's internal sensors or a wearable device, and take various other measurements using the iPhone [50]. The premise was to take advantage of proliferation of smartphones in daily lives and around the globe to perform scientific studies with a much larger number of subjects that was possible to date and thus help medical research move ahead faster. Simultaneously with the release of the ResearchKit, Apple announced five research studies that were lead by several prominent medical institutions around the country. The initial ResearchKit apps included: (1) *Asthma Health* app (Mt. Sinai, Weill Cornell Medical College, and LifeMap) for collecting asthma related markers, (2) *mPower* app (University of Rochester and Sage Bionetworks) for tracking symptoms in Parkinson's Diseases, (3) *Share the Journey* app (Dana-Farber Cancer Institute, UCLA Fielding School of Public Health, Penn Medicine, and Sage Bionetworks) to study quality of life of patients treated for breast

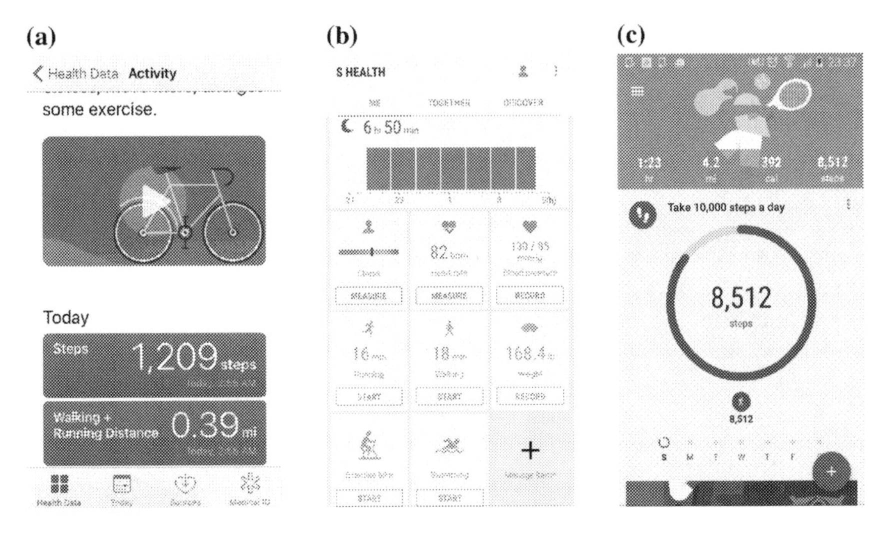

Fig. 2 **a** A screenshot of the Apple Health activity tracking screen; **b** a screenshot of the Samsung S Health summary screen; and **c** a screenshot of the Google Fit activity tracking screen

cancer, (4) *GlucoSuccess* app (Massachusetts General Hospital) to track diet, physical activity, and medication in persons with diabetes, and (5) *MyHeart Counts* app (Stanford University and American Heart Association) to study risk factors for cardiovascular disease [72]. Since the release, several other studies have been in progress, including *Autism & Beyond ResearchKit* app for autism, *CTracker* to understand impacts of hepatitis C in daily life, *Mind Share* app for studying Alzheimer's disease, and others.

ResearchKit is aimed to lower the barriers to development, integration, data storage, and distribution of such apps for clinical research. To simplify the development, the framework is composed of three pre-defined modules which can be further customized, including: (1) informed consent, (2) surveys, and (3) active tasks [50].

By providing electronic version of the informed consent for research studies, scientists using ResearchKit have much greater outreach to potential subjects across the country (and across the globe) while also simplifying and accelerating the enrollment process. When MyHeart Counts ResearchKit app lead by Stanford University was first released in March 2015, over 10,000 participants signed up within the first 24 h [5]. Such wide scale medical research however raised several ethical concerns, including privacy, research on minors, and potential issues with the informed consent process [47].

Survey modules provide pre-defined layouts to create different type of surveys that include a sequence of questions with various answering modes. The surveys can use ordered tasks where the steps are always the same or navigable ordered task where tasks can change or branch out. ResearchKit offers various answer formats, including scale, boolean, multiple choice, and location. In addition to these, the ResearchKit framework provides special answer formats for asking questions about quantities or characteristics that the user might already have stored in the Health app [3].

Finally, the active tasks modules include several pre-defined activities that are performed under semi-controlled conditions (e.g., time limited) while iPhone sensors actively collect data. The collected data are in the raw form passed on to the app. The ResearchKit framework currently includes six predefined active task categories, including motor activities, fitness, cognition, voice, audio, and hole peg. The motor activities are focused on (a) *gait and balance* and (b) *tapping speed*. Fitness active tasks include (a) *general fitness activity* and (b) *timed walk*. Cognition active tasks include (a) *Spatial memory*, (b) *Paced Serial Addition Test (PSAT)*, (c) *Tower of Hanoi*, and (d) *Reaction time measurement*. Voice active task is focused on *sustained phonation*, while audio includes *tone audiometry*. Hole peg is the latest active, which evaluates hand dexterity via multi-touch display. The developers can further extend the set of tasks by defining their own active tasks that collect simultaneous data from a set of iPhone sensors.

One of the important features of Apple ResearchKit is that it protects user privacy by giving users controls on what health information they would like to provide for each study they are enrolled in. Although ResearchKit provides encryption for data transmission and storage, it is up to the investigators to ensure that their apps are compliant with regulatory requirements (e.g., HIPAA in the United States) [68].

From the success of ResearchKit to be able to conduct large-scale studies, Apple realized that the same principles could help with individual care (Jeff Williams, Apple COO). In March 2016, Apple released *CareKit*, an open-source framework designed specifically for patient-centered disease self-management [4]. The CareKit framework is available for developers to build apps that would encourage users to take more active role in their care and share the data with their doctor. The CareKit framework was initially released with four modules that included (1) *Care Card* to help people track individual care plans and action items (e.g., taking medications), (2) *Symptom and Measurement Tracker* to let users record their symptoms via notes, measurements, and photos, (3) *Insight Dashboard* to graphically map symptoms against the action items in the Care Card to show effects of treatments, and (4) *Connect* to easily share health information with their doctor, care teams or family members [4]. The first two CareKit apps released were *Parkinson's Central* (by National Parkinson Foundation, Inc.) aimed to empower people with Parkinson's and their caregivers to track symptoms and medications and *One Drop* (Informed Data Systems, Inc.) app for managing diabetes. Several other CareKit apps are in development at the time of writing (September 2016), including apps for post-surgery progress, home health monitoring, diabetes management, mental health, and maternal health.

The open source model of Apple ResearchKit and CareKit allows the researchers and developers to continue expanding the existing set of modules and adding new ones. Some of the recent contributions include incorporation of genetic data and lab test results. Although several research studies are on-going, to date only the *mPower* study on Parkinson's Disease has published a report in a scientific journal by releasing their mobile data of subjects who opted to share their data broadly [17]. The released data includes demographics, monthly survey responses for Parkinson

Disease Questionnaire 8 (PDQ-8) and Universal Parkinson Disease Rating Scale (MDS-UPDRS), and data from four activities on memory, tapping, voice, and walking, which were completed three times a day, of over 9,000 subjects.

3.2 Samsung Digital Health and S Health[3]

Samsung launched the health platform *S Health* in July 2012 with the release of their Android phone Galaxy S III. The initial intention was to create a wellness platform that is compatible with a number of healthcare sensors such as blood glucose meters, blood pressure monitors, and body composition scales. The S Health platform was intended as the Andorid counterpart to Apple's iPhone HealthKit. Over the years, the S Health platform created an ecosystem for tracking fitness and health by providing their development platform, Samsung Digital Health software development kit (SDK), to third-party developers.

The S Health platform thus provides a mechanism for data sharing between data-sensing devices and various consumer applications for analysis, coaching, and social interaction. One of the important components of S Health is the dashboard which integrates the results obtained from various apps and provides different ways to track and visualize health data as graphs or tables. An example screenshot is depicted in Fig. 2b. The basic building block of the S Health platform is a *tracker*. The platform comprises of various pre-defined trackers, including step, weight, sleep, heart rate, oxygen saturation (SpO2), blood glucose, blood pressure, food, water and caffeine intake, and several exercise trackers. Some of the trackers can take advantage of the smartphone's internal sensors to provide values directly, such as step tracking and heart rate, while others connect to wearables or third-party apps to obtain the data for a particular tracker. Users have various privacy controls to select which data can be shared between the apps or with the platform itself.

Initially, S Health was limited only to Samsung Galaxy devices. In September 2015, S Health support was extended to all devices running Andorid 4.4 (KitKat) or higher. The latest release of S Health (v. 5.0) added various features such as vital signs tracking, creating training plans, setting goals for workouts or sleep, weekly summaries, and social interaction with the feature 'Together' where users can challenge their friends in various fitness activity competitions. Furthermore, the security of health data is now being addressed through Samsung Knox,[4] an enterprise-grade security platform that provides a level of protection and encryption with hardware-backed credential storage. The S Health app can thus detect unauthorized changes on the smartphone via the Knox framework and render the data inaccessible if a security threat is determined.

[3]Samsung renamed "S Health" to "Samsung Health" in April 2017.

[4]https://www.samsungknox.com.

Although S Health has been primarily geared towards fitness and individualized health self-monitoring, Samsung has established several collaborations with health care researchers that would "accelerate the validation and commercialization of new sensors, algorithms, and digital health technologies" for preventive medicine.[5] Samsung partnered with University of California San Francisco (UCSF) in 2014 and established the UCSF-Samsung Digital Health Innovation Lab. Within the announcement of this collaboration, Samsung also released a new open hardware platform *Simband*. Simband was intended to provide a design blueprint for developing wearable devices which would incorporate various advanced sensors, including measurements of galvanic skin response, ECG, heart rate, and others. In collaboration with UCSF, these sensors were also being clinically validated [16]. To facilitate large-scale clinical trials, the health researchers can now take advantage of Samsung ARTIK Cloud [6] (formerly known as SAMI), which is a device-agnostic cloud-based data exchange platform that aggregates measurements from a variety of sources (including smartphones, smart-watches, IoT devices, etc.). This framework can provide researchers with capabilities to collect, securely store, view, and analyze data in real-time. At the time of writing, Samsung does not have a publicly available equivalent of Apple's ResearchKit that would specifically target clinical trials.

3.3 Google Fit

Google Fit health-tracking platform was released in October 2014 for the Android operating system. The platform is intended to collect and aggregate data from popular fitness trackers and health-related apps into a central repository. Google Fit can take advantage of the smartphone's sensors or wearable devices to count steps and record exercise activities (e.g., walking, running, cycling). Google Fit consists of the following components: (1) *fitness store* for storing data from various fitness devices and apps in a cloud-based repository, (2) *sensor framework* which defines high-level representations for sensors, fitness data types, data points, and sessions, (3) *permissions and user controls* that implements a mechanism for user-controlled access to collected data, and (4) *Google Fit APIs* which include Android API for access and recording from sensors and REST API for storing and access of user data in the fitness store.[7] An example screenshot is depicted in Fig. 2.

Following the announcements by Apple and Samsung to enter the clinical research, Google announced in June 2015 that their Google X research division developed a health-tracking wristband that can be used for clinical and drug trials [23]. The wearable device would measure pulse, heart rhythm, skin temperature, light exposure, and noise levels, providing researchers with minute-by-minute

[5] https://www.ucsf.edu/news/2014/02/111976/samsung-ucsf-partner-accelerate-new-innovations-preventive-health-technology.

[6] https://www.artik.cloud/.

[7] https://www.developers.google.com/fit/.

patient data. To date, no further information has been released, however Google continues to show interest in health research with the founding of their company *Verily*[8] and their effort *DeepMind Health*.[9]

3.4 Other Commercial Platforms

Aside from the big players in the mobile market, Microsoft in October 2014 released the smart wearable device Microsoft Band and the health-tracking platform Microsoft Health. The two products enable users to collect and view their data about step counts, workouts, and sleep quality. Since its release, Microsoft Health has been updated to support several other wearable devices and connects to partner apps, such as *MyFitnessPal*, *Strava*, *RunKeeper*, and *MapMyFitness*. The Microsoft Band SDK and Microsoft Health Cloud API provide developers with tools to access measurements on the smartband and to create new health apps that take advantage of Microsoft's ecosystem.

Several other health and fitness platforms that collect data from smartphone and wearable devices have been developed over the years. Under Armour recently released their fitness platform *Under Armour Connected Fitness*[10] and the accompanying app *UA Record*. The platform aggregates collected data on activity, sleep, and workouts from mobile sensors and third party devices. Through their app, members can share their data and compete with their friends in various customized health and fitness challenges. Under Armour provides an SDK for developers as well as access to the platform with free and paid subscriptions. In addition, Under Armour released *UA HealthBox* which includes a scale, wristband, and chest heart rate monitor to measure, track, and manage sleep, fitness, activity, and nutrition.

Finally, several of the wearable smart device manufacturers also provide apps that are geared towards collecting fitness activity data and tracking progress over time, while being able to share these data with other users. Some of these applications can be used independently or they can connect to one or more major health frameworks, such as Apple Health, Samsung S Health, and Google Fit. Examples of such wearable smart-bands include FitBit,[11] Pebble watch,[12] Nike FuelBand,[13] and JawBone.[14]

---

[8]https://www.verily.com/.

[9]https://www.deepmind.com/applied/deepmind-health/.

[10]https://www.underarmour.com/en-us/ua-record.

[11]https://www.fitbit.com/.

[12]https://www.pebble.com/.

[13]https://www.nike.com/us/en_us/c/nike-plus.

[14]https://www.jawbone.com/.

3.5 The Berkeley Telemonitoring Project

The Berkeley Telemonitoring Project at University of California, Berkeley has recently released an open source framework for the development of research-oriented telemonitoring systems.[15] The development of this framework was preceded by a pilot study of telemonitoring patients with CHF using a smartphone. The study was conducted between University of California at Berkeley, Northwestern Medical Faculty Foundation (Chicago, IL), and New York University [9, 10]. Fifteen patients, who were recruited for the study, were remotely monitored for a period of three months using a smartphone app that collected information about their vital signs, physical activity, symptoms, and health behavior. The goal of the study was to evaluate the feasibility and acceptability of telemonitoring via a smartphone under real-world conditions. Specifically, the study aimed to examine the usability, privacy implications, and technical requirements of telemonitoring as encountered by patients and healthcare providers. The study findings guided the design and implementation of the aforementioned framework [8].

The Berkeley Telemonitoring framework consists of a set of libraries that can be used to build a distributed real-time health-monitoring system comprised of telemonitoring servers and Andorid-based telemonitoring nodes (e.g., smartphone, smartwatch, tablet, etc.). For the remainder of this section, we will refer to the telemonitoring node as a smartphone for simplicity. The choice to support Android thus complements the efforts carried out by Apple ResearchKit for the iOS devices. The share of Android operating system (OS) in the smartphone market, as of June 2016, was 83.7% (versus 15.3% for Apple iOS), making it an attractive choice for a telemonitoring platform. To the best of our knowledge, there are no similar general frameworks for research currently available for Android. A systematic review of the mHealth research by Hussain et al. reveals that the majority of the first medical apps targeted iOS (since its release predated Android); however, most of the health research apps available now, based on the surveyed sample, target either Android alone or both platforms [48].

In the next few paragraphs we outline some of the design objectives that were followed to develop this framework.

There are several disadvantages in using smartphones as telemonitoring nodes. For starters, smartphones are limited in their battery, computational, and connectivity resources. As a result, smartphone apps are more susceptible to interruptions than software running on personal computers. For instance, if resources are needed, the Android OS may choose to kill an app that is running in the background. Subsequently, telemonitoring apps have to be able to recover from faults in a tolerant way, including retaining any collected data which were not delivered to the server before the fault. Thus, one goal is to elevate the responsibility of fault-tolerance from the app layer to the framework.

---

[15] https://www.telemonitoring.berkeley.edu.

Second, telemonitoring apps, particularly those running continuously in the background, need to be mindful of their battery consumption. High battery consumption may ultimately entice users to uninstall the app from their smartphone [9, 10]. Therefore, another design objective is to (i) design the different modules in an energy-aware manner; and (ii) provide tools to allow the delegation of computationally-intensive tasks from the smartphones to remote servers (distributed computing).

Moreover, telemonitoring systems curate health data, which are privacy-sensitive by nature. As such, it is vital to design the framework with privacy in mind. For example, in order to assess a subject's risk of clinical deterioration in certain chronic health conditions, the analysis may rely on the subject's relative parameters compared to the rest of the population. Therefore, by utilizing distributed computation on the cloud, the system can request this analysis to take place on a trusted server where the population data reside, and by that mitigate the privacy risks of sharing the population data (or statistics based on them) with the smartphone of the subject. However, distributed computation, in conjunction with data access controls, is not sufficient to protect patient privacy. More sophisticated privacy threats need to be addressed within the framework, such as for example statistical inference attacks.

Since the framework is aimed at non-technical developers, the programing interface has to be simple enough; while being at the same time flexible enough to allow more seasoned developers to extend its functionality. To achieve this goal, a simple API is provided that hides the complex implementation details. The different modules included in the framework can be further extended using Object-Oriented Programming (OOP) principles.

Finally, health telemonitoring systems must be able to collect health-related data from various sources at different scales. These sources include self-reported data by patients through survey-like instruments, such as for examples various symptoms that a patient may be experiencing. Other sources of health-related data are external sensors, wearable devices, and stationary devices. Similarly, any internal sensor available on the smartphone may serve as a source of health-related data. For example, accelerometer data can be used to estimate step counts and energy expenditure. Therefore, the framework needs to include tools that facilitate data collection from all of these sources in an easy-to-use way.

A summary of the objectives can be found in Table 1.

Framework Structure

The Berkeley Telemonitoring framework consists of three main libraries: *client library*, *server library*, and *core library*. The client library, written in Java as a natural selection for Android-based system, is used by the smartphone app. Similarly, the server library deployed on the server is also implemented in Java in order to reduce the development overhead. The uniformity of implementing both libraries in Java enables them to share certain data structures that can be placed in a common library, the core library. This consistency also allows telemonitoring apps and servers to communicate data structures seamlessly via serialization (i.e., the process of translating data structures into a format that can be transmitted or stored).

Table 1 Objectives and principles in designing the Berkeley Telemonitoring framework

Identified issue	Design objective
Fault-tolerance	Embedded fault telerance in the framework's modules
Battery consumption	Provide tools for delegating computation to a server (distributed computing) and for monitoring battery consumption
Privacy	Design privacy-preserving data structures, access controls, and data analysis and communication technologies
Flexibility	The framework should enable developers to extend its functionality
Ease of use	The API should be easy to use and should hide any technical details that are not health-related
Access to vital signs and symptoms	The framework should facilitate the collection of health data (i) by implementing algorithms that estimate vital signs from internal sensors; (ii) by supporting the collection of data from external devices, wearables and sensors; and (iii) by supporting the collection of self-reported data by patients, which can take the form of surveys

Serialization is useful because it is typically independent of the communication protocol, security and privacy layers or data-storage paradigm.

To be concrete, the core library supplies data structures for data storage, privacy and security, surveys, and fault tolerance. The client library supplies tools to (i) connect to external devices for data acquisition; (ii) estimate health-related variables from internal smartphone sensors; (iii) delegate computation; (iv) communicate with the server; and (v) render surveys on the smartphone screen. Consequently, the server library includes tools to (i) manage data collection and retention; (ii) analyze data; (iii) perform delegated computation; and (iv) communicate with the smartphones. The architecture of the Berkeley Telemonitoring framework is depicted in Fig. 3.

Event-Based Programming

The Berkeley Telemonitoring framework adopts the event-based programming paradigm. In this paradigm, the app requests a service from the framework and immediately resumes control of the CPU. The framework in return, will attempt to provide the requested service and will inform the app through callbacks whenever a change to the status of the requested service occurs. These changes are referred to as *events*, and the constructs that are used by the app to implement the actions performed when an event occurs are referred to as *listeners*.

Data Storage Paradigm

As mentioned previously, oftentimes the Andorid OS may need to free resources by killing apps that are not actively being used in the foreground. This means that the

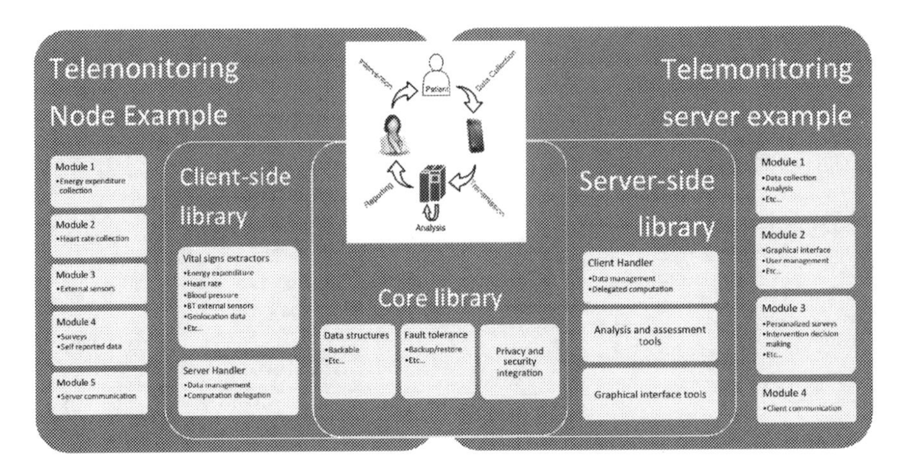

Fig. 3 The architecture of the Berkeley Telemonitoring framework

telemonitoring app has to be developed in such a way to be able to recover from such situations gracefully. The naive approach is to dismiss any datapoints that were collected prior to such an event but not yet submitted to the server. Another option is to design data structures in a fault-tolerant way by ensuring that a copy of every datapoint is stored in some non-volatile storage (e.g., built-in storage) upon its collection. This copy can then be retrieved after such a hiatus. Altough this enables a more reliable data collection process, it normally requires careful implementation from the developer of the telemonitoring app, increasing the complexity of the development cycle.

The Berkeley Telemonitoring framework achieves fault-tolerance by providing *backables*, data structures that are able to be immediately backed up on non-volatile storage whenever their content changes. Another component related to fault-tolerant data storage is called a *backup cabinet*. Each backup cabinet has designated location on the internal storage for data storage. Backup cabinets allow backables to be registered inside them for automatic backup services as described earlier. Upon registration of a backable, the backup cabinet retrieves any previously backed-up copy of that backable if it exists. Afterwards, the backup cabinet creates (if necessary) and updates the backup copy whenever the contents of the backable change.

Privacy and Security

To ensure that the collected data are secure, backup cabinets utilize the Android OS storage options to store the data in a space only accessible to the app that generated them. Further mechanisms that would allow storing, recovering, and communicating data structures in a secure and privacy-preserving manner are currently being implemented in the Berkeley Telemonitoring framework. Those technologies are being implemented over backables and backup cabinets for easy and seamless integration. For example, privacy-preserving measures against statistical inference attacks are being incorporated in the framework. These measures are based on the Private Disclosure of Information framework that is discussed in Sect. 4.

Bluetooth and BLE
The Berkeley Telemonitoring framework extends the Android Bluetooth and Bluetooth Low Energy (BLE) stacks in an effort to unify their behaviors [13]. Originally, Android's stack for Bluetooth is polling based; that is, the app layer has to actively check whether any change in the status of any connection occurs (e.g., message received, connection established, etc.). On the other hand, Android's BLE stack is event-based; which makes it fundamentally different than the Bluetooth stack. The framework's extended Bluetooth and BLE stacks both conform with the event-based paradigm. For example, when the app requests from the framework's Bluetooth stack to connect to an external device, the app regains control over the CPU immediately after placing the request. The framework, on the other hand will inform the app through the app's listeners upon the occurrence of any event.

Moreover, the Berkeley Telemonitoring framework provides an extension to natively support data collection from Bluetooth or BLE devices that are compliant with the ISO/IEEE 11073 Personal Health Device (PHD) standard [38]. That is, the app only needs to define an object representing a PHD device and request to connect and collect data from it. The framework, in turn, will connect to the device and start collecting data from it and delivering the data to the app through listeners, complying with the event-based programming paradigm. Note that the app does not need to implement the PHD standard protocols or know what type of device it is connecting to beforehand (e.g., blood pressure monitor vs thermometer). For example, consider an app that wants to support data collection from any PHD-compliant thermometer as well as any PHD-compliant blood pressure monitor. The app can initialize a backable for the thermometer data and another one for the blood pressure data. In addition, if the app has an object representing a PHD-compliant device (as returned by the Bluetooth/BLE stack to the app), it can register both backables with it and request to start collecting data. The framework in turn will fill the applicable backable(s) depending on the type of the device, and the app can be notified when data are added to the backable(s) using listeners as described earlier. Figure 4a depicts a screenshot of an app using the Bluetooth stack to scan for nearby devices.

Estimators and Extractors
In addition to the ability of the Berkeley Telemonitoring framework to collect data from IEEE 11073 compliant devices, it also provides the ability to use data from internal smartphone sensors to estimate health-related variables. These components are referred to as *estimators*. Similarly, the framework provides the app the ability to extract raw sensory data from internal sensors available on the phone through components that are referred to as *extractors*. An estimator or an extractor uses a backable to store the data it estimates or extracts in. The estimation or extraction process starts upon request from the app and remains active until the app requests to stop it.

At the time of writing, the following estimators and extractors were supported: (1) Heart rate estimator from a face video: the estimator calculates an estimate of

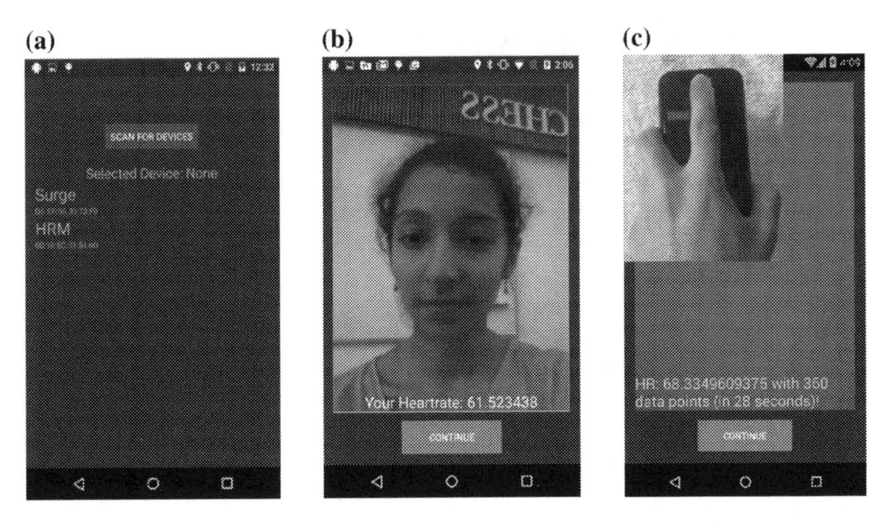

Fig. 4 **a** Bluetooth/BLE stack example: scanning for nearby devices; **b** Face-based heart rate estimator example; and **c** finger-based heart rate estimator example (*top* positioning of the finger on the smartphone camera; *bottom* video frame captured by the camera with the estimator's output)

the heart-beat rate in real-time from a video feed of the subject's face. This estimator is a real-time implementation of the algorithm described by Poh et al. [13, 66]. An example of the estimator in action is depicted in Fig. 4b; (2) Heart rate estimator from a finger video: the estimator calculates an estimate of the heart-beat rate in real-time from a video feed of the subject's index finger that is placed over the camera [13]. An example of the estimator in action is depicted in Fig. 4c; (3) Energy expenditure estimator: the estimator calculates an estimate of energy expenditures in a real-time from tri-axial accelerometer data [24, 33]; (4) Cadence estimator: the estimator calculates an estimate of cadence (steps per minute) in real-time from tri-axial accelerometer data [11, 59]; (5) Speed estimator: the estimator calculates an estimate of walking speed in real-time from tri-axial accelerometer data [13, 63]; (6) Global Positioning System (GPS) extractor: the extractor allows the app to collect the GPS data as provided by the phone; (7) Battery extractor: the extractor allows the app to collect selected battery status information, including whether the phone is charging and the current battery level; and (8) Call status extractor: the extractor allows the app to collect information about whether the phone is currently in a phone call or not.

Surveys
In addition to the sensor-facilitated data collection, the Berkeley Telemonitoring framework also provides the ability to represent, render, and collect data from surveys that can be delivered to the patient through the smartphone. In the framework, a *survey* is a list of *survey nodes*; and each survey node is composed of a *question* and an *answer* pair. The node question describes the question component (e.g., text question, picture question, etc.) and the node answer describes the answer component

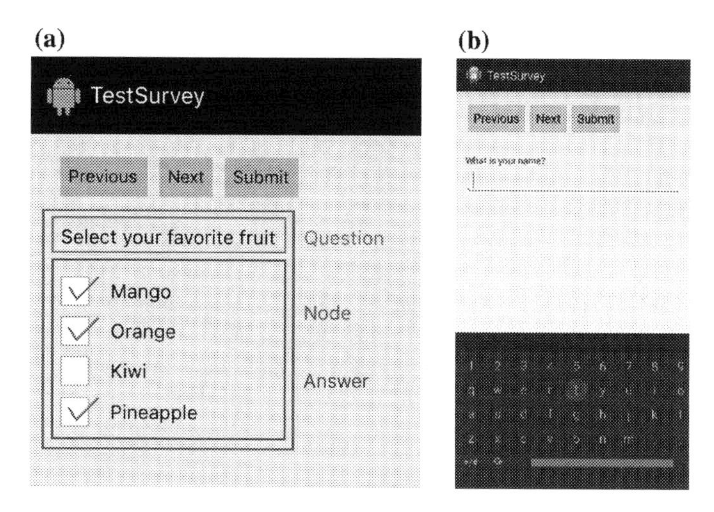

Fig. 5 **a** The survey components; and **b** an example of a survey node composed of a text question and a text answer

(e.g., check list, radio list, text box, etc.). See Fig. 5a for a depiction of this design. An example of a survey node with a text question and a text answer is depicted in Fig. 5b.

In addition to the survey construct, the framework also includes a *survey renderer* module that automatically renders any given survey node and returns an Android fragment that can be placed anywhere in the app. This design (a) enables mHealth apps to deploy surveys that include any combination of question type and answer type; (b) enables developers to extend the framework in order to include new types of questions and answers; and (c) allows apps to easily include the surveys (both designing surveys and displaying them).

Client-Server Communication
The Berkeley Telemonitoring framework provides modules facilitating the smartphones-servers communication. The burden of implementing these modules traditionally falls on the app developer. Similar to previously discussed constructs, the communication modules need to be implemented in a manner that is tolerant to faults. The Berkeley Telemonitoring framework abstracts the communication by defining the *job* construct as the atomic communication unit. We describe the following two types of jobs.

Data Jobs: Jobs that describe the intent to transmit data from the smartphone to the server. The most common use of these jobs is to transmit the health-related data collected during monitoring (e.g., vital signs and surveys).

Request Jobs: Jobs that describe the smartphone's intent to delegate computation to a server. As discussed earlier, there are mainly two important benefits of allowing delegation of computation:

1. Computational power: Delegating heavier computations allows the smartphone to obtain their results in a quicker manner, without incurring a cumbersome consumption of battery on the smartphone; and
2. Privacy: The server has access to information about the rest of the monitored population. Delegation of computation allows telemonitoring apps to complete computations that may require access to data other than those pertaining to the smartphone's owner in a privacy-preserving way. The classical example of such computation is estimating a patient's risk of clinical deterioration. This computation may need to compare the patient's data to the rest of the population. Sending relevant statistics of the population data to the smartphone presents a privacy risk [36, 37]. Therefore, instead of bringing the data to the computation, this mechanism allows the computation to be delivered to the data (where it is trusted to reside), potentially better protecting the privacy of the other patients.

The Berkeley Telemonitoring framework includes the design of the jobs and the infrastructure to implement specific protocols that can communicate these jobs. This specification in the framework is referred to as *meta-protocol*; i.e., the set of requirements for a protocol in terms of handling jobs. Any implementation that satisfies these requirements is considered a valid telemonitoring communication protocol. This design allows developers to implement their own protocols by satisfying the requirements dictated by the meta-protocol [8]. The meta-protocol also natively facilitates distributed computing by allowing a server to have multiple physical addresses for distribution of load and data as needed (similar to SMTP servers for mail). The framework also includes an off-the-shelf fault-tolerant protocol, *Tele-interfacing (TI)* protocol, that performs communication using Transport Layer Security (TLS), or its predecessor, Secure Socket Layer (SSL)—if desired—over Transmission Control Protocol (TCP).

Example App: MarathonCoach

Figure 6 depicts screenshots from an example fitness app, *MarathonCoach*, that was built using the Berkeley Telemonitoring framework. The app takes advantage of several of the aforementioned functionalities. MarathonCoach aims to provide personalized coaching to long-distance runners through the runner's physical parameters and monitoring during runs [11]. The model adopted for marathon-running training is to try to optimize the cadence of the runner during a set time frame. That is, once the runner's physical parameters are provided to the app (Fig. 6a), the runner's cadence is obtained (during the initial run), the target cadence is set and the target date to reach the target cadence is set, the app will develop an exercise regimen that helps the runner achieve his or her target cadence (Fig. 6b). MarathonCoach starts by showing a list of the past runs by the runner using the app. When the runner triggers the start of a new run, the app requests to take heart-beat rate measurements from a face video or a finger video (Figs. 4b, c). The user in turn can opt to take these measurements or skip them, after which the run starts and the monitoring app begins to collect data about the runner's speed, cadence, GPS location, and heart rate via an any ISO/IEEE 11073 compliant external heart rate monitor (Fig. 6c). During the run, the app gives the runner feedback about his or her run, such as for example cadence

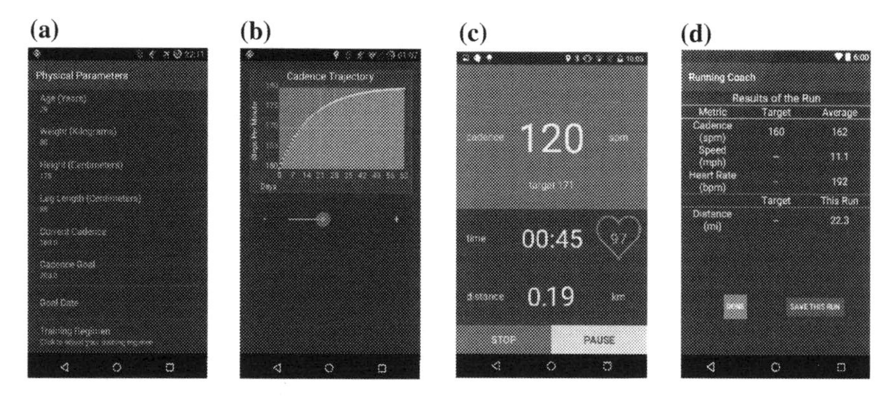

Fig. 6 Screenshots from the MarathonCoach app that was built using the Berkeley Telemonitoring framework: **a** the main screen for the runner's physical parameters; **b** a runner's exercise regimen for cadence as a function of time; **c** the screen that is displayed during a run; and **d** the screen that is displayed after the run is completed

being too high or too low. The feedback is delivered to the runner through vibration and audio cues (and on the screen). Once the run is completed, the app will again request to take heart-beat rate measurements from a face video and a finger video. Similarly to the pre-run case, the user can choose to take these measurements or skip them. This is done in order to further validate the accuracy and usability of the face-based and finger-based heart-beat rate estimation algorithms as used by individuals in a non-controlled environment (outside of the lab). We achieve this validation by comparing the estimates from the algorithms with the data obtained from the external heart rate monitor. Afterwards, the app displays the summary of the run (Fig. 6d). At the time of writing, the app was being studied for efficacy and usability at University of California, Berkeley.

3.6 Intervention

One of the important aspects of proactive health care is the *intervention*. The goal of health-behavioral intervention is to initiate and sustain health-improving activities; similarly, the preventive interventions are intended to discourage unhealthy behaviors before they start [70]. Health behavioral interventions originate from social science theories which primarily relied on observational and self-reported data. The goal of the intervention process is to assess the health risk from the data by using predictive health-behavior models [25]. Furthermore, one needs to also monitor the response to the intervention and modify it appropriately in order to be effective. According to Spring et al. this process can be characterized by "4 Ms": monitoring, modeling, motivating, and modifying [70].

Availability of real-time data through smartphone monitoring provides new opportunities to revisit health-behavioral modeling. The high granularity and multi-modal nature of the observations can help build better models and facilitate more effective interventions. As mentioned previously, the observations can include objective measurements, such as physical activity, vital signs, location, phone usage, and subjective information such as pain, energy level, emotional state, etc. Based on these data, we can create models that capture the health-behavior to various degrees of fidelity. The models, which are typically based on control systems engineering, are aimed to determine the level of intervention that would maximize the effect on the individual's behavior. The models have to be dynamically adapted as the behavior of the user changes over time. In the context of changing health-behavior, motivation is the driving force of understanding, changing, and maintaining health behavior [70]. Since different people are motivated differently, it is important that the entire process is individualized in order to keep the users engaged. In addition to technological features (e.g., intuitive interaction, appealing design, variety in incentives, etc.), health intervention needs to activate effective behavior change mechanisms that will initiate the change and sustain the positive behavior over a longer time period.

There have been a handful of studies evaluating mobile intervention via smartphones in various populations, including in patients with depression [19] and schizophrenia [14], and to promote weight loss [57] and physical activity [19].

3.7 Challenges

In spite of the efforts described thus far to advance the potential of health and fitness monitoring and intervention, many challenges remain open. On the clinical side, designing monitoring and intervention systems and studies requires the involvement of qualified professionals in healthcare, which is currently lacking [48]. Moreover, there is a lack of evidence of clinical effectiveness, efficacy and objective research to evaluate clinical outcomes of mHealth systems [10, 39]. A better understanding of the negative effects of mHealth apps and systems is also needed, and the development of predictive models that take behavior into consideration is required (dubbed *physio-behavioral models*) [10, 39, 48]. Another challenge related to the clinical aspects of mHealth is that there is a considerable amount of mHealth systems, apps, devices, and frameworks that facilitate collection of data; however, there is a lack of autonomous expert systems that can provide effective feedback and timely intervention based on these data [8, 10]. The *proper authorship* of data can also be a challenge; that is, are we able to identify when the data collected through telemonitoring are authored by the someone other than patient being monitored? [10].

From a systems and standardization point of view, there is an absence of a regulatory framework for design and development of mHealth systems [48]. Moreover, for mHealth systems to be adopted in healthcare institutions, there is a need to integrate them in existing healthcare delivery and/or reimbursement systems [39, 48]. Particularly, technical challenges arise from the lack of seamless interfaces between app platforms and existing information technology systems used by healthcare providers (e.g., integration with electronic health records) [48]. An additional challenge in this category is the user experience and usability of mHealth systems for patients. A few examples include (a) commitment of patients to use a specific mHealth system on a daily basis; (b) achieving user engagement that does not diminish over time (*usage fatigue*); (c) remembering to recharge the devices involved in the mHealth system; (d) the consumers' learning curve in using new mHealth systems; and (e) getting reliable access to the mHealth systems in rural areas due to poor or lack of signal [10, 48]. Moreover, some of the frameworks provide capabilities of collecting the data related to selected tasks but do not provide any post-processing capabilities to calculate relevant medical quantities based on the collected data. For example, they enable apps to collect accelerometer data or step counts, but do not provide tools to estimate energy expenditures based on such data. Furthermore, many commercial platforms implement proprietary solutions for processing the sensor data, making the comparison of the same quantity between different apps and platforms difficult. The lack of standardization and transparency therefore also limits the medical professionals and researchers to unify the data collection processes, share data, and draw reliable conclusions from different studies since each study may have calculated the values using a different method or algorithm. This problem is apparent even in simple quantities such as step counting [20]. With higher-level inferences from these measurements, such as energy expenditure, there are even more variables that affect the accuracy and reliability of the extracted feature. Apple's ResearchKit, for example, allows for the researchers to calculate energy expenditure from given step counts and raw accelerometer data instead. In such scenario different researchers may implement the calculation not only using a different algorithm but a different code which may be prone to errors. With this example, it is clear that for the health research there is a need to standardize and provide open source methods for calculation of health markers that can be affirmed and maintained by the scientific community [8, 10, 48].

In addition to these challenges, legal and ethical concerns are being raised in the mHealth literature. For example, it is not clear what is the best way of obtaining informed consent for studies based on mobile apps in healthcare. This challenge is particularly interesting in studies that target a large number of participants, such as in the case of the studies conducted with Apple ResearchKit [47, 48]. To that end, as of September 2016, a clinical study is being conducted by Duke University to compare the standard informed consent process in medical practice to the process featured in Apple's ResearchKit.[16] Although the use of mHealth technologies, such as Apple ResearchKit, provides unprecedented opportunity for large scale clinical trials, there is also a significant lack for population coverage and a potential bias due to differences between the user bases of specific platforms and smartphones in general [50].

There are also challenges on the administrative side. For instance, the financial costs of developing new mHealth systems and/or interfacing them to existing health IT system may hinder their wide adoption [18, 48]. Another example of challenges in this category is privacy and security. Health data are privacy-sensitive data and as such, need to be stored, transmitted, analyzed and retained carefully. Currently, there

[16]https://www.clinicaltrials.gov/ct2/show/NCT02799407.

Table 2 Taxonomy summary of the different health and fitness frameworks

Framework	Target use	Features and contributions	Disadvantages
Apple HealthKit	Consumer health and fitness tracking	Aggregation, exchange, and visualization of health data collected from apps and external sensors	Missing support for other ecosystems (Andorid, Windows)
		Health provider information sharing and future integration with electronic medical records	
Apple ResearchKit	Medical research; Clinical trials	Open-source framework for large-scale data collection for medical research	As clinical research tool limited to only one platform (iOS), there is potential bias for clinical research [50]
		Provides modules for (1) informed consent, (2) surveys, and (3) active tasks that include motor activities, cognition, voice, audio, etc.	Potential ethical issues regarding electronic consent [47, 48]
Apple CareKit	Patient self-management	Open-source framework for development of patient-centered disease self-management apps	Missing support for other ecosystems (Android, Windows) limits accessibility to patients
		Ability to share data with care takers, family, and doctors	
Samsung S Health SDK	Consumer health and fitness tracking	Android-based platform featuring data collection and aggregation from health apps and various sensors	Limited to Android operating system and until recently only to Samsung phones
		Includes mechanisms for data analysis, coaching, and social interaction while ensuring security via Samsung Knox supported encryption	

(continued)

Table 2 (continued)

Framework	Target use	Features and contributions	Disadvantages
Google Fit	Consumer health and fitness tracking	Android-based platform for data collection from popular fitness trackers and health-related apps	Primary focused on fitness data, less on health data
		Sensor framework for high-level representation of sensors, fitness data types, data points and sessions	Privacy concerns regarding data sharing with 3rd parties
Microsoft Health	Consumer health and fitness tracking	Cross-platform (Windows, Android, iOS) health-tracking framework with support for popular trackers and health-related apps	Not widely popular
		Features data aggregation, storage, analytics	
Under Armour Connected Fitness	Consumer health & fitness tracking	Platform for aggregating data on activity, sleep, and workouts from sensors and third-party devices. ncludes social networking component for athletes and fitness users	Primary focused on fitness data, less on health data.
Berkeley Telemonitoring	Medical research; Clinical trials; Consumer health and fitness tracking	Android-based open-source framework for development of health-monitoring apps	Limited to Android operating system
		Provides libraries for server and client, distributed computation, secure and robust data storage, and modules for survey administration, connectivity to medical devices, and several validated algorithms for vital signs	

is little research on privacy-aware methods that are geared towards mHealth relative to the amount of privacy-related research being performed in other fields of healthcare information technology such as electronic health records [6, 10, 18, 47, 48]. For example, Apple HealthKit and ResearchKit provide the consumer the ability to grant permissions to the different mobile health apps to access her or his health data. This approach provides access control but does not protect against other types of privacy leaks such as inference attacks [6]. Moreover, compliance of mHealth systems with governmental regulations such as the Health Insurance Portability and Accountability Act (HIPAA) is an open challenge. A taxonomy summary of the different health and fitness frameworks presented in this section can be found in Table 2.

4 Private Disclosure of Information

4.1 Introduction

Telemonitoring is one example of an emerging area with growing interest to collect sensitive personal and private data. Warner argues that the lack of privacy guarantees can cause individuals to be reluctant to share their data with data collectors (such as doctors, government agencies, researchers, etc.) or instead provide false information [74]. Therefore, users need to be assured that their privacy will be preserved throughout the whole process of data collection and use. Since the data involved in the telemonitoring setting are sensitive from a privacy point of view, privacy-preserving technologies are needed in order to protect patients' privacy and increase compliance and adoption.

In order to achieve this goal, we first have to identify the stages in the life cycle of data in telemonitoring. These stages include (i) the disclosure (or submission) of the data by the users to the data collector; (ii) the processing of the data; (iii) the analysis; and/or (iv) the publishing of (often a sanitized version of) the data or relevant findings based on them. In this section we discuss the framework for Private Disclosure of Information (PDI), which aims to prevent an adversary from inferring certain sensitive information about patients—typically diagnosis—using the data that were disclosed during health telemonitoring communication with their doctors [6]. This threat is usually referred to as *inference attack*.

In traditional encryption approaches to maintaining privacy, it is often implicitly assumed that the data themselves *are* the private information. However, in some scenarios, the data *can be used* to infer certain private information about the subjects from the given data. For example, respiration rate by itself might not be considered private information. However, if the data from the collected respiration rate are used to infer whether the individual is a smoker or not, they become sensitive information. One can argue that because the information about whether someone smokes is private, the respiration rate data become private *by implication*.

Under such circumstances, one should sanitize the transmitted data in a way that reveals as little as possible about the private information to an adversary. In summary, our objective is to encode the transmitted data in order to hide another private piece of information that can be derived from these data. In the words of Sweeney: "Computer security is not privacy protection" [71]. The converse is also true, privacy does not replace security. The discussed approach is therefore to be viewed as complementary to classical security approaches. For example, data can be first sanitized then encrypted.

4.2 Problem Formulation

Notation

We use the following shorthand notation for probability density (mass) functions. We always use a pair of a capital and a small symbols of the same letter for a random variable and a realization of it, respectively. For notation simplicity and conciseness, given random variables X and Y, instead of writing $p_X(x)$ for the marginal density (mass) function of X we simply write $p(x)$, and instead of writing $p_{X|Y}(x|y)$ for the conditional density (mass) function of X given Y, we simply write $p(x|y)$.

Setting and Threat Model

Consider a setting in which a patient, Bob, is diagnosed with a health condition c. Bob's doctor, Alice, offers Bob a telemonitoring technology in order to stay updated about his vital signs, symptoms and other health-related variables. Note that for the purposes of this section, the goal is not to provide or update the diagnosis, but to merely remotely monitor Bob's health status *after* a diagnosis is obtained.

The information that Bob would like to share with Alice, x, is of sensitive nature. That is because if x fell in the hands of an adversary, Eve, it can be used to learn Bob's diagnosis through statistical reasoning. It is therefore desirable to devise an information disclosure process that would protect Bob against Eve's inference attack. This process is desired to work in conjunction with the traditional techniques that protect the disclosed message itself (e.g., encryption). Finally, we denote the encoded information that Bob actually discloses to Alice through the telemonitoring system by z (the sanitized version of x).

The threat model can be described as follows. Eve does not originally know Bob's diagnosis c, and therefore treats it as a random variable C (Note that the diagnosis c is known to Alice beforehand and is therefore not part of the transmission). Eve wants to update her belief about Bob's diagnosis $p(C|Bob)$ to $p(C|Bob, z)$ after observing Bob's disclosed information z. We will assume in this setting, that both Eve and Alice know that the sender of the message z is Bob. That is, we assume that Bob's identity is attached to his disclosed messages in the system. The threat model is depicted in Fig. 7. We therefore are defending Bob against an inference attack by a passive eavesdropper, Eve.

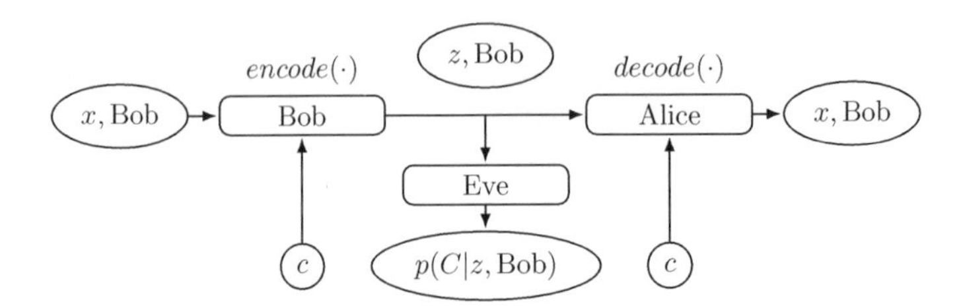

Fig. 7 The threat model which PDI is addressing: a passive eavesdropper performing a statistical inference attack on a piece of private information c (diagnosis) from a disclosed message z

Based on this, our goal is to encode the information x to z in a way that minimizes Eve's ability to gain information about the diagnosis c from z. In contrast, traditional encryption techniques aim to limit Eve's ability to reason about the original message x—not c—from z. Using our notation, if Eve treats the original message as a random variable X, the goal of traditional encryption is to limit Eve's ability to update her belief $P(X|Bob)$ to $p(X|Bob, z)$. Although these two goals are related, they are also different as has been demonstrated in inference attacks relying on encrypted messages (for example see [58, 75]).

In summary, if we denote the subject identifier of the patient using the telemonitoring system by s (which is Bob in the discussion above), the goal is to devise an information disclosure process that delivers the following premises:

DECODING Alice can make full use of the sent information z, i.e. obtain the original message x from the transmitted message z; and

HIDING CLASS Eve's ability to make inference about c given s, based on the sent information z is minimized.

Definitions

Formally, we use $\mathbb{S}$ for the set of identifiers of patients using the telemonitoring system. We use $\mathbf{I}$ for the information space from which the health data is drawn and $\mathbb{C}$ for the set of possible diagnoses of patients which we would like keep private. Similarly, we define the random variables S for the identity of the patient disclosing the information. We define the random variable C for the private diagnosis. Finally we define the random variables X and Z for the piece of health information that the patient would like to disclose and the piece of information that the patient actually discloses (after encoding), respectively. We call Z the sanitized information. In our treatment, we will consider encoding mechanisms of the following form.

Definition 1 A privacy mapping function (PMF) is a function $R : \mathbb{C} \rightarrow \mathbf{I}^{\underline{\mathbf{I}}}$ where $\mathbf{I}^{\underline{\mathbf{I}}}$ is the set of injective functions $\mathbf{I} \rightarrow \mathbf{I}$.

A simple way to think about a PMF, R, is as an encoding scheme. That is, for every diagnosis $c \in \mathbb{C}$, $R(c)$ is an encoding function. Recall that Alice knows the diagnosis of her patient s, and that the patient identity s is attached to every (sanitized) message that is disclosed. Since $R(c)$ is injective by definition, there exists a left inverse

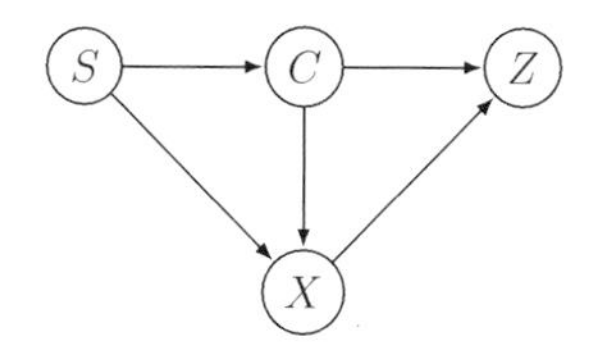

Fig. 8 The statistical graphical model of PDI. S: the patient's identity; C: the patient's diagnosis; X: the original data to be disclosed; and Z: the sanitized data actually disclosed

$[R(c)]^l$ that Alice can use to decode any disclosed message back to the original message.[17] This ensures the satisfaction of the premise (DECODING) above. Our encoding process (encode(·) from Fig. 7) is therefore $z = [R(c)](x)$ and the decoding process (devode(·) from Fig. 7), is therefore $x = [R(c)]^l(z)$. From this, it follows that the random variables Z, X and C are related as $Z = [R(C)](X)$. The statistical graphical model relating the random variables is depicted in Fig. 8.

Illustrating Example

To illustrate the concepts presented thus far, we consider the following example of a telemonitoring scenario for the purpose of monitoring the weight of patients who are of ages 19 or younger. Let the information space be $\mathbf{I} \triangleq \{(bmi, w) \in \mathbb{R}^2\}$ where bmi and w represent the patient's body mass index (BMI) $[\frac{\text{kg}}{\text{m}^2}]$ and weight [kg], respectively.[18] Let the set of diagnosis be $\mathbb{C} \triangleq \{UW, HW, OW, OB\}$ for underweight, health weight, overweight, and obese, respectively. These categories are consistent with the definitions of the Center for Disease Control and Prevention (CDC) for weight categories. According to these definitions, the weight category of a child or a teen is classified based on the individual's BMI percentile among the same age and gender group as described in Table 3. Note that since the age and gender of the patient are not part of the information space, the adversary's inference of the weight status category of a patient based on BMI and weight is not perfect.

From these definitions, the distribution of diagnoses is $p(UW) = 0.05, p(HW) = 0.8, p(OW) = 0.1$ and $p(OB) = 0.05$ among individuals from our patient population. If Eve has no extra knowledge about any particular patient, her prior belief $p(c|s)$ is simply equal to $p(c)$ for all $c \in \mathbb{C}$ and $s \in \mathbb{S}$. However, if Eve observes the message $x = (50, 120) \in \mathbf{I}$ without encoding (i.e., $z = x$) coming from the patient Bob (corresponding to Bob weighing 120 kg and being about 155 cm tall), her posterior belief $p(C = OB|Z = (50, 120), S = Bob)$ will substantially increase, compared to her prior belief of 0.05. The reason this was possible is that $p(Z = (50, 120)|C = OB, S = Bob)$ is much larger than $p(Z = (50, 120)|C = c, S = Bob)$ for any $c \neq OB$. To see this, consider the Bayesian update $p(c|z, s) = \frac{p(z|c,s)}{p(z|s)} p(c|s)$. A high ratio of

[17]We say that $g : D_2 \to D_1$ is a left inverse of a function $f : D_1 \to D_2$ if for all $x \in D_1$ we have $g(f(x)) = x$.

[18]BMI is a measure of relative weight based on an individual's mass and height. Defined as $BMI \triangleq \frac{mass(kg)}{height(m)^2}$.

Table 3 BMI-for-age weight status categories and the corresponding BMI percentiles within the same age and gender group. Definitions corresponding to individuals of age 19 or less

Weight category	BMI Percentile range
Underweight	$BMI < 5\%$
Healthy weight	$5\% \leq BMI < 85\%$
Overweight	$85\% \leq BMI < 95\%$
Obese	$95\% \leq BMI$

$\frac{p(z|c,s)}{p(z|s)}$ will increase the posterior confidence that Eve has in the diagnosis c for the patient s.

What happens if we, alternatively, encode the message $x = (50, 120) \in \mathbb{I}$ in a way that yields a ratio $\frac{p(z|c,s)}{p(z|s)}$ close to one for all $c \in \mathbb{C}$, $s \in \mathbb{S}$ and $z \in \mathbf{I}$? Eve's Bayesian update will yield a posterior belief $p(c|z, s)$ that is very close to her prior belief $p(c|s)$, as desired.

Satisfying the HIDING CLASS Premise

Recall that the requirement (DECODING) is satisfied by construction. We would now like to address the second premise (HIDING CLASS). For the model in Fig. 8, one needs to supply the following probability distributions. $p(s)$, the prior of patients transmitting messages in the system. $p(c|s)$, Eve's prior of patients' diagnoses—based on auxiliary knowledge. $p(x|c, s)$, the generative model of health data given a diagnosis and a patient. Finally, $p(z|x, c)$ is simple and can be modeled as $\mathbb{P}(Z = z|X = x, C = c) = 1$ if and only if $z = [R(c)](x)$ and 0 otherwise, for all $z, x \in \mathbb{I}$ and $c \in \mathbb{C}$.

From the example discussion in the previous subsection, we see that it is desirable to choose a PMF, R, that yields a posterior belief $p(C|s, z)$ that is as close as possible to the prior belief $p(C|s)$ for all $s \in \mathbb{S}$ and $z \in \mathbf{I}$. For that purpose, we elect to utilize the Conditional Mutual Information measure, defined as follows.

Definition 2 [28, c.f. Definition 8.49] Let X, Y and Z be random variables. The *conditional mutual information of X and Y given Z, $I(X, Y|Z)$*, is defined as

$$I(X, Y|Z) \triangleq \mathbb{E}_{p(x,y,z)} \left[\log \frac{p(x, y|z)}{p(x|z)p(y|z)} \right]$$

The use of Mutual Information as a measure of privacy for side information channels was axiomatically justified by Jiao et al. and is applicable to our setting [52]. Formally, we choose a PMF that minimizes the conditional mutual information measure between Z and C, given S—which is a function of the PMF R:

$$R^* = \arg\min_{R \text{ is a PMF}} I(Z, C|S; R) \tag{1}$$

Once a PMF R is chosen—which can be made public, even to Eve—the disclosure process can be carried as follows.

Sending The transaction of disclosing a piece of information $x \in \mathbf{I}$ by a patient with diagnosis $c \in \mathbb{C}$ is performed by applying the following transformation $z \leftarrow [R(c)](x)$ and sending z (or some encrypted version of it).

Receiving The transaction of receiving a piece of information $z \in \mathbf{I}$ sent by patient with diagnosis $c \in \mathbb{C}$ is performed by applying $x \leftarrow [R(c)]^l(z)$. Where $[R(c)]^l$ is a left inverse of $R(c)$.

Note that the problem in Eq. 1 is not convex. Furthermore, it is of interest to study how to learn the model in Fig. 8 and find an optimal PMF R from data. For that purpose, a MATLAB toolbox was developed by the Berkeley Telemonitoring Project [7]. We briefly mention a result and refer the reader to [6] for more formal and thorough analysis and further properties of the presented information disclosure process. The result states that if a PMF maps all data from the different diagnosis onto the same distribution, then (i) the PMF is an optimal solution to Eq. 1; and (ii) the PMF achieves perfect privacy (i.e., the eavesdropper's belief about the patient's diagnosis *does not* improve after observing the sanitized data). An example of this result on a simple case is presented below in Equation Theorem 1, which states that if data are distributed uniformly per diagnosis, then a PMF exists that achieves perfect privacy. Furthermore, Theorem 1 provides a closed-form formula for said PMF, which maps the data from the different diagnosis onto the standard uniform distribution, making them look identical to an eavesdropper; thus eliminating the ability of an eavesdropper to perform statistical inference based on the sanitized data.

Theorem 1 *If $X|C = c, S = s \sim U(a_c, b_c)$ (Continuous Uniform distribution) for every $c \in \mathbb{C}$ and $s \in \mathbb{S}$, then $[R(c)](x) = \frac{x-a_c}{b_c-a_c}$ is an optimal solution to Eq. 1 achieving $I(Z, C|S; R) = 0$.*

The intuition set forth here is further empirically demonstrated in Sect. 4.3 where the data from each diagnosis, after sanitization, are mapped onto a distribution that is similar to that of the data from the other diagnoses (Fig. 10) to limit inference attacks.

4.3 Experimentation

In this section we walk the reader through an example that aims to motivate and demonstrate PDI. The example is in line with the one given in the Illustrating Example Subsection. In this example we use data that are published by the Center for Disease Control and Prevention (CDC) as part of the National Health and Nutrition

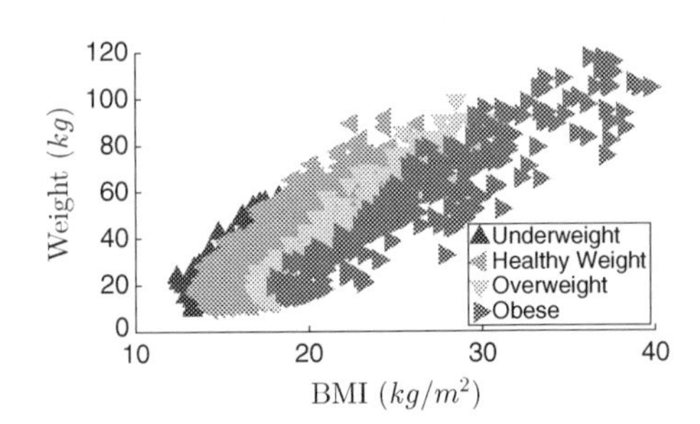

Fig. 9 BMI and weight for the different weight status groups. Note the regularity of the clusters for the different weight groups

Examination Survey of 2012.[19] Specifically, we use the Body Measures (BMX_G) portion of the data.[20]

Setting
In our setting, we consider the disclosed information to be both Body Mass Index (BMI) and weight. Our patients are assumed to be individuals of both genders that are 19 years of age or less. We consider the private information to be the weight status category of the subject. The CDC considers the following four standard weight status categories for the aforementioned age group (i) underweight; (ii) healthy weight; (iii) overweight; and (iv) obese. There are 3, 355 data points in the data set with subjects of 19 years of age or less.

Recall that according to the definitions of the CDC, the weight category of a child or a teen is classified based on the individual's BMI percentile among the same age and gender group as described in Table 3. Since the age of the patient is not part of the information space, the inference of the weight status category of the patient based on BMI and weight is not perfect. The data for the different classes (diagnoses) are depicted in Fig. 9.

Inference Based on Original Data Using the data, we trained 3 SVM classifiers with Gaussian kernels. The classifiers are aggregate in terms of the "positive" class in the following sense. The first classifier treats the "positive" class as the Underweight category (and so the "negative" class is the rest of the categories). The second classifier treats the "positive" class as either the underweight or healthy weight category. Finally, the third classifier treats the "positive" class as any category except the obese category. We used a 40–60 split for training-testing. In numbers, we used 1, 371 data points for training and 1, 984 data points for testing.

The training for all SVMs was done using 10-fold cross-validation among the data in the training set to pick the best σ of the Gaussian kernels and the best box boundaries of the classifiers. The classification phase is done by taking a majority vote from the three classifiers and the output is the class which most classifiers agree

[19] https://www.n.cdc.gov/nchs/nhanes/search/nhanes11_12.aspx.

[20] https://wwwn.cdc.gov/nchs/nhanes/2011-2012/BMX_G.htm.

Table 4 Confusion matrix before sanitizing. UW = Underweight, HW = Healthy Weight, OW = Overweight, OB = Obese

		True category			
		UW	HW	OW	OB
Predicted category	UW	47	20	0	0
	HW	14	1203	66	1
	OW	0	45	194	47
	OB	0	2	37	308

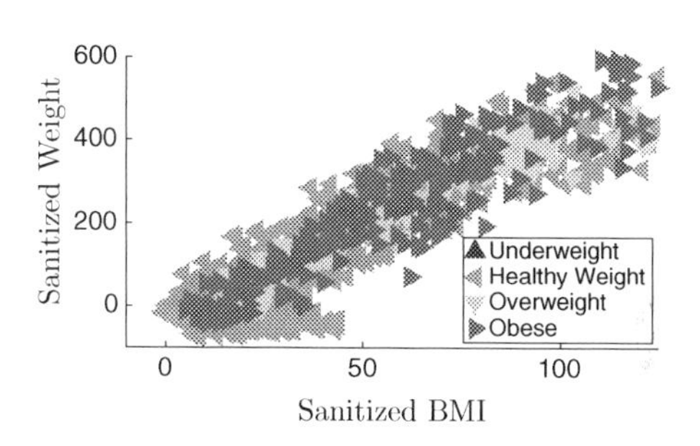

Fig. 10 BMI and weight for the different weight status groups after sanitization. Note how the clusters for the different weight groups are now less distinguishable

on. The results of the classifier are described in Table 4 in terms of the confusion matrix of the different categories. The total accuracy of the classifier is 88.31%.[21]

Inference Based on Sanitized Data We would like to sanitize the information at hand (BMI and weight) in order to maintain the weight status category as private as possible (based on the training set only). Therefore, we aim to utilize PDI in order to sanitize the data as discussed earlier. In order to learn the PMF from the training data, we use the MATLAB toolbox [7]. The code snippet that achieves this is listed in Algorithm 1. The distribution of the resultant sanitized data is depicted in Fig. 10. In order to evaluate the quality of the sanitization, we now train three new SVM classifiers with the same training procedure as in the Inference Based on Original Data Subsection, but this time using the sanitized data (and of course, encoding the test set too for evaluation). Same as before, we then use a majority vote from the three classifiers to predict the class of any data point. The resultant confusion matrix is described in Table 5.

It is clear that the classification results would degrade after sanitizing the information. The total accuracy dropped to 66.03% (from 88.31%). Given that the data from different classes are highly indistinguishable, the classifier now classifies most data points as "healthy weight". This is to be expected since most of the data points are in the "healthy weight" category. In informal words, if a classifier would have to make

[21]The adopted total accuracy measure is $trace(M)/N$ where M is the confusion matrix and N is the cardinality of the test set. This is the percentage of true classifications over the test set.

Table 5 Confusion matrix after sanitizing. UW = Underweight, HW = Healthy Weight, OW = Overweight, OB = Obese

		True category			
		UW	HW	OW	OB
Predicted category	UW	48	14	0	5
	HW	13	1217	276	290
	OW	0	25	13	29
	OB	0	14	0	32

a "bet", it would bet on the class with the most amount of data points. Formally, a lower bound on the total accuracy can be achieved by considering the trivial classifier that always predicts "healthy weight" (deterministic), which has total accuracy of $1,270/1,948 = 64.01\%$. This shows that our result of 66.03% is not much further from a lower-bound guaranteed accuracy.

Algorithm 1 The MATLAB code for learning the PMF from the BMX_G data using the toolbox [7].

```
pdi_begin % Begin the definition of a PDI problem
    % Declare data dimensions of the data
    pdi_dimension weight 0:5:180; % Weight is discretized by 5 kg
    pdi_dimension BMI 0:2:60; % BMI is discretized by 2 kg/(m^2)

    % Declare diagnoses
    pdi_class UW HW OW OB % Underweight; Healthy Weight; Overweight; Obese
    % Provide data for the different diagnoses
    pdi_datapoints UW UW_DATA
    pdi_datapoints HW HW_DATA
    pdi_datapoints OW OW_DATA
    pdi_datapoints OB OB_DATA

    % Declare parameters for PMF (affine transformations)
    pdi_var shift(pdi_nrdimensions, pdi_nrclasses); % Shift parameters
    pdi_var scale(pdi_nrdimensions, pdi_nrclasses); % Scale parameters

    % Constraints on the parameters
    scale(:,1) == 1; % Don't scale the data from the Underweight diagnosis
    shift(:,1) == 0; % Don't shift the data from the Underweight diagnosis
    scale >= 0.1; % Don't scale by 0 (to insure left inverse)

    % PMF: function of the parameters and diagnosis (affine transformations)
    pdi_reference f(x, c) bsxfun(@times, ...
                           bsxfun(@minus, x, shift(:,c)), scale(:,c));
pdi_end % End the definition of the PDI problem and solve
```

Note that the data set is biased in size against the "underweight" category. There are only 126 data points with weight category "underweight" out of the 3,355 total data points (3.76%). This makes sanitizing that class particularly hard, especially because the modeling in the toolbox is based on n-dimensional histograms and is not parametric. For this reason the classification results before and after sanitization for the "underweight" category are comparable.

To intuitively demonstrate how privacy is preserved, we take a piece of sanitized information at random from our data set, $z = [77.17, 296.45]^T$, without looking at its ground truth weight category. If we decode this data point using the decoding function of "healthy weight", we get $x = [21, 53.8]^T$, which is a legitimate "healthy weight" BMI and weight data point. If we use the decoding function of "overweight", we get $x = [25.12, 62.4]^T$, which is also a legitimate "overweight" BMI and weight data point. Similarly, if we use the decoding function of "obese", we get $x = [30.42, 69.08]^T$, which is also a legitimate "obese" BMI and weight data point. Simply put, if Eve decodes a sanitized datapoint z using a hypothesized diagnosis c, she will get a decoded message that cannot be used to rule out c as the diagnosis, since $[R(c)]^I(z)$ will look like a valid datapoint from the class c according to the generative model $p(x|c, s)$. This is, in essence, how the privacy of the diagnosis c gets protected even after disclosing the sanitized data z.

5 Discussion and Future Research Directions

In this chapter we have explored real-time health monitoring that can be accomplished using a smartphone in combination with other connected mHealth technologies. There are currently numerous smartphone apps pertaining to fitness, health management, and medical applications. Initial fragmentation in this space gave rise to development of more general frameworks, such as Apple Health and Samsung S Health, that would provide a more concise way to track the health data as well as to exchange the data between different apps and support sharing. Apple ResearchKit now facilitates several large scale clinical trials that use smartphone to collect various health-related data. The smartphone thus opened new opportunities to improve health and healthcare delivery for individuals. The distributed nature of the telemonitoring can, in connection with big data analytics, such as predictive modeling, provide new insights into prevention and management of existing diseases, improve support for patients and their care takers, lead to discovery of new drugs, protect patient privacy, and reduce overall cost of health care.

Adoption of smartphone-based health monitoring however still faces several challenges that were discussed in this chapter. These challenges include: (i) lack of evidence of clinical effectiveness, efficacy and objective research to evaluate clinical outcomes; (ii) the absence of a regulatory framework that standardizes development; (iii) lack of integration into existing healthcare IT systems; (iv) usability; (v) financial costs of development, integration and testing; (vi) lack of automated intervention technologies based on the data being collected; (vii) proper delivery of informed consent; (viii) objectiveness of authored data (can the data be trusted, and when?); (ix) standardization of health measures obtained from smartphone and wearable sensors; (x) proper authorship (were the data authored by the patient being monitored?); (xi) battery consumption of devices; (xii) usage fatigue (patients' willingness to use the technology wears out with time); (xiii) understanding negative effects and development of physio-behavioral models; and (xiv) privacy. Some of the remaining issues are addressed by The Berkeley Telemonitoring Framework, an open source framework that enables development of research telemonitoring smartphone applications with security and privacy in mind. In this chapter we also included a novel approach to privacy based on Private Disclosure of Information (PDI) which is aimed to prevent an adversary from inferring certain sensitive information from data that are being collected during telemonitoring. With commercial entities entering the health telemonitoring, we believe the privacy will become an increasingly important issue for patients.

Acknowledgements Many people have directly and indirectly helped in preparing the manuscript of this chapter, both their support and feedback are greatly appreciated. The authors would like to thank David M. Liebovitz, MD for his continued support in telemonitoring and mHealth research. The Berkeley Telemonitoring Project would not have been possible without the dedication of every member of its team—their contributions are greatly appreciated and valued. Many thanks go to Katherine Driggs-Campbell for the initial conversation that spurred the idea of Private Disclosure of Information (PDI). The authors are also greatly indebted to Yusuf Erol, Michael Carl Tschantz, Arash Nourian and John F. Canny for their fruitful discussions and feedback that significantly improved the quality of the work on PDI. This work was supported in part by TRUST, Team for Research in Ubiquitous Secure Technology, which receives funding support for the National Science Foundation (NSF award number CCF-0424422). The publication of this chapter was made possible by Grant Number HHS 90TR0003/01. Any opinions, findings, conclusions, views or recommendations expressed in this chapter are those of the authors and do not necessarily reflect the views of the National Science Foundation or the official views of the United States Department of Health and Human Services.

References

1. N. R. Adam and J. C. Worthmann. Security-control methods for statistical databases: A comparative study. *ACM Computing Surveys (CSUR)*, 21(4):515–556, 1989.
2. N. Alshurafa, J.-A. Eastwood, S. Nyamathi, J. J. Liu, W. Xu, H. Ghasemzadeh, M. Pourhomayoun, and M. Sarrafzadeh. Improving compliance in remote healthcare systems through smartphone battery optimization. *Biomedical and Health Informatics, IEEE Journal of*, 19(1):57–63, Jan 2015.
3. Apple Inc. ResearchKit programming guide - Creating surveys at http://www.researchkit.org/docs/docs/Survey/CreatingSurveys.html.
4. Apple Inc. Apple Advances Health Apps with CareKit at http://www.apple.com/pr/library/2016/03/21Apple-Advances-Health-Apps-with-CareKit.html, 2016.
5. AppleInsider Staff. Over 10K participants sign up for Stanford medical trial after ResearchKit debut at http://www.appleinsider.com/articles/15/03/11/over-10k-participants-sign-up-for-stanford-medical-trial-after-researchkit-debut, 2015.
6. D. Aranki and R. Bajcsy. Private disclosure of information in health tele-monitoring. *arXiv preprint* arXiv:1504.07313, 2015.
7. D. Aranki and R. Bajcsy. Private disclosure of information matlab toolbox at https://www.telemonitoring.berkeley.edu/PDI/, 2016.
8. D. Aranki, G. Kurillo, A. Mani, P. Azar, J. van Gaalen, Q. Peng, P. Nigam, M. P. Reddy, S. Sankavaram, Q. Wu, and R. Bajcsy. A telemonitoring framework for android devices. In

2016 IEEE First International Conference on Connected Health: Applications, Systems and Engineering Technologies (CHASE), pages 282–291. IEEE, 2016.
9. D. Aranki, G. Kurillo, P. Yan, D. M. Liebovitz, and R. Bajcsy. Continuous, real-time, tele-monitoring of patients with chronic heart-failure: lessons learned from a pilot study. In *Proceedings of the 9th International Conference on Body Area Networks*, pages 135–141. ICST (Institute for Computer Sciences, Social-Informatics and Telecommunications Engineering), 2014.
10. D. Aranki, G. Kurillo, P. Yan, D. M. Liebovitz, and R. Bajcsy. Real-time tele-monitoring of patients with chronic heart-failure using a smartphone: Lessons learned. *IEEE Transactions on Affective Computing*, 2016.
11. C. Asuncion, U. Balakrishnan, H. Sarver, L. Serven, and E. Song. A telemonitoring solution to long-distance running coaching. Master's thesis, EECS Department, University of California, Berkeley, May 2016.
12. F. Axisa, A. Dittmar, and G. Delhomme. Smart clothes for the monitoring in real time and conditions of physiological, emotional and sensorial reactions of human. In *Engineering in Medicine and Biology Society, 2003. Proceedings of the 25th Annual International Conference of the IEEE*, volume 4, pages 3744–3747. IEEE, 2003.
13. P. Azar, A. Mani, Q. Peng, and J. van Gaalen. Expanded telehealth platform for android. Master's thesis, EECS Department, University of California, Berkeley, May 2015.
14. D. Ben-Zeev, S. M. Schueller, M. Begale, J. Duffecy, J. M. Kane, and D. C. Mohr. Strategies for mHealth Research: Lessons from 3 Mobile Intervention Studies. *Administration and Policy in Mental Health and Mental Health Services Research*, 42:157–167, 2015.
15. L. Bishop, B. J. Holmes, and C. M. Kelley. National consumer health privacy survey 2005. *California HealthCare Foundation, Oakland, CA*, 2005.
16. R. Bloss. Wearable sensors bring new benefits to continuous medical monitoring, real time physical activity assessment, baby monitoring and industrial applications. *Sensor Review*, 35(2):141–145, 2015.
17. B. M. Bot, C. Suver, E. C. Neto, M. Kellen, A. Klein, C. Bare, M. Doerr, A. Pratap, J. Wilbanks, E. R. Dorsey, S. H. Friend, and A. D. Trister. The mPower study, Parkinson disease mobile data collected using ResearchKit. *Scientific Data*, 3:160011, 2016. doi:10.1038/sdata.2016.11
18. M. N. K. Boulos, A. C. Brewer, C. Karimkhani, D. B. Buller, and R. P. Dellavalle. Mobile medical and health apps: state of the art, concerns, regulatory control and certification. *Online Journal of Public Health Informatics*, 5(3), 2014.
19. M. N. Burns, M. Begale, J. Duffecy, D. Gergle, C. J. Karr, E. Giangrande, and D. C. Mohr. Harnessing context sensing to develop a mobile intervention for depression. *Journal of Medical Internet Research*, 13(3):1–17, 2011.
20. M. A. Case, H. A. Burwick, K. G. Volpp, and M. S. Patel. Accuracy of smartphone applications and wearable devices for tracking physical activity data. *JAMA*, 313(6):625–626, 2015.
21. Centers for Medicare & Medicaid Services. National health expenditures 2014 highlights at https://www.cms.gov/Research-Statistics-Data-and-systems/Statistics-Trends-and-reports/NationalHealthExpendData/Downloads/highlights.pdf, 2014.
22. S. I. Chaudhry, J. A. Mattera, J. P. Curtis, J. A. Spertus, J. Herrin, Z. Lin, C. O. Phillips, B. V. Hodshon, L. S. Cooper, and H. M. Krumholz. Telemonitoring in patients with heart failure. *New England Journal of Medicine*, 363(24):2301–2309, 2010.
23. C. Chen and B. Womack. Google reveals health-tracking wristband at http://www.bloomberg.com/news/articles/2015-06-23/google-developing-health-tracking-wristband-for-health-research.
24. K. Y. Chen and M. Sun. Improving energy expenditure estimation by using a triaxial accelerometer. *Journal of Applied Physiology*, 83(6):2112–2122, 1997.
25. M. Y. Chih, T. Patton, F. M. McTavish, A. J. Isham, C. L. Judkins-Fisher, A. K. Atwood, and D. H. Gustafson. Predictive modeling of addiction lapses in a mobile health application. *Journal of Substance Abuse Treatment*, 46(1):29–35, 2014.
26. R. A. Clark, S. C. Inglis, F. A. McAlister, J. G. Cleland, and S. Stewart. Telemonitoring or structured telephone support programmes for patients with chronic heart failure: systematic review and meta-analysis. *BMJ*, 334(7600):942, 2007.

27. G. Cormode. Personal privacy vs population privacy: Learning to attack anonymization. In *Proceedings of the 17th ACM SIGKDD International Conference on Knowledge Discovery and Data Mining*, pages 1253–1261. ACM, 2011.
28. T. M. Cover and J. A. Thomas. *Elements of Information Theory*. John Wiley & Sons, 2 edition, 2006.
29. R. B. D'Agostino, R. S. Vasan, M. J. Pencina, P. A. Wolf, M. Cobain, J. M. Massaro, and W. B. Kannel. General cardiovascular risk profile for use in primary care the framingham heart study. *Circulation*, 117(6):743–753, 2008.
30. K. L. Dannecker, S. A. Petro, E. L. Melanson, and R. C. Browning. Accuracy of fitbit activity monitor to predict energy expenditure with and without classification of activities. *Medicine & Science in Sports & Exercise*, 43(5):62, 2011.
31. D. E. Denning and J. Schlorer. Inference controls for statistical databases. *Computer*, 16(7):69–82, 1983.
32. N. V. Dhurandhar, D. A. Schoeller, A. W. Brown, S. B. Heymsfield, D. M. Thomas, T. I. Sørensen, J. R. Speakman, M. M. Jeansonne, and D. B. Allison. Energy balance measurement: when something is not better than nothing. *International Journal of Obesity*, 2014.
33. D. Donaire-Gonzalez, A. de Nazelle, E. Seto, M. Mendez, M. J. Nieuwenhuijsen, and M. Jerrett. Comparison of physical activity measures using mobile phone-based calfit and actigraph. *Journal of Medical Internet Research*, 15(6), 2013.
34. G. Duncan and D. Lambert. The risk of disclosure for microdata. *Journal of Business & Economic Statistics*, 7(2):207–217, 1989.
35. G. T. Duncan and D. Lambert. Disclosure-limited data dissemination. *Journal of the American Statistical Association*, 81(393):10–18, 1986.
36. C. Dwork. Differential privacy. In *Automata, Languages and Programming*, pages 1–12. Springer, 2006.
37. C. Dwork. Differential privacy: A survey of results. In *Theory and Applications of Models of Computation*, pages 1–19. Springer, 2008.
38. EMB/11073. ISO/IEEE health informatics – personal health device communication part 00103: Overview. *ISO/IEEE Std 11073-00103:2012*, 2012.
39. D. S. Eng and J. M. Lee. The promise and peril of mobile health applications for diabetes and endocrinology. *Pediatric diabetes*, 14(4):231–238, 2013.
40. C. Farkas and S. Jajodia. The inference problem: A survey. *SIGKDD Explor. Newsl.*, 4(2):6–11, Dec. 2002.
41. B. Fung, K. Wang, R. Chen, and P. S. Yu. Privacy-preserving data publishing: A survey of recent developments. *ACM Computing Surveys (CSUR)*, 42(4):14, 2010.
42. A. D. Galbreath, R. A. Krasuski, B. Smith, K. C. Stajduhar, M. D. Kwan, R. Ellis, and G. L. Freeman. Long-term healthcare and cost outcomes of disease management in a large, randomized, community-based population with heart failure. *Circulation*, 110(23):3518–3526, 2004.
43. G. Giamouzis, A. Kalogeropoulos, V. V. Georgiopoulou, S. Laskar, A. L. Smith, S. B. Dunbar, F. Triposkiadis, and J. Butler. Hospitalization epidemic in patients with heart failure: risk factors, risk prediction, knowledge gaps, and future directions. *Journal of Cardiac Failure*, 17(1):54–75, 2011.
44. G. Giamouzis, D. Mastrogiannis, K. Koutrakis, G. Karayannis, C. Parisis, C. Rountas, E. Adreanides, G. E. Dafoulas, P. C. Stafylas, J. Skoularigis, S. Giacomelli, Z. Olivari, and F. Triposkiadis. Telemonitoring in chronic heart failure: a systematic review. *Cardiology Research and Practice*, 2012, 2012.
45. A. Gkoulalas-Divanis, G. Loukides, and J. Sun. Publishing data from electronic health records while preserving privacy: A survey of algorithms. *Journal of Biomedical Informatics*, 50:4–19, 2014.
46. C.-J. Hsiao and E. Hing. *Use and characteristics of electronic health record systems among office-based physician practices, United States, 2001-2012*. US Department of Health and Human Services, Centers for Disease Control and Prevention, National Center for Health Statistics, 2012.

47. D. L. Hunter. An Apple a day keeps the research ethics committee away? *Research Ethics*, 11(1):2–3, 2015.
48. M. Hussain, A. Al-Haiqi, A. Zaidan, B. Zaidan, M. Kiah, N. B. Anuar, and M. Abdulnabi. The landscape of research on smartphone medical apps: Coherent taxonomy, motivations, open challenges and recommendations. *Computer Methods and Programs in Biomedicine*, 122(3):393–408, 2015.
49. S. Inglis. Structured telephone support or telemonitoring programmes for patients with chronic heart failure. *Journal of Evidence-Based Medicine*, 3(4):228–228, 2010.
50. J. Jardine, J. Fisher, and B. Carrick. Apple's ResearchKit: smart data collection for the smartphone era? *Journal of the Royal Society of Medicine*, 108(8):294–296, 2015.
51. S. F. Jencks, M. V. Williams, and E. A. Coleman. Rehospitalizations among patients in the medicare fee-for-service program. *New England Journal of Medicine*, 360(14):1418–1428, 2009.
52. J. Jiao, T. Courtade, K. Venkat, and T. Weissman. Justification of logarithmic loss via the benefit of side information. In *Information Theory (ISIT), 2014 IEEE International Symposium on*, pages 946–950. IEEE, 2014.
53. R. Klaassen, R. op den Akker, and H. op den Akker. Feedback presentation for mobile personalised digital physical activity coaching platforms. In *Proceedings of the 6th International Conference on PErvasive Technologies Related to Assistive Environments*, PETRA '13, pages 64:1–64:8, New York, NY, USA, 2013. ACM.
54. Y.-D. Lee and W.-Y. Chung. Wireless sensor network based wearable smart shirt for ubiquitous health and activity monitoring. *Sensors and Actuators B: Chemical*, 140(2):390–395, 2009.
55. N. Li, T. Li, and S. Venkatasubramanian. t-closeness: Privacy beyond k-anonymity and l-diversity. In *IEEE International Conference on Data Engineering*, volume 7, pages 106–115, 2007.
56. A. Machanavajjhala, D. Kifer, J. Gehrke, and M. Venkitasubramaniam. L-diversity: Privacy beyond k-anonymity. *ACM Trans. Knowl. Discov. Data*, 1(1), Mar. 2007.
57. C. K. Martin, A. C. Miller, D. M. Thomas, C. M. Champagne, H. Han, and T. Church. Efficacy of SmartLoss (SM), a smartphone-based weight loss intervention: Results from a randomized controlled trial. *Obesity*, 23(5):935–42, 2015.
58. B. Miller, L. Huang, A. D. Joseph, and J. D. Tygar. I know why you went to the clinic: Risks and realization of https traffic analysis. In *Privacy Enhancing Technologies: 14th International Symposium, PETS 2014, Amsterdam, The Netherlands, July 16-18, 2014. Proceedings*, pages 143–163. Springer International Publishing, 2014.
59. M. Mladenov and M. Mock. A step counter service for java-enabled devices using a built-in accelerometer. In *Proceedings of the 1st International Workshop on Context-Aware Middleware and Services: Affiliated With the 4th International Conference on Communication System Software and Middleware (COMSWARE 2009)*, pages 1–5. ACM, 2009.
60. B. Obama. United States health care reform: Progress to date and next steps. *JAMA*, 316(5):525–532, 2016.
61. A. Pande, Y. Zeng, A. K. Das, P. Mohapatra, S. Miyamoto, E. Seto, E. K. Henricson, and J. J. Han. Energy expenditure estimation with smartphone body sensors. In *Proc. of the 8th International Conference on Body Area Networks*, pages 8–14, 2013.
62. G. Paré, K. Moqadem, G. Pineau, and C. St-Hilaire. Clinical effects of home telemonitoring in the context of diabetes, asthma, heart failure and hypertension: a systematic review. *Journal of Medical Internet Research*, 12(2), 2010.
63. J.-g. Park, A. Patel, D. Curtis, S. Teller, and J. Ledlie. Online pose classification and walking speed estimation using handheld devices. In *Proceedings of the 2012 ACM Conference on Ubiquitous Computing*, pages 113–122. ACM, 2012.
64. M. S. Patel, D. A. Asch, and K. G. Volpp. Wearable devices as facilitators, not drivers, of health behavior change. *JAMA*, 313(5):459–460, 2015.
65. Patient Protection and Affordable Care Act. Patient Protection and Affordable Care Act. *Public Law*, (111–148), 2010.

66. M.-Z. Poh, D. J. McDuff, and R. W. Picard. Advancements in noncontact, multiparameter physiological measurements using a webcam. *Biomedical Engineering, IEEE Transactions on*, 58(1):7–11, 2011.
67. N. M. Rickles, B. L. Svarstad, J. L. Statz-Paynter, L. V. Taylor, and K. A. Kobak. Pharmacist telemonitoring of antidepressant use: effects on pharmacist–patient collaboration. *Journal of the American Pharmacists Association*, 45(3):344–353, 2005.
68. S. Ritter. Apple's Research Kit Development Framework for Iphone Apps Enables Innovative Approaches to Medical Research Data Collection. *Clinical Trials*, 5(2):1000e120, 2015.
69. R. S. Sandhu. Lattice-based access control models. *Computer*, 26(11):9–19, Nov 1993.
70. B. Spring, M. Gotsis, A. Paiva, and D. Spruijt-Metz. Healthy apps: Mobile devices for continuous monitoring and intervention. *IEEE Pulse*, 4(6):34–40, 2013.
71. L. Sweeney. k-anonymity: A model for protecting privacy. *International Journal of Uncertainty, Fuzziness and Knowledge-Based Systems*, 10(05):557–570, 2002.
72. A. G. Taylor. The ResearchKit Health Projects. In *Get Fit with Apple Watch*, chapter 8, pages 111–117. Apress, 2015.
73. D. E. R. Warburton, C. W. Nicol, and S. S. D. Bredin. Health benefits of physical activity: the evidence. *CMAJ: Canadian Medical Association Journal = Journal de l'Association medicale canadienne*, 174(6):801–9, 2006.
74. S. L. Warner. Randomized response: A survey technique for eliminating evasive answer bias. *Journal of the American Statistical Association*, 60(309):63–69, 1965.
75. A. M. White, A. R. Matthews, K. Z. Snow, and F. Monrose. Phonotactic reconstruction of encrypted voip conversations: Hookt on fon-iks. In *Security and Privacy (SP), 2011 IEEE Symposium on*, pages 3–18. IEEE, 2011.

Exploiting Physiological Sensors and Biosignal Processing to Enhance Monitoring Care in Mental Health

Gaetano Valenza and Enzo Pasquale Scilingo

Abstract In this chapter, we describe how it is possible to exploit physiological sensors and related signal processing methods to enhance monitoring care mental health. Specifically, focusing on wearable sensors for Autonomic Nervous System (ANS) dynamics, we report on recent progresses in monitoring mood swings associated with bipolar disorder through the so-called PSYCHE system. Current clinical practice in diagnosing patients affected by this psychiatric disorder, in fact, is based only on verbal interviews and scores from specific questionnaires. Furthermore, no reliable and objective psycho-physiological markers are currently taken into account. We particularly describe a pervasive, wearable, and personalized system based on a comfortable t-shirt with integrated fabric electrodes and sensors able to acquire electrocardiogram, respirogram, and body posture information. In order to identify a pattern of objective physiological parameters to support the diagnosis, we describe ad-hoc methodologies of advanced biosignal processing able to effectively recognize four possible clinical mood states in bipolar patients (i.e., depression, mixed state, hypomania, and euthymia) who underwent long-term (up to 24 h) monitoring. Mood assessment is here intended as an intra-subject evaluation in which the patient's states are modeled as a stochastic process with time dependency, i.e., in the time domain, each mood state refers to the previous one(s). Experimental results are reported in terms of statistical analysis, as well as confusion matrices from automatic mood state recognition, and demonstrate that wearable and comfortable ANS monitoring could be a viable solution to enhance monitoring care in mental health. We conclude the chapter describing a methodology predicting mood changes in bipolar disorder using heartbeat nonlinear dynamics exclusively.

G. Valenza (✉) · E.P. Scilingo
Bioengineering and Robotics Research Centre "E. Piaggio" & Department of Information Engineering, School of Engineering, University of Pisa, Largo Lucio Lazzarino 1, 56122 Pisa, Italy
e-mail: g.valenza@ing.unipi.it

E.P. Scilingo
e-mail: e.scilingo@ing.unipi.it

© Springer International Publishing AG 2017

S.U. Khan et al. (eds.), *Handbook of Large-Scale Distributed Computing in Smart Healthcare*, Scalable Computing and Communications,
DOI 10.1007/978-3-319-58280-1_19

Keywords PSYCHE platform · Autonomic nervous system monitoring · Hearth rate variability · Respiration · Wearable textile system · Multilayer perceptron · Mood recognition · Bipolar disorder · Nonlinear dynamics · Support vector machines

1 Introduction

In this section, we briefly report on symptoms, prevalence, current clinical practice, and diagnosis and treatment limitations related to bipolar disorder. Then, recent finding linking autonomic nervous system dynamics with pathological mood changes follow below.

1.1 The Bipolar Disorder

Bipolar disorder, formerly known as manic-depressive illness, is a psychiatric condition in which patients experience dramatic mood shifts. Typically, the disorder is cyclic passing from episodes of pathological low moods (depression) to pathological high moods (mania or hypomania) through episodes of co-presence of depressive and maniacal symptoms (mixed state). Sometime, in the middle, patients experience periods of relatively good affective balance (euthymia). Depression is characterized by symptoms of sadness a desperation with a lack of interest together with other several neurovegetative symptoms including loss of appetite and sleep. Other symptoms such as cognitive retardation, somatic pain or functional symptoms (headache, dyspepsia etc.) are frequent as well. Moreover, thoughts of ruin, guilt or death including suicidal thoughts that might end in suicide attempts can be experienced by depressed patients. On the other hand, patients with mania experience an increased activity and an acceleration of thoughts. Hyperactivity is often not finalized and patients switching from task to task are not able to complete any activity. In the maniac phase patients also experience a reduction of the necessity to sleep, sleeping a few hours per night without feeling tired. Finally, mania is characterized by an iperexcited mood with the idea of grandiosity and hypertrophic self-esteem. Maniacs often believe of being a descendent of some important historical character. In the mixed state, patients experience shared symptoms of both mania and depression. For instance, patients can be hyperactive but have insomnia, have an increased self-esteem but also thoughts of inadequacy, and so on.

Bipolar disorder is very common in western population [1–4]. Almost 15% of the population in the United States has suffered from at least one episode of mood disorder [1], and more than two million Americans have been specifically diagnosed with bipolar disorder. Furthermore, it has been estimated that about 27% (equals 82.7

million; 95% confidence interval: 78.5–87.1) of the adult European population, from 18 to 65 years of age, is or has been affected by at least one mental disorder [2, 3]. A recent worldwide survey in 11 countries has found an overall lifetime prevalence of 1% for the typical forms of bipolar disorder and 1.4% for milder sub-threshold disorders [5].

Although this important prevalence and high cost of treatment, the clinical management of mood disorders is still controversial.

First of all, bipolar disorder is often undetected for years before it is diagnosed and treated. Secondly, bipolar patients are extremely heterogeneous in terms of phenomenology, severity of the symptoms, number and duration of the episodes, as well as the time interval between them. Even during euthymic periods (i.e., after remission from maniacal or depressive episodes), patients tend to experience sub-threshold mood alterations over time. In spite of the non-specific symptoms, the diagnosis of bipolar disorders and, more in general, of psychiatric pathological conditions is based only on interviews with the clinicians who evaluate symptoms self-reported by the patients themselves relying on scores obtained from rating scales. Although these interviews are 'structured' (i.e. questions and question order are established and defined in specific manuals) and high rates of consensus can be achieved among specialists (psychiatrists and clinical psychologists), the diagnosis is subjected to personal and often arbitrary interpretation of the clinicians. Indeed, there are no objective clinical exams are envisaged in current clinical practice [6–8].

Clinical diagnosis is based on the criteria proposed by the Diagnostic Statistic Manual of Mental Disorders (DSM-IV-TR) [9] edited by the American Psychiatric Association. According to this manual, the diagnosis of depression is made if 5 symptoms out of 9 are present. Similar cut-offs are applied for the diagnosis of other episodes. In line with this approach, a patient who has had only 4 symptoms of depressive episodes is considered remitted (although partially remitted). These clearly can bring to biased interpretation and inconsistency [6–8].

The above description portrays a dramatic scenario in which research and technological advances could (and should) greatly contribute and bridge the current gaps. Despite the fact that many studies have been carried out on several biomarkers, e.g. sleep quality, circadian heart rate rhythms, cortisol dynamics, as well as dysfunctions of the central and autonomic nervous systems, none of them has attained an acceptable level of accuracy in clinical use in order to evaluate and predict the development of mental disorders.

Next, after reporting on recent findings linking bipolar disorder and autonomic nervous system (ANS) dynamics, we briefly describe a textile-based, ANS and behavioural monitoring platform (see Sect. 2). Then, we describe the experimental setup (see Sect. 3.2) of three exemplary studies involving patients with bipolar disorder, whose mood changes are characterized and predicted through advanced signal processing methods (see Sect. 3.3). Experimental results (Sect. 4) and Discussion (Sect. 5) of the main achievements close the chapter.

1.2 Bipolar Disorder and Autonomic Nervous System Dynamics

Mood disorders have been previously associated with alterations in Autonomic Nervous System (ANS) functioning [10, 11]. Depressed subjects frequently present clinical symptoms related to autonomic dysfunction such as sleep pattern alterations, decreased appetite, gastrointestinal paresthesia and increased sweating [12]. In addition, multiple studies have reported decreased Heart Rate Variability (HRV) and baroreflex sensitivity in these subjects [13].

Several studies have been performed on proposing biomarkers that consider sleep quality [14–16], circadian heart rate rhythms [17, 18], cortisol dynamics, [19–21], as well as ANS functionality [22–27]. However, none of these studies is sufficiently reliable to have a translational application in the current clinical practice. A possible explanation for these negative results can be that mood disorders are more heterogeneous, in terms of psychophysiological, neuroendocrine and neurobiological correlates, than relatively simple clinical phenotypes usually adopted for clinical and also for research purposes. In other words, patients, although homogeneous from a clinical descriptive point of view, are extremely dishomogeneous in terms of endophenotypes.

2 The PSYCHE Platform

A collaborative European research project called PSYCHE, PerSonalized monitoring sYstems for Care in mental HEalth, aims to overcome the above mentioned limitations [24, 28–35]. The scope of the PSYCHE project is to identify a personalized, pervasive, cost-effective, and multi-parametric platform for long-term monitoring of mental disorders. Patients were monitored by means of sensorized clothes and could interact with user-friendly interfaces on smartphones to communicate with clinicians, who, in turn, could check the mental status of patients by means of professional web-based interfaces.

More specifically, PSYCHE acquired a wide set of behavioral and physiological parameters that were continuously monitored through a smartphone and a sensorized t-shirt. The sensorized t-shirt (developed by Smartex s.r.l, Pisa, Italy) is able to comfortably evaluated the cardiac activity by recording the electrocardiogram (ECG) through dry textile-based electrodes, the respiration activity by means of textile piezoresistive sensors, and the physical activity using a three-axial accelerometer. More specifically, the inter-beat interval series (hereinafter RR) extracted from the ECG, i.e. the series constituted by the distance of two consecutive peaks of the ECG, and the respiratory dynamics were considered in the biosignal analysis strategy. A wide set of physiological features, both in the time and frequency domain, both through standard and non linear techniques, were extracted from the RR and the respiration signals in order to evaluate mood changes.

The smartphone collects these data sending it out to a remote data server. Moreover, the smartphone includes digital agendas, digitalized questionnaires, voice analysis, and scheduling of dedicated affective elicitation protocols. Accordingly, the aim is to support the standard clinical practice, which as a whole remains unchanged, continuing to use questionnaires and interviews for diagnosis, through an appropriate unobtrusive system which continuously collects physiological and behavioral data to be further analyzed and used as decision support to clinical diagnosis.

Other physiological signals as well as behavioral parameters were taken into account as part of the PSYCHE project (e.g. voice, activity index, sleep pattern alteration, electrodermal response, biochemical markers), but they are not reported in this chapter. A user-friendly device such as a smartphone for monitoring environmental information such as light, temperature and noise further completes the PSYCHE platform.

The PSYCHE concept of decision support system for bipolar disorder and a system prototype are shown in Figs. 1 and 2, respectively.

It is worth noting that the use of dry textile-based electrodes provides several advantages. First, the system is easy to use because sensors are automatically located and allows maximizing comfort. Second, a special multilayer structure increases the amount of sweat and reduces the rate of evaporation reaching electrochemical equilibrium between the skin and electrodes after a couple of minutes. Therefore, the signal quality [36] is remarkably improved and kept as constant as possible. When skin-electrode contact is not satisfactory, the quality of the signals is remarkably worsened. Accordingly, a preliminary check on the quality of data is necessary. The shirt, in male or female version, is made of elastic fibers enabling tight adhesion to the body and metallic knitted fibers to form the electrodes. Moreover, respiration activity is recorded through piezoresistive fiber stretching. These materials are knitted

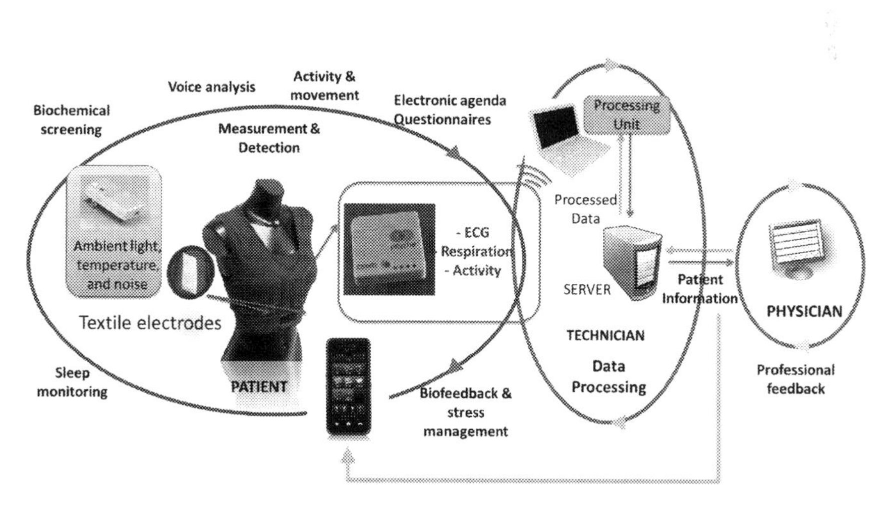

Fig. 1 Overview of the PSYCHE system as global platform serving as decision support system for bipolar disorder management

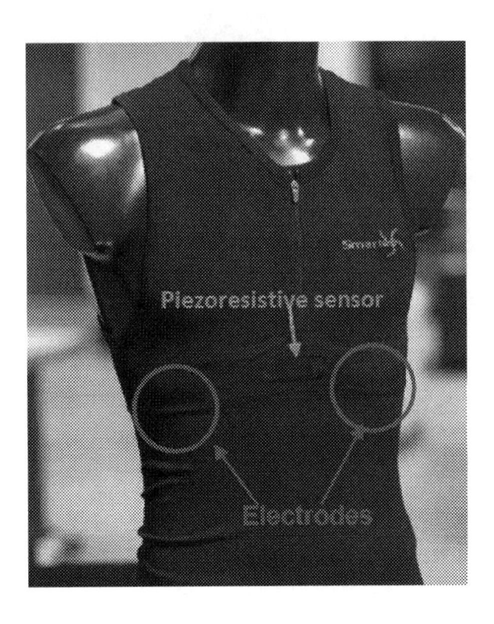

Fig. 2 Wearable system prototype

together and are fully integrated in the garment without any mechanical and physical discontinuity, creating areas with different functionalities. The shirt was designed to appear as a usual and ordinary underwear garment. It is thermally comfortable and includes a polyamide yarn with antibacterial properties. Garments, indeed, are made of commercial yarns, to be easily washed and disinfected, which are already tested (and certified) to come into contact with human skin. The fabric electrodes for ECG recording and the piezoresistive sensors for respiration activity acquisition are finally connected through conductive fabric wires to a portable electronics inserted into a small pocket. Connection between garment and electronics is made by means of a simple plug, easily removable.

Technical specifications of the PSYCHE wearable monitoring platform are reported in Table 1.

Throughout this chapter, we demonstrate that a single-variable approach, as proposed by previous literature, is not sufficient to robustly characterize mood episodes in bipolar disorder [24]. Instead, a multi-parametric and personalized approach, i.e., mood episodes are identified as an intra-subject analysis, is much more effective.

Furthermore, our personalized approach identifies mood states as an intra-subject analysis taking into account the temporal dynamics of the illness. From a signal processing point of view, patients' mood changes are modeled as a discrete-time stochastic process in which each recording, associated to a specific mood state, also depends on the previous state respecting the so-called Markov property [37]. We demonstrate that mood changes in bipolar disorders can be modeled as a Markov chain, in which each state is characterized by ANS-HRV features extracted over long periods of time (up to 18 hours). Multi-class recognition of these mood states achieved an accuracy as high as 99%.

Table 1 Technical specifications of the wearable monitoring platform (provided by Smartex s.r.l.)

Characteristics	
Power supply	Litium battery (life up to 18 h)
Data storage	MicroSD card
Data communication	Micro USB, bluetooth
Electrocardiogram	
Measurement principle	Bio-potentials on the thorax
Sensors	Textile electrodes
Number of leads	1
Input auto configurable analog filter	0.67–40 Hz
Analog-to-digital conversion	16 bits
Sampling rate	250 Hz
Respiration signal	
Measurement principle	Piezoresistive method
Range of electrical resistance	$20k\Omega$–$10M\Omega$
Bandwidth	DC to 10 Hz
Resolution	12 bits
Sampling rate	25 Hz

Finally, we propose a methodology predicting mood changes using heartbeat linear and nonlinear dynamics. Such changes are intended as transitioning between euthymic state (EUT), i.e., the good affective balance, and non-euthymic state (non-EUT)—which means fulfilled the criteria for one of the mood states defined above -, and vice-versa.

3 Materials and Methods

This chapter aims at presenting methods and results on the identification of mood swings on bipolar patients by acquiring and processing peripheral physiological signals. Specifically, a set of features, i.e. commonly-used standard features and features extracted through nonlinear dynamic methods, were extracted from the peripheral signals and used to implement the automatic mood-tracking system. Experimental results are shown by means of confusion matrices [38].

3.1 The Mood Model

As mentioned above, the diagnosis of bipolar disorder in the current clinical practice is made through clinician-administered rating scales and questionnaires, namely the Bauer internal mood scale (IMS) [39], the profile of mood states (POMS) [40], the 16th items version of the quick inventory of depressive symptomatology (QIDS) [41], and the Young mania scale (YMS) [42]. Concerning the Italian versions of these scales, IMS and YMS can be found in [43]. The Italian version of POMS was published by Farné et al. [44]. Finally, the Italian version of QIDS can be found in the web-page https://www.ids-qids.org/tr-italian.html. Bipolar disorder can be conceptualized through two main dimensions, i.e. mania and depression, onto a cartesian plane as shown in Fig. 3. This model of mood states describes all of the possible states of the mental disorder. During each clinical visit, each patient was diagnosed as belonging to a class of this model according to outcomes of the clinical rating scales.

Unlike some commonly used mood agendas, this model considers mania and depression not as opposite sides of a unique dimension, but as two different dimensions, whose linear combination allows for the identification of mixed states. Three levels with two degrees of severity for each of the two dimensions were considered in order to approximate the mixed clinical severity. This model has to be intended as a preliminary approach to categorize the mood states. In the literature other studies exploring the mood assessment (e.g. Mehrabian et al. [45]) consider other basic dimensions. However, this preliminary clinical model fitted the needs of the PSYCHE project, which were to classify different clinical states. Moreover, the algorithm for datamining, which is part of the PSYCHE project, might allow for multiple classes with a higher number of subjects. The model will be enriched with other dimensions (e.g. anxiety levels) when the enrollment of the patients will be sufficient to increase the complexity of the analysis.

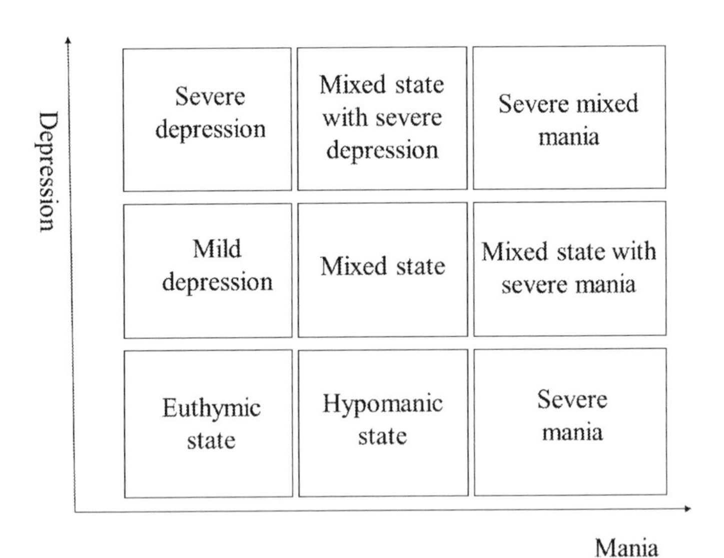

Fig. 3 The mania-depression model for bipolar mood assessment

3.2 *Recruitment of Eligible Subjects and Experimental Protocol*

Patients were recruited according to the following general inclusion/exclusion criteria:

- Age 18–65.
- Diagnosis of bipolar disorder (I or II).
- Presence of a mood episode at the moment of the recruitment of any polarity (depression, hypomania, mixed).
- Low risk of suicidality (as assessed as no thoughts of death and no previous attempts).
- No somatic or neurologic disorders that might be related to bipolar disorders (e.g. thyroid alterations).
- Absence of cognitive impairment.
- Absence of substance abuse disorders.
- Necessity of a change in treatment (treatment change is defined as a augmentation of doses, introduction of or switch to new drugs, introduction of physical treatments).
- Willingness of all patients to sign the informed consent for the PSYCHE project approved by the ethical committee of the University of Pisa and Strasbourg.
- Absence of delusions or hallucinations at the moment of the recruitment.

Before being recruited, the patient was introduced by a clinician to the purpose of the study and was asked to sign an informed consent approved by the ethical committee of the University of Pisa and Strasburg University Hospital. Once enrolled, the patients were asked to fill out severa questionnaires and rating scales in order to assess the current clinical mood at the hospital. All clinical states were evaluated by clinicians according to DSM-IV-TR criteria [9]. In this way four possible clinical mood labels (depression, hypomania, mixed-state, and euthymic state) were assigned. The mood label associated to each patient's evaluation was assigned independently of the previous ones. Each patient, moreover, was assigned to a specific class of the previously described mania-depression model.

During the clinical interview two questionnaires are administered in order to identify the mood state: Quick Inventory of Depressive Symptomatology Clinician Rating (QIDS-C16) and Young Mania Rating Scale (YMRS). More specifically, depression was diagnosed when QIDS-C16 score was greater than or equal to 8, hypomania when YMRS score was greater than or equal to 6, and mixed state when QIDS-C16 score was greater than or equal to 8 and YMRS score was greater than or equal to 6. The cut-off for the QIDS-C16 was set at 8 as it is considered equivalent to an HDRS-17 (Hamilton Depression Rating Scale 17 items) score of 10. Such a score on the HDRS has been proposed as a threshold to define recurrence or relapse [46]. For the YMRS, the score of 6 for hypomania is quite a standard threshold to quantify the lack of hypomanic symptoms. Such a value is in between the strict threshold definition at 4 [47], and the less stringent definition at 8 [48]. Euthymic state, i.e., clinical remission, was defined by having a score below the thresholds above mentioned for both the scales.

During the study, treatment choice remained at the discretion of the clinician as well as the change of treatment in case of lack of response.

After the interview, each patient was asked to wear the sensing shirt and keep it as long as the battery ran out, i.e. approximately for 18 h after leaving the hospital. They are free to perform daily activities at home or elsewhere while the aforementioned physiological signals are monitored and stored in a microSD card. As soon as the subject gave the t-shirt back, data were downloaded and stored in the database for further analysis.

3.2.1 Study 1: Characterization of Pathological Mood States in Bipolar Disorder

In this preliminary study, three bipolar patients were monitored for a period between the enrollment and the reaching of euthymia condition. The study can achieve up to a maximum of 6 evaluations for each patient, over a period of 90 days. More specifically, the protocol was defined so as to evaluate the patient at the enrollment time repeat the clinical assessment after one, two, four, eight, and twelve weeks.

The first three consecutive patients enrolled for the preliminary validation phase of the PSYCHE project were included in this study.

Patient 1 (hereinafter BP1) is a 38 year-old female, patient 2 (hereinafter BP2) is a 55 year-old male, and patient 3 is a 37 year-old female (hereinafter BP3). The mood state diagnosed by the clinician corresponded to a class label, which in turn was associated to a point in the feature space, according to the model described in Sect. 3.1 and schematically reported in Fig. 3. According to this model, Table 2 reports the mood states of the patients during each acquisition. The mood states evaluated in this study are the remission- euthymia, (ES), mild depression (MD), severe depression (SD), and mild mixed state (MS).

Table 2 Clinical labels associated to each patient during each acquisition

ID	ACQ. 1	ACQ. 2	ACQ. 3	ACQ. 4	ACQ. 5	ACQ. 6
BP1	MD	SD	MD	ES		
BP2	MD	MD	MD	MD	MD	ES
BP3	MS	ES				

3.2.2 Study 2: Temporal Characterization of Pathological Mood States in Bipolar Disorder

In order to study the temporal dynamics of mood swings in bipolar disorder, a total of 15 patients were recruited: 7 in Pisa and 8 in Strasbourg. Among these, we used for our study 8 subjects for a total of 42 acquisitions (2 from Pisa and 6 from Strasbourg) because they had more than one long-term acquisition and at least one mood change. Patients BP1, BP2, BP3, BP4, BP5, and BP6 were recruited in the out- patient University clinic of Strasbourg, France. Patients BP7 and BP8 were recruited in high intensity clinical facilities (psychiatric ward and day-hospital) at the University Hospital of Pisa, Italy.

Each patient was evaluated and monitored over a period starting from the day of the enrollment up to remission, i.e. when the patient reaches an euthymic state within an observation window of 3 months. In any case, each patient cannot exceed six evaluations over the whole monitoring period.

Details on the patients' acquisitions as well as mood state information are reported in Table 3.

3.2.3 Study 3: Prediction of Pathological Mood States in Bipolar Disorder

This study was designed to test the ability of the proposed methodology, using the PSYCHE system, to predict mood changes in cyclothymic and rapid-cycling bipolar disorders subjects. Specifically, 14 patients were enrolled (age: 33.43 ± 9.76, age range: 23–54; 6 females) including 6 rapid-cycling bipolar patients, 4 patients with cyclothymic disorders, and 4 subjects with cyclothymic temperament. At the enrollment time, 8 patients were not taking any psychotropic medication. None of the subjects suffers from cardiac arrhythmia or significant cardiovascular disease needing pharmacological treatment. The following psychotropic medications were prescribed at inclusion: Antidepressants (fluoxetine): 1 subject (P1); mood stabilizers (lamotrigine 4; lithium 2; pregabaline 1): 5 subjects (P5, P6, P10, P12, P14);

Table 3 Clinical labels associated to each patient during each acquisition

ID	ACQ. 1	ACQ. 2	ACQ. 3	ACQ. 4	ACQ. 5	ACQ. 6
BP1	HY	HY	HY	ES	ES	
BP2	HY	MS	HY	HY		
BP3	HY	HY	HY	ES	ES	
BP4	DP	DP	DP	DP	DP	ES
BP5	DP	DP	HY	DP	HY	
BP6	HY	HY	HY	ES	ES	
BP7	DP	DP	ES			
BP8	MS	MS	DP	DP	DP	ES

antipsychotics (quetiapine 4; aripiprazole 2; cyamemazine 1): 5 subjects (P5, P6, P11, P12, P14); benzodiazepine-like: 2 subjects (P5 and P11). The study took place in the psychiatry department of the University Hospital of Strasbourg and Geneva.

Patients with cyclothymia and cyclothymic temperament, or with rapid cycling bipolar disorder were recruited in the general population via ads in newspapers and universities and in the clinical population (patients followed by the clinical investigators). First interview with the participants was made on the phone. During this preliminary phone interview they were asked to fill out the 12-item cyclothymic subscale from the short version of the Temperamental Evaluation of Memphis, Pisa, Paris and San Diego or TEMPS-A. If the screening outcome was positive the patients were recruited. Cyclothymia had to be confirmed by a clinical assessment based on the DSM-IV-TR criteria of cyclothymic disorder and the Akiskal criteria of cyclothymia.

Patients were monitored for a period of 14 weeks and they were required to wear the sensorized shirt just a few hours before going to bed and keep it overnight twice a week. They were not constrained to stay still, but they were free to perform daily activities at home or elsewhere while the aforementioned physiological signals were monitored. Participants were asked to use the system during the night from early evening, e.g. 8 p.m. until morning, after wake-up time. The patients could take the system off when they take a shower and/or want to get dressed. Then, patients were asked to bring the system back to their clinician, while the recorded data was manually sent to a central database. Accordingly, each patient can be associated with a sequence of consecutive mood states.

3.3 Biomedical Signal Processing Methodology

Details on the pre-processing, feature extraction and reduction, and classification follow below.

A general scheme of the proposed mood recognition system is shown in Fig. 4.

3.3.1 Preprocessing

Signals were acquired from the wearable system and preprocessed. A specific segmentation of 5 min wide windows has been made on each signal in order to achieve conditions of stationarity [49]. A tenth order band-pass finite impulse response filter with cut-off frequencies of 0.05–35 Hz realized through the Butterworth polynomial has been applied to ECG signal. Next the well-known automatic algorithm developed by Pan-Tompkins [50] has been applied to the ECG signal in order to detect the R peaks from each QRS complex. The temporal distance between two consecutive R peaks is referred to as RR interval (t_{RR}), consequently the HR (beats per minute) is estimated as the following ratio: $HR = \frac{60}{t_{RR}}$. Moreover, as the obtained time series

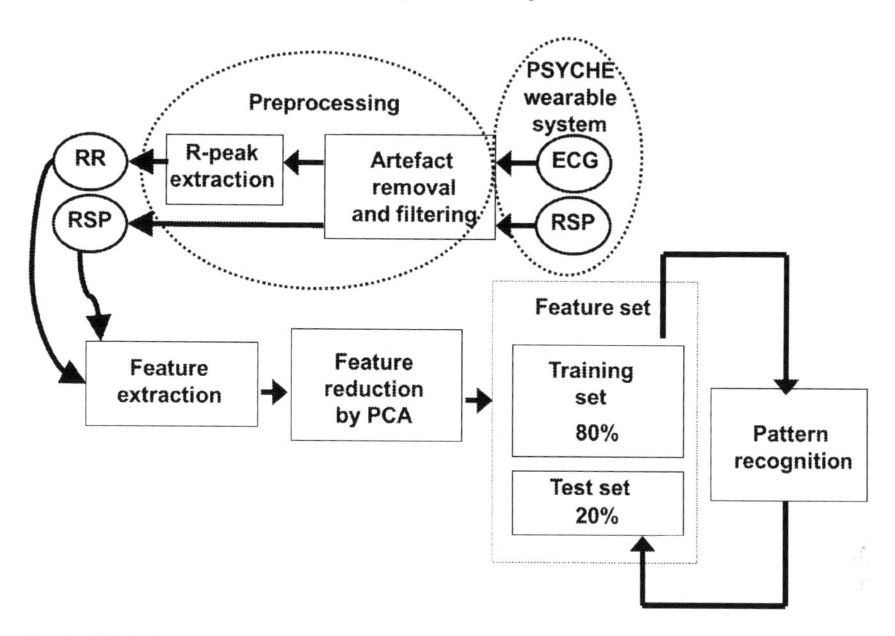

Fig. 4 Block diagram representing the acquisition and processing chain

sequence of RR intervals is non-uniform, this sequence was further re-sampled in agreement with the algorithm of Berger et al. [51]. The respiration (RSP) signal was filtered as well in order to detrend the baseline and reject possible movement artifacts. More specifically, baseline is removed by applying a band-pass filter with a bandwidth 0.05–1 Hz. Generally, when signals come from wearable systems the issue of movement artifacts is very crucial, as mismatch between skin and fabric electrode is intrinsically present. Accordingly, the signals need to be carefully filtered removing artifact movements. Specifically, a specific artifact movement removal (AMR) algorithm has been applied before the feature extraction process. It is a simple and robust algorithm consisting of four steps as shown in Fig. 5. The first step is to filter the ECG within the bandwidth in which the artifact movements were strongest, i.e. from 0.1 to 4 Hz [52]. Then, the filtered signal is treated in order to extrapolate the maximum and the minimum envelopes thus extracting the smoothed mean envelope. Finally, a simple statistical threshold, i.e. 95th percentile, has been applied in order to identify the portions of the signal affect by movement artifacts. More specifically, when the threshold is exceed the signal is considered to be affected by artifacts. The relative parts of the signals with artifacts were discarded.

3.3.2 Feature Extraction

The feature extraction phase of the signals require the non-stationary condition. Accordingly, features were extracted within moving time windows of length W of the

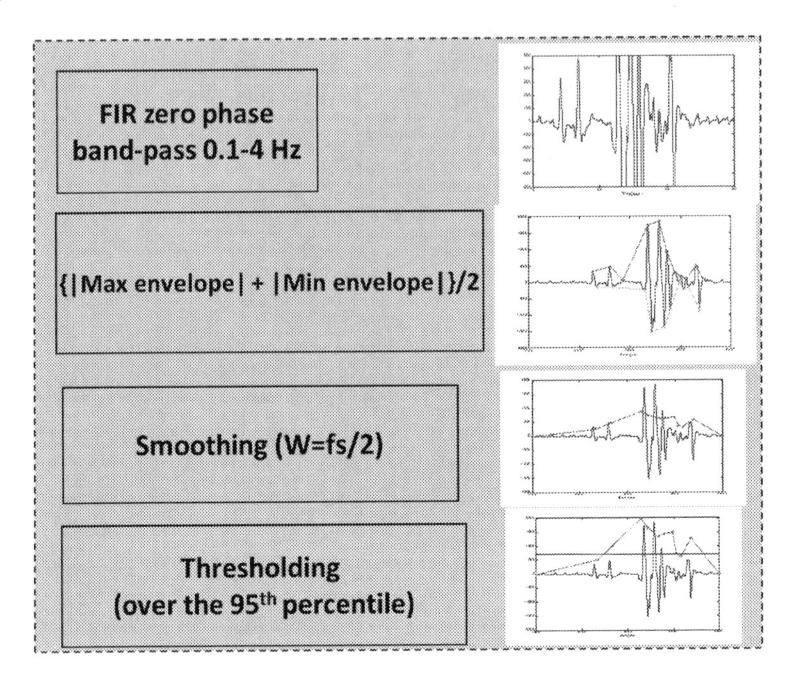

Fig. 5 Artifact movement removal algorithm

artifact-free signal. Each acquisition (see Table 8) can be considered as a concatenation of equally-long (i.e. W) segments of biosignals. The feature space is built by associating each multidimensional point with each acquisition having the same class label. A set of general statistics and specific features (hereinafter called *standard features*) has been extracted along with features extracted from nonlinear dynamic techniques (e.g. entropy measures, recurrence plot, etc.). The feature set is extracted using techniques well-known in the literature, which here are briefly described. Standard features were extracted from time series analysis, statistics, frequency domain transformation and geometric evaluation. The selected features extracted from the RR and RSP signals are reported in Table 4. These measures have been identified according to guidelines and previous outcomes from psycho-physiological and bioengineering studies reported in the current literature. Specifically, the RR standard features were extensively reported in [49, 53], and the nonlinear measures were already treated and used in a previous study of the authors [54].

RR interval series: standard features Concerning the RR signal, the traditional approach proposed in the current literature (see [49, 53] for review) was applied. Time domain features included statistical indices such as the mean (μ_{RR}) and the standard deviation (σ_{RR}) value of the RR intervals, the root mean square of successive differences of intervals (RMSSD), and the number of successive differences of intervals which differ by more than 50 ms (pNN50% expressed as a percentage of the total number of heartbeats analyzed). Referring to the morphological patterns of RR,

Table 4 Selected features extracted from RR and RSP signals

Typology	Biosignal	Feature	Typology	Biosignal	Feature
Standard measures	RR	μ_{RR} σ_{RR} RMSSD pNN50% TINN LF HF LF/HF	High order spectra	RR & RSP	MBI VBI MMB PEB NBE NBSE
	RSP	RSPR MFD SDFD MSD SDSD MAXRSP MINRSP DMMRSP Skewness Kurtosis Power in 0–0.1 Hz Power in 0.1–0.2 Hz Power in 0.2–0.3 Hz Power in 0.3–0.4 Hz	Nonlinear dynamics	RR	DLE ApEn RecR DET LAM TT AV ENTR L_{max} DFA α_1 DFA α_2

the triangular index was calculated. It was derived from the histogram of RR intervals into the NN window (TINN) in which a triangular interpolation was performed. All extracted features in the frequency domain were based on the power spectral density (PSD) of the RR. An auto-regressive (AR) model was used to estimate the PSD in order to provide a better frequency resolution than the nonparametric method. The optimal order p was estimated according to the Akaike information criterion [55]. The Burg method was used to get the AR model parameters. Two main spectral components were distinguished in a spectrum calculated from short-term recordings: the low frequency (LF), 0.04–0.15 Hz, and the high frequency (HF), 0.15–0.4 Hz. The distribution of the power changes was in agreement with the ANS modulation. In the literature, the LF/HF ratio is considered to mirror sympatho/vagal balance or to reflect sympathetic modulations [49].

Respiration activity: standard features Regarding the RSP signal, several features were calculated following the same time-domain segmentation defined for the RR. Specifically, the mean and the standard deviation of the first (MFD and SDFD, respectively) and second derivative (MSD and SDSD, respectively), i.e. variation of the respiration signal, and the standard deviation of the amplitude were evaluated for each segment of length W of each acquisition. The respiration rate (RSPR) was calculated as the frequency corresponding to the maximum spectral magnitude. Other statistical parameters such as the maximum (MAXRSP) and the minimum

(MINRSP) values of breathing amplitude and their difference (DMMRSP) were estimated. Moreover, the skewness, which quantifies the asymmetry of the probability distribution, and the kurtosis, which was a measure of the peakedness of the probability distribution, were evaluated. Concerning the RSP features in the frequency domain, spectral power in the bandwidths 0–0.1 Hz, 0.1–0.2 Hz, 0.2–0.3 Hz, 0.3–0.4 Hz, [56] was calculated as well.

High order spectra and nonlinear analysis: For both RR and RSP signals, high order spectra (HOS) features were also evaluated. HOS refers to the Fourier transform of moments or cumulants of an order grater than two. In particular, the two dimensional third order cumulant Fourier transform, called bispectrum [57, 58] was calculated. It measures the correlation among three spectral peaks, ω_1, ω_2 and $(\omega_1 + \omega_2)$ and also estimates the phase coupling among frequencies. In this work, the bispectral feature set was comprised of: mean and variance of bispectral invariants (MBI and VBI, respectively), mean magnitude of the bispectrum (MMB) and the phase entropy (PEB), normalized bispectral entropy (NBE) and normalized bispectral squared entropy (NBSE). For a detailed review of these features, please refer to [59]). Several nonlinear RR measures were also extracted along with the standard morphological and spectral features [49, 53]. Even if the physiological meaning of these features is still unclear, they resulted to be an important quantifier of cardiovascular control dynamics mediated by the ANS [60–66]. Finally, nonlinear measures related to ANS modulation were estimated. Specifically, the dominant Lyapunov exponent (DLE) [67, 68], the approximate entropy (ApEn) [69, 70], features from the recurrence plot [71] by means of the recurrence quantification analysis (RQA) [72], and the detrended fluctuation analysis (DFA) [73, 74] were evaluated. DLE was calculated through the approach proposed by Rosenstein et al. [75], which ensures reliable values even in short data sets. In fact, it is easy and fast to implement because it uses a simple measure of exponential divergence that circumvents the need of approximating the tangent map. In this way, the convergence, if negative, or divergence, if positive, of trajectories in each dimension of the RR attractor could be easily described. ApEn is a common measure of dynamical systems [76], even in terms of complexity or irregularity of the signal [69, 70]. Large values of ApEn indicate high irregularity while smaller values suggests a more regular signal. RQA quantifies the number and the duration of recurrences of a dynamical system. The following features were calculated [72]: recurrence rate (RecR), determinism (DET), laminarity (LAM), trapping time (TT), average diagonal line length (AV), entropy (ENTR), and longest diagonal line (L_{max}). Finally, in the nonlinear analysis, the statistical self-affinity of a signal is determined by the DFA. It is commonly used to analyze time series for long-memory processes [77] (as we think for mood disorders). DFA was introduced by Peng et. al. 1994 [73] and represents an extension of the (ordinary) fluctuation analysis, which is affected by non-stationarities. DFA features are constituted by the two scaling exponents α_1 and α_2, which are related to the short-term and long-term fluctuations.

3.3.3 History-Dependent Analysis

Once all HRV features are extracted for each patient, the feature set related to the k-th acquisition can be defined as a multidimensional vector $X_{nk}(\mathrm{T_m})$ representing n features evaluated within the time window T_m. Therefore, $X_{nk}(\mathrm{T_m})$ is a matrix of features consisting of m rows (each of the rows corresponds to one of the time windows T_m within the acquisition) and n columns (each of the columns contains one of the HRV features). In order to consider the process of mood states such as the Markov chain, i.e., $\Pr\{X_{nk} = x|(X_{n(k-1)} = x_{k-1})\}$, a simple rescaling procedure is applied. Specifically, for each column of the matrix $X_{nk}(\mathrm{T_m})$, the matrix $Y_{nk}(\mathrm{T_m}) = [X_{nk}(\mathrm{T_m}) - \mathrm{Median}(X_{n(k-1)}(\mathrm{T_m}), m)]/\mathrm{MAD}(X_{n(k-1)}(\mathrm{T_m}))$ is calculated, where $\mathrm{MAD}(X) = \mathrm{Median}(|X - \mathrm{Median}(X)|)$. The quantity $\mathrm{Median}(X_{n(k-1)}(\mathrm{T_m}), m)$ is intended as a vector of the median values of the features calculated through all the rows m of the matrix $X_{nk}(\mathrm{T_m})$, thus over all the time windows T_m of the acquisition $k-1$).

This model is based on the hypothesis that the transition between two clinical mood states is dependent on the past history of mood fluctuations. In other words, the current clinical status of a patient is influenced by the previous status, and therefore also the neurovegetative balance should be rescaled by a factor taking into account the previous clinical status. A simplified block scheme representing such a rescaling procedure over multiple mood states of a patient is shown in Fig. 6. Because of the absence of preceding recordings, the first observation of each patient was used exclusively to obtain the rescaling values useful for the characterization of the observation which followed in time.

3.3.4 Biosignal Processing for Mood State Prediction

A general block scheme of the signal processing chain for mood prediction is shown in Fig. 7. From each acquisition the longest artifact-free segment of signal was selected through the previously developed methodology for artifact detection and removal described above [24], including visual inspection. Sub-segments of 5 min of this segment were used to calculate informative features, which were defined in

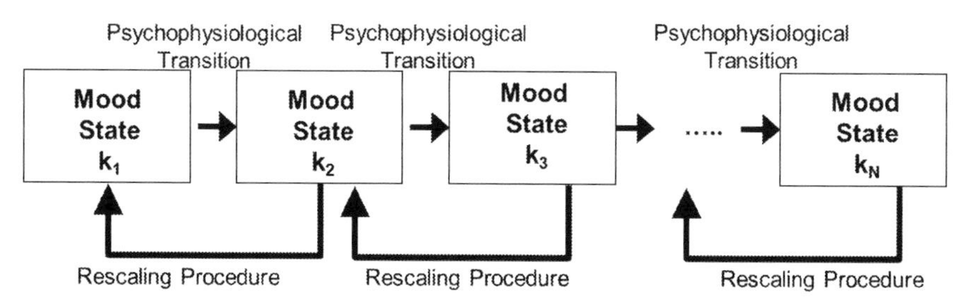

Fig. 6 Simplified block scheme over multiple mood states representing the Markov modeling of the mood recognition procedure

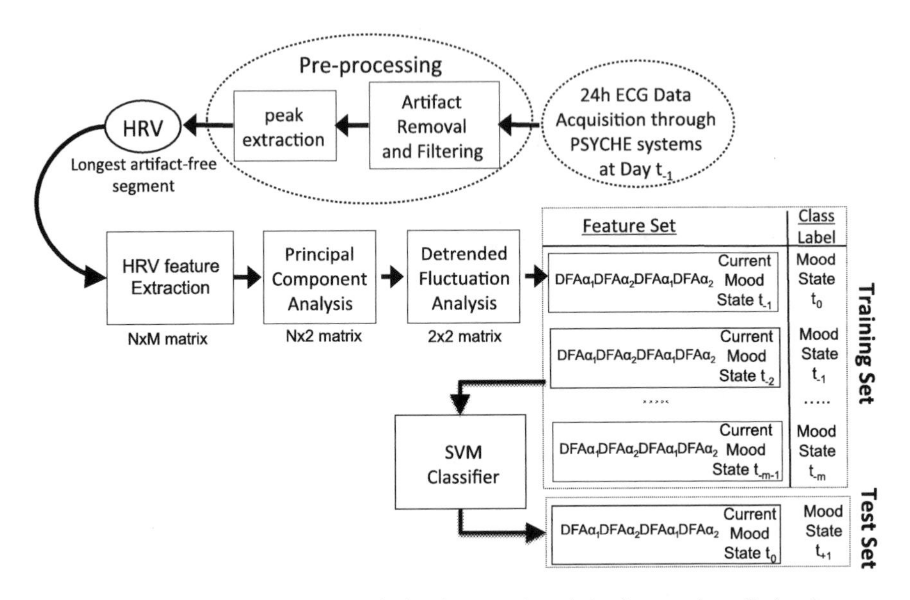

Fig. 7 Block scheme of the proposed signal processing chain for mood prediction between EUT/non-EUT class

the time and frequency domains, as well as from nonlinear analysis (see [53] for calculation details and related literature review).

Each acquisition of each patient is represented in a NxM matrix (N: number of windows x M: number of features), describing the evolution over time of the feature space. A method of size reduction, i.e. Principal Component Analysis, was then applied to this matrix, and the first two dimensions were retained for further analyses. This approach is justified by the fact that, in most cases, such first two dimensions explained more than 90% of data variance. The evolution over time of these two dimensions is synthesized through DFA, taking the α_1 and α_2 parameters as estimates for the short- and long-term correlation, respectively. In addition to the features coming from DFA analysis, also the current mood state was also included as an input feature. This choice is motivated by the fact that, in a previous study [31], it has been demonstrated that mood changes in bipolar patients can be modeled as a stochastic process with Markovian properties. In other words, starting from a current observation at day t_0, and considering past observations at days (t_{-1}, t_{-2},...,), it is possible to predict through a personalized approach the mood state between EUT/non-EUT at day t_{+1}. A graphical representation of this concept is shown in Fig. 8.

3.3.5 Feature Reduction and Classification

A suitable feature reduction strategy, i.e. PCA, has been applied in order to reduce the high number of features and promote an effective pattern recognition. It allows

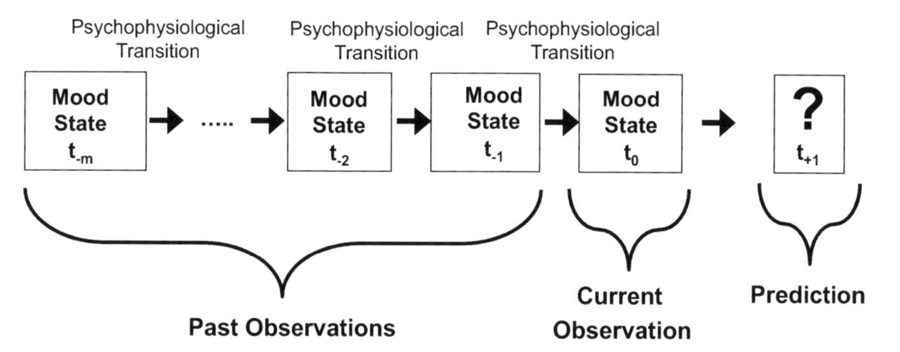

Fig. 8 Graphical representation of mood state temporal dynamics of a given patient with BD

to project high-dimensional data to a lower dimensional space with a minimal loss of information. This method does not select a feature subset, but creates new features by a linear combination of the original values.

In the study 1, the standard Multi-Layer Perceptron (MLP) algorithm was used to classify mood states. The MLP [78] with the integrate-and-fire neuron model is one of the possible network used in the pattern recognition. It was trained through a supervised learning method, i.e. input and output values are specified and the relations between them learnt. The MLP provided the highest statistically-significative accuracy concerning the considered intra-subject recognition. Accordingly, only results from MLP and, briefly, the theory behind will be reported and discussed.

Specifically, in the training phase, for each data record, each activation function of the artificial neurons is calculated. The weight w_{ij} of a generic neuron i at time T for the input vector $\overline{f_n^k} = f_{n1}^k, \ldots, f_{nF}^k$ is modified on the basis of the well-established back propagation of the resulting error between the input and the output values. The output from the MLP is a boolean vector; each element represents the activation function of an output neuron. In this study, an MLP having three layers of neurons has been implemented. The first layer, the input one, was comprised of 7 neurons, one for each of the reduced dimension of the feature space. The third layer, the output one, was comprised of 2 neurons, one for each of the considered classes to be recognized. The second layer, the hidden one, was comprised of an empirically estimated number of neurons. Specifically, this number was chosen as the superior limit of the half difference between the number of the input and output neurons, i.e. 5.

Classification for Study 2 and Study 3 was carried out through a Leave-One-Out (LOO) procedure applied on a Support Vector Machine (SVM)-based pattern recognition. More specifically, we used a nu-SVM (nu = 0.5) having a radial basis kernel function with $\gamma = n^{-1}$.

All of the classification results were expressed as recognition accuracy in detailed confusion matrices. The generic element r_{ij} of the confusion matrix indicated the percentage of how many times a pattern belonging to the class i was classified as belonging to the class j. A more diagonal confusion matrix corresponded to a higher degree of classification. The matrix must be read by columns.

4 Experimental Results

In this section, we report experimental results regarding the characterization of pathological mood states in bipolar disorder (Study 1), the temporal characterization of pathological mood states in bipolar disorder (Study 2), and the prediction of pathological mood states in bipolar disorder (Study 3).

4.1 *Study 1*

According to the developed mania-depression model, the goal was to test the ability of the classifiers of discriminating the mood state. Table 8 reports for each patient the initial and final time of each acquisition along with the percentages of the signal cleaned from the movement artifacts. After the AMR step, each signal was visually checked in order to identify physiological (ectopic or arrhythmic beats) or algorithmic artifacts (i.e. errors due to misdetection of the R-peaks). As it can be seen, good percentages of the retained signals were achieved, thus confirming the robustness of the wearable system even during long-term monitoring in a natural environment. The training phase was carried out on 80% of the feature dataset, while the testing phase was on the remaining 20%. Moreover, a 40-fold cross-validation steps has been performed. This latter method is done in order to obtain unbiased classification results, i.e. to consider a gaussian distribution of the classification results, which can therefore be described as mean and standard deviation among the 40 confusion matrices obtained. According to the processing chain reported in Sect. 3.3, the feature set was constructed by using the segmented and filtered signals. Some descriptive statistics about the most relevant indexes, also used for the classification, are reported in Tables 5, 6 and 7. To average among all the values, the median values over all the acquisitions for each class were considered according to the outcome of the Kolmogorov-Smirnov test for normality ($p < 0.05$, i.e. data are not normally distributed). The values are expressed as median and its respective absolute deviation (i.e. for a feature X, $X = median(X) \pm MAD(X)$ where $MAD(X) = |X - median(X)|$). The dimension of this dataset was reduced by applying the PCA algorithm. Since each principal component accounts for a given amount of the total variance, we found that a reduced dimension of 7 components gives the cumulative variance equal to 95% at least. In this study, due to the small number of patients as well as the small number of examples for some classes, only an intra-subject classification was performed. We collected the confusion matrices from several commonly-used algorithms such as LDC, QDC, MOG, k-NN, KSOM, MLP, and PNN. Taking into account the elements of the main diagonal, i.e. r_{ij} with $i = j$, a statistical analysis was performed for each $i = j = \{1, 2\}$ by means of the ANOVA test. Concerning BP1 and BP2, the *post-hoc* analysis, using the Bonferroni correction, gave a significative p-value ($p < 0.05$) for both elements r_{11} and r_{22} showing that the best accuracy was obtained by means of the MLP neural network and, thus, it is the most suitable classifier for the con-

Table 5 Selected descriptive statistics of the features from the bipolar patient BP1

BP1 features	MD	SD	ES
μ_{RR}	0.7559 ± 0.0615	0.7507 ± 0.0826	0.8224 ± 0.1267
σ_{RR}	0.0317 ± 0.0172	0.0350 ± 0.0120	0.0685 ± 0.0250
RMSSD	0.0340 ± 0.0168	0.0424 ± 0.0181	0.0446 ± 0.0104
pNN50%	4.8128 ± 3.8649	3.9537 ± 2.4831	20.3980 ± 8.4363
TINN	0.2100 ± 0.1150	0.2825 ± 0.0975	0.3100 ± 0.1000
LF	2.6900 ± 2.2989	2.8248 ± 2.4202	0.0026 ± 0.0021
HF	3.6341 ± 2.9069	4.1721 ± 3.6044	8.4589 ± 3.1042
LF/HF	0.7388 ± 0.3289	0.6517 ± 0.2305	3.0415 ± 2.2429
ApEn	0.8640 ± 0.1186	0.8624 ± 0.1076	0.7077 ± 0.1145
DFA α_1	0.9758 ± 0.1691	0.8489 ± 0.1670	1.3865 ± 0.2047
DFA α_2	0.8288 ± 0.1798	0.6992 ± 0.1522	0.9661 ± 0.1615

Values are expressed as $X = median(X) \pm MAD(X)$

Table 6 Selected descriptive statistics of the features from the bipolar patient BP2

BP2 features	MD	ES
μ_{RR}	0.7687 ± 0.0661	0.8192 ± 0.0988
σ_{RR}	0.0313 ± 0.0107	0.0319 ± 0.0136
RMSSD	0.0364 ± 0.0150	0.0274 ± 0.0129
pNN50%	3.4424 ± 2.3524	4.3256 ± 3.4817
TINN	0.2575 ± 0.0825	0.1800 ± 0.0650
LF	2.6926 ± 1.7427	4.4200 ± 3.2629
HF	2.4233 ± 2.0904	1.9436 ± 1.6271
LF/HF	1.0468 ± 0.5698	2.9063 ± 1.9288
ApEn	0.7891 ± 0.1226	0.7902 ± 0.1030
DFA α_1	0.9322 ± 0.2053	1.2849 ± 0.2125
DFA α_2	0.8364 ± 0.1575	0.7839 ± 0.1537

Values are expressed as $X = median(X) \pm MAD(X)$

sidered application, i.e. mood recognition/discrimination. Regarding the three confusion matrices of BP3, the MLP gave comparable results ($p > 0.05$) in terms of r_{11} values obtained by means of KSOM, and in terms of r_{22} values obtained by means of QDC. Otherwise, significative p-values ($p < 0.05$) were obtained pointing out the MLP better accuracy. We also report that the k-NN, LDC, MOG and PNN gave poor results for all of the patients. In fact, at least one of the two elements of the main diagonal of the confusion matrix was <67% (Table 8).

The MLP results are shown in Tables 9, 10, 11, 12 and 13. Insufficient recognition was obtained by considering the 3-class problem (i.e. ES vs. MD vs. SD) on patient BP1.

Table 7 Selected descriptive statistics of the features from the bipolar patient BP3

BP3 features	MS	ES
μ_{RR}	0.9698 ± 0.0244	0.7505 ± 0.0653
σ_{RR}	0.0979 ± 0.0108	0.0218 ± 0.0072
RMSSD	0.0606 ± 0.0062	0.0221 ± 0.0108
pNN50%	33.9872 ± 5.2543	1.0959 ± 1.0959
TINN	0.4375 ± 0.0500	0.1650 ± 0.0850
LF	0.0062 ± 0.0019	13.4740 ± 8.9033
HF	0.0013 ± 0.0006	7.6230 ± 4.9012
LF/HF	5.4873 ± 2.5745	1.7222 ± 0.9657
ApEn	0.6399 ± 0.0517	0.8115 ± 0.0922
DFA α_1	1.5118 ± 0.0914	1.0785 ± 0.2299
DFA α_2	0.9476 ± 0.1344	0.8489 ± 0.1629

Values are expressed as $X = median(X) \pm MAD(X)$

Table 8 Percentage of biosignals retained after the AMR step

Subj. ID	Original signal length	Retained signal length	% Retained
BP1-ACQ. 1	15h40m33s	10h20m8s	82,3453
BP1-ACQ. 2	16h30m6s	12h54m30s	70,3354
BP1-ACQ. 3	13h22m52s	11h36m24s	94,7302
BP1-ACQ. 4	15h17m29s	12h40m33s	79,1542
BP2-ACQ. 1	12h15m39s	8h22m16s	68,2755
BP2-ACQ. 2	15h14m3s	11h48m35s	77,5215
BP2-ACQ. 3	11h59m31s	10h5m36s	84,1692
BP2-ACQ. 4	10h16m26s	7h5m2s	68,9507
BP2-ACQ. 5	12h54m12s	10h40m42s	82.7556
BP2-ACQ. 6	16h19m50s	8h56m1s	54.7045
BP3-ACQ. 1	17h36m7s	15h51m40s	90,1105
BP3-ACQ. 2	14h49m5s	11h24m28s	76,9848

The *original signal length* column refers to the amount of data recorded for each acquisition until the wearable system battery ran out. The *retained signal length* column refers to the amount of artifact-free data retained for the post-processing analyses

Table 9 Intra-subject BP3

Conf. mat. MLP	Class ES	Class MS
Class ES	**97.96 ± 2.27**	3.24 ± 3.06
Class MS	2.04 ± 2.27	**96.76 ± 3.06**

Class ES: 126 examples. Class MS: 162 examples. Total: 288 examples

Table 10 Intra-subject BP2

Conf. mat. MLP	Class ES	Class MD
Class ES	**68.31 ± 6.49**	11.13 ± 3.23
Class MD	31.69 ± 6.49	**88.87 ± 3.23**

Class ES: 216 examples. Class MD: 412 examples. Total: 628 examples

Table 11 Intra-subject BP1

Conf. mat. MLP	Class ES	Class MD-SD
Class ES	**74.58 ± 7.34**	7.65 ± 2.05
Class MD-SD	25.42 ± 7.34	**92.35 ± 2.05**

Class ES: 131 examples. Class MD: 415 examples. Total: 546 examples

Table 12 Intra-subject BP1

Conf. mat. MLP	Class ES	Class MD
Class ES	**79.00 ± 7.12**	12.00 ± 3.82
Class MD	21.00 ± 7.12	**88.00 ± 3.82**

Class ES: 131 examples. Class MD: 283 examples. Total: 414 examples

Table 13 Intra-subject BP1

Conf. mat. MLP	Class ES	Class SD
Class ES	**93.75 ± 3.81**	5.25 ± 3.84
Class SD	6.25 ± 3.81	**94.75 ± 3.84**

Class ES: 131 examples. Class MD: 132 examples. Total: 263 examples

4.2 Study 2

Classifications were performed according to the methodology described in Sect. 3.3.3 and reported as intra-subject evaluations. Tables 14, 15, 16, 17, 18, 19, 20 and 21 show the recognition accuracy in terms of confusion matrices as well as the total average accuracy obtained through the LOO procedure on nu-SVMs. *Standard* dataset refers to an independently-processed feature set, i.e., the feature set belonging to a specific acquisition of a patient is taken as an input for the LOO-SVM clas-

Table 14 Confusion matrix of SVM classifier for BP1. Values are expressed as percentages

	Dataset	Hypomania	Euthymia
Hypomania	Standard	**91.99**	8.01
	Markov	88.64	11.36
Euthymia	Standard	80.40	19.60
	Markov	29.20	**70.80**

Total Accuracies: Standard 55.79%; Markov 79.72%
Bold values indicate the best correct classification results for each mood state

Table 15 Confusion matrix of SVM classifier for BP3. Values are expressed as percentages

	Dataset	Hypomania	Euthymia
Hypomania	Standard	96.70	3.30
	Markov	**97.78**	2.22
Euthymia	Standard	64.44	35.56
	Markov	11.11	**88.89**

Total Accuracies: Standard 66.13%; Markov 93.33%
Bold values indicate the best correct classification results for each mood state

Table 16 Confusion matrix of SVM classifier for BP2. Values are expressed as percentages

	Dataset	Hypomania	Mixed-State
Hypomania	Standard	**97.03**	2.97
	Markov	86.46	13.54
Mixed-State	Standard	62.5	37.5
	Markov	3.75	**96.25**

Total Accuracies: Standard 67.26%; Markov 91.35%
Bold values indicate the best correct classification results for each mood state

Table 17 Confusion matrix of SVM classifier for BP4. Values are expressed as percentages

	Dataset	Depression	Euthymia
Depression	Standard	98.53	1.47
	Markov	**99.68**	0.32
Euthymia	Standard	83.91	16.09
	Markov	8.05	**91.95**

Total Accuracies: Standard 57.31%; Markov 95.81%
Bold values indicate the best correct classification results for each mood state

Table 18 Confusion matrix of SVM classifier for BP5. Values are expressed as percentages

	Dataset	Depression	Hypomania
Depression	Standard	**85.44**	14.56
	Markov	74.87	25.13
Hypomania	Standard	23.02	76.98
	Markov	3.77	**96.23**

Total Accuracies: Standard 81.21%; Markov 85.55%
Bold values indicate the best correct classification results for each mood state

sification without performing any rescaling procedure. *Markov* dataset refers to the proposed methodology, i.e., feature set is processed ad-hoc in order to consider information from the previous mood state (see details on Sect. 3.3.3).

According to the description of data processing reported in Sect. 3.3.3, $n = 24$ features constituted the feature space dimension of both standard and Markov datasets. No dimensionality reduction techniques were applied to reduce such a dimension.

Since no patients had a maniac episode, we assigned four labels: hypomania, depression, mixed state and euthymia.

Table 19 Confusion matrix of SVM classifier for BP6. Values are expressed as percentages

	Dataset	Hypomania	Euthymia
Hypomania	Standard	88.75	11.25
	Markov	**93.98**	6.02
Euthymia	Standard	27.27	72.73
	Markov	7.49	**92.51**

Total Accuracies: Standard 80.74%; Markov 93.24%
Bold values indicate the best correct classification results for each mood state

Table 20 Confusion matrix of SVM classifier for BP7. Values are expressed as percentages

	Dataset	Depression	Euthymia
Depression	Standard	96.34	3.66
	Markov	**97.47**	2.53
Euthymia	Standard	45.56	54.44
	Markov	13.33	**86.67**

Total Accuracies: Standard 75.39%; Markov 92.07%
Bold values indicate the best correct classification results for each mood state

Patients BP1 and BP3 underwent five visits alongside long-term ANS monitoring. Starting from a period of hypomania, patients reached the euthymic state. As shown in Tables 14 and 15, considering the proposed Markov dataset, the subjective ANS patterns are well-distinguished reaching more than 88% of accuracy in recognizing the hypomaniac state. Concerning the results obtained from data gathered from BP1, we report that higher classification accuracy on hypomania class was achieved adopting a standard dataset. However, when using the same dataset, high mis-classification accuracy was obtained for the euthymia class.

Likewise to BP1 and BP3, patient BP2 began the study showing hypomaniacal psychosis. Then, depressive behaviors were diagnosed changing the mood state to mixed-state. Afterwards, the previous observed hypomania state was observed twice. In this case, more than 86 and 96% accuracy was reached in distinguishing hypomania from mixed-state patterns.

BP4 experienced depressive psychosis for the whole course of the illness, reaching good affective balance after five monitoring sessions. In order to take into account the unbalanced number of available examples per class, two different learning rates were considered in the SVM training phase, giving the euthymic examples four times more penalty with respect to the depressive examples. As the two considered states are very different in clinical terms, the two patterns resulted strongly distinguished with a recognition accuracy as high as 99.68%.

BP5 showed mood swings between depressive and hypomaniacal psychosis. Despite the fact that about 25% of the depressive patterns were confused with the hypomaniacal ones, the hypomania states were recognized with more than 96% accuracy. Likewise for BP1, results obtained on data gathered from BP2 and BP5 show that in using the standard approach, a higher classification accuracy for one class is associated to a very low and insufficient accuracy on another one. Like BP4, patients

Table 21 Confusion matrix of SVM classifier for BP8. Values are expressed as percentages

	Dataset	Mixed-State	Depression	Euthymia
Mixed-State	Standard	65.86	26.42	7.72
	Markov	**78.08**	13.70	8.22
Depression	Standard	13.79	78.52	7.69
	Markov	4.51	**93.90**	1.59
Euthymia	Standard	22.60	24.66	52.74
	Markov	7.53	8.22	**84.25**

Total Accuracies: Standard 65.71%; Markov 85.41%
Bold values indicate the best correct classification results for each mood state

BP6 and BP7 displayed severe pathological behavior before reaching the euthymic condition. Accordingly, accuracy greater than 86% was obtained in recognizing such states.

BP8 showed mood swings among three states such as the mixed-state, depression, and euthymia. This case is very interesting for this work as we obtained interesting performance, considering a three-class pattern recognition problem (see Table 21).

For each patient, higher total accuracy was obtained considering mood states as a Markov chain rather than using a standard approach. Although a further statistical analysis revealed that there are no differences between the sensitivity values given by the two methodologies, significant differences were found concerning the specificity values ($p < 0.02$) and total accuracies ($p < 0.01$) according to the non-parametric Wilcoxon signed rank test for paired data performed on all the subjects. Moreover, in order to generalize these results, it is worthwhile mentioning that we tested the classifier also when data were normalized with respect to a casual mood status achieving also lower performances than the proposed Markovian approach.

4.3 Study 3

In this study, results were achieved considering data gathered from 14 patients. As mentioned in the previous section, from each acquisition of each patient, the longest artifact-free segment of signal was selected. Table 22 reports average lengths, across all observations of each patients, of acquired signals and longest artifact-free segments.

During the acquisitions in Strasbourg, P_3 interrupted the study for 5 weeks between acquisition number 21 and number 22 due to summer holidays. For three other patients, P_1, P_5 and P_8, study duration has to be shortened respectively to 13, 12 and 11.5 weeks due to different factors (P_1: leaving for summer holidays; P_5: delay in study inclusion due to personal unavailability; P_8: delay in enrolling the patient due to the prolongation of the participation of P_3 in the study). Personalized prediction accuracies in forecasting the mood state (EUT/non-EUT) at time t_{+1} are shown

Table 22 Average lengths of acquired and longest artifact-free signals an expressed in seconds

Patient ID	Acquired signal	Longest Artifact-free segment
P1	26120.37 ± 7149.69	22350 ± 11400
P2	5889.30 ± 5990.24	5700 ± 6000
P3	22743.92 ± 19339.44	11400 ± 4800
P4	10990.78 ± 15108.46	10800 ± 5625
P5	9007.48 ± 4661.27	6150 ± 2400
P6	25492.20 ± 6865.27	16950 ± 14700
P7	28077.65 ± 4320.94	27600 ± 3900
P8	6957.64 ± 7864.32	5400 ± 3975
P9	25924.71 ± 12516.53	17400 ± 6600
P10	29916.71 ± 9192.53	22800 ± 11925
P11	30468.44 ± 5604.22	25200 ± 9675
P12	31165.16 ± 3654.47	12600 ± 3300
P13	20242.29 ± 5790.03	10500 ± 2250
P14	30400.33 ± 9032.32	14700 ± 4575

Ranges are expressed in seconds as $median \pm interquartile - range$

Table 23 Experimental Results expressed as prediction accuracy for each patient. The total number of available acquisitions ('N. Acq.', second column), and the number of acquisitions taken as initial training set ('Training Acq.', third column) are also reported

Patient ID	N. Acq.	Training Acq.	Prediction Acc. (%)
P_1	22	1:5	70.6
P_2	18	1:3	75
P_3	14	1:3	60
P_4	15	1:3	83.3
P_5	8	1:3	60
P_6	19	1:4	73.33
P_7	22	1:4	77.78
P_8	10	1:2	42.85
P_9	18	1:5	70
P_{10}	12	1:3	80
P_{11}	18	1:3	66.67
P_{12}	8	1:3	66.67
P_{13}	16	1:9	71.43
P_{14}	8	1:3	66.67

in Table 23. In this table, the second column reports the total number of acquisitions used for the accuracy estimation, whereas the third column reports the number of acquisitions used for the initial training set ($x : y$ means that the initial training set was considered from acquisition x to acquisition y).

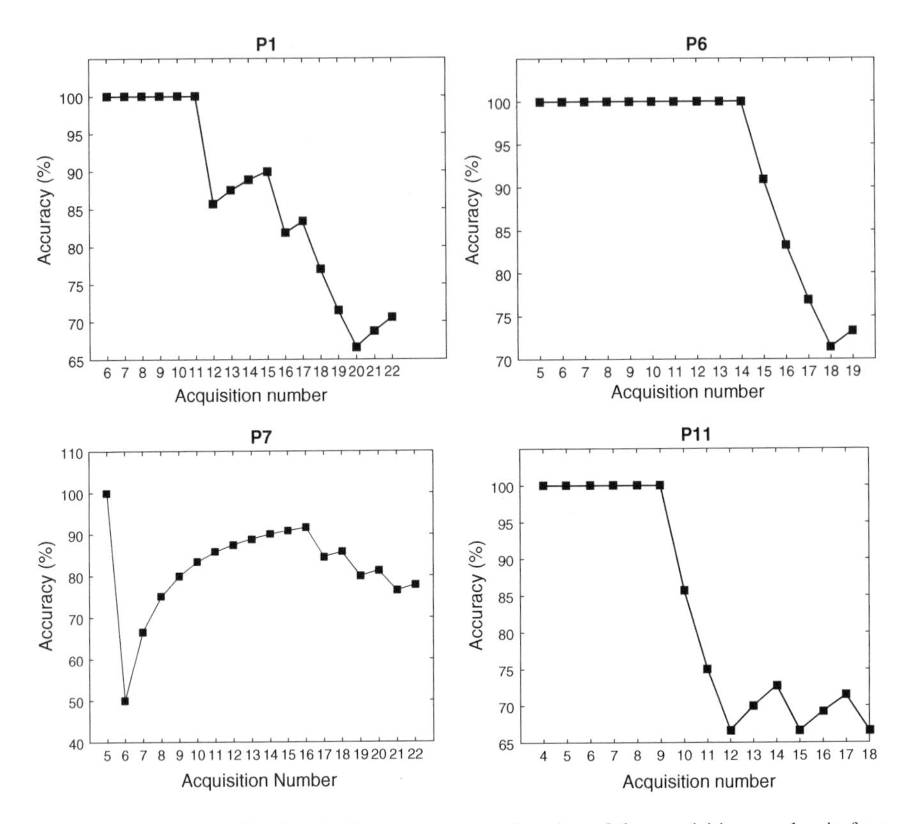

Fig. 9 Exemplary trends of prediction accuracy as a function of the acquisition number in four patients

In addition to accuracy, reported in Table 23, the classifier performance was evaluated also in terms of sensitivity, specificity, positive predictive value and negative predictive value. Results are reported in Table 3.

Importantly, prediction accuracies reported in Table 23 should be considered as a snapshot of all possible prediction accuracies related to a given patient. As an example, we report in Fig. 9 trends of the prediction accuracy as a function of different observations, considering data gathered from 4 patients. It is possible to recognize trends in which higher accuracy is associated with the first predictions and, then, the accuracy decreases, as well as trends in which the lower recognition accuracy is associated with first the predictions.

In order to investigate which feature could provide a major contribution in forecasting the next mood state, a further analysis based on the circle of correlation of the PCA transformation matrix was performed. Table 24 shows the first 5 mostly correlated features for each patient.

Table 24 Experimental Results expressed as percentage among patients

Accuracy	69%
Sensitivity	57%
Specificity	78%
Positive predictive value	60%
Negative predictive value	76%

Table 25 First 5 mostly correlated features among patients, predicting mood changes

HRV Feature	Frequency
Std RR	12/14
RMSSD	11/14
Poincaré SD1	11/14
Poincaré SD2	11/14
HF power	8/14

This analysis was performed considering the PCA calculation on all the acquisitions of each patient, and suggests that the HRV features reported in Table 25 are the most informative in forecasting the next mood state.

5 Conclusions and Discussion

In this chapter, an effective mood recognition system in bipolar patients has been presented [24, 28–35]. There are several studies in the literature that have shown how mood disorders are correlated with several dysfunctions of the ANS [19–21].

Bipolar disorder is widespread and has a high impact on the society [1–4], therefore an effective and reliable decision support system to clinical diagnosis is crucial. Clinicians, indeed, currently rely their diagnosis on rating scales and questionnaire scores [6–8] with no objective exams.

Accordingly, a wearable system able to detect and predict mood fluctuation could provide important clinical information even without physician. This will improve the medical treatment as well as shorten the symptomatic period. Although there are several studies reporting biomarkers that statistically discriminate different mood states [14–23], a single-variable approach is not sufficient to robustly characterize mood swings [24, 35]. In this frame, the PSYCHE platform is a wearable, comfortable and unobtrusive monitoring systems which apply a multi-parametric approach to give decision support system for the diagnosis of bipolar disorder. Specifically, the platform uses heart rate variability as a good non-invasive marker of the ANS activity [49, 53], especially effective in emotion recognition systems [54, 79–83].

In this chapter, results have been presented through confusion matrices. This approach allows showing values for the straightforward calculation of widely used statistical measures such as the sensitivity, specificity, ROC curves, area under the curve etc. Nevertheless, results only emphasize the whole cardio-respiratory pattern of the different mood states instead of identifying the actual biomarkers.

The proposed multi-parametric biomedical signal processing approach also accounts for clinical course during a mood fluctuation. The onset of a new mood state brings the past clinical history along, and the identification of the next state is more accurate if the previous one is considered. From a point of view purely speculative our approach goes beyond the rigid application of DSM-IV-TR labels, but introduces the new concept that the clinical diagnosis is looking backward. Better understanding of the patient's mood status can be achieved considering the dynamics of the disorder rather than the single observation treated as completely independent. For instance, patients with bipolar disorders present different clinical signs whether a depressive episode follows or precedes a maniac status [84].

Experimental results were very satisfactory. Considering patients with a mood label such as depression, hypomania, mixed-state, and euthymic state, we are able to distinguish subjective mood states with high accuracy, especially when a pathological clinical status is compared with the reference euthymic status (e.g. euthymic versus depressed, and euthymic versus mixed-state). Moreover, the comparison of the obtained findings through Markov mood state modeling with a standard approach further confirms the crucial role played by the long-term dynamics of pathological mental states. A further statistical analysis, in fact, revealed that a reliable and significantly higher specificity values are achieved only when the temporal dynamics of the illness is taken into account. The translational clinical application of the proposed methodology is not a challenging task, as ECG monitoring systems are widely available even in a portable fashion (e.g. standard ECG holter). However, as the proposed methodology focuses on the intra-subject classification, the new training phase has to be performed for every new patient. Ideally, such a training phase requires at least four acquisitions of physiological data that covers all the possible mood states, although a minimum switch of two mood states is strongly needed. Moreover, during such a training phase, doctors have to determine the mood states during each of the acquisitions. Then, these labels together with physiological data can be used to train the classifier. Only after this training phase, the proposed system will be able to diagnose the patient without an input from doctors. Major improvements of the system are expected to solve the inter-subject variability issue for the mood classification.

Furthermore, we reported promising results suggesting that it is possible to forecast mood states in bipolar disorder and in cyclothymic temperament subjects using heartbeat dynamics exclusively, gathered from ECG. To this extent, we reduced the problem predicting two possible mental states: the euthymic state, i.e., the good affective balance, and non-euthymic state, i.e., every mood state among depression, hypomania, and mixed state. From a clinical point of view, outcomes of this mood prediction study are very relevant. Knowing in advance whether the patient is getting better or not could effectively help clinicians to optimize the therapy and make changes in time, if necessary. On the other hand, understanding if the patient is going to have a relapse is very important and informative to perform a more accurate clinical monitoring, and plan a treatment at very early stage.

While the proposed experimental procedure provides for carrying out normal life activities, it is worthwhile mentioning that different life activities could be easily associated to different HRV dynamics. Using the methodology proposed in this work, such changes are minimized considering long-term, history-dependent dynamics referred to as one of the four possible pathological mood states. Given the high classification accuracy, it is indeed possible to hypothesize that the few misclassified samples can be interpreted as either algorithmic/mathematical artifacts or physiological outliers, i.e. events not related to mood markers for any reason (including also misleading daily activities).

The impact of this research can open new opportunities to create a closed loop between patients and clinicians through continuous communication and feedback that facilitates disease management by fostering a new collaboration, with more autonomy and empowerment for the patient. Constant monitoring and feedback (to both patients and physicians) are the new keys to managing the illness, to helping patients, to facilitating interaction between patient and physician, as well as to alerting professionals in case of relapse and depressive or manic episodes, and as a ultimate goal, to identifying signal trends in order to predict critical events. Moreover, the possibility of introducing other past mood states to the analysis and mood state labeling features is intriguing also from a clinical point of view. This is because it introduces the idea that mood disorders cannot be considered to be a series of independent and stand alone states, but rather a chronological sequence of mood states that are related each other. Previous studies have been limited to not considering this issue and may be one of the possible reasons for their lack of ability to discriminate mood status at single subject levels.

It is necessary to mention some limitations of our studies. In fact, the whole PSYCHE system relies on the patient mood label given by the physician during the training phase. Therefore, an error in such an evaluation could be crucial for the further assessment biasing the decision support. In addition, more data coming from a statistical representative and homogeneous population of a bipolar patient is needed for the validation of the system in terms of generalization, robustness and reliability. As mentioned in the method section, another possible limitation of the study is the fact that it relies on an ad-hoc mood model without a clinical validation. The model is a summarized pattern sets of mood states relying on clinical observations. It resulted to be an effective and viable means to fulfill the PSYCHE project mission, which is to predict and classify the clinical status. A more detailed and validated model will be defined when a higher number of participants will be available for the analysis. However, it is worthwhile underlining that diagnosis in psychiatry still suffers, in general, from a lack of validity, i.e. clinical diagnoses are not supported by the evidence of neurobiological changes. Therefore, a validated model for clinical assessment is quite far from being achieved. We are aware that more acquisitions, possibly with more frequent transitions, can remarkably improve prediction performance and may help to generalize our results to the wider clinical presentation and phenotypes of bipolar disoder. Another limitation of this study is a potentially confounding effect of the psychotropic medication in subjects including antidepressants, mood stabilizers, antipsychotics and benzodiazepine-like medication prescribed regularly. Common side effects of psychotropic drugs include anticholinergic and autonomic effects. These effects might have diminished the predictive power of our study. However, in psychiatric practice, patients with mood disorders are very frequently treated with psychotropic medications. Therefore, our results are very encouraging regarding the clinical usability of the PSYCHE system. Additional studies are needed to assess the impact of psychotropic drugs on its predictive power.

Further analyses, in fact, highlighting the most relevant features for classification will better clarify the psychophysiological correlates of bipolar disorders. The future study will investigate if these specific features can be used as a preclinical marker, meaning that they start to change even before the subject mood changes. In this case, it would be possible to use the PSYCHE platform to have an early, presymptomatic diagnosis of mood episodes. Further studies with a larger number of recruited patients will be provided a more complete understanding and knowledge of HRV and ANS alterations in bipolar disorder, therefore allowing for the assessment of the most important features related to pathological mental states.

References

1. R. Kessler, K. McGonagle, S. Zhao, C. Nelson, M. Hughes, S. Eshleman, *et al.*, "Lifetime and 12-month prevalence of dsm-iii-r psychiatric disorders in the united states: results from the national comorbidity survey," *Archives of general psychiatry*, vol. 51, no. 1, p. 8, 1994.
2. H. Wittchen and F. Jacobi, "Size and burden of mental disorders in europe–a critical review and appraisal of 27 studies," *European neuropsychopharmacology*, vol. 15, no. 4, pp. 357–376, 2005.
3. S. Pini, V. de Queiroz, D. Pagnin, L. Pezawas, J. Angst, G. Cassano, *et al.*, "Prevalence and burden of bipolar disorders in european countries," *European Neuropsychopharmacology*, vol. 15, no. 4, pp. 425–434, 2005.
4. Y. Chen and S. Dilsaver, "Lifetime rates of suicide attempts among subjects with bipolar and unipolar disorders relative to subjects with other axis i disorders," *Biological Psychiatry*, vol. 39, no. 10, pp. 896–899, 1996.
5. K. R. Merikangas, R. Jin, J.-P. He, R. C. Kessler, S. Lee, N. A. Sampson, M. C. Viana, L. H. Andrade, C. Hu, E. G. Karam, *et al.*, "Prevalence and correlates of bipolar spectrum disorder in the world mental health survey initiative," *Archives of general psychiatry*, vol. 68, no. 3, p. 241, 2011.
6. E. Vieta, M. Reinares, and A. Rosa, "Staging bipolar disorder," *Neurotoxicity research*, vol. 19, no. 2, pp. 279–285, 2011.
7. A. Andreazza, M. Kauer-Sant'Anna, B. Frey, D. Bond, F. Kapczinski, L. Young, and L. Yatham, "Oxidative stress markers in bipolar disorder: a meta-analysis," *Journal of affective disorders*, vol. 111, no. 2, pp. 135–144, 2008.
8. M. Phillips and E. Vieta, "Identifying functional neuroimaging biomarkers of bipolar disorder: toward dsm-v," *Schizophrenia bulletin*, vol. 33, no. 4, pp. 893–904, 2007.
9. A. P. Association, *Diagnostic and statistical manual of mental disorders: DSM-IV-TR*. American Psychiatric Publishing, Inc., 2000.
10. R. M. Carney, K. E. Freedland, and R. C. Veith, "Depression, the autonomic nervous system, and coronary heart disease," *Psychosomatic medicine*, vol. 67, pp. S29–S33, 2005.
11. J. M. Gorman and R. P. Sloan, "Heart rate variability in depressive and anxiety disorders," *American heart journal*, vol. 140, no. 4, pp. S77–S83, 2000.
12. A. Tylee and P. Gandhi, "The importance of somatic symptoms in depression in primary care," *Primary care companion to the Journal of clinical psychiatry*, vol. 7, no. 4, p. 167, 2005.
13. A. H. Kemp, D. S. Quintana, M. A. Gray, K. L. Felmingham, K. Brown, and J. M. Gatt, "Impact of depression and antidepressant treatment on heart rate variability: a review and meta-analysis," *Biological psychiatry*, vol. 67, no. 11, pp. 1067–1074, 2010.

14. H. G. Stampfer, "The relationship between psychiatric illness and the circadian pattern of heart rate," *Australian and New Zealand journal of psychiatry*, vol. 32, no. 2, pp. 187–198, 1998.
15. G. Iverson, H. Stampfer, and M. Gaetz, "Reliability of circadian heart pattern analysis in psychiatry," *Psychiatric quarterly*, vol. 73, no. 3, pp. 195–203, 2002.
16. G. Iverson, M. Gaetz, E. Rzempoluck, P. McLean, W. Linden, and R. Remick, "A new potential marker for abnormal cardiac physiology in depression," *Journal of behavioral medicine*, vol. 28, no. 6, pp. 507–511, 2005.
17. J. Taillard, P. Sanchez, P. Lemoine, and J. Mouret, "Heart rate circadian rhythm as a biological marker of desynchronization in major depression: A methodological and preliminary report," *Chronobiology international*, vol. 7, no. 4, pp. 305–316, 1990.
18. J. Taillard, P. Lemoine, P. Boule, M. Drogue, and J. Mouret, "Sleep and heart rate circadian rhythm in depression: The necessity to separate," *Chronobiology International*, vol. 10, no. 1, pp. 63–72, 1993.
19. R. Carney, K. Freedland, M. Rich, and A. Jaffe, "Depression as a risk factor for cardiac events in established coronary heart disease: a review of possible mechanisms," *Annals of Behavioral Medicine*, vol. 17, no. 2, pp. 142–149, 1995.
20. A. Glassman, "Depression, cardiac death, and the central nervous system," *Neuropsychobiology*, vol. 37, no. 2, pp. 80–83, 1998.
21. L. Watkins, J. Blumenthal, and R. Carney, "Association of anxiety with reduced baroreflex cardiac control in patients after acute myocardial infarction," *American Heart Journal*, vol. 143, no. 3, pp. 460–466, 2002.
22. A. Fagiolini, K. Chengappa, I. Soreca, and J. Chang, "Bipolar disorder and the metabolic syndrome: causal factors, psychiatric outcomes and economic burden," *CNS drugs*, vol. 22, no. 8, pp. 655–669, 2008.
23. K. Latalova, J. Prasko, T. Diveky, A. Grambal, D. Kamaradova, H. Velartova, J. Salinger, and J. Opavsky, "Autonomic nervous system in euthymic patients with bipolar affective disorder.," *Neuro endocrinology letters*, vol. 31, no. 6, p. 829, 2010.
24. G. Valenza, C. Gentili, A. Lanatà, and E. P. Scilingo, "Mood recognition in bipolar patients through the psyche platform: preliminary evaluations and perspectives," *Artificial intelligence in medicine*, vol. 57, no. 1, pp. 49–58, 2013.
25. B. Levy, "Autonomic nervous system arousal and cognitive functioning in bipolar disorder," *Bipolar disorders*, vol. 15, no. 1, pp. 70–79, 2013.
26. B. L. Henry, A. Minassian, M. P. Paulus, M. A. Geyer, and W. Perry, "Heart rate variability in bipolar mania and schizophrenia," *Journal of psychiatric research*, vol. 44, no. 3, pp. 168–176, 2010.
27. A. Voss, V. Baier, S. Schulz, and K. Bar, "Linear and nonlinear methods for analyses of cardiovascular variability in bipolar disorders," *Bipolar disorders*, vol. 8, no. 5p1, pp. 441–452, 2006.
28. G. Valenza, L. Citi, C. Gentili, A. Lanatá, E. Scilingo, and R. Barbieri, "Point-process nonlinear autonomic assessment of depressive states in bipolar patients.," *Methods of information in medicine*, vol. 53, no. 4, 2014.
29. A. Greco, G. Valenza, A. Lanata, G. Rota, and E. P. Scilingo, "Electrodermal activity in bipolar patients during affective elicitation," *IEEE journal of biomedical and health informatics*, vol. 18, no. 6, pp. 1865–1873, 2014.
30. G. Valenza, M. Nardelli, G. Bertschy, A. Lanata, and E. Scilingo, "Mood states modulate complexity in heartbeat dynamics: A multiscale entropy analysis," *EPL (Europhysics Letters)*, vol. 107, no. 1, p. 18003, 2014.
31. G. Valenza, M. Nardelli, A. Lanata, C. Gentili, G. Bertschy, R. Paradiso, and E. P. Scilingo, "Wearable monitoring for mood recognition in bipolar disorder based on history-dependent long-term heart rate variability analysis," *Biomedical and Health Informatics, IEEE Journal of*, vol. 18, no. 5, pp. 1625–1635, 2014.
32. A. Lanata, G. Valenza, M. Nardelli, C. Gentili, and E. P. Scilingo, "Complexity index from a personalized wearable monitoring system for assessing remission in mental health," *Biomedical and Health Informatics, IEEE Journal of*, vol. 19, no. 1, pp. 132–139, 2015.

33. G. Valenza, M. Nardelli, C. Gentili, G. Bertschy, M. Kosel, E. P. Scilingo, *et al.*, "Predicting mood changes in bipolar disorder through heartbeat nonlinear dynamics,"
34. G. Valenza, L. Citi, C. Gentili, A. Lanatá, E. P. Scilingo, and R. Barbieri, "Characterization of depressive states in bipolar patients using wearable textile technology and instantaneous heart rate variability assessment," *IEEE journal of biomedical and health informatics*, vol. 19, no. 1, pp. 263–274, 2015.
35. G. Valenza and E. P. Scilingo, *Autonomic Nervous System Dynamics for Mood and Emotional-State Recognition: Significant Advances in Data Acquisition, Signal Processing and Classification*. Springer Science & Business Media, 2014.
36. E. Scilingo, A. Gemignani, R. Paradiso, N. Taccini, B. Ghelarducci, and D. De Rossi, "Performance evaluation of sensing fabrics for monitoring physiological and biomechanical variables," *Information Technology in Biomedicine, IEEE Transactions on*, vol. 9, no. 3, pp. 345–352, 2005.
37. C. W. Gardiner *et al.*, *Handbook of stochastic methods*, vol. 3. Springer Berlin, 1985.
38. R. Kohavi and F. Provost, "Glossary of terms," *Machine Learning*, vol. 30, pp. 271–274, 1998.
39. M. Bauer, C. Vojta, B. Kinosian, L. Altshuler, and H. Glick, "The internal state scale: replication of its discriminating abilities in a multisite, public sector sample," *Bipolar Disorders*, vol. 2, no. 4, pp. 340–346, 2000.
40. D. McNair, M. Lorr, and L. Droppleman, "Poms: profile of mood states," *Educational and Industrial Testing Service publisher, San Diego (CA), USA*, 1971.
41. A. Rush, M. Trivedi, H. Ibrahim, T. Carmody, B. Arnow, D. Klein, *et al.*, "The 16-item quick inventory of depressive symptomatology (qids), clinician rating (qids-c), and self-report (qids-sr): a psychometric evaluation in patients with chronic major depression," *Biological psychiatry*, vol. 54, no. 5, pp. 573–583, 2003.
42. R. Young, J. Biggs, V. Ziegler, and D. Meyer, "A rating scale for mania: reliability, validity and sensitivity.," *The British Journal of Psychiatry*, vol. 133, no. 5, pp. 429–435, 1978.
43. L. Conti, *Repertorio delle scale di valutazione in psichiatria*. SEE, Florence, Italy, 1999.
44. M. Farné, A. Sebellico, D. Gnugnoli, and A. Corallo, *Profile Of Mood States: versione italiana*. Giunti OS, Florence, Italy., 1991.
45. A. Mehrabian and E. O'Reilly, "Analysis of personality measures in terms of basic dimensions of temperament.," *Journal of Personality and Social Psychology*, vol. 38, no. 3, p. 492, 1980.
46. E. Frank, R. F. Prien, R. B. Jarrett, M. B. Keller, D. J. Kupfer, P. W. Lavori, A. J. Rush, and M. M. Weissman, "Conceptualization and rationale for consensus definitions of terms in major depressive disorder: remission, recovery, relapse, and recurrence," *Archives of general psychiatry*, vol. 48, no. 9, pp. 851–855, 1991.
47. M. Berk, F. Ng, W. V. Wang, J. R. Calabrese, P. B. Mitchell, G. S. Malhi, and M. Tohen, "The empirical redefinition of the psychometric criteria for remission in bipolar disorder," *Journal of affective disorders*, vol. 106, no. 1, pp. 153–158, 2008.
48. S. Gopal, D. C. Steffens, M. L. Kramer, and M. K. Olsen, "Symptomatic remission in patients with bipolar mania: results from a double-blind, placebo-controlled trial of risperidone monotherapy.," *Journal of Clinical Psychiatry*, vol. 66, no. 8, pp. 1016–1020, 2005.
49. A. Camm, M. Malik, J. Bigger, G. Breithardt, S. Cerutti, R. Cohen, *et al.*, "Heart rate variability: standards of measurement, physiological interpretation, and clinical use," *Circulation*, vol. 93, no. 5, pp. 1043–1065, 1996.
50. J. Pan and W. Tompkins, "A real-time QRS detection algorithm," *IEEE Transactions on Biomedical Engineering*, pp. 230–236, 1985.
51. R. Berger, S. Akselrod, D. Gordon, and R. Cohen, "An efficient algorithm for spectral analysis of heart rate variability," *Biomedical Engineering, IEEE Transactions on*, no. 9, pp. 900–904, 2007.
52. J. Webster *et al.*, *Medical instrumentation: application and design*. John Wiley, New York, USA, 1998.
53. U. Rajendra Acharya, K. Paul Joseph, N. Kannathal, C. Lim, and J. Suri, "Heart rate variability: a review," *Medical and Biological Engineering and Computing*, vol. 44, no. 12, pp. 1031–1051, 2006.

54. G. Valenza, A. Lanata, and E. P. Scilingo, "The role of nonlinear dynamics in affective valence and arousal recognition," *Affective Computing, IEEE Transactions On*, vol. 3, no. 2, pp. 237–249, 2012.
55. H. Akaike, "Fitting autoregressive models for prediction," *Annals of the Institute of Statistical Mathematics*, vol. 21, no. 1, pp. 243–247, 1969.
56. S. Koelstra, A. Yazdani, M. Soleymani, C. Mühl, J. Lee, A. Nijholt, *et al.*, "Single Trial Classification of EEG and Peripheral Physiological Signals for Recognition of Emotions Induced by Music Videos," *Brain Informatics*, pp. 89–100, 2010.
57. J. Mendel, "Tutorial on higher-order statistics (spectra) in signal processing and system theory: Theoretical results and some applications," *Proceedings of the IEEE*, vol. 79, no. 3, pp. 278–305, 1991.
58. C. Nikias, "Higher-order spectral analysis: A nonlinear signal processing framework," *PTR Prentice-Hall, Inc., Englewood Cliffs, NJ, USA*, 1993.
59. K. Chua, V. Chandran, U. Acharya, and C. Lim, "Application of higher order statistics/spectra in biomedical signals–a review," *Medical engineering & physics*, vol. 32, no. 7, pp. 679–689, 2010.
60. F. Atyabi, M. Livari, K. Kaviani, and M. Tabar, "Two statistical methods for resolving healthy individuals and those with congestive heart failure based on extended self-similarity and a recursive method," *Journal of Biological Physics*, vol. 32, no. 6, pp. 489–495, 2006.
61. L. Glass, "Introduction to controversial topics in nonlinear science: Is the normal heart rate chaotic?," *Chaos: An Interdisciplinary Journal of Nonlinear Science*, vol. 19, no. 2, p. 028501, 2009.
62. L. Glass, "Synchronization and rhythmic processes in physiology," *Nature*, vol. 410, no. 6825, pp. 277–284, 2001.
63. A. Goldberger, C. Peng, and L. Lipsitz, "What is physiologic complexity and how does it change with aging and disease?," *Neurobiology of aging*, vol. 23, no. 1, pp. 23–26, 2002.
64. C. Poon and C. Merrill, "Decrease of cardiac chaos in congestive heart failure," *Nature*, vol. 389, no. 6650, pp. 492–495, 1997.
65. M. Tulppo, A. Kiviniemi, A. Hautala, M. Kallio, T. Seppanen, T. Makikallio, *et al.*, "Physiological background of the loss of fractal heart rate dynamics," *Circulation*, vol. 112, no. 3, p. 314, 2005.
66. G. Wu, N. Arzeno, L. Shen, D. Tang, D. Zheng, N. Zhao, *et al.*, "Chaotic signatures of heart rate variability and its power spectrum in health, aging and heart failure," *PloS one*, vol. 4, no. 2, p. e4323, 2009.
67. A. Lyapunov, "Problem general de la stabilite du mouvement," *Ann. Math. Stud*, vol. 17, 1949.
68. D. Ruelle, "Where can one hope to profitably apply the ideas of chaos?," *Physics Today*, vol. 47, p. 24, 1994.
69. Y. Fusheng, H. Bo, and T. Qingyu, "Approximate Entropy and its application in biosignal analysis," *Nonlinear biomedical signal processing*, p. 72, 2000.
70. J. S. Richman and J. R. Moorman, "Physiological time-series analysis using approximate entropy and sample entropy," *American Journal of Physiology-Heart and Circulatory Physiology*, vol. 278, no. 6, pp. H2039–H2049, 2000.
71. N. Marwan, M. Carmen Romano, M. Thiel, and J. Kurths, "Recurrence plots for the analysis of complex systems," *Physics Reports*, vol. 438, no. 5–6, pp. 237–329, 2007.
72. J. Zbilut and C. Webber Jr, *Recurrence quantification analysis*. Wiley Online Library, New York, USA, 2006.
73. C. Peng, S. Buldyrev, S. Havlin, M. Simons, H. Stanley, and A. Goldberger, "Mosaic organization of dna nucleotides," *Physical Review E*, vol. 49, no. 2, p. 1685, 1994.
74. C.-K. Peng, S. Havlin, H. E. Stanley, and A. L. Goldberger, "Quantification of scaling exponents and crossover phenomena in nonstationary heartbeat time series," *Chaos: An Interdisciplinary Journal of Nonlinear Science*, vol. 5, no. 1, pp. 82–87, 1995.
75. M. Rosenstein, J. Collins, and C. De Luca, "A practical method for calculating largest lyapunov exponents from small data sets," *Physica D: Nonlinear Phenomena*, vol. 65, no. 1–2, pp. 117–134, 1993.

76. S. M. Pincus, "Approximate entropy as a measure of system complexity.," *Proceedings of the National Academy of Sciences*, vol. 88, no. 6, pp. 2297–2301, 1991.
77. C. Peng, S. Havlin, H. Stanley, and A. Goldberger, "Quantification of scaling exponents and crossover phenomena in nonstationary heartbeat time series," *Chaos An Interdisciplinary Journal of Nonlinear Science*, vol. 5, no. 1, p. 82, 1995.
78. W. KinneBrock, *Neural Networks*. Oldenburg Verlag, Munchen, Germany, 1992.
79. L. Ivonin, H.-M. Chang, W. Chen, and M. Rauterberg, "Automatic recognition of the unconscious reactions from physiological signals," in *Human Factors in Computing and Informatics*, pp. 16–35, Springer, 2013.
80. L. Ivonin, H.-M. Chang, W. Chen, and M. Rauterberg, "Unconscious emotions: quantifying and logging something we are not aware of," *Personal and ubiquitous computing*, vol. 17, no. 4, pp. 663–673, 2013.
81. R. Calvo and S. D'Mello, "Affect detection: An interdisciplinary review of models, methods, and their applications," *Affective Computing, IEEE Transactions on*, vol. 1, no. 1, pp. 18–37, 2010.
82. G. Valenza, A. Lanatá, and E. P. Scilingo, "Improving emotion recognition systems by embedding cardiorespiratory coupling," *Physiological measurement*, vol. 34, no. 4, p. 449, 2013.
83. G. Valenza, P. Allegrini, A. Lanatà, and E. Scilingo, "Dominant lyapunov exponent and approximate entropy in heart rate variability during emotional visual elicitation," *Frontiers in Neuroengineering*, vol. 5, 2012.
84. A. Koukopoulos, D. Reginaldi, L. Tondo, C. Visioli, and R. Baldessarini, "Course sequences in bipolar disorder: depressions preceding or following manias or hypomanias," *Journal of affective disorders*, vol. 151, no. 1, pp. 105–110, 2013.

Part V
Resource Allocation, Quality of Service (QoS), and Context-Awareness in Smart Healthcare

Resource Allocation in Body Area Networks for Energy Harvesting Healthcare Monitoring

Shiyang Leng and Aylin Yener

1 Introduction

Health monitoring body area networks (BANs) have the potential to create a paradigm shift in providing personal healthcare [1]. A BAN consists of multiple wireless body sensors attached to or implanted in the human body to continuously monitor the patient's vital signs. The goal of BANs is to gather and analyze real-time health information by delivering and computing data collected at the sensors to physicians via wireless networking and mobile or cloud computing. Due to the short communication range of BAN nodes, gateway devices such as smartphones are usually exploited to relay the connection to remote stations.

One major challenge for health monitoring BANs is sustainable energy supply. Body sensors are desired to be unobtrusive and small in size, and are thus envisioned to employ energy storage devices with very limited storage capacity, which leads to the energy-constrained scenarios. Such scarcity of energy is a potential road block for perpetual and pervasive health monitoring. Energy harvesting has recently emerged as a promising solution [2–4] that enables energy-constrained wireless body sensors to scavenge energy from ambient energy sources such as sunlight, electromagnetic waves and so on. In particular, the human body has been confirmed to be an eligible energy source candidate for energy harvesting [1, 2]. Body motion, heat, or biochemical energy can be utilized to generate electrical energy powering up wireless devices. Thanks to the significant progress on hardware implementation, energy harvesting has been integrated into energy-constrained wireless body sensors to realize self-sustainable BANs [5, 6].

S. Leng (✉) · A. Yener
Electrical Engineering Department, School of EECS,
The Pennsylvania State University, University Park, PA 16802, USA
e-mail: sfl5154@psu.edu

A. Yener
e-mail: yener@ee.psu.edu

© Springer International Publishing AG 2017

S.U. Khan et al. (eds.), *Handbook of Large-Scale Distributed Computing in Smart Healthcare*, Scalable Computing and Communications,
DOI 10.1007/978-3-319-58280-1_20

Unlike conventional battery energy supply that is stable and controllable, energy harvesting is a time-varying process which largely depends on the environment. Due to the intermittent nature of energy harvesting, energy harvesting devices require careful management of energy expenditure to meet the quality of service (QoS) requirement and energy efficient operation. In recent years, resource allocation in energy harvesting communication networks has been studied extensively [7–10]. A few works have investigated BANs with energy harvesting in terms of energy harvesting modeling, physical layer optimization, and protocol design [11–16].

In this chapter, we review recent progress on resource allocation for BANs with energy harvesting. Data and energy scheduling with practical constraints in different types of systems are summarized. The remainder of the chapter is organized as follows. In Sect. 2, energy harvesting sources and techniques for BANs are introduced. Section 3 discusses resource allocation issues in fundamental point-to-point communications. In Sect. 4, data and energy scheduling in multi-node communication networks are presented. Section 5 summarizes the chapter.

2 Energy Harvesting Sources and Techniques

In this section, we introduce energy harvesting sources that are used to power the body area sensors. The characteristics of different types of energy harvesting sources and the associated energy harvesting techniques are discussed.

2.1 Photovoltaic Energy Harvesting

Photovoltaic energy harvesting is the process of converting light from the sun or artificial illumination into electricity using photovoltaic (PV) cells. When illuminated, PV cells absorb light and result in photovoltaic effect. Specifically, incoming photons excite the electrons into higher energy states and enable them to form an electric current that is proportional to the illuminance. Due to the abundant and highly accessible source of light, photovoltaic energy harvesting is widely applied in a variety of wireless devices in BANs from wearable sensors to implantable sensors [17–20].

For outdoor environments, sunlight is the obvious energy source, although its availability could vary depending on weather condition, daytime duration, and location. Generally, the PV panel generates 100 mW/cm^2 in standard outdoor conditions [21]. For indoor environments, illumination from either artificial light or natural light can be utilized to photovoltaic energy harvesting. The most common light source is the overhead fluorescent lights in office, hospital, and residential environments. In a typical room with windows, energy can also be harvested from the natural external light source. Unlike outdoor natural irradiance of sunlight, the energy density of the indoor light is inherently limited. Indoor illumination depending on the duration and the intensity of the artificial and natural irradiance generally ranges from 100 lux to 1000 lux which is one or two orders of magnitude lower than the outdoor illumination [22]. The outcome power density of the PV panel under indoor conditions is about 100–1000 μW/cm^2 which is about 100–1000 times less than that of the outdoor case [20, 21].

The energy conversion efficiency of a PV panel is influenced by many factors, such as the material used for the PV panel, the amount of illumination, and the spectra of light [22]. In particular, for wearable and implantable wireless sensors, bending and shadowing of the PV panel caused by uncontrollable human body movements and gestures also affect the generated power level, as less surface of the panel is exposed perpendicularly to the light. Toh et al. [20] reports that the power produced from the flexible PV panel with 30 ° of bending, decreases about 4.85% compared to that of a flat PV panel. To enable the PV panel to operate at the maximum power point, a power/voltage management circuit, which is called Maximum Power Point Tracking (MPPT), is typically implemented to optimize the current and voltage on the panel [22].

2.2 Thermoelectric Energy Harvesting

Thermoelectric energy harvesting is to generate electrical energy from thermal energy using the thermoelectric generator (TEG). A TEG is composed of two dissimilar thermoelectric semiconductors, *p*-type and *n*-type, connected in series between the hot and cold sides. It works as the energy converter based on the principle of Seebeck effect, which states that a voltage gradient is stimulated when there is a temperature difference between the two types of semiconductors [23]. Thermoelectric energy harvesting is widely used thanks to the ubiquitous availability of thermal energy, especially for wearable applications [24–30]. The human body continuously releases heat to maintain a normal body temperature. An adult typically dissipates power about 119 W, burning about 10.3 MJ a day when sitting in an office [24]. By exposing the hot side of the TEG to the skin and the cold side to the environment, the temperature gradient between the human body and the environment triggers the Seebeck effect, generating energy proportional to the temperature difference.

The power density generated by thermoelectric energy harvesting on the human body can be influenced by many factors, including the material and the structure of the TEG, the attachment location, clothing thermal insulation, and the wearer's activity. For instance, the TEG attached on the human leg with normal temperature 35.5 °C generates less energy than that attached to the human palm with normal temperature 38 °C [27]. The human body in a static state produces a relatively low power compared with walking, in which state the temperature gradient is increased by cooling via the wind [31]. As shown in [31], the produced power density is 20–60 μW/cm^2 when the room temperature is 18–25 °C, and 600 μW/cm^2 when the ambient temperature is 0 °C. However, the output voltage of a thermoelectric energy harvesting module is typically too low to power up the body sensor. A boost circuit, which is usually a DC-DC (direct current) converter, is developed to amplify the weak output to higher voltage [30].

2.3 Kinetic Energy Harvesting

Kinetic energy harvesting is a form of mechanical energy harvesting exclusively applied to the human body. It produces electrical energy from human motion and vibration via transduction methods [23]. The human body generates abundant kinetic energy through daily activities, including macro motions like the movements of limbs and joints and micro motions such as the natural vibration of the human chest during breathing [32]. Kinetic energy harvesting has garnered significant research interest and has become a popular energy harvesting technique for autonomous wearable sensors [23, 30, 33–35].

Conventional mechanical energy harvesting, that converts the energy of displacements and oscillations of a transducer into electrical energy, falls into three categories: electromagnetic, electrostatic, and piezoelectric. Electromagnetic transduction is normally applied to macro-scale energy harvesting due to its large material size [33]. In contrast, electrostatic and piezoelectric energy harvesting are more practical for small-scale applications. Electrostatic transduction can be implemented in microelectronic devices via integrated circuits [23], while piezoelectric transduction is suitable for harvesting energy from periodic movements, which are typical in human activities, like walking and running. Thus, piezoelectric energy harvesting is largely utilized in wearable sensors for health monitoring [30, 34, 35]. The piezoelectric energy harvester can produce a power density of 7.4 $\mu W/cm^3$ when the user running at 7 mile/h [30]. The generated power depends on the user's running speed.

2.4 Electromagnetic Energy Harvesting

Electromagnetic energy harvesting refers to the wireless energy transfer via electromagnetic (EM) waves. Due to the broadcast nature of EM waves, electromagnetic energy is ubiquitously available either from existing ambient waves or dedicated radio frequency (RF) energy transfer. This enables the electromagnetic energy harvesting to be a promising solution for self-sustaining wireless BANs [36–40].

Electromagnetic energy harvesting can be categorized into resonant energy harvesting and RF energy harvesting. Resonant energy harvesting is usually applied to near-field recharging, where the energy transmitter and the receiver are closely located. The energy is transferred via resonant inductive coupling between two magnetically coupled coils that resonant at the same frequency. Resonant energy harvesting can achieve an energy transfer efficiency higher than 80% [40]. The implantable device designed in [36] incorporates a resonant energy harvester that can supply 1.7 mA at 3.3 V over a distance up to 25 mm between the coupling coils.

For far-field recharging, RF energy harvesting is utilized to scavenge energy via a rectifying antenna (rectenna) from existing ambient electromagnetic waves such as radio and WiFi signals or from dedicated electromagnetic energy beams. The RF energy is collected by the antenna and rectified to DC output. However, the energy transfer efficiency is relatively low as the electromagnetic waves are attenuated promptly in propagation. In order to mitigate this, beamforming for energy transfer is developed [41]. On the other hand, in order to improve the RF-DC conversion efficiency, the multi-band rectenna is proposed to collect ambient RF energy from multiple frequency bands [39, 40]. In [40], a dual-band RF energy harvester harvesting cellular and WiFi sources that are of power densities about 1 $\mu W/cm^3$ achieves RF-DC conversion efficiency of 37% at 915 MHz and 20% at 2.45 GHz.

2.5 *Biochemical Energy Harvesting*

Biochemical energy harvesting, used exclusively in human-powered BANs, extracts energy from chemical energy sources in the human body [42–44]. Biochemical energy harvesting benefits from biocompatibility and is more suitable to be used in implantable devices. Biofuel cells are used to convert chemical energy into to electrical energy via electrochemical reactions. A typical biofuel cell consists of two electrodes, anode and cathode, that are located in separate chambers and connected via an external circuit. Chemical substances are oxidized at the anode and release electrons, which are conducted to the cathode via the external circuit. The protons generated in oxidation travel from the anode to the cathode through the solution so that a current is formed in a closed loop [42, 44].

Two major classes of biofuel cells are enzyme-based biofuel cells and microbial-based biofuel cells. Enzyme-based biofuel cells use catalytic enzymes to facilitate the oxidation of chemical substances to generate electrical energy [45]. On the other hand, microorganisms are utilized by microbial-based biofuel cells in the energy producing process. Among different types of potential chemical substances, glucose is the most commonly considered chemical energy source. 24 electrons are released from a single glucose molecule in oxidation and are conducted to form a current by the biofuel cell [44]. In the recent implementations [42, 43], biofuel cells using glucose fuels generate power densities 10–1000 $\mu W/cm^2$ to supply low-power implantable microelectronic systems.

In Table 1, we summarize these energy harvesting sources and techniques applied to BANs. For each energy harvesting technique, we list its energy harvesters and energy sources. The energy harvesting amounts of specific application examples are shown as well for each category.

Table 1 Energy harvesting sources and techniques for BANs

Energy harvesting techniques	Energy harvesters	Energy sources	Amount
Photovoltaic	PV cells	Outdoor sunlight	100 mW/cm^2 [21]
		Indoor illumination	100–1000 μW/cm^2 [20, 21]
Thermoelectric	TEG	Body heat	20–60 μW/cm^2 (18–25 °C) [31] 600 μW/cm^2 (0 °C) [31]
Kinetic	Piezoelectric transducers	Body motion	7.4 μW/cm^3 (7 mile/h)[30]
Electromagnetic	Resonant coupling coils	EM induction	3.3 V at 1.7 mA (25 mm) [36]
	Rectifying antennas	RF harvesting	RF-DC efficiency 37% (915 MHz) 20% (2.45 GHz) [40]
Biochemical	Biofuel cells	Glucose	10–1000 μW/cm^2 [42, 43]

3 Data and Energy Scheduling in Point-to-Point Communications

So far, we have seen that there are a number of potential energy sources to power and sustain the operation of BANs via energy harvesting. In this section, we detail efficient allocation of the harvested energy for perpetual operation. In particular, we consider point-to-point data and energy scheduling in BANs with energy harvesting.

In point-to-point communications, a single body sensor transmits data directly to a gateway device via a single link. For such a system with energy-constrained nodes that are solely powered by energy harvesting, efficient energy allocation strategy has to be carefully designed. We discuss both offline and online settings. In the offline setting, perfect knowledge of the channel state, data state, and energy state in the scheduling period is known a priori at the transmitter. For the online setting, only causal knowledge and the statistics of either channel state, data state, or energy state are available at the transmitter. In the sequel, both settings are introduced with the system models of channel, data acquisition, and energy harvesting. Next, typical system performance metrics including throughput, transmission completion time, and generalized utility functions are specified. Lastly, resource allocation problems and their solutions are presented.

3.1 *Offline Scheduling*

In this setting, the channel state, energy harvesting state, and the data queuing state, are known prior to transmission. Considerable effort has focused on resource allocation in point-to-point communications with offline approach [7, 8, 46–56]. Offline resource allocation problems are commonly formulated as convex optimization problems and analytical solutions can typically be obtained by convex optimization techniques. They serve as a benchmark for online cases, as well as an accurate performance indicator for predictable energy sources like sunlight.

3.1.1 System Model

The system consists of a transmitter and a receiver as shown in Fig. 1. Energy is harvested by the transmitter to be used for data transmission. Throughout the chapter, we will consider models which take into account the energy expended for data transmission only, noting that other processing costs can be and have been considered in follow up works [54]. We will also limit our discussion to models where the transmitter can adjust its transmission power instantaneously so as to accommodate data rate to its available energy, noting that recent work considers discrete rate adaptation [49]. Throughout the chapter, we adopt a discrete time model, i.e., a time-slotted system, without loss of generality.

Consider data transmission from the energy harvesting transmitter to the receiver via a fading additive white Gaussian noise (AWGN) channel and a time-slotted model. Assume that the duration of each time slot is L seconds within which the channel fading level, energy harvesting state, and data queuing state are static. For a transmission period of T time slots, the received signal at slot t is given by

$$y_t = \sqrt{h_t}x_t + n_t,\ t = 1, 2, \ldots, T, \tag{1}$$

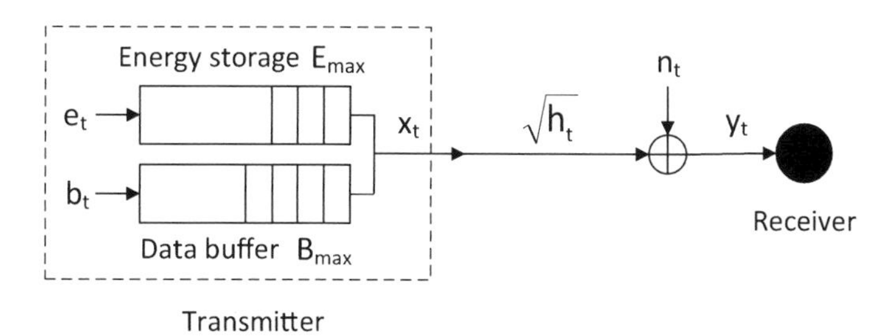

Fig. 1 System model for point-to-point communications. The transmitter harvests energy of amount e_t at time slot t and stores in its energy storage unit of capacity $E_{\max}$. b_t represents the data arrival at t. The data buffer has capacity $B_{\max}$. Signal x_t is transmitted over an AWGN channel with gain h_t. The receiver receives signal y_t corrupted by noise n_t

where h_t is the channel gain, x_t is the channel input signal, and n_t is the white Gaussian noise with zero mean and unit variance. The transmission power is p_t at time slot t, i.e., $|x_t|^2 = p_t$. Hence, the instantaneous rate in bits per channel use is

$$r_t = \frac{1}{2}\log_2(1 + h_t p_t),\ t = 1, 2, \ldots, T. \tag{2}$$

In this setting, channel state information (CSI) is assumed available at the transmitter before transmission.

Energy Harvesting Model At the transmitter, energy harvesting occurs in an intermittent manner. Energy harvesting amounts and arrival instants are known a priori. At the beginning of time slot t, energy $e_t \geq 0$ is harvested. The unused portion of harvested energy can be stored in an energy storage device such as a supercapacitor or a battery. In this chapter, we review studies which assume that there is no energy loss in recharging or discharging the storage device, noting that the extension of the framework handling such losses has been studied in [55]. During the transmission period, energy consumption up to a certain time should be no larger than the total harvested energy by that time. This *energy causality* constraint is thus given by [7, 46]

$$\sum_{t=1}^{n} Lp_t \leq \sum_{t=1}^{n} e_t,\ \ n = 1, 2, \ldots, T. \tag{3}$$

More specifically, the consumed energy by the end of time slot n is no larger than the total harvested energy up to time slot n.

In practice, the energy storage device has finite capacity, which is small for body sensors. Let $E_{\max}$ denote the energy storage capacity. Any excess energy beyond the storage capacity has to be discarded. Since waste of energy is not desired, we also impose the no-energy-overflow constraint [7, 8]:

$$\sum_{t=1}^{n} e_t - \sum_{t=1}^{n} Lp_t \leq E_{\max},\ \ n = 1, 2, \ldots, T, \tag{4}$$

that is, the residual stored energy is no larger than the storage capacity at any time slots.

Data Acquisition Model The transmitter has a data buffer of size $B_{\max}$. While recent work [48] addressed the impact of finite data buffers, here we consider simply that a sufficiently large data buffer is available, i.e., $B_{\max} \to \infty$. There are two scenarios for data acquisition. One is that the total required data of B bits are available at the beginning of transmission, namely, data ready before transmission (DBT). The other scenario is that data packets arrive intermittently during the course of transmission, namely, data during transmission (DDT), with a full knowledge of data amounts and arrival instants available before transmission. For DDT model, $b_t \geq 0$ bits of data enter the data buffer at slot t. Similar to energy causality, the intermittent data arrivals result in data causality constraints, i.e.,

$$\sum_{t=1}^{n} Lr_t \leq \sum_{t=1}^{n} b_t, \quad n = 1, 2, \ldots, T. \tag{5}$$

3.1.2 Performance Metrics and Problem Formulations

The various metrics for resource allocation considered here includes throughput, transmission completion time, and generalized system utility functions. The associated resource allocation optimization problems are introduced based on the aforementioned system model.

Throughput Maximization [7, 8] Consider an AWGN block fading channel with DBT data acquisition model, i.e., backlogged data is assumed. The objective is to maximize transmitted data within T slots, namely, throughput maximization. The problem is formulated subject to the energy causality constraint and the no-energy-overflow constraint given as
Problem 1

$$\max_{\mathbf{p}\geq 0} \quad \sum_{t=1}^{T} \frac{L}{2} \log_2(1 + h_t p_t) \tag{6a}$$

$$\text{s.t.} \quad \sum_{t=1}^{n} Lp_t \leq \sum_{t=1}^{n} e_t, \quad n = 1, 2, \ldots, T, \tag{6b}$$

$$\sum_{t=1}^{n} e_t - \sum_{t=1}^{n} Lp_t \leq E_{\max}, \quad n = 1, 2, \ldots, T, \tag{6c}$$

where $\mathbf{p} = \{p_1, p_2, \ldots, p_T\}$ and $\mathbf{p} \geq 0$ means that $\mathbf{p}$ is nonnegative elementwise.

Transmission Completion Time Minimization [7, 8, 46] For the transmission completion time minimization problem, the aim is to find an optimal transmission strategy that sends the required data of B bits in the shortest period under the energy constraints. Here, the simple DBT data model is considered, where $B < \infty$ bits need to be delivered. The problem is formulated as
Problem 2

$$\min_{\mathbf{p}\geq 0, T} \quad T \tag{7a}$$

$$\text{s.t.} \quad \sum_{t=1}^{T} \frac{L}{2} \log_2(1 + h_t p_t) = B, \tag{7b}$$

$$\sum_{t=1}^{n} Lp_t \leq \sum_{t=1}^{n} e_t, \quad n = 1, 2, \ldots, T, \tag{7c}$$

$$\sum_{t=1}^{n} e_t - \sum_{t=1}^{n} Lp_t \leq E_{\max}, \; n = 1, 2, \ldots, T. \tag{7d}$$

System Utility Maximization [56] System utility function $U : \mathbb{R}_+ \rightarrow \mathbb{R}$ is assumed to be a nondecreasing, concave function of resource level $\mathbf{p} = \{p_1, p_2, \ldots, p_T\}$. For instance, the rate-power function in (2) is a commonly used utility function, where the resource is the transmission power and the utility is the rate. A general utility maximization problem can be formulated as

Problem 3

$$\max_{\mathbf{p} \geq 0} \quad \sum_{t=1}^{T} U(p_t) \tag{8a}$$

$$\text{s.t.} \quad p_t \in \mathcal{F}, \; t = 1, 2, \ldots, T, \tag{8b}$$

where $\mathcal{F}$ is the feasible region of the relevant resource allocation constraints.

3.1.3 Resource Allocation Algorithm

In this part of the chapter, the solution to throughput maximization problem, i.e., Problem 1 described in (6), is presented. In particular, in the remainder of Sect. 3.1, we summarize the results from [7, 8].

Let us define a change in either channel fading level, energy level, or data queuing state as an *event*, and the time interval between two consecutive event as an *epoch* [7]. For Problem 1, let K be the number of changes of channel fading within a finite period of T slots, and J be the number of energy harvests. Then, there are $K + J$ epochs beginning at time instant s_i and of length τ_i for $i = 1, 2, \ldots, K + J$ and $s_1 = 0$, as shown in Fig. 2.

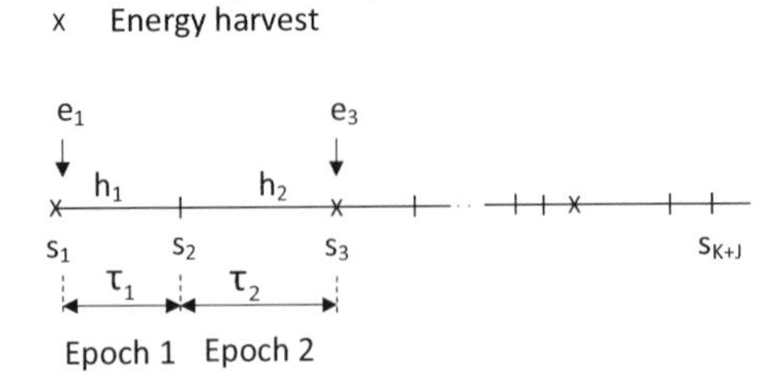

Fig. 2 Events and epochs on the time axis. Events happen at time instants $s_1, s_2, s_3, \ldots$. At s_1, energy harvesting occurs, i.e., energy of amount $e_1 > 0$ is harvested. At s_2, a channel fading event occurs, i.e., $h_1 \neq h_2$. At s_3, an energy harvest $e_3 > 0$ takes place. The time intervals from s_1 to s_2 and from s_2 to s_3 are epoch 1 and epoch 2 with length $\tau_1 = s_2 - s_1$ and $\tau_2 = s_3 - s_2$, respectively

As proved in [8, 46], the optimal transmission power that maximizes the throughput must be constant in each epoch. Based on this observation, one can formulate the equivalent optimization problem that finds the per epoch power. For epoch i, the channel fading level is denoted by h_i, the amount of energy harvest by e_i, and the transmission power by p_i. Note that $e_i > 0$ for some i if event i is an energy harvest, while $e_i = 0$ if event i is a change in the fading state. The throughput maximization problem can thus be equivalently expressed as

$$\max_{\mathbf{p}\geq 0} \quad \sum_{i=1}^{K+J} \frac{\tau_i}{2} \log_2(1 + h_i p_i) \tag{9a}$$

$$\text{s.t.} \quad \sum_{i=1}^{n} \tau_i p_i \leq \sum_{i=1}^{n} e_i, \; n = 1, 2, \ldots, K + J, \tag{9b}$$

$$\sum_{i=1}^{n} e_i - \sum_{i=1}^{n} \tau_i p_i \leq E_{\max}, \; n = 1, 2, \ldots, K + J, \tag{9c}$$

where $\mathbf{p} = \{p_1, p_2, \ldots, p_{K+J}\}$ and $\mathbf{p} \geq 0$, i.e., $\mathbf{p}$ is nonnegative elementwise.

Note that (9) is a strictly convex optimization problem, since the objective function (9a) is strictly concave, and the feasible region that is restricted by a set of linear constraints is convex [57]. The Lagrangian is given as

$$\begin{aligned} \mathcal{L}(\mathbf{p}, \boldsymbol{\lambda}, \boldsymbol{\delta}, \boldsymbol{\gamma}) = & \sum_{i=1}^{K+J} \frac{\tau_i}{2} \log_2(1 + h_i p_i) - \sum_{n=1}^{K+J} \lambda_n \Big(\sum_{i=1}^{n} \tau_i p_i - \sum_{i=0}^{n} e_i \Big) \\ & - \sum_{n=1}^{K+J} \delta_n \Big(\sum_{i=1}^{n} e_i - \sum_{i=1}^{n} \tau_i p_i - E_{\max} \Big) + \sum_{n=1}^{K+J} \gamma_i p_i, \end{aligned} \tag{10}$$

where $\boldsymbol{\lambda} = \{\lambda_n\}_{n=1}^{K+J}$, $\boldsymbol{\delta} = \{\delta_n\}_{n=1}^{K+J}$, and $\boldsymbol{\gamma} = \{\gamma_n\}_{n=1}^{K+J}$ are sequences of Lagrangian multipliers that are associated with energy causality constraints in (9b), no-energy-overflow constraints in (9c), and nonnegative transmission power constraint, respectively. The unique optimal solution satisfies the Karush-Kuhn-Tucker (KKT) conditions that are

$$\frac{\partial \mathcal{L}}{\partial p_i} = \frac{\tau_i h_i}{(2 \ln 2)(1 + h_i p_i)} - \tau_i \sum_{n=i}^{K+J} \lambda_n + \tau_i \sum_{n=i}^{K+J} \delta_n + \gamma_i = 0, \tag{11}$$

$$\sum_{i=1}^{n} \tau_i p_i - \sum_{i=1}^{n} e_i \leq 0, \tag{12}$$

$$\sum_{i=1}^{n} e_i - \sum_{i=1}^{n} \tau_i p_i - E_{\max} \leq 0, \tag{13}$$

$$p_i \geq 0, \tag{14}$$
$$\lambda_n, \delta_n, \gamma_n \geq 0, \tag{15}$$

for $i = 1, 2, \ldots, K + J$, $n = 1, 2, \ldots, K + J$. Equation (11) is the first-order stationarity condition. Equations (12)–(14) give the primal feasibility conditions. Equation (15) is the dual feasibility condition. Furthermore, the associated complementary slackness conditions are

$$\lambda_n \Big(\sum_{i=1}^{n} \tau_i p_i - \sum_{i=1}^{n} e_i \Big) = 0, \tag{16}$$
$$\delta_n \Big(\sum_{i=1}^{n} e_i - \sum_{i=1}^{n} \tau_i p_i - E_{\max} \Big) = 0, \tag{17}$$
$$\gamma_n p_n = 0, \tag{18}$$

for $n = 1, 2, \ldots, K + J$. Conforming to (11) and (16)–(18), the optimal transmission power is given by

$$p_i^* = \left[\frac{1}{(2 \ln 2) \sum_{n=i}^{K+J} (\lambda_n - \delta_n)} - \frac{1}{h_i} \right]^+, \ \forall i, \tag{19}$$

where $[x]^+ = \max\{0, x\}$. As shown in (19), the optimal power is given in a form of water-filling solution with water level $\mu_i \triangleq \frac{1}{(2 \ln 2) \sum_{n=i}^{K+J} (\lambda_n - \delta_n)}$ and base level the reciprocal channel gain $\frac{1}{h_i}$. Formally, the structure of the optimal power allocation is given by the following theorem.

Theorem 1 ([7, Theorem 1]) *When $E_{\max} = \infty$, the optimal water levels μ_i^* is a monotonically increasing sequence: $\mu_{i+1}^* \geq \mu_i^*$. Moreover, if the energy causality constraint (9b) holds with inequality for some m, i.e., $\sum_{i=1}^{m} \tau_i p_i < \sum_{i=1}^{m} e_i$, then $\mu_{m+1}^* = \mu_m^*$.*

Proof [7] When $E_{\max} = \infty$, the no-energy-overflow constraint (9c) always holds with inequality, which results in $\delta_n = 0$, $\forall n$. Then, the water level is $\mu_i^* = \frac{1}{(2 \ln 2) \sum_{n=i}^{K+J} \lambda_n}$. Since $\lambda_n \geq 0$ for all n, μ_i^* is a monotonically increasing sequence. Furthermore, if for some m, $\sum_{i=1}^{m} \tau_i p_i < \sum_{i=1}^{m} e_i$, this implies that $\lambda_m = 0$ by the slackness condition in (16). Hence, $\mu_{m+1}^* = \mu_m^*$. In particular, $\mu_m^* = \mu_n^*$ for all epochs m and n between two consecutive energy arrivals. Since only the changes of channel fading occur in these epochs, it necessitates (9b) holding with inequality and results in the equalized water level. ■

Theorem 1 implies that energy is allowed to flow only from present to the future for optimal energy allocation, i.e., energy can be stored to be expended in the future. More specifically, (9b) holding with inequality means that the energy is not depleted.

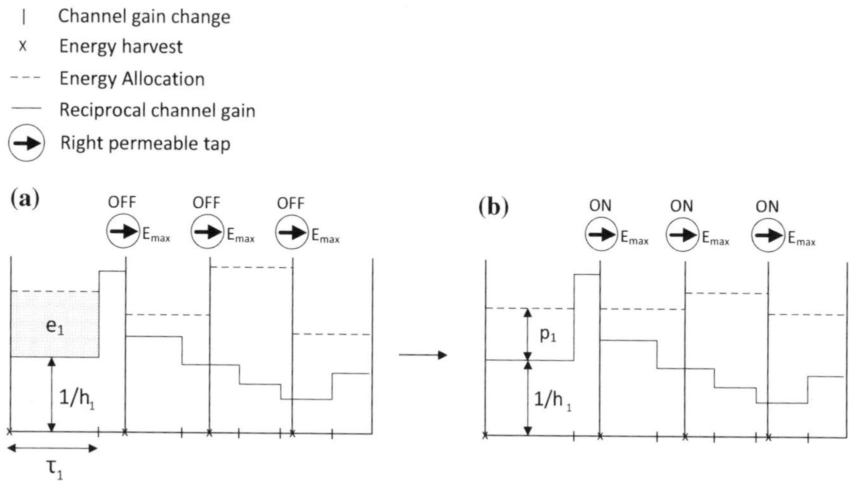

| Channel gain change
x Energy harvest
--- Energy Allocation
— Reciprocal channel gain
Right permeable tap

(a) OFF OFF OFF E_{max} E_{max} E_{max} e_1 $1/h_1$ τ_1

(b) ON ON ON E_{max} E_{max} E_{max} p_1 $1/h_1$

Fig. 3 Illustration of the directional water-filling algorithm. The first bin (epoch) has width τ_1 and base level $1/h_1$. The permeable walls located at the 4 energy harvesting instants divides the bins into 4 blocks. The first block has available water (energy) e_1. **a** Water level is equalized between bins within each block. **b** Water level is further equalized between blocks. Water (energy) flows from block 1 to block 2 and from block 3 to block 4, i.e., is stored to be used in the future. The right permeable taps limit the water (energy) flow up to $E_{\max}$. The optimal transmission power in epoch 1 is p_1

That is, some energy is available, but not used for current epoch, which will be transferred to future epochs to improve throughput. In this case, the optimal transmission strategy is to equalize the water level. However, when (9b) holds with equality, energy is depleted for the current epoch so that no energy is transferred for future use and the water level must change with an increase.

If $E_{\max}$ is finite, there may not be monotonicity of the water levels when the no-energy-overflow constraint (9c) holds with equality and the associated Lagrangian multiplier δ_n is nonzero. In fact, the no-energy-overflow constraint restricts the energy that can be transferred from the current epoch i to future epochs to no larger than $E_{\max}$. Thus, the water levels are only equalized to the extent that no-energy-overflow constraint allows.

The above observation of optimal transmission power allocation can be interpreted as *directional water-filling algorithm* as termed in [7]. That is, the process of energy allocation is modeled as pouring water into a vessel with a number of bins. The width of the ith bin is the length of epoch i, τ_i, and the base level is the reciprocal channel gain $\frac{1}{h_i}$ as shown in Fig. 3. The bins are divided into blocks by permeable walls at the instants of energy arrivals. Each nonzero energy harvest initializes one block and becomes the available water (energy) for this block. The optimal energy allocation policy tends to equalize the water level as much as possible subject to the energy causality constraints and the no-energy-overflow constraints. The water level for the ith bin is $\frac{e_i}{\tau_i}$. According to the energy causality constraint, the energy is transferred only from the past to the future. Correspondingly, the permeable walls allow water flowing between blocks only from left to right. If the water level of block k is larger than the water level of block $k+1$, the water level tends to be equalized between these two blocks by flowing water to the right. Simultaneously, the no-energy-overflow constraint imposes an upper bound $E_{\max}$ to the amount of flowing water (transferred energy) from the kth block to the subsequent blocks. This is indicated in Fig. 3 with taps that control the water flow to the right. Finally, the allocated power p_i for epoch i is the height difference between the water level μ_i and the reciprocal channel gain $\frac{1}{h_i}$.

The following theorem states that the solutions of the throughput maximization and transmission completion time minimization problems are closely related.

Theorem 2 ([8, Theorem 2]) *For a given energy harvesting scenario in Problems 1 and 2, the two optimization problems yield identical power allocation policies for given transmission duration of T slots and data B. In other words, if the maximum throughput power allocation policy for T time slots departs a total B bits, then the minimum transmission completion time policy for B bits completes the transmission at slot T, and vice versa.*

Proof [8] The Lagrangian dual problem of transmission completion time minimization in Problem 2 is formulated as

$$\max_{\theta} \left\{ \min_{\mathbf{p}\in\mathcal{P},T} T + \theta\big(B - \sum_{t=1}^{T} \frac{L}{2} \log_2(1 + h_t p_t)\big) \right\}, \tag{20}$$

where θ is the Lagrangian multiplier associated with the data transmission completion constraint (7b). $\mathcal{P}$ is the feasible region formed by constraints (7c), (7d) and $\mathbf{p} \geq 0$. For each given T, $\mathbf{p}$ can be solved. Thus, the dual problem can be written as

$$\max_{\theta} \left\{ \min_{T} \left\{ \min_{\mathbf{p}\in\mathcal{P}} T + \theta\big(B - \sum_{t=1}^{T} \frac{L}{2} \log_2(1 + h_t p_t)\big) \right\} \right\}, \tag{21}$$

which is equivalent to

$$\max_{\theta} \left\{ \min_{T} T + \theta\Big(B - \big\{ \max_{\mathbf{p}\in\mathcal{P}} \sum_{t=1}^{T} \frac{L}{2} \log_2(1 + h_t p_t)\big\}\Big) \right\}. \tag{22}$$

It can be observed that the optimal transmission power $\mathbf{p}^*$ for transmission completion time minimization Problem 2 arises from the solution of the inner throughput maximization problem which is Problem 1. Since both problems are strictly convex and each has a unique optimal solution, they have identical optimal power allocation solution. Thus, the minimum transmission slots T^* in Problem 2 is the time constraint T in Problem 1. ■

By Theorem 2, the transmission completion time minimization Problem 2 can be solved iteratively by solving the inner throughput maximization problem in (22) for each given T.

3.2 *Online Scheduling*

Online scheduling in point-to-point communications develops transmission policies in terms of energy allocation and data management based on causal information and statistical knowledge of the system state. Online resource allocation problems have received significant interest in recent literature [11–13, 58–66]. Online formulations are more suitable for more dynamic energy harvesting scenarios where treating future energy arrival times and amounts as a random process is more fitting. Below, we first provide a summary of the different stochastic models and then focus on one specific model and provide the results to characterize the online power allocation policy from [63–65].

3.2.1 System Models

In the online setting, a stochastic process that models energy harvesting can be time-uncorrelated or time-correlated.

In time-uncorrelated models, the channel fading level, the energy harvesting process, and the data arrival process are typically described as random processes composed of independent channel changes, energy harvests, and data arrivals in time, respectively. For instance, in a time-slotted system, the energy arrival in each time slot can be modeled as an identical and independent distributed (i.i.d.) Bernoulli process with parameter ρ [63–65]. That is, in each time slot, either energy of amount e is harvested with probability ρ, or no energy is harvested with probability $1-\rho$. In another example [7], the stochastic energy harvesting process is modeled as a Poisson counting process with rate λ_e such that energy is harvested independently at t_i with amount e_i, $i = 1, 2, \ldots, \infty$. By the Poisson property, the energy inter-arrival time follows exponential distribution with mean $1/\lambda_e$.

In time-correlated models, the channel fading level, the energy harvesting process, and the data arrival process are modeled as a correlated random process. A Markov decision process (MDP) is widely applied [12, 58–62] to characterize the online resource allocation. An MDP is used to model a decision making problem for time-correlated random processes. An MDP is generally defined by the quadruplet $\langle \mathcal{S}, \mathcal{A}, \mathbb{P}(\mathbf{s}'|\mathbf{s}, a), R(\mathbf{s}, a)\rangle$ [61], where $\mathcal{S}$ represents the set of system states consisting of continuous or discrete channel, energy, and data states, $\mathcal{A}$ is the set of action, which could refer to the transmission power or the energy expenditure, $\mathbb{P}(\mathbf{s}'|\mathbf{s}, a)$ denotes the state transition probability from state $\mathbf{s}$ to state $\mathbf{s}'$ given that action $a \in \mathcal{A}$ is taken, and $R(\mathbf{s}, a)$ is the reward yielded when action a is taken at state $\mathbf{s}$, which could be data throughput. An MDP is formulated to maximize the expected reward, for instance, the expected throughput, by deriving the optimal policy $\pi(\cdot) : \mathcal{S} \rightarrow \mathcal{A}$. MDP problems are generally solved numerically by dynamic programming. However, as indicated in [65], this approach often requires large computation load, high dependence on the exact model of the stochastic process of channel fading, energy harvesting, and data collection, which is hard to obtain in practice, and little insight into the structure of the resource allocation policy. This makes it less than ideal for body sensors which have limited computational capabilities.

In the following, we focus on online point-to-point communications with energy harvesting by employing the time-uncorrelated system model. In particular, the remainder of Sect. 3.2 summarizes references [63–65].

Consider the transmission of backlogged data from an energy harvesting transmitter to a receiver over an AWGN channel. Just as in Sect. 3.1.1, a discrete-time system model is used. Assume for simplicity that the duration of each time slot is 1 second. At slot t, the received signal is

$$y_t = \sqrt{h}x_t + n_t,\ t = 1, 2, \dots, T, \tag{23}$$

where x_t is the transmitted signal and n_t is the white Gaussian noise with zero mean and unit variance. h is the channel gain that is assumed to be static throughout the transmission period of T time slots. The transmitter is equipped with a sufficiently large data buffer and an energy storage device with finite capacity $E_{\max}$. DBT data acquisition model is employed. The energy harvesting process is modeled as an i.i.d. Bernoulli random process denoted by $\mathbf{e} = \{e_t\}_{t=1}^{T}$, where e_t is the random variable denoting the energy harvest at time slot t. With the causal knowledge of the energy harvesting process, the transmitter knows the harvested energy e_i for $i = 1, \dots, t$. Energy harvest e_t is a Bernoulli random variable given as

$$e_t = \begin{cases} E_{\max} & \text{with probability } \rho, \\ 0 & \text{with probability } 1-\rho, \end{cases} \quad t = 1, 2, \dots, T, \tag{24}$$

which means that at each time slot the energy storage device is either fully charged to $E_{\max}$ or harvesting no energy with probability ρ and $1-\rho$, respectively. Let S_t denote the available energy beginning at slot t and $\mathbf{p} = \{p_t\}_{t=1}^{T}$ be the transmission policy throughout T slots, where p_t is the transmission power of slot t. The energy storage state S_t is given as

$$S_t = \min\{S_{t-1} - p_{t-1} + e_t,\ E_{\max}\},\ t = 1, 2, \dots, T, \tag{25}$$

where $S_1 = E_{\max}$ is assumed without loss of generality. The instantaneous data rate is

$$r_t = \frac{1}{2}\log_2(1 + hp_t),\ t = 1, 2, \dots, T. \tag{26}$$

3.2.2 Problem Formulation and Solution

For a transmission period of T time slots, the T-horizon expected throughput is defined as

$$\mathcal{T}(\mathbf{p}) = \frac{1}{T}\sum_{t=1}^{T}\mathbb{E}[r_t], \tag{27}$$

where the expectation $\mathbb{E}[\cdot]$ is taking on the energy harvest random variables $e_1, \ldots,$ e_T. The aim is to maximize the long-term expected throughput Ψ under energy constraints. The problem is formulated as

Problem 4

$$\max_{\mathbf{p}} \quad \Psi = \liminf_{T\to\infty} \mathcal{T}(\mathbf{p}) \tag{28a}$$

$$\text{s.t.} \quad 0 \le p_t \le S_t,\ t = 1, 2, \ldots, T, \tag{28b}$$

$$S_t = \min\{S_{t-1} - p_{t-1} + e_t, E_{\max}\},\ t = 1, 2, \ldots, T. \tag{28c}$$

Recall that an epoch is defined as the inter-arrival time between two consecutive nonzero energy harvests. It is shown in [63] that the optimal transmission policy that solves Problem 4 has the same structure in each epoch, thereby, Problem 4 is equivalent to maximizing the expected number of transmitted bits in each epoch. Let J_T be the number of epochs in T slots. Note that J_T is a random variable following geometric distribution due to the i.i.d. Bernoulli energy harvesting process. By the strong law of large numbers, it is given that

$$\lim_{T\to\infty}\frac{T}{J_T} = \lim_{T\to\infty}\frac{T}{\frac{1}{E_{\max}}\sum_{t=1}^{T} e_t} = \frac{E_{\max}}{\mathbb{E}[e_t]} = \frac{E_{\max}}{\rho E_{\max}} = \frac{1}{\rho}, \tag{29}$$

almost surely. Let Q_j be the number of transmitted bits in epoch j, $j = 1, \ldots, J_T$. The objective function in Problem 4 can be written as [63]

$$\begin{aligned}\Psi &= \liminf_{T\to\infty}\frac{1}{T}\sum_{t=1}^{T}\mathbb{E}[r_t] \\ &= \liminf_{T\to\infty}\frac{\sum_{j=1}^{J_T}\mathbb{E}[Q_j]/J_T}{T/J_T} \\ &= \liminf_{T\to\infty}\frac{1}{J_T}\sum_{j=1}^{J_T}\rho\mathbb{E}[Q_j].\end{aligned} \tag{30}$$

Note that $T \to \infty$ implies $J_T \to \infty$ almost surely. From (30), it is observed that in order to maximize the long-term average throughput Ψ, it is sufficient to maximize the expected transmitted data in each epoch, i.e., $\mathbb{E}[Q_j]$. Since the energy storage device is fully charged at the start of each epoch and the channel is static, the transmission policy that maximizes $\mathbb{E}[Q_j]$ also maximizes $\mathbb{E}[Q_k]$, $k \neq j$. This fact reveals that the optimal long-term transmission policy that solves Problem 4 consists of an identical optimal *epoch transmission policy* for each epoch and results in an identical epoch expected throughput. Denote the epoch transmission policy by $\mathbf{p}^{\mathrm{ep}} = \{p_1^{\mathrm{ep}}, p_2^{\mathrm{ep}}, \ldots\}$. Then, the epoch expected throughput $\mathbb{E}[Q^{\mathrm{ep}}]$ can be explicitly written as

$$\mathbb{E}[Q^{\mathrm{ep}}] = \sum_{n=1}^{\infty}\sum_{i=1}^{n}\frac{1}{2}\log_2(1+hp_i^{\mathrm{ep}})\rho(1-\rho)^{n-1} = \sum_{i=1}^{\infty}\frac{1}{2}\log_2(1+hp_i^{\mathrm{ep}})(1-\rho)^{i-1}. \tag{31}$$

Consequently, Problem 4 can be transformed to the following epoch expected throughput maximization problem:

$$\max_{\mathbf{p}^{\mathrm{ep}}} \quad \mathbb{E}[Q^{\mathrm{ep}}] \tag{32a}$$

$$\text{s.t.} \quad 0 \le p_i^{\mathrm{ep}},\ i = 1, 2, \ldots, \tag{32b}$$

$$\sum_{i=1}^{\infty} p_i^{\mathrm{ep}} \le E_{\max}, \tag{32c}$$

where the constraint (32c) is because the consumed energy in each epoch is limited to the harvested energy $E_{\max}$ at the beginning of the epoch.

It can be seen that (32) is strictly convex. By formulating the Lagrangian and solving the KKT conditions, the optimal epoch transmission policy is obtained as

$$p_i^{\mathrm{ep}*} = \begin{cases} \frac{(1-\rho)^{i-1}}{(2\ln 2)\upsilon} - \frac{1}{h}, & \text{if } \upsilon \le \frac{h(1-\rho)^{i-1}}{2\ln 2} \\ 0, & \text{otherwise}, \end{cases} \tag{33}$$

where υ is the nonnegative Lagrangian multiplier associated with constraint (32c). Note that $(1-\rho)^{i-1} \to 0$ as i increases, which implies that $p_i^{\mathrm{ep}*}$ vanishes to zero for $i > M$, where M is the smallest integer that satisfies $\upsilon > h(1-\rho)^M/(2\ln 2)$. By the optimal transmission power $p_i^{\mathrm{ep}*}$, (32c) must hold with equality. Then, υ can be solved as

$$\upsilon = \frac{h[1-(1-\rho)^M]}{(2\ln 2)\rho(M+hE_{\max})}, \tag{34}$$

where M is the smallest integer that satisfies $[\rho(M+hE_{\max})+1](1-\rho)^M < 1$. Hence, the optimal epoch transmission policy is given as

$$p_i^{\mathrm{ep}*} = \begin{cases} \frac{1}{h}\left(\frac{M+hE_{\max}}{1-(1-\rho)^M}\rho(1-\rho)^{i-1} - 1\right), & \text{if } 1 \le i \le M \\ 0, & \text{otherwise.} \end{cases} \tag{35}$$

Further, the optimal long-term transmission policy can be expressed as [65]

$$p_t^* = \begin{cases} \frac{1}{h}\left(\frac{M+hE_{\max}}{1-(1-\rho)^M}\rho(1-\rho)^{t-j_t}-1\right), & \text{if } t-j_t \le M \\ 0, & \text{otherwise,} \end{cases} \quad (36)$$

where j_t is the time slot index of the most recent energy harvest for current slot t.

3.2.3 Resource Allocation Algorithm

This section presents the extension of the above optimal transmission policy of an i.i.d. Bernoulli energy harvesting process to general i.i.d. energy harvesting processes summarizing the results in references [64, 65]. In a general i.i.d. energy harvesting process denoted by $\mathbf{E} = \{E_t\}_{t=1}^T$, the energy harvest E_t at time slot t for $t = 1, 2, \ldots, T$ are assumed to be nonnegative i.i.d. random variables with mean $\mathbb{E}[E_t] > 0$. In the following, a *fixed fraction policy* and its near-optimality are presented from [65].

From (36), it can be observed that the optimal transmission policy has an exponentially decaying structure. The following fixed fraction policy is proposed in [65] by preserving the exponentially decaying structure of the optimal policy:

$$\Pi = \left\{\pi_t : \pi_t = \rho S_t, \text{ where } S_t = (1-\rho)^{t-j_t}E_{\max}, \ t = 1, \ldots, T\right\}. \quad (37)$$

More specifically, in each time slot, ρ portion of the residual energy is allocated for transmission. It is obvious that transmission policy Π satisfies the energy constraints in (28b) and (28c). Intuitively, this transmission policy is motivated as follows. Since $\log(\cdot)$ is concave, the throughput is maximized by uniformly allocating energy. In other words, if it is known that the available energy is S_t currently and the next energy harvest will arrive in m slots, allocating S_t/m energy to each slot maximizes the throughput. For the online setting of a Bernoulli energy harvesting process, the expected time to the next energy harvest is $1/\rho$ for each time slot. Thus, ρ portion of the residual energy is allocated.

In order to characterize the near-optimal property of the fixed fraction policy, the following proposition is first presented to provide an upper bound on the achievable throughput.

Proposition 1 ([65, Proposition 2]) *The optimal throughput under any i.i.d. harvesting process* $\mathbf{E}$ *is bounded by*

$$\Psi^* \le \frac{1}{2}\log(1 + h\mu),$$

where $\mu \triangleq \mathbb{E}[\min\{E_t, E_{\max}\}]$.

Proof [65] Without loss of generality, the energy harvest variable E_t can be replaced with $\tilde{E}_t \triangleq \min\{E_t, E_{\max}\}$. This is from the fact that whenever the harvested energy E_t

is larger than $E_{\max}$, it will clipped to at most $E_{\max}$ due to the limited energy storage capacity. The average harvested energy is $\mu = \mathbb{E}[\min\{E_t, E_{\max}\}]$. Then, for any T and any transmission policy $\mathbf{p}$, the long-term throughput is given as

$$\begin{aligned}
\Psi &= \liminf_{T\to\infty} \frac{1}{T}\sum_{t=1}^{T} \mathbb{E}\left[\frac{1}{2}\log_2(1+hp_t)\right] \\
&\overset{(1)}{\leq} \liminf_{T\to\infty} \frac{1}{2}\log_2\left(1+\frac{h}{T}\mathbb{E}\left[\sum_{t=1}^{T} p_t\right]\right) \\
&\overset{(2)}{\leq} \liminf_{T\to\infty} \frac{1}{2}\log_2\left(1+\frac{h}{T}\mathbb{E}\left[E_{\max}+\sum_{t=2}^{T} \tilde{E}_t\right]\right) \\
&= \liminf_{T\to\infty} \frac{1}{2}\log_2\left(1+\frac{h}{T}E_{\max}+h\frac{T-1}{T}\mu\right) \\
&= \frac{1}{2}\log_2(1+h\mu)
\end{aligned}$$

where (1) is because log is a concave function, and (2) is because the total consumed energy up to slot T is no larger than the total harvested energy plus the initially available energy, i.e., $\sum_{t=1}^{T} p_t \leq E_{\max} + \sum_{t=2}^{T} \tilde{E}_t$. ■

Applying the fixed fraction policy Π to an i.i.d. Bernoulli energy harvesting process $\mathbf{E}$ with mean $\mu = \mathbb{E}[\min\{E_t, E_{\max}\}]$, the performance can be characterized as follows.

Proposition 2 ([65, Proposition 3, 4]) *For an i.i.d. Bernoulli energy harvesting process* $\mathbf{E}$ *with mean* $\mu = \mathbb{E}[\min\{E_t, E_{\max}\}]$, *the throughput achieved by the transmission policy* Π *is bounded as*

$$\begin{aligned}
\frac{1}{2}\log(1+h\mu) &\geq \liminf_{T\to\infty} \mathcal{T}(\Pi) \geq \frac{1}{2}\log(1+h\mu) - 0.72, \\
\frac{1}{2}\log(1+h\mu) &\geq \liminf_{T\to\infty} \mathcal{T}(\Pi) \geq \frac{1}{2}\cdot\frac{1}{2}\log(1+h\mu).
\end{aligned}$$

As proved in [65], applying this transmission policy Π to any i.i.d. processes with mean $\mu = \mathbb{E}[\min\{E_t, E_{\max}\}]$, an i.i.d. Bernoulli harvesting process gives the worst performance. This results in a lower bound of the throughput for any i.i.d. harvesting process with mean $\mu = \mathbb{E}[\min\{E_t, E_{\max}\}]$, which is the throughput achieved by the Bernoulli energy harvesting process. The following theorem states the conclusion.

Theorem 3 ([65, Theorem 2]) *For any i.i.d. nonnegative energy harvesting process* $\mathbf{E}$ *with mean* $\mu = \mathbb{E}[\min\{E_t, E_{\max}\}]$, *the throughput achieved by the transmission policy* Π *is bounded as*

$$\frac{1}{2}\log(1+h\mu) \geq \liminf_{T\to\infty} \mathcal{T}(\Pi) \geq \frac{1}{2}\log(1+h\mu) - 0.72,$$
$$\frac{1}{2}\log(1+h\mu) \geq \liminf_{T\to\infty} \mathcal{T}(\Pi) \geq \frac{1}{2}\cdot\frac{1}{2}\log(1+h\mu).$$

The detailed proofs of Proposition 2 and Theorem 3 can be found in [65].

4 Data and Energy Scheduling in Multi-Node Communications

In this section, data and energy scheduling in multi-node communication networks are investigated. In contrast with point-to-point communications, multi-node communications employ more complicated network topologies and present opportunities for efficient resource utilization by means of cooperation across multiple wireless nodes. Here we focus on offline resource allocation design for energy harvesting systems in some canonical models that are building blocks of BANs, namely, the two-hop channel, the broadcast channel (BC), and the multiple access channel (MAC).

4.1 Two-Hop Channel

Wireless communications with relays extend communication ranges and lower energy consumptions by multiple short hops instead of one single long hop [67, 68]. This model is especially fitting for health monitoring BANs where the sensor nodes are small with limited energy storage and communication range. The challenge of operating an energy harvesting multi-node network is to coordinate the transmission and reception of wireless nodes subject to the energy and data causality over each hop. In this section, we provide the treatment of the two-hop energy harvesting communications with half-duplex relays summarizing the results of [68]. The structure of optimal data and energy scheduling in terms of throughput maximization are discussed.

4.1.1 System Model

Consider transmitting backlogged data from an energy harvesting source (S) to a destination (D) via an energy harvesting relay (R) in T time slots as shown in Fig. 4. The relay employs the decode-and-forward as in [68]. There is no direct link between the source and the destination. The link between the source and the relay and the link between the relay and the destination are modeled as independent AWGN channels with channel gain h^{SR} and h^{RD}, respectively, which are assumed to be static for

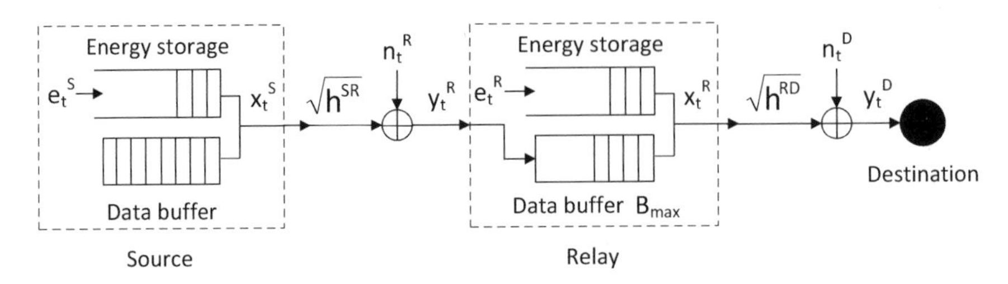

Fig. 4 System model of multi-node communications in the two-hop channel. The source and the relay harvest energy e_t^S and e_t^R respectively at time slot t. The source transmits signal x_t^S over an AWGN channel with gain h^{SR} and the relay receives signal y_t^R. A finite data buffer with capacity B_{max} is equipped at the relay. The relay decodes the received signal and forwards it to the destination by transmitting signal x_t^R over an AWGN channel with gain h^{RD}. The destination receives signal y_t^D. n_t^R and n_t^D are the noise at the relay and the destination, respectively

simplicity. Then, in terms of the transmitted signal x_t^S at the source in time slot t, the received signals at the relay and the destination are given by

$$y_t^R = \sqrt{h^{SR}} x_t^S + n_t^R, \; t = 1, 2, \ldots, T, \tag{38}$$

$$y_t^D = \sqrt{h^{RD}} x_t^R + n_t^D, \; t = 1, 2, \ldots, T, \tag{39}$$

respectively. n_t^R and n_t^D are the additive white Gaussian noise at the relay and the destination with zero mean and unit variance. The relay first decodes the source signal x_t^S based on the received y_t^R, then forwards it to the destination by transmitting signal x_t^R. The source and the relay signals, x_t^S and x_t^R, are transmitted with power p_t^S and p_t^R, respectively, i.e., $|x_t^S|^2 = p_t^S$, $|x_t^R|^2 = p_t^R$.

Assume that the source and the relay are capable to change their transmission data rate instantaneously by adapting the transmission power. The rate-power function of the SR link and the RD link at slot t are given by

$$r_t^S = \frac{1}{2} \log_2(1 + h^{SR} p_t^S), \; t = 1, 2, \ldots, T, \tag{40}$$

$$r_t^R = \frac{1}{2} \log_2(1 + h^{RD} p_t^R), \; t = 1, 2, \ldots, T. \tag{41}$$

DBT data acquisition model with a sufficiently large data buffer is applied at the source. In particular, the relay is equipped with a finite data buffer with capacity B_{max}. The source and the relay harvest energy independently in the transmission period of T time slots. Energy of amount e_t^S and e_t^R are harvested respectively at the source and the relay at time slot t. Assume that the energy harvesting profiles are known to all nodes prior to transmission. Both nodes are assumed to have infinite energy storage capacity, i.e., $E_{max} = \infty$. Energy loss caused by recharging and discharging is not considered.

4.1.2 Problem Formulation

The aim is to maximize the data transmitted to the destination in T time slots. An optimal transmission strategy is desired, by which power allocation and transmission time scheduling for each node are optimally designed. Note that the optimality of constant transmission power in epochs holds here, as for the single link point-to-point transmission, due to the concavity of the rate-power function [68]. In the sequel, epoch-indexed notation is used for the transmission power and the data rate.

For notation simplification, energy harvests at the source and the relay are combined in a single time series $s_1, s_2, \ldots, s_J$ by allowing zero energy arrivals to the source or the relay at some instants when only the other node harvests energy, where $s_1 = 0$ and J is the total number of energy harvests. Energy of amount e_i^{S} and e_i^{R} are harvested respectively at the source and the relay at time instant s_i, $i = 1, 2, \ldots, J$. The inter-arrival time between consecutive energy harvests is denoted by τ_i for epoch i. In each epoch, the half-duplex scheme necessitates the source and the relay to transmit alternatively. Let l_i^{S} and l_i^{R} be the transmission durations of the source and the relay in epoch i with corresponding transmission power p_i^{S} and p_i^{R}, respectively. Due to the intermittent energy arrivals over time, energy causality constraint has to be fulfilled by any feasible power allocation policy. Furthermore, data causality and finite data buffer at the relay have to be taken into account. The data causality implies that the transmitted data by the relay by a certain time cannot exceed its received data by that time. The finite data buffer constrains the data buffered at the relay is no larger than $B_{\max}$. Based on these arguments, the transmission power and duration sequences, $\mathbf{p}^{\mathrm{S}} = \{p_1^{\mathrm{S}}, \ldots, p_J^{\mathrm{S}}\}$, $\mathbf{p}^{\mathrm{R}} = \{p_1^{\mathrm{R}}, \ldots, p_J^{\mathrm{R}}\}$, $\mathbf{l}^{\mathrm{S}} = \{l_1^{\mathrm{S}}, \ldots, l_J^{\mathrm{S}}\}$, and $\mathbf{l}^{\mathrm{R}} = \{l_1^{\mathrm{R}}, \ldots, l_J^{\mathrm{R}}\}$ are optimized by solving the following throughput maximization problem as was done in [68].

Problem 5

$$\max_{\mathbf{p}^{\mathrm{S}},\mathbf{p}^{\mathrm{R}},\mathbf{l}^{\mathrm{S}},\mathbf{l}^{\mathrm{R}}} \quad \sum_{i=1}^{J} \frac{l_i^{\mathrm{R}}}{2} \log_2(1 + h^{\mathrm{RD}} p_i^{\mathrm{R}}) \tag{42a}$$

$$\text{s.t.} \quad \sum_{i=1}^{n} l_i^{\mathrm{R}} p_i^{\mathrm{R}} \leq \sum_{i=1}^{n} e_i^{\mathrm{R}}, \; n = 1, 2, \ldots, J, \tag{42b}$$

$$\sum_{i=1}^{n} l_i^{\mathrm{S}} p_i^{\mathrm{S}} \leq \sum_{i=1}^{n} e_i^{\mathrm{S}}, \; n = 1, 2, \ldots, J, \tag{42c}$$

$$\sum_{i=1}^{n} l_i^{\mathrm{R}} r_i^{\mathrm{R}} \leq \sum_{i=1}^{n} l_i^{\mathrm{S}} r_i^{\mathrm{S}}, \; n = 1, 2, \ldots, J, \tag{42d}$$

$$\sum_{i=1}^{n} l_i^{\mathrm{S}} r_i^{\mathrm{S}} \leq \sum_{i=1}^{n} l_i^{\mathrm{R}} r_i^{\mathrm{R}} + B_{\max}, \; n = 1, 2, \ldots, J, \tag{42e}$$

$$l_i^{\mathrm{S}} + l_i^{\mathrm{R}} \leq \tau_i, \; i = 1, 2, \ldots, J, \tag{42f}$$

$$p_i^{\mathrm{S}}, \; p_i^{\mathrm{R}}, \; l_i^{\mathrm{S}}, \; l_i^{\mathrm{R}} \geq 0, \; i = 1, 2, \ldots, J. \tag{42g}$$

Constraints (42b) and (42c) state the energy causality at the relay and the source, respectively. Constraints (42d) expressed the data causality and constraint (42e) is due to the finite data buffer at the relay. Constraint (42f) describes the half-duplex relaying scheme.

4.1.3 Resource Allocation Algorithm

Problem 5 as it is stated is not convex. However, it can be expressed in a form that is convex in its variables [68]. To do so, first, note that the transmitted bits by the source and the relay in epoch i are given by

$$d_i^{\mathrm{S}} = \frac{l_i^{\mathrm{S}}}{2}\log_2(1 + h^{\mathrm{SR}} p_i^{\mathrm{S}}), \tag{43}$$

$$d_i^{\mathrm{R}} = \frac{l_i^{\mathrm{R}}}{2}\log_2(1 + h^{\mathrm{RD}} p_i^{\mathrm{R}}). \tag{44}$$

Then, the transmission power can be expressed as

$$p_i^{\mathrm{S}} = \frac{1}{h^{\mathrm{SR}}}\left(e^{(2\ln 2)d_i^{\mathrm{S}}/l_i^{\mathrm{S}}} - 1\right), \tag{45}$$

$$p_i^{\mathrm{R}} = \frac{1}{h^{\mathrm{RD}}}\left(e^{(2\ln 2)d_i^{\mathrm{R}}/l_i^{\mathrm{R}}} - 1\right). \tag{46}$$

To obtain a convex formulation, the problem is rewritten in terms of $\mathbf{d}^{\mathrm{S}} = \{d_1^{\mathrm{S}}, \ldots, d_J^{\mathrm{S}}\}$, $\mathbf{d}^{\mathrm{R}} = \{d_1^{\mathrm{R}}, \ldots, d_J^{\mathrm{R}}\}$, $\mathbf{l}^{\mathrm{S}}$, and $\mathbf{l}^{\mathrm{R}}$, which is given as

$$\max_{\mathbf{d}^{\mathrm{S}},\mathbf{d}^{\mathrm{R}},\mathbf{l}^{\mathrm{S}},\mathbf{l}^{\mathrm{R}}} \quad \sum_{i=1}^{J} d_i^{\mathrm{R}} \tag{47a}$$

$$\text{s.t.} \quad \sum_{i=1}^{n} \frac{l_i^{\mathrm{R}}}{h^{\mathrm{RD}}}\left(e^{(2\ln 2)d_i^{\mathrm{R}}/l_i^{\mathrm{R}}} - 1\right) \le \sum_{i=1}^{n} e_i^{\mathrm{R}},\ n = 1, 2, \ldots, J, \tag{47b}$$

$$\sum_{i=1}^{n} \frac{l_i^{\mathrm{S}}}{h^{\mathrm{SR}}}\left(e^{(2\ln 2)d_i^{\mathrm{S}}/l_i^{\mathrm{S}}} - 1\right) \le \sum_{i=1}^{n} e_i^{\mathrm{S}},\ n = 1, 2, \ldots, J, \tag{47c}$$

$$\sum_{i=1}^{n} d_i^{\mathrm{R}} \le \sum_{i=1}^{n} d_i^{\mathrm{S}},\ n = 1, 2, \ldots, J, \tag{47d}$$

$$\sum_{i=1}^{n} d_i^{\mathrm{S}} \le \sum_{i=1}^{n} d_i^{\mathrm{R}} + B_{\max},\ n = 1, 2, \ldots, J, \tag{47e}$$

$$l_i^{\mathrm{S}} + l_i^{\mathrm{R}} \le \tau_i,\ i = 1, 2, \ldots, J, \tag{47f}$$

$$d_i^{\mathrm{S}},\ d_i^{\mathrm{R}},\ l_i^{\mathrm{S}},\ l_i^{\mathrm{R}} \ge 0,\ i = 1, 2, \ldots, J. \tag{47g}$$

Note that $l_i^{\mathrm{R}} e^{(2\ln 2)d_i^{\mathrm{R}}/l_i^{\mathrm{R}}}$ is the perspective of the convex function $e^{(2\ln 2)d_i^{\mathrm{R}}}$, thus, it is a convex function of l_i^{R} and d_i^{R} [57]. Similarly, $l_i^{\mathrm{S}} e^{(2\ln 2)d_i^{\mathrm{S}}/l_i^{\mathrm{S}}}$ is a convex function jointly of l_i^{S} and d_i^{S}. This makes the reformulated problem convex so that a solution can be identified. By taking derivatives of the Lagrangian with respect to d_i^{R} and d_i^{S} and setting them to zero, and further exploiting the rate-power function, the optimal transmission power for the source and the relay are expressed as

$$p_i^{\mathrm{S}^*} = \left[\frac{\sum_{n=i}^{J} \theta_{3,n} - \sum_{n=i}^{J} \theta_{4,n}}{(2\ln 2)\sum_{n=i}^{J} \theta_{2,n}} - \frac{1}{h^{\mathrm{SR}}}\right]^+, \ \forall i, \tag{48}$$

$$p_i^{\mathrm{R}^*} = \left[\frac{1 - \sum_{n=i}^{J} \theta_{3,n} + \sum_{n=i}^{J} \theta_{4,n}}{(2\ln 2)\sum_{n=i}^{J} \theta_{1,n}} - \frac{1}{h^{\mathrm{RD}}}\right]^+, \ \forall i, \tag{49}$$

respectively. $\theta_{k,i}$ for $k = 1, \ldots, 4$ are the nonnegative Lagrangian multipliers corresponding to constraints (47b)–(47e). Based on the associated complementary slackness conditions, the following lemmas that state the properties of the optimal transmission policy can be proved.

Lemma 1 ([68, Lemma 4]) *Whenever $p_i^{\mathrm{R}^*}$ strictly increases from epoch i to $i+1$, either the energy storage or the data buffer of the relay must be depleted at s_{i+1}. And whenever $p_i^{\mathrm{R}^*}$ strictly decreases from epoch i to $i+1$, the data buffer of the relay must be full at s_{i+1}.*

Proof [68] From the complementary slackness condition, it is argued that whenever $\theta_{1,i} > 0$, constraint (47b) must hold with equality, i.e., the energy storage of the relay must be depleted at time instant s_{i+1}, and whenever $\theta_{3,i} > 0$, constraint (47d) must hold with equality, which implies the depletion of the data buffer at s_{i+1}. From (49), $p_i^{\mathrm{R}^*} < p_{i+1}^{\mathrm{R}^*}$ results in either $\theta_{1,i} > 0$ or $\theta_{3,i} > 0$ or both. Similarly, by the complementary slackness conditions, whenever $\theta_{4,i} > 0$, constraint (47e) must hold with equality, i.e., the relay's data buffer must be full at s_{i+1}. From (49), $p_i^{\mathrm{R}^*} > p_{i+1}^{\mathrm{R}^*}$ implies $\theta_{4,i} > 0$. Therefore, the lemma is proved. ■

Lemma 2 ([68, Lemma 5]) *The optimal transmission power of the source is non-decreasing. Whenever $p_i^{\mathrm{S}^*}$ strictly increases form epoch i to $i+1$, either the energy storage of the source must be depleted or the data buffer of the relay must be full, or both the energy storage of the source and the data buffer of the relay must be depleted at s_{i+1}.*

Proof [68] By the complementary slackness condition, $\theta_{2,i} > 0$ implies the energy storage of the source must be depleted at s_{i+1}. Similarly, $\theta_{3,i} > 0$ results that the data buffer at the relay must be depleted at s_{i+1}, and $\theta_{4,i} > 0$ results that the data buffer at the relay must be full at s_{i+1}. Now different possible cases are investigated for $\theta_{2,i}$, $\theta_{3,i}$, and $\theta_{4,i}$, in which ($\theta_{2,i} = 0, \theta_{3,i} > 0, \theta_{4,i} > 0$) and ($\theta_{2,i} > 0, \theta_{3,i} > 0, \theta_{4,i} > 0$) can never happen as the data buffer cannot be empty and full at the same time.

(i) For the case of $(\theta_{2,i} = 0, \theta_{3,i} = 0, \theta_{4,i} = 0)$, from (48), $p_i^{S*} = p_{i+1}^{S\ \ *}$.

(ii) For the cases of $(\theta_{2,i} > 0, \theta_{3,i} = 0, \theta_{4,i} = 0)$, $(\theta_{2,i} = 0, \theta_{3,i} = 0, \theta_{4,i} > 0)$, and $(\theta_{2,i} > 0, \theta_{3,i} = 0, \theta_{4,i} > 0)$, it is obtained $p_i^{S*} < p_{i+1}^{S\ \ *}$.

(iii) For the cases of $(\theta_{2,i} > 0, \theta_{3,i} > 0, \theta_{4,i} = 0)$ and $(\theta_{2,i} = 0, \theta_{3,i} > 0, \theta_{4,i} = 0)$, it is argued by contradiction that $p_i^{S*} \leq p_{i+1}^{S\ \ *}$. Suppose $p_i^{S*} > p_{i+1}^{S\ \ *}$. A new transmission policy $\bar{p}_i^S, \bar{p}_{i+1}^S$ can be obtained by equalizing the transmission power, i.e., $\bar{p}_i^S = \bar{p}_{i+1}^S = \frac{l_i p_i^{S*} + l_{i+1} p_{i+1}^{S\ \ *}}{l_i + l_{i+1}}$, such that same energy is consumed but more data is sent to the relay because of the concavity of the rate-power function. Based on this observation, another feasible policy can be deduced by decreasing the transmission duration of the source and increasing the transmission duration of the relay such that the extra data sent to the relay can be forwarded to the destination, in which way the total throughput is improved. Thus, the transmission policy with $p_i^{S*} > p_{i+1}^{S\ \ *}$ cannot be optimal.

■

It is shown in [68] that one can schedule the transmission between the source and the relay within the feasible region. In each epoch, the source transmits until the data buffer of the relay is full, or it approaches the optimal transmission duration, then the relay starts transmitting until all data queuing in the buffer is departed, or it reaches its optimal transmission duration in the current epoch [68].

4.2 *Broadcast Channel*

In a broadcast setting, data transmission occurs within T time slots from an energy harvesting transmitter to two receivers as shown in Fig. 5. This setting is considered in reference [68] whose results we summarize in this section. The scenario with more than 2 receivers can be extended to as indicated in [69, 70]. The backlogged data is buffered in a sufficiently large data buffer at the transmitter ready before transmission, i.e., DBT data acquisition model. Energy is harvested to maintain the operation at the transmitter, where, like the other models we have described so far, energy consumption only on transmission is taken into account. Assume that the transmitter has infinite energy storage capacity.[1] Energy of amount e_t is harvested by the transmitter at time slot t. The link between the transmitter and receiver k, $k = 1, 2$, is modeled as an AWGN channel with static channel gain h_k^{BC}. At time slot t, the received signal is

$$y_{k,t} = \sqrt{h_k^{BC}} x_t + n_{k,t},\ k = 1, 2,\ t = 1, \ldots, T, \tag{50}$$

where x_t is the transmit signal and $n_{k,t}$ is the white Gaussian noise at receiver k with zero mean and unit variance. Without loss of generality, assume that $h_1^{BC} \geq h_2^{BC}$,

[1] Finite storage capacity extension has been studied in [70].

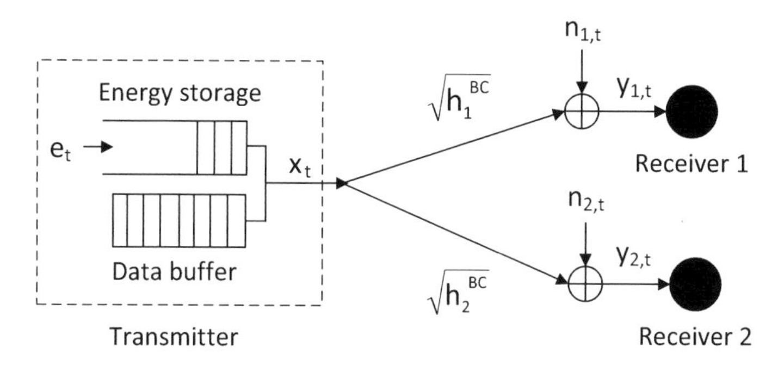

Fig. 5 System model of multi-node communications in the broadcast channel. The transmitter harvests energy e_t at time slot t. It transmits signal x_t simultaneously to receiver 1 and receiver 2 over two different AWGN channels with gain h_1^{BC} and h_2^{BC}, respectively. Receiver 1 receives signal $y_{1,t}$ and receiver 2 receives signal $y_{2,t}$. $n_{1,t}$ and $n_{2,t}$ are the noise at receiver 1 and receiver 2, respectively

thus, receiver 1 has a stronger channel than receiver 2. The capacity region for this two-user broadcast channel is given by [71]

$$r_{1,t}^{\mathrm{BC}} \leq \frac{1}{2}\log_2\left(1+\eta h_1^{\mathrm{BC}} p_t\right),\ t=1,\ldots,T, \tag{51}$$

$$r_{2,t}^{\mathrm{BC}} \leq \frac{1}{2}\log_2\left(1+\frac{(1-\eta)h_2^{\mathrm{BC}} p_t}{\eta h_2^{\mathrm{BC}} p_t+1}\right),\ t=1,\ldots,T, \tag{52}$$

where p_t is the transmission power for signal x_t and $\eta \in (0,1)$ represents the power sharing parameter denoting that η portion of the transmission power is dedicated to receiver 1. With respect to the rate pair $(r_{1,t}^{\mathrm{BC}}, r_{2,t}^{\mathrm{BC}})$ on the boundary of the capacity region, the transmission power p_t can be expressed as a function of $r_{1,t}^{\mathrm{BC}}$ and $r_{2,t}^{\mathrm{BC}}$ given as

$$p_t = f(r_{1,t}^{\mathrm{BC}}, r_{2,t}^{\mathrm{BC}}) = \left(\frac{1}{h_2^{\mathrm{BC}}}-\frac{1}{h_1^{\mathrm{BC}}}\right)2^{2r_{2,t}^{\mathrm{BC}}}+\frac{1}{h_1^{\mathrm{BC}}}2^{2(r_{1,t}^{\mathrm{BC}}+r_{2,t}^{\mathrm{BC}})}-\frac{1}{h_2^{\mathrm{BC}}}. \tag{53}$$

Note that p_t is convex with respect to $r_{1,t}^{\mathrm{BC}}$ and $r_{2,t}^{\mathrm{BC}}$.

The aim is to maximize the sum number of bits transmitted to the two receivers within T time slots. An optimal transmission policy that maximizes the sum channel throughput in a period of T time slots is desired. Once again, by the optimality of constant transmission power in epochs [68], policies with epoch-indexed transmission power p_i and corresponding rate $r_{k,i}^{\mathrm{BC}}$ for $k=1,2$, $i=1,2,\ldots,J$ are considered. J is the number of energy harvests, thus, the number of epochs. Denote the length of epoch i by τ_i. Energy harvests occur at time instants s_i with amount e_i, $i=1,2,\ldots,J$. Now the sum throughput maximization problem subject to the energy causality constraint is formulated as follows.

Problem 6

$$\max_{\mathbf{r}_1^{\mathrm{BC}},\mathbf{r}_2^{\mathrm{BC}},\mathbf{p}_1,\mathbf{p}_2} \quad \sum_{i=1}^{J} \tau_i (r_{1,i}^{\mathrm{BC}} + r_{2,i}^{\mathrm{BC}}) \tag{54a}$$

$$\text{s.t.} \quad \sum_{i=1}^{n} \tau_i f(r_{1,i}^{\mathrm{BC}}, r_{2,i}^{\mathrm{BC}}) \le \sum_{i=1}^{n} e_i, \; n = 1, 2, \ldots, J, \tag{54b}$$

$$r_{1,i}^{\mathrm{BC}} \ge 0, \; i = 1, 2, \ldots, J, \tag{54c}$$

$$r_{2,i}^{\mathrm{BC}} \ge 0, \; i = 1, 2, \ldots, J. \tag{54d}$$

Here the maximization is over $\mathbf{r}_k^{\mathrm{BC}} = \{r_{k,1}^{\mathrm{BC}}, \ldots, r_{k,J}^{\mathrm{BC}}\}$ and $\mathbf{p}_k = \{p_{k,1}, \ldots, p_{k,J}\}$, $k = 1, 2$. Since $f(r_{1,i}^{\mathrm{BC}}, r_{2,i}^{\mathrm{BC}})$ is a convex function with respect to $r_{1,i}^{\mathrm{BC}}$ and $r_{2,i}^{\mathrm{BC}}$, Problem 6 is convex. Then, by formulating the Lagrangian, equating its derivatives with respect to $r_{1,i}^{\mathrm{BC}}$ and $r_{2,i}^{\mathrm{BC}}$ to zero, and exploiting the relationship between p_i and $r_{k,i}^{\mathrm{BC}}$, $k = 1, 2$, in (53), it is obtained that

$$p_i = \frac{1 + \beta_{3,i}/\tau_i}{(2 \ln 2) \sum_{n=i}^{J} \beta_{1,n}} - \frac{1}{h_2^{\mathrm{BC}}}, \; \forall i, \tag{55}$$

where $\beta_{1,n}$, $\beta_{2,i}$, and $\beta_{3,i}$ are the Lagrangian multipliers with respect to constraints (54b)–(54d), respectively. Since $0 < \eta < 1$ and $p_i > 0$ must hold, $r_{k,i}^{\mathrm{BC}} > 0, k = 1, 2$, is always true. Then, $\beta_{3,i}$ must be zero to satisfy the complementary slackness condition $\beta_{3,i} r_{2,i}^{\mathrm{BC}} = 0$. Hence, the optimal transmission power is given as

$$p_i^* = \frac{1}{(2 \ln 2) \sum_{n=i}^{J} \beta_{1,n}} - \frac{1}{h_2^{\mathrm{BC}}}, \; \forall i. \tag{56}$$

The optimal transmission power p_i^* has the same form as the single user transmission power in Sect. 3.1.3. Thus, it can be solved by directional water-filling algorithm in Sect. 3.1.3 and preserving the monotonically increasing property stated in Theorem 1.

4.3 *Multiple Access Channel*

In this section, data transmission is considered within T time slots from two energy harvesting transmitters to one receiver over a multiple access channel as shown in Fig. 6, and results from [68, 72] are summarized. DBT data acquisition model with a sufficiently large data buffer is applied at the transmitters. Two transmitters harvest energy independently during the transmission period of T slots with infinite energy storage devices. Similar notation of energy arrivals as in Sect. 4.1.1 is applied, that

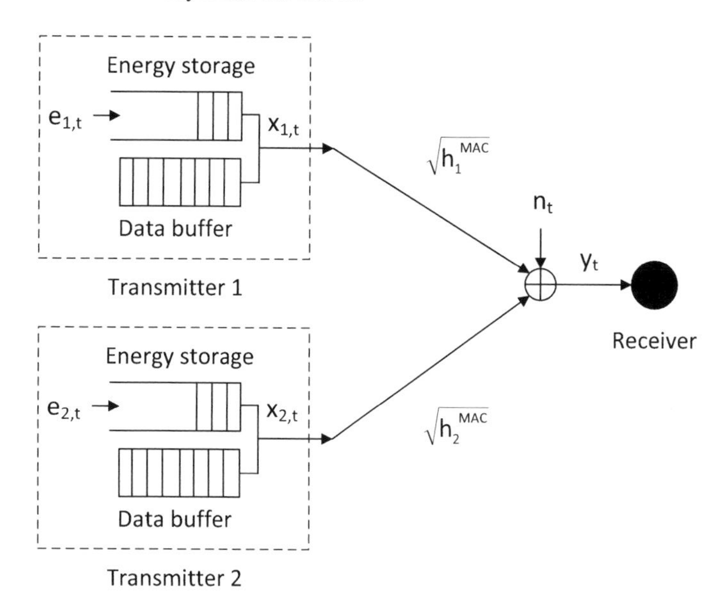

Fig. 6 System model of multi-node communications in the multiple access channel. Transmitter 1 harvests energy $e_{1,t}$ at time slot t and transmits signal $x_{1,t}$ over an AWGN channel with gain h_1^{MAC}. Simultaneously, transmitter 2 harvests energy $e_{2,t}$ and transmits signal $x_{2,t}$ over an AWGN channel with gain h_2^{MAC}. The receiver receives signal y_t. n_t is the noise at the receiver

is, the energy arrival instants are combined in a single sequence allowing zero energy harvests for some instants when only one of the transmitters has energy arrival. Energy of amount $e_{k,t}$ is harvested by transmitter k at time slot t.

The backlogged data at the transmitters is sent to the receiver. The links from transmitter 1 and transmitter 2 to the receiver are modeled as AWGN channels with static channel gain h_1^{MAC} and h_2^{MAC}, respectively. Then, the received signal at the receiver in slot t is given as

$$y_t = \sqrt{h_1^{\text{MAC}}} x_{1,t} + \sqrt{h_2^{\text{MAC}}} x_{2,t} + n_t, \ t = 1, \dots, T, \tag{57}$$

where $x_{k,t}$ is the signal sent by transmitter k and n_t is the white Gaussian noise with zero-mean and unit-variance. Denote the transmission power for $x_{k,t}$ by $p_{k,t}$. The capacity region for this two-user multiple access channel is [71]

$$r_{1,t}^{\text{MAC}} \leq \frac{1}{2} \log_2(1 + h_1^{\text{MAC}} p_{1,t}), \ t = 1, \dots, T, \tag{58}$$

$$r_{2,t}^{\text{MAC}} \leq \frac{1}{2} \log_2(1 + h_2^{\text{MAC}} p_{2,t}), \ t = 1, \dots, T, \tag{59}$$

$$r_{1,t}^{\text{MAC}} + r_{2,t}^{\text{MAC}} \leq \frac{1}{2} \log_2(1 + h_1^{\text{MAC}} p_{1,t} + h_2^{\text{MAC}} p_{2,t}), \ t = 1, \dots, T, \tag{60}$$

where $r_{1,t}^{\mathrm{MAC}}$ and $r_{2,t}^{\mathrm{MAC}}$ are the data rates on the two links.

By the optimality of constant transmission power in epochs [68], the aim is to find the transmission power $p_{k,i}$ and rate $r_{k,i}^{\mathrm{MAC}}$ for transmitter k in the ith epoch for $i = 1, 2, \ldots, J$, where J is the number of energy harvests, thus, the number of epochs. The length of epoch i is denoted by τ_i. At time instant s_i, energy of amount e_i is harvested, $i = 1, 2, \ldots, J$. The throughput maximization problem under the energy causality constraint and the MAC capacity region constraint is formulated as [68]

Problem 7

$$\max_{\mathbf{r}_1^{\mathrm{MAC}}, \mathbf{r}_2^{\mathrm{MAC}}, \mathbf{p}_1, \mathbf{p}_2} \quad \sum_{i=1}^{J} \tau_i (r_{1,i}^{\mathrm{MAC}} + r_{2,i}^{\mathrm{MAC}}) \tag{61a}$$

$$\text{s.t.} \quad \sum_{i=1}^{n} \tau_i p_{k,i} \leq \sum_{i=1}^{n} e_{k,i}, \; k = 1, 2, \; n = 1, 2, \ldots, J, \tag{61b}$$

$$r_{1,i}^{\mathrm{MAC}} \leq \frac{1}{2} \log_2(1 + h_1^{\mathrm{MAC}} p_{1,i}), \; i = 1, 2, \ldots, J, \tag{61c}$$

$$r_{2,i}^{\mathrm{MAC}} \leq \frac{1}{2} \log_2(1 + h_2^{\mathrm{MAC}} p_{2,i}), \; i = 1, 2, \ldots, J, \tag{61d}$$

$$r_{1,i}^{\mathrm{MAC}} + r_{2,i}^{\mathrm{MAC}} \leq \frac{1}{2} \log_2(1 + h_1^{\mathrm{MAC}} p_{1,i} + h_2^{\mathrm{MAC}} p_{2,i}), \; i = 1, 2, \ldots, J, \tag{61e}$$

$$r_{k,i}^{\mathrm{MAC}} \geq 0, \; k = 1, 2, \; i = 1, 2, \ldots, J, \tag{61f}$$

$$p_{k,i} \geq 0, \; k = 1, 2, \; i = 1, 2, \ldots, J, \tag{61g}$$

where $\mathbf{r}_k^{\mathrm{MAC}} = \{r_{1,1}^{\mathrm{MAC}}, \ldots, r_{1,J}^{\mathrm{MAC}}\}$ and $\mathbf{p}_k = \{p_{k,1}, \ldots, p_{k,J}\}$ for $k = 1, 2$. Note that Problem 7 is convex. Therefore, the optimal solution can be attained by considering its Lagrangian and KKT conditions. Formulating the Lagrangian $\mathcal{L}$ with multipliers $\omega_{k,n}$, $\kappa_{1,i}$, $\kappa_{2,i}$, $\kappa_{3,i}$, $\xi_{k,i}$ and $\phi_{k,i}$ associated with constraints (61b)–(61g), taking derivatives with respect to each optimization variable and setting them to zero, it is obtained that [68]

$$\frac{\partial \mathcal{L}}{\partial r_{1,i}^{\mathrm{MAC}}} = \tau_i - \kappa_{1,i} - \kappa_{3,i} + \xi_{1,i} = 0, \tag{62}$$

$$\frac{\partial \mathcal{L}}{\partial r_{2,i}^{\mathrm{MAC}}} = \tau_i - \kappa_{2,i} - \kappa_{3,i} + \xi_{2,i} = 0, \tag{63}$$

$$\frac{\partial \mathcal{L}}{\partial p_{1,i}} = -\tau_i \sum_{n=i}^{J} \omega_{1,n} + \frac{\kappa_{1,i} h_1^{\mathrm{MAC}}}{(2 \ln 2)(1 + h_1^{\mathrm{MAC}} p_{1,i})} + \frac{\kappa_{3,i} h_1^{\mathrm{MAC}}}{(2 \ln 2)(1 + h_1^{\mathrm{MAC}} p_{1,i} + h_2^{\mathrm{MAC}} p_{2,i})} + \phi_{1,i} = 0, \tag{64}$$

$$\frac{\partial \mathcal{L}}{\partial p_{2,i}} = -\tau_i \sum_{n=i}^{J} \omega_{2,n} + \frac{\kappa_{2,i} h_2^{\mathrm{MAC}}}{(2 \ln 2)(1 + h_2^{\mathrm{MAC}} p_{2,i})} + \frac{\kappa_{3,i} h_2^{\mathrm{MAC}}}{(2 \ln 2)(1 + h_1^{\mathrm{MAC}} p_{1,i} + h_2^{\mathrm{MAC}} p_{2,i})} + \phi_{2,i} = 0. \tag{65}$$

Without loss of generality, both transmitters are delivering data to the the receiver such that $r_{k,i}^{\mathrm{MAC}} > 0$ and $p_{k,i} > 0$ for $k = 1, 2$. Thus, $\xi_{k,i} = 0$ and $\phi_{k,i} = 0$, $k = 1, 2$, must hold to satisfy the associated complementary slackness conditions. By (62) and (63), $\kappa_{1,i} = \kappa_{2,i}$ for $\forall i$. Due to the MAC capacity region constraints in (61c)–(61e), (61c) and (61d) cannot hold with equality simultaneously. This implies that $\kappa_{1,i} = \kappa_{2,i} = 0$ must hold to satisfy the corresponding complementary slackness conditions. As a result, the optimal transmission power can be expressed as follows [68].

$$p_{1,i}{}^{*} = \left[\frac{1}{(2\ln 2)\sum_{n=i}^{J}\omega_{1,n}} - \frac{h_2^{\mathrm{MAC}}}{h_1^{\mathrm{MAC}}}p_{2,i}{}^{*} - \frac{1}{h_1^{\mathrm{MAC}}}\right]^{+}, \ \forall i, \tag{66}$$

$$p_{2,i}{}^{*} = \left[\frac{1}{(2\ln 2)\sum_{n=i}^{J}\omega_{2,n}} - \frac{h_1^{\mathrm{MAC}}}{h_2^{\mathrm{MAC}}}p_{1,i}{}^{*} - \frac{1}{h_2^{\mathrm{MAC}}}\right]^{+}, \ \forall i. \tag{67}$$

5 Conclusion

In this chapter, we studied resource allocation in BANs with energy harvesting. Multiple viable energy sources for BANs and the corresponding energy harvesting techniques were introduced. Apart from conventional energy sources like photovoltaic, thermoelectric, and electromagnetic energy harvesting applicable to BANs, we also discussed the human-powered energy sources like kinetic and biochemical energy harvesting.

In order to efficiently allocate the harvested energy from these potential sources, optimal resource allocation policies have been studied in the literature in terms of energy and data scheduling in both point-to-point and multi-node energy harvesting communications. We have provided a detailed review of these recent developments. The point-to-point transmission is the most common form of transmitting health monitoring data from the wearable or implantable sensors to the gateway device. We have provided the problem formulations and solutions in both offline and online settings of energy and data scheduling in detail for different performance metrics. In the offline setting, the full knowledge of the channel state and energy harvesting profile is utilized to optimally allocate the limited harvested energy. This idealized setting is applicable to BANs with predictable energy harvesting sources, for instance, solar. Its system performance serves as a benchmark for the online settings. On the other hand, more dynamic energy harvesting process such as kinetic energy harvesting is difficult to precisely predict. For such scenarios, the online setting can be applied to solve resource allocation in BANs when only causal knowledge and the statistics of the energy harvesting process are available. Online resource allocation can be employed to facilitate real-time health monitoring data transmission in an energy-efficient manner.

We have also reviewed multi-node communications with energy harvesting for large-scale BANs that employs complicated network structures. Optimal offline strategies for data transmission between energy harvesting nodes have been studied for the two-hop channel, the broadcast channel, and the multiple access channel. As building blocks of large-scale BANs, resource allocation problems addressed in these canonical models shed some light on the overall energy-efficient system design.

Health monitoring sensors, in particular implantable sensors, are small in size and may have very limited computational capabilities. Thus, it may be necessary to look for near-optimal policies with very low computational complexity in practice. The optimal energy allocation policies discussed in this chapter can be viewed as performance benchmarks for such applications.

References

1. B. Johny and A. Anpalagan, "Body area sensor networks: Requirements, operations, and challenges," *IEEE Potentials*, vol. 33, no. 2, pp. 21–25, 2014.
2. T. Starner, "Human-powered wearable computing," *IBM systems Journal*, vol. 35, no. 3.4, pp. 618–629, 1996.
3. F. Goodarzy, E. S. Skafidas, and S. Gambini, "Feasibility of energy-autonomous wireless microsensors for biomedical applications: Powering and communication," *IEEE Reviews in Biomedical Engineering*, vol. 8, pp. 17–29, 2015.
4. M.-L. Ku, W. Li, Y. Chen, and K. R. Liu, "Advances in energy harvesting communications: Past, present, and future challenges," *IEEE Communications Surveys & Tutorials*, vol. 18, no. 2, pp. 1384–1412, 2016.
5. Y. Zhang, F. Zhang, Y. Shakhsheer, J. D. Silver, A. Klinefelter, M. Nagaraju, J. Boley, J. Pandey, A. Shrivastava, E. J. Carlson, A. Wood, B. H. Calhoun, and B. P. Otis, "A batteryless 19 μW MICS/ISM-band energy harvesting body sensor node SoC for ExG applications," *IEEE Journal of Solid-State Circuits*, vol. 48, no. 1, pp. 199–213, 2013.
6. V. Misra, A. Bozkurt, B. Calhoun, T. Jackson, J. S. Jur, J. Lach, B. Lee, J. Muth, O. Oralkan, M. Ozturk, S. Trolier-McKinstry, D. Vashaee, D. Wentzloff, and Y. Zhu, "Flexible technologies for self-powered wearable health and environmental sensing," *Proceedings of the IEEE*, vol. 103, no. 4, pp. 665–681, 2015.
7. O. Ozel, K. Tutuncuoglu, J. Yang, S. Ulukus, and A. Yener, "Transmission with energy harvesting nodes in fading wireless channels: Optimal policies," *IEEE Journal on Selected Areas in Communications*, vol. 29, no. 8, pp. 1732–1743, 2011.
8. K. Tutuncuoglu and A. Yener, "Optimum transmission policies for battery limited energy harvesting nodes," *IEEE Transactions on Wireless Communications*, vol. 11, no. 3, pp. 1180–1189, 2012.
9. O. Ozel, K. Tutuncuoglu, S. Ulukus, and A. Yener, "Fundamental limits of energy harvesting communications," *IEEE Communications Magazine*, vol. 53, no. 4, pp. 126–132, 2015.
10. S. Ulukus, A. Yener, E. Erkip, O. Simeone, M. Zorzi, P. Grover, and K. Huang, "Energy harvesting wireless communications: A review of recent advances," *IEEE Journal on Selected Areas in Communications*, vol. 33, no. 3, pp. 360–381, 2015.
11. A. Seyedi and B. Sikdar, "Modeling and analysis of energy harvesting nodes in body sensor networks," in *Proc. 5th International Summer School and Symposium on Medical Devices and Biosensors*, 2008, pp. 175–178.
12. A. Seyedi and B. Sikdar, "Energy efficient transmission strategies for body sensor networks with energy harvesting," *IEEE Transactions on Communications*, vol. 58, no. 7, pp. 2116–2126, 2010.
13. J. Ventura and K. Chowdhury, "Markov modeling of energy harvesting body sensor networks," in *Proc. IEEE 22nd International Symposium on Personal, Indoor and Mobile Radio Communications*, 2011, pp. 2168–2172.

14. Y. He, W. Zhu, and L. Guan, "Optimal resource allocation for pervasive health monitoring systems with body sensor networks," *IEEE Transactions on Mobile Computing*, vol. 10, no. 11, pp. 1558–1575, 2011.
15. S. Manfredi, "Congestion control for differentiated healthcare service delivery in emerging heterogeneous wireless body area networks," *IEEE Wireless Communications*, vol. 21, no. 2, pp. 81–90, 2014.
16. E. Ibarra, A. Antonopoulos, E. Kartsakli, J. J. Rodrigues, and C. Verikoukis, "QoS-aware energy management in body sensor nodes powered by human energy harvesting," *IEEE Sensors Journal*, vol. 16, no. 2, pp. 542–549, 2016.
17. S. Ayazian, V. A. Akhavan, E. Soenen, and A. Hassibi, "A photovoltaic-driven and energy-autonomous CMOS implantable sensor," *IEEE Transactions on Biomedical Circuits and Systems*, vol. 6, no. 4, pp. 336–343, 2012.
18. Y. K. Tan and S. K. Panda, "Energy harvesting from hybrid indoor ambient light and thermal energy sources for enhanced performance of wireless sensor nodes," *IEEE Transactions on Industrial Electronics*, vol. 58, no. 9, pp. 4424–4435, 2011.
19. A. Liberale, E. Dallago, and A. L. Barnabei, "Energy harvesting system for wireless body sensor nodes," in *Proc. IEEE Biomedical Circuits and Systems Conference (BioCAS) Proceedings*, 2014, pp. 416–419.
20. W. Y. Toh, Y. K. Tan, W. S. Koh, and L. Siek, "Autonomous wearable sensor nodes with flexible energy harvesting," *IEEE Sensors Journal*, vol. 14, no. 7, pp. 2299–2306, 2014.
21. J. A. Paradiso and T. Starner, "Energy scavenging for mobile and wireless electronics," *IEEE Pervasive computing*, vol. 4, no. 1, pp. 18–27, 2005.
22. W. S. Wang, T. O'Donnell, N. Wang, M. Hayes, B. O'Flynn, and C. O'Mathuna, "Design considerations of sub-mW indoor light energy harvesting for wireless sensor systems," *ACM Journal on Emerging Technologies in Computing Systems (JETC)*, vol. 6, no. 2, p. 6, 2010.
23. S. Basagni, M. Y. Naderi, C. Petrioli, and D. Spenza, "Wireless sensor networks with energy harvesting," *Mobile Ad Hoc Networking: The Cutting Edge Directions*, pp. 701–736, 2013.
24. D. C. Hoang, Y. K. Tan, H. B. Chng, and S. K. Panda, "Thermal energy harvesting from human warmth for wireless body area network in medical healthcare system," in *Proc. International Conference on Power Electronics and Drive Systems (PEDS)*, 2009, pp. 1277–1282.
25. R. Kappel, W. Pachler, M. Auer, W. Pribyl, G. Hofer, and G. Holweg, "Using thermoelectric energy harvesting to power a self-sustaining temperature sensor in body area networks," in *Proc. IEEE International Conference on Industrial Technology (ICIT)*, 2013, pp. 787–792.
26. G. Wu and X. Yu, "System design on thermoelectic energy harvesting from body heat," in *Proc. 39th Annual Northeast Bioengineering Conference (NEBEC)*, 2013, pp. 157–158.
27. H. P. Wong and Z. Dahari, "Human body parts heat energy harvesting using thermoelectric module," in *Proc. IEEE Conference on Energy Conversion (CENCON)*, 2015, pp. 211–214.
28. S. Jo, M. Kim, M. Kim, and Y. Kim, "Flexible thermoelectric generator for human body heat energy harvesting," *Electronics letters*, vol. 48, no. 16, pp. 1013–1015, 2012.
29. A. Ghosh, Meenakshi, S. Khalid, V. P. Harigovindan, "Performance analysis of wireless body area network with thermal energy harvesting," in *Proc. Global Conference on Communication Technologies (GCCT)*, 2015, pp. 916–920.
30. M. Wahbah, M. Alhawari, B. Mohammad, H. Saleh, and M. Ismail, "Characterization of human body-based thermal and vibration energy harvesting for wearable devices," *IEEE Journal on Emerging and Selected Topics in Circuits and Systems*, vol. 4, no. 3, pp. 354–363, 2014.
31. V. Leonov, "Thermoelectric energy harvesting of human body heat for wearable sensors," *IEEE Sensors Journal*, vol. 13, no. 6, pp. 2284–2291, 2013.
32. N. B. Amor, O. Kanoun, A. Lay-Ekuakille, G. Specchia, G. Vendramin, and A. Trotta, "Energy harvesting from human body for biomedical autonomous systems," *Sensors, 2008 IEEE*, 2008, pp. 678–680.
33. P. D. Mitcheson, E. M. Yeatman, G. K. Rao, A. S. Holmes, and T. C. Green, "Energy harvesting from human and machine motion for wireless electronic devices," *Proceedings of the IEEE*, vol. 96, no. 9, pp. 1457–1486, 2008.

34. G. De Pasquale and A. Somà, "Energy harvesting from human motion with piezo fibers for the body monitoring by MEMS sensors," in *Proc. Symposium on Design, Test, Integration and Packaging of MEMS/MOEMS (DTIP)*, 2013, pp. 1–6.
35. L. Xie and M. Cai, "Human motion: Sustainable power for wearable electronics," *IEEE Pervasive Computing*, vol. 13, no. 4, pp. 42–49, 2014.
36. C. Sauer, M. Stanacevic, G. Cauwenberghs, and N. Thakor, "Power harvesting and telemetry in CMOS for implanted devices," *IEEE Transactions on Circuits and Systems I: Regular Papers*, vol. 52, no. 12, pp. 2605–2613, 2005.
37. J. Cheng, L. Xia, C. Ma, Y. Lian, X. Xu, C. P. Yue, Z. Hong, and P. Y. Chiang, "A near-threshold, multi-node, wireless body area sensor network powered by RF energy harvesting," in *Proc. IEEE Custom Integrated Circuits Conference*, 2012, pp. 1–4.
38. N. Barroca, H. M. Saraiva, P. T. Gouveia, J. Tavares, L. M. Borges, F. J. Velez, C. Loss, R. Salvado, P. Pinho, R. Gonçalves, N. B. Carvalho, R. Chavez-Santiago, I. Balasingham, "Antennas and circuits for ambient RF energy harvesting in wireless body area networks," in *Proc. IEEE 24th Annual International Symposium on Personal, Indoor, and Mobile Radio Communications (PIMRC)*, 2013, pp. 532–537.
39. Z. Liu, Z. Zhong, and Y. X. Guo, "High-efficiency triple-band ambient RF energy harvesting for wireless body sensor network," in *Proc. IEEE MTT-S International Microwave Workshop Series on RF and Wireless Technologies for Biomedical and Healthcare Applications (IMWS-Bio)*, 2014, pp. 1–3.
40. S. Kim, R. Vyas, J. Bito, K. Niotaki, A. Collado, A. Georgiadis, and M. M. Tentzeris, "Ambient RF energy-harvesting technologies for self-sustainable standalone wireless sensor platforms," *Proceedings of the IEEE*, vol. 102, no. 11, pp. 1649–1666, 2014.
41. R. Zhang and C. K. Ho, "MIMO broadcasting for simultaneous wireless information and power transfer," *IEEE Transactions on Wireless Communications*, vol. 12, no. 5, pp. 1989–2001, 2013.
42. B. I. Rapoport, J. T. Kedzierski, and R. Sarpeshkar, "A glucose fuel cell for implantable brain-machine interfaces," *PloS one*, vol. 7, no. 6, p. e38436, 2012.
43. A. Zebda, S. Cosnier, J.-P. Alcaraz, M. Holzinger, A. Le Goff, C. Gondran, F. Boucher, F. Giroud, K. Gorgy, H. Lamraoui, P. Cinquin, "Single glucose biofuel cells implanted in rats power electronic devices," *Scientific reports*, vol. 3, p. 1516, 2013.
44. C.-Y. Sue and N.-C. Tsai, "Human powered MEMS-based energy harvest devices," *Applied Energy*, vol. 93, pp. 390–403, 2012.
45. F. Davis and S. P. Higson, "Biofuel cells - recent advances and applications," *Biosensors and Bioelectronics*, vol. 22, no. 7, pp. 1224–1235, 2007.
46. J. Yang and S. Ulukus, "Optimal packet scheduling in an energy harvesting communication system," *IEEE Transactions on Communications*, vol. 60, no. 1, pp. 220–230, 2012.
47. M. Gregori and M. Payaró, "Energy-efficient transmission for wireless energy harvesting nodes," *IEEE Transactions on Wireless Communications*, vol. 12, no. 3, pp. 1244–1254, 2013.
48. B. Varan and A. Yener, "Delay constrained energy harvesting networks with limited energy and data storage," *IEEE Journal on Selected Areas in Communications*, vol. 34, no. 5, pp. 1550–1564, 2016.
49. F. Shan, J. Luo, W. Wu, M. Li, and X. Shen, "Discrete rate scheduling for packets with individual deadlines in energy harvesting systems," *IEEE Journal on Selected Areas in Communications*, vol. 33, no. 3, pp. 438–451, 2015.
50. S. Wei, W. Guan, and K. R. Liu, "Power scheduling for energy harvesting wireless communications with battery capacity constraint," *IEEE Transactions on Wireless Communications*, vol. 14, no. 8, pp. 4640–4653, 2015.
51. C. Huang, R. Zhang, and S. Cui, "Optimal power allocation for outage probability minimization in fading channels with energy harvesting constraints," *IEEE Transactions on Wireless Communications*, vol. 13, no. 2, pp. 1074–1087, 2014.
52. F. M. Ozcelik, G. Uctu, and E. Uysal-Biyikoglu, "Minimization of transmission duration of data packets over an energy harvesting fading channel," *IEEE Communications Letters*, vol. 12, no. 16, pp. 1968–1971, 2012.

53. N. Roseveare and B. Natarajan, "An alternative perspective on utility maximization in energy-harvesting wireless sensor networks," *IEEE Transactions on Vehicular Technology*, vol. 63, no. 1, pp. 344–356, 2014.
54. O. Orhan, D. Gündüz, and E. Erkip, "Energy harvesting broadband communication systems with processing energy cost," *IEEE Transactions on Wireless Communications*, vol. 13, no. 11, pp. 6095–6107, 2014.
55. K. Tutuncuoglu, A. Yener, and S. Ulukus, "Optimum policies for an energy harvesting transmitter under energy storage losses," *IEEE Journal on Selected Areas in Communications*, vol. 33, no. 3, pp. 467–481, 2015.
56. K. Tutuncuoglu and A. Yener, "Communicating with energy harvesting transmitters and receivers," in *Proc. Information Theory and Applications Workshop (ITA)*, 2012, pp. 240–245.
57. S. Boyd and L. Vandenberghe, *Convex optimization*. Cambridge university press, 2004.
58. R. Srivastava and C. E. Koksal, "Basic performance limits and tradeoffs in energy-harvesting sensor nodes with finite data and energy storage," *IEEE/ACM Transactions on Networking*, vol. 21, no. 4, pp. 1049–1062, 2013.
59. V. Sharma, U. Mukherji, V. Joseph, and S. Gupta, "Optimal energy management policies for energy harvesting sensor nodes," *IEEE Transactions on Wireless Communications*, vol. 9, no. 4, pp. 1326–1336, 2010.
60. N. Michelusi, K. Stamatiou, and M. Zorzi, "Transmission policies for energy harvesting sensors with time-correlated energy supply," *IEEE Transactions on Communications*, vol. 61, no. 7, pp. 2988–3001, 2013.
61. P. Blasco, D. Gunduz, and M. Dohler, "A learning theoretic approach to energy harvesting communication system optimization," *IEEE Transactions on Wireless Communications*, vol. 12, no. 4, pp. 1872–1882, 2013.
62. S. Mao, M. H. Cheung, and V. W. Wong, "Joint energy allocation for sensing and transmission in rechargeable wireless sensor networks," *IEEE Transactions on Vehicular Technology*, vol. 63, no. 6, pp. 2862–2875, 2014.
63. A. Kazerouni and A. Ozgur, "Optimal online strategies for an energy harvesting system with Bernoulli energy recharges," in *Proc. 13th International Symposium on Modeling and Optimization in Mobile, Ad Hoc, and Wireless Networks (WiOpt)*, 2015, pp. 235–242.
64. Y. Dong, F. Farnia, and A. Ozgur, "Near optimal energy control and approximate capacity of energy harvesting communication," *IEEE Journal on Selected Areas in Communications*, vol. 33, no. 3, pp. 540–557, 2015.
65. D. Shaviv and A. Ozgur, "Universally near optimal online power control for energy harvesting nodes," *IEEE Journal on Selected Areas in Communications*, vol. 34, no. 12, pp. 3620–3631, 2016.
66. S. Zhang, A. Seyedi, and B. Sikdar, "An analytical approach to the design of energy harvesting wireless sensor nodes," *IEEE Transactions on Wireless Communications*, vol. 12, no. 8, pp. 4010–4024, 2013.
67. I. Krikidis, G. Zheng, and B. Ottersten, "Harvest-use cooperative networks with half/full-duplex relaying," in *Proc. IEEE Wireless Communications and Networking Conference (WCNC)*, 2013, pp. 4256–4260.
68. O. Orhan and E. Erkip, "Energy harvesting two-hop communication networks," *IEEE Journal on Selected Areas in Communications*, vol. 33, no. 12, pp. 2658–2670, 2015.
69. J. Yang, O. Ozel, and S. Ulukus, "Broadcasting with an energy harvesting rechargeable transmitter," *IEEE Transactions on Wireless Communications*, vol. 11, no. 2, pp. 571–583, 2012.
70. O. Ozel, J. Yang, and S. Ulukus, "Optimal broadcast scheduling for an energy harvesting rechargeable transmitter with a finite capacity battery," *IEEE Transactions on Wireless Communications*, vol. 11, no. 6, pp. 2193–2203, 2012.
71. T. M. Cover and J. A. Thomas, *Elements of Information Theory*. New York: Wiley, 1991.
72. J. Yang and S. Ulukus, "Optimal packet scheduling in a multiple access channel with energy harvesting transmitters," *Journal of Communications and Networks*, vol. 14, no. 2, pp. 140–150, 2012.

Medical-QoS Based Telemedicine Service Selection Using Analytic Hierarchy Process

Ali Hassan Sodhro, Faisal K. Shaikh, Sandeep Pirbhulal, Mir Muhammad Lodro and Madad Ali Shah

Abstract An emerging breakthrough paradigm shift in health industry and wearable devices, large scale and distributed mobile cloud computing technologies have led to new opportunities for medical healthcare systems. Telemedicine service selection and management of Medical-Quality of Service (m-QoS) in large-scale and distributed medical health system (e.g. medical data centers, hospitals, medical servers and medical clouds, etc.) is a key challenge for both industry and academia. The aim of this chapter is to improve and manage m-QoS by prioritizing Telemedicine service by using decisive and intelligent tool called Analytic Hierarchy Process (AHP). This service will be provided on urgency basis from the pool of medical services with the help of AHP. In this connection, four telemedicine services are considered i.e. Tele-surgery, Tele-Consultation, Tele-Education and Tele-Monitoring. In this research, three m-QoS parameters are considered i.e. throughput, jitter and delay. These services are evaluated by potential doctors and patients. We propose an AHP based decision making algorithm for selecting urgent and important service for the fast and cost-effective treatment of the emergency patients at the remote location in the hospital, because AHP is the significantly fast decision making technique used to assess, select and manage the emergency services at various priority levels in large scale and distributed medical health systems.

A.H. Sodhro (✉) · M.M. Lodro · M.A. Shah
Sukkur Institute of Business Administration, Sukkur, Sindh, Pakistan
e-mail: ali.hassan@iba-suk.edu.pk

M.M. Lodro
e-mail: mir.lodro@iba-suk.edu.pk

M.A. Shah
e-mail: madad@iba-suk.edu.pk

F.K. Shaikh
Mehran University of Engineering and Technology, Jamshoro, Sindh, Pakistan
e-mail: faisal.shaikh@faculty.muet.edu.pk

S. Pirbhulal
Shenzhen Institutes of Advanced Technology, Chinese Academy of Sciences, Shenzhen, China
e-mail: sandeep@siat.ac.cn

© Springer International Publishing AG 2017

S.U. Khan et al. (eds.), *Handbook of Large-Scale Distributed Computing in Smart Healthcare*, Scalable Computing and Communications,
DOI 10.1007/978-3-319-58280-1_21

The comprehensive purpose is indicated in the first level of the strategy. The decisive entities are presented in the intermediate level and the target-based alternatives are located at the lowest level. MATLAB is used for experimental results to measure and evaluate goal, decision making parameters and options from both qualitative and quantitative aspect. The proposed AHP algorithm is simulated for three decision parameters and four different Telemedicine services in which highest priority is given to decision parameter, throughput and Telemedicine service, Tele-Surgery for large scale and distributed medical health systems.

Keywords Medical-QoS · Telemedicine · Analytic hierarchy process

Main Goals of this Chapter

The main goal of this chapter is to manage medical Quality of Service (m-QoS) by selecting Telemedicine service from the pool of medical services on the priority and urgency basis for emergency patients at remote location in the hospital on the basis of three decision parameters such as, throughput, delay and jitter with the help of decision making mathematical tool known as AHP. Moreover, we construct a hierarchy of Telemedicine service selection problem by dividing that into three levels. In Level1 there is an objective, Level2 shows decision parameters or criteria and Level3 contains Telemedicine services or alternatives. An AHP pair-wise comparison matrix is constructed then weights and composite weights of Level2 and Level3 elements are calculated. However, the quality and quantity of multiple entities such as, objective, decision parameters and alternatives is determined and measured with the help of AHP. The algorithm is simulated for three decision parameters and four different Telemedicine services in which highest priority is given to decision parameter Throughput and Telemedicine service Tele-Surgery respectively. In near future, we intend to optimize the m-QoS.

Contribution of this Chapter

The main contribution of this chapter is that we propose an AHP based algorithm in order to manage m-QoS based on Telemedicine service selection, evaluation, and assessment on the priority and urgency basis by randomly selecting three decision parameters such as, throughput, delay and jitter, to provide cost-effective and quality life to emergency patients at remote location in the hospital.

1 Introduction

Conventional healthcare services have seamlessly been integrated with pervasive computing paradigm and consequently cost-effective and dependable smart healthcare services and systems have emerged. Currently, the smart healthcare systems use joint Telemedicine and Wireless Body Sensor Networks (WBSNs) and wearable devices for ubiquitous health monitoring and Ambient Assisted Living. For better Telemedicine service selection and m-QoS measurement a large scale and emerging breakthrough in wearable devices, large scale and distributed mobile cloud computing technologies plays an important role. The Telemedicine system uses smart-phones and several handheld devices to ensure ubiquitous access to the healthcare information and services. However, due to the intrinsic architectural limitations in terms of CPU speed, storage, and memory, the mobile and other computing devices seem inadequate to handle huge volumes of medical data being generated unceasingly. In addition, the sensor data is highly complex and multi-dimensional. Therefore, integrating the Telemedicine with large-scale and distributed computing paradigms, such as the cloud, cluster, and grid computing is inevitable to handle the processing and storage needs to select Telemedicine services and measuring m-QoS.

Moreover, the contemporary research efforts mostly focus on health information delivery methods to ensure the information exchange within a Telemedicine service selection. Consequently, the efforts have been very limited in interconnecting several Telemedicine services remotely through the servers. This chapter aims to concentrate the myriad research efforts appropriate to the large-scale distributed computing, smart healthcare systems, Telemedicine service selection and m-QoS measurement for healthcare.

Medical-Quality of Service (m-QoS) is relatively different from conventional wireless QoS in terms of desired needs of the medical healthcare society. The main quality evaluation ingredients for Telemedicine are the throughput, delay, and, packet loss ratio, etc. In addition Telemedicine is integrated with multiple emerging and state-of-the art technologies to facilitate users at cost-effective level. Telemedicine applications are categorized in large scale such as; surgery, consultation, education and training and homecare etc. So, in order to choose and decide about best one requires intelligent and effective decision making tool. In this regard AHP is considered as a prominent and decisive technique to establish trade-off between cost and benefits of the medical service. One of the pioneers and founders of AHP proposal is T.L. Saaty. It is observed that AHP gives an impressive results and structured approach to obtain individual weights of various attributes of a service so that they can be compared in an easy and simple way then simplify decision making in the selection process.

Moreover, AHP is a mathematical method and decision making tool that dissolves and synthesis a complex problem into a simple and understandable one with unique and best decision strategy. In addition, the decision parameters and performance indicators with inter-relationship between them at different levels to present big picture of AHP is shown in Fig. 1. The relative values of service factors and sub-factors with respect to their parents are approximated with the help of matched comparison results according to the perception, knowledge and experience of users. The compared results within each parent are shown in a matrix, and then changed into a ratio scale by calculating the eigenvector of the matrix. The AHP intelligently decides on the basis of ranking and ratio scale of elements and to be integrated with other different methods e.g., linear programming, artificial intelligence and quality function deployment etc. This enables physicians and patients to get facility from all the integrated techniques and thus to be aware about the targeted outcome on time. There has not been much work done on m-QoS management with the help of AHP by considering and prioritizing Telemedicine services on the basis of urgency and emergency.

Many previous researches show that, large scale and distributed computing plays an important role in massive medical data monitoring and management but do not discuss the relationship of Telemedicine service selection, m-QoS and large scale and distributed computing, that combination presents vital role in medical health and provides many benefits to the patients and physicians as compared to traditional medical care.

Althebyan et al. [1], develop the clod based medical health platform for large scale and distributed telemedicine system. Trobec et al. [2], propose energy-efficient algorithm for the large scale and distributed computing system to monitor the patient's health. Chung et al. [3], present large scale and distributed computing scenario for the telemedicine system. Krivitski et al. [4], develop an algorithm for dealing with large scale and distributed system for medical health monitoring. Von Wangenheim et al. [5], design the medical image based large scale telemedicine networks for medical health monitoring. Kovendhan et al. [6], propose a distributed file transfer system for the large scale Telemedicine system.

Fouad [7], propose a joint framework of WBSN and Telemedicine system for health monitoring from physician and patient-centric point of view. Kailasam et al. [8], present a typical telemedicine system for providing cost-effective and easy healthcare services in rural areas of developing countries with clear and big picture. However, in developing nations like Pakistan where majority live in remote areas, and it is hard to provide easy access and medical to emergency patients. In this regard, large-scale and web-based telemedicine set-up is considered as viable option to effectively entertain many users (i.e. patients and doctors) and whole population from available health centers and medical operation theaters. Hsieh et al. [9],

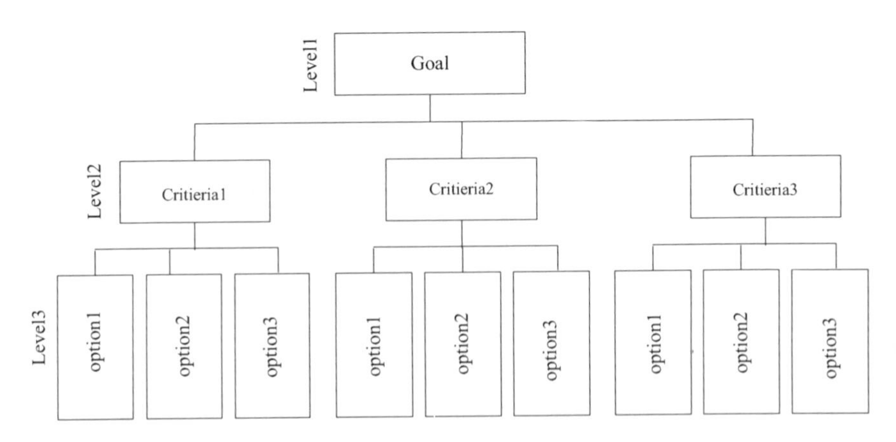

Fig. 1 Structural representation of Analytic Hierarchy Process

develop a 12 lead ECG based medical health monitoring system which improve m-QoS and efficiency, especially for patients in rural areas. Topacan et al. [10], present AHP in health service. Sharna et al. [11] and Tawil et al. [12] examine performance of vertical handoff algorithms by differentiating QoS parameters using AHP. Yeh et al. [13] discuss device selection for Telemedicine system. Alharthi et al. [14] present AHP based method to rank different factors for pharmacy system. Ajami et al. [15] design AHP-based approach for evaluating records of medical departments. Sri Kavya [16], present how to select suitable wireless technology for rural areas. Schiltz [17] analyse the e-health system from the business perspective using AHP. Gao [18] discuss the AHP-based web service selection method. Mirchandani [19] present the energy management technique for LTE system using AHP. Al-Qurishi [20] present cloud based eHealth framework using AHP. Gülçin [21] design fuzzy-AHP based strategy for analyzing healthcare service. Pecchia [22] examine the physician's assessment in healthcare using AHP. Oltés [23] compare the functionality of healthcare systems based on AHP. Fengou [24], present AHP-based approach for group profile creation in ubiquitous healthcare.

Saaty [25] develop AHP based decision making technique for leaders. Fortino et al. [26], propose framework for medical health applications, body sensor networks for focusing on the main health problems. Ghasemzadeh et al. [27], develop human activity monitoring using wearable devices for large scale health monitoring system. Fortino et al. [28], discuss the blood pressure measurement techniques for the healthcare monitoring system. Grayina et al. [29, 30], develop sensor fusion mechanism and cardiac system for large scale BSNs. Galzarno et al. [31], present a large scale wearable computing networks for medical applications, but they did not consider the analytic hierarchy mechanism for Telemedicine services. Smart et al. [32], design central channel shifting strategy for ad hoc networks. Fortino et al. [33, 34], discuss the IoT and programming based management systems for the healthcare applications, but AHP is not considered in their approach.

None of the existing works have focused on m-QoS management based on Telemedicine service selection. Also no one discussed about the selection of critical Telemedicine service from the pool of medical services on urgency and priority basis with the help of AHP. To the best of knowledge our work is the first step to achieve this goal.

The main contribution of this research is that we manage m-QoS based on Telemedicine service selection, evaluation, and assessment on the priority and urgency basis by randomly selecting three decision parameters to provide cost-effective and quality life to patients.

The rest of the chapter is organized as follows; Sect. 2 discusses AHP in detail, Sect. 3 describes AHP algorithm, Sect. 4 develops Telemedicine service selection procedure. Section 5 presents results and chapter is concluded in Sect. 6.

AHP strategically lay-outs a problem into various distinct levels. In addition, it is a structural procedure of modeling the decision at hand and consists of overall target or goal, several options for reducing the objective, and a decision making parameters that relate the alternatives to the goal as shown in the Fig. 1.

2 Analytic Hierarchy Process

A decision making tool named AHP is considered as a viable approach for several areas such as, medical health, education, and industry etc. The ultimate aim is in the top-most priority level, whereas, decision making entities are placed in the middle-level and options are kept in the last/final level.

An AHP has particular applications in decision making and is used in various fields such as government, business, industry, healthcare and education etc. The overall objective is the first level of the hierarchy. The decision parameters are presented in the intermediate level and the alternatives are located at the lowest level. For instance, a group of physicians and patients choose desired service among the given pool of Telemedicine services. The performance indicators are throughput, delay and jitter. The Fig. 2 presents the step-by-step service selection procedure. In second step the main goals are compared with each other to determine relative importance according to Table 1. The numbers 1, 3, 5, 7 and 9 are used to show equal, moderate, strong, very strong and extreme levels respectively. While 2, 4, 6 and 8 shows the compromise between above values. The smaller one in a pair is selected as a unit and larger one is estimated as a multiple of that unit. Similarly, the complenteries of these numbers represent the inverted comparison results. In the last step, the composite weights of the all decision parameters are obtained by computing the values of AHP matrix. For instance, we fixed throughput to 1 and vary delay from 1 to 9. i.e. 1_1 shows that throughput and delay are equally important to the target and 1_2 shows that throughput have two times more priority

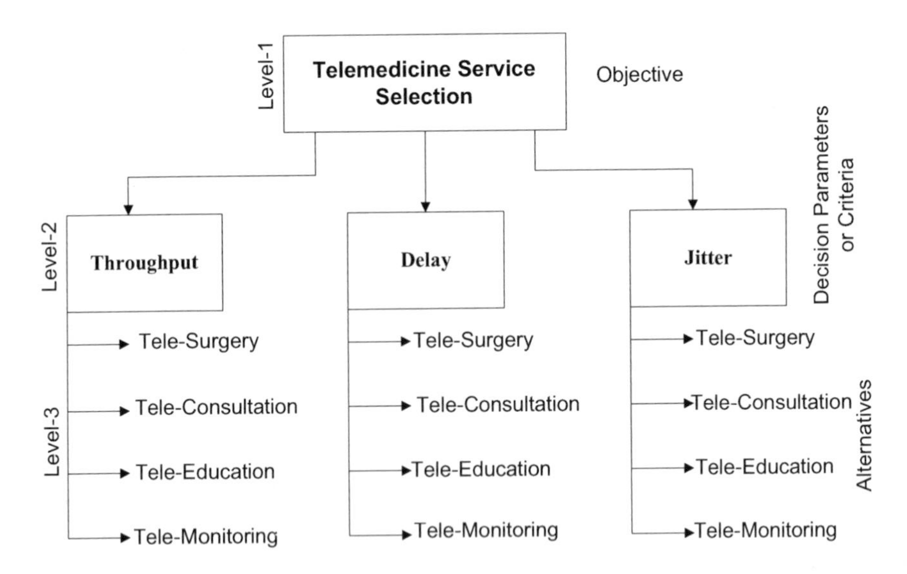

Fig. 2 Proposed AHP hierarchy for Telemedicine service selection

Table 1 Saaty's scale for matched Similarity [25]

Comparison	Value of a_{ij}
A and B have same importance	1
A has relatively less valuable than B	3
A has more significance compared B	5
A is very strongly significant in comparison to B	7
A is precisely essential than B	9
To establish agreement between above values	2, 4, 6, 8
complementary	1/3, 1/5, 1/7, 1/9

than delay. Hence, 1_1–1_9 scale show different weight levels for decision making entities and available services as given in Table 1.

Suppose, that n components to be compared, from these $a1, \ldots, an$ denote relative significance of ai with respect to aj by aij and form a square matrix $M = (aij)$ of order n with the constraints that $aij = 1/aji$, for $i \neq j$, and $aii = 1$, such a matrix is said to be complementary one. The weights are persistent if they are transitive, that is $aik = aij \times ajk$ for all i, j and k. Such a matrix might exist if the aij is calculated exactly from measured data. Then find a vector V of order n like as, $MV = \lambda \times V$. For aforesaid matrix, V is considered to be an eigenvector and λ is an eigenvalue.

For a regular matrix, $\lambda = n$. In addition for matrices involving human analysis, the condition $aik = aij \times ajk$ does not hold because of inconsistency in human judgment to a greater or lesser extent. In such a case the V vector satisfies the equation $MV = \lambda_{\max} \times V \geq n$. Any difference between $\lambda_{\max}$ and n, is an indication of the discrepancy in people's perception. If $\lambda_{\max} = n$ then the prudence have turned out to be steady. Finally, a consistency index (CI) can be computed from $(\lambda_{\max} - n)/(n-1)$ that needs to be assessed against experience made completely at random. Furthermore, Saaty has determined large samples at random matrices of increasing order and consistency indices of those matrices. A true consistency ratio (CR) is calculated by dividing CI for the set of perceptions by the index for the corresponding random matrix. Saaty [25] suggests that if that ratio exceeds 0.1 the set of judgments may be too deviated to be reliable. In practice, CR of more than 0.1 sometimes has to be accepted. A CR of zero 0 means that the judgments are perfectly uniform.

3 Analytic Hierarchy Process Algorithm

The AHP algorithm in Fig. 3 is used to resolve very challenging and complex issue of selecting best Telemedicine service among the presented options based on a set of distinct decision parameters. For further information interested readers can see [25].

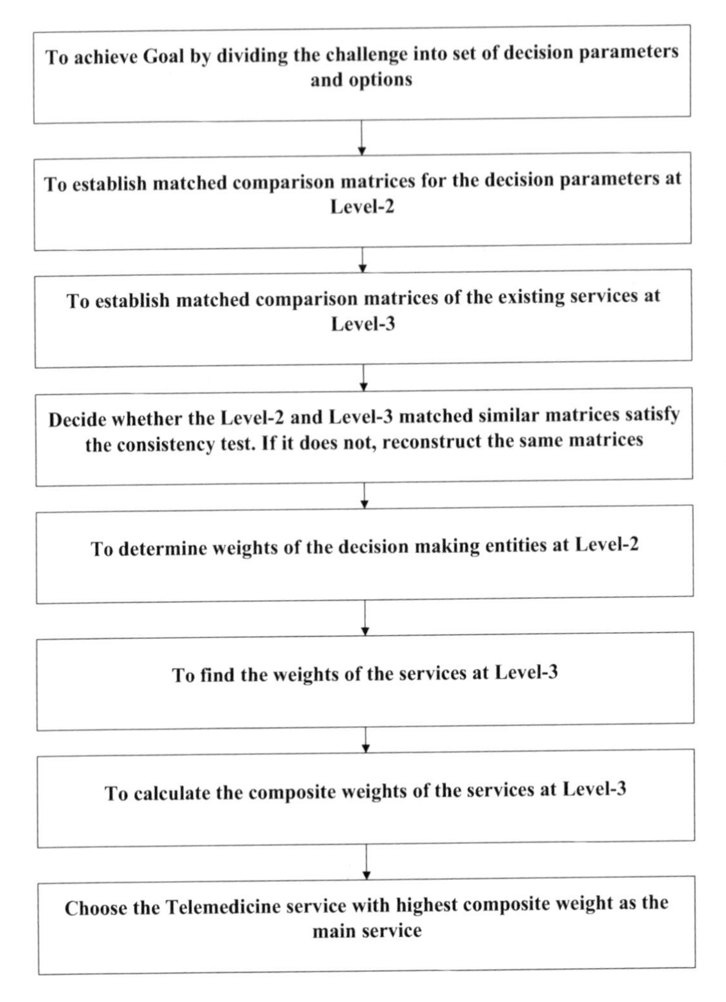

Fig. 3 Flowchart of the AHP Algorithm [25]

4 Analytic Hierarchy Process for Telemedicine Service Selection

In this section a Telemedicine service is chosen step-by-step from the pool of basic medical services of large scale and distributed healthcare system with the help of AHP.

4.1 Decision Making Hierarchy

Main goal of this sub-section is to manage the m-QoS by selecting critical Telemedicine service on priority and urgency basis. This establishes a strategic procedure at Level-1 as shown in Fig. 2. The performance metrics e.g., throughput, delay and Jitter are treated as the decision making components, while Telemedicine services are considered as the set of options, placed at Level-2 and Level-3 of the hierarchy, respectively.

4.2 Formation of Similarity Matrix

The decisive entities are arranged into rows and columns format. Decision making components are compared and evaluated based on the range of values from 1 to 9 as shown in Table 1. Suppose, the diagonal elements in the range from top-left to bottom-right are supposed to be 1. Initially, the upper triangular matrix is filled according to the priority level of row parameter A and correlation level of column parameter (B) with the help of Table 1. Equation (1) builds and fills upper triangular matrix, which finally gives lower triangular matrix.

$$aji = \frac{1}{aij} \tag{1}$$

aji, is the pair-wise similarity matrix in the *ith* row and *jth* column. Building the matched comparison and matched similarity matrices of the decision options at Level-2 and Level-3 respectively. Therefore, 3×3 matrices at Level-2 and 4×4 matrices at Level-3 are possible. A square AHP matrix with similar outcome of two choices is used to carry these results under one parent.

$$\begin{matrix} \\ Throughput \\ Delay \\ Jitter \end{matrix} \begin{bmatrix} Throughput & Delay & Jitter \\ 1 & 2/1 & 3/1 \\ 1/2 & 1 & 2/1 \\ 1/3 & 1/2 & 1 \end{bmatrix}$$

4.3 Calculation of Eigenvector and Consistency

An AHP matrix *M*, has the complementary formula as, $MV = \lambda \times V$, whereas, *V* and λ are the non-zero eigenvector, and scalar eigenvalue respectively. As each element in *M* is the ratio of the weight of one decisive indicator to another according to their parents. When M is persistency matrix, i.e. $mij = mik \times mkj$ $(i, j, k = 1, 2, \ldots, n)$, then $n \times n$ matrix M is represented as

$$M = \begin{bmatrix} m_{11} & m_{12} \ldots & m_{1n} \\ \vdots & \vdots & \vdots \\ m_{n1} & m_{n2} \ldots & m_{nn} \end{bmatrix} = \begin{bmatrix} w_1/w_1 & w_1/w_2 \ldots & w_1/w_n \\ \vdots & \vdots & \vdots \\ w_n/w_1 & w_n/w_2 \ldots & w_n/w_n \end{bmatrix}$$

whereas, n is the number of decision parameters and $wi(i = 1, 2, \ldots, n)$ shows the weight of the decision making entities. If all wi are arranged into a weight matrix i.e. $(W)^T = [w_1 \quad w_2 \quad \ldots \quad w_n]$, then $MW = n \times W$. Thus, the weight vector and number of elements of M become its eigenvector and eigenvalue respectively. However, the AHP matrices are usually not exactly regular due to user's random perception. As a result, the eigenvector with the maximum eigenvalue $\lambda_{\max}$ is chosen as the weight matrix. The total value of each column of the pair-wise similarity matrix is computed and kept in the final row. The last obtained matrix is averaged by making the elements of the entire row as 1 and this matrix is known as normalized comparison matrix. Normalized predominant eigenvector is acquired by finding average value of each row of the normalized comparison matrix. Now $\lambda_{\max}$ can be achieved by using Eq. (2).

$$\lambda_{\max} = \sum_{i=1}^{n} a_i \times b_i \tag{2}$$

whereas, a_i and b_i represents the elements in the *ith* row of the normalized desired eigenvector and sum row in the *ith* column of the similarity matrix before normalization, accordingly.

The persistency of an AHP matrix can be analyzed by consistency ratio (CR), which is defined as the ratio of consistency index (CI) to random index (RI) based on the size of n, as shown in Table 2. CI is computed by using Eq. (3)

$$CI = \frac{\lambda_{\max} - n}{n - 1} \tag{3}$$

where, n depicts the size of the similarity matrix.

The consistency ratio (CR) is acquired by using Eq. (4)

$$CR = \frac{CI}{RI} \tag{4}$$

When CR < 0.1 then matched comparison matrix is uniform and adaptable.

Table 2 Consistency Index [25]

n	1	2	3	4	5	6	7	8	9	10	11
RI	0	0	0.58	0.9	1.12	1.24	1.32	1.41	1.45	1.49	1.51

4.4 Determining Weight of Decision Parameters

The Eq. (5) determines the weight of each decision making entity.

$$WDP = \frac{NEV_n}{309.9385} \tag{5}$$

WDP is the weight of decision parameters and $NEV_n (n = 1, 2, 3)$ is the normalized eigenvector at Level-2.

4.5 Determining Weight of Telemedicine Services

An Eq. (6) determines the weight of available Telemedicine services at Level-3 with respect to decision making parameters.

$$WasrvDP = \frac{NEVDP}{SNEVDP} \tag{6}$$

whereas, *WaservDP*, *NEVDP* and *SNEVDP* are the weight of existing service, normalized eigenvector and the Sum of normalized eigenvector according to decision parameters, respectively.

4.6 Composite Weights of Available Telemedicine Services

The composite weights in Level-3 can be found with the help of Eq. (7)

$$CWaserv = \sum_{p=1}^{n} WDP \times WasrvDP \tag{7}$$

CWaserv is the composite weight of pre-defined services with number of decision making components *n*.

5 Experimental Performance and Discussion

An Intelligent Decision Analysis (IDA) technique is used to elect the random data for establishing pair-wise comparison matrices to prioritize critical Telemedicine service.

First we will find decision making parameters or criteria in Level-2.

Step-1: Determining the pair-wise comparison Matrix

$$M = \begin{matrix} \\ Throughput \\ Delay \\ Jitter \end{matrix} \begin{bmatrix} Throughput & Delay & Jitter \\ 1 & 2/1 & 3/1 \\ 1/2 & 1 & 2/1 \\ 1/3 & 1/2 & 1 \end{bmatrix}$$

Or Matrix M can be written as

$$M = \begin{bmatrix} 1.0 & 2.0 & 3.0 \\ 0.5 & 1.0 & 2.0 \\ 0.3333 & 0.5 & 1.0 \end{bmatrix}$$

Step-2: squaring the Matrix M

$$\begin{bmatrix} 1.0 & 2.0 & 3.0 \\ 0.5 & 1.0 & 2.0 \\ 0.3333 & 0.5 & 1.0 \end{bmatrix} \begin{bmatrix} 1.0 & 2.0 & 3.0 \\ 0.5 & 1.0 & 2.0 \\ 0.3333 & 0.5 & 1.0 \end{bmatrix} = \begin{bmatrix} 3.0 & 5.5 & 10 \\ 1.6666 & 3.0 & 5.5 \\ 0.9166 & 1.6666 & 3.0 \end{bmatrix}$$

Step-3: To calculate the eigenvector by sum of rows (SoR) of Matrix (to first four decimal places)

$$M = \begin{bmatrix} 3.0 + & 5.5 + & 10 \\ 1.6666 + & 3.0 + & 5.5 \\ 0.9166 + & 1.6666 + & 3.0 \end{bmatrix}$$

$$M = \frac{SoR \begin{bmatrix} 18.5 \\ 10.1666 \\ 5.5832 \end{bmatrix}}{SoR\_total\; 34.2498}$$

$$\begin{bmatrix} 18.5/34.2498 \\ 10.1666/34.2498 \\ 5.5832/34.2498 \end{bmatrix} = \begin{bmatrix} 0.5401 \\ 0.2968 \\ 0.1630 \end{bmatrix} \rightarrow \text{Eigenvector} = \text{E0}$$

$$\frac{\begin{bmatrix} 0.5401 \\ 0.2968 \\ 0.1630 \end{bmatrix}}{1.0}$$

Again step-1: Establishing pair-wise square Matrix

$$M = \begin{bmatrix} 3.0 & 5.5 & 10 \\ 1.6666 & 3.0 & 5.5 \\ 0.9166 & 1.6666 & 3.0 \end{bmatrix}$$

Again step-2: Squaring the Matrix

$$M = \begin{bmatrix} 3.0 & 5.5 & 10 \\ 1.6666 & 3.0 & 5.5 \\ 0.9166 & 1.6666 & 3.0 \end{bmatrix} \begin{bmatrix} 3.0 & 5.5 & 10 \\ 1.6666 & 3.0 & 5.5 \\ 0.9166 & 1.6666 & 3.0 \end{bmatrix} = \begin{bmatrix} 27.3326 & 49.666 & 90.25 \\ 15.0409 & 27.3326 & 49.666 \\ 8.2772 & 15.0409 & 27.3323 \end{bmatrix}$$

Again step-3: Compute the eigenvector

$$\begin{bmatrix} 27.3326+ & 49.666+ & 90.25 \\ 15.0409+ & 27.3326+ & 49.666 \\ 8.2772+ & 15.0409+ & 27.3323 \end{bmatrix} = \begin{bmatrix} 167.2486 \\ 92.0395 \\ 50.6504 \end{bmatrix} = \begin{bmatrix} 0.5396 \\ 0.2969 \\ 0.1634 \end{bmatrix} \rightarrow \text{Eigenvector} = \text{E1}$$

$$\frac{\begin{bmatrix} 0.5396 \\ 0.2969 \\ 0.1634 \end{bmatrix}}{1.0}$$

Now we will compute difference (D) of eigenvectors E1 and E0.

$$D = E1 - E0 = \begin{bmatrix} 0.5396 \\ 0.2969 \\ 0.1634 \end{bmatrix} - \begin{bmatrix} 0.5401 \\ 0.2968 \\ 0.1630 \end{bmatrix} = \begin{bmatrix} -0.0005 \\ 0.0001 \\ 0.0004 \end{bmatrix} \rightarrow \text{Almost zero}$$

So, E1 or V eigenvector is suitable for calculating maximum eigenvalue ($\lambda_{\max}$), CI, RI and CR for decision parameters at Level-2.

Step-4: Measure Consistency Index (CI)

CI is calculated by using formula $MV = \lambda_{\max} \times V$, M is an AHP matrix, V is the eigenvector and $\lambda_{\max}$ is the maximum eigenvalue.

$$\begin{bmatrix} 1.0 & 2.0 & 3.0 \\ 0.5 & 1.0 & 2.0 \\ 0.3333 & 0.5 & 1.0 \end{bmatrix} \begin{bmatrix} 0.5396 \\ 0.2969 \\ 0.1634 \end{bmatrix} = \lambda\text{max} \begin{bmatrix} 0.5396 \\ 0.2969 \\ 0.1634 \end{bmatrix}$$

$$\begin{bmatrix} 0.5396+ & 0.5938+ & 0.4902 \\ 0.2698+ & 0.2969+ & 0.3268 \\ 0.1798+ & 0.1484+ & 0.1634 \end{bmatrix} = \lambda\text{max} \begin{bmatrix} 0.5396 \\ 0.2969 \\ 0.1634 \end{bmatrix}$$

$$\begin{bmatrix} 1.6236 \\ 0.8935 \\ 0.4916 \end{bmatrix} = \lambda\text{max} \begin{bmatrix} 0.5396 \\ 0.2969 \\ 0.1634 \end{bmatrix}, \quad \lambda\text{max} = \begin{bmatrix} 1.6236/0.5396 \\ 0.8935/0.2969 \\ 0.4916/0.1634 \end{bmatrix} = \begin{bmatrix} 3.0088 \\ 3.0094 \\ 3.0085 \end{bmatrix}$$

Therefore, Average value of these maximum eigenvalues at $n = 3$ is.

$$\lambda_{\max} = \frac{3.0088 + \quad 3.0094 + \quad 3.0085}{3} = \frac{9.0262}{3} = 3.0087$$

Now, from Eq. (3) we have

$$CI = \frac{\lambda_{\max} - n}{n - 1} = \frac{3.0087 - 3}{3 - 1} = \frac{0.0087}{2} = 0.0043 < 0.1$$

As CI value 0.0043 is <0.1 so pair-wise comparison matrices are consistent and adjusted.

Now from Eq. (4) and Table 2 (RI = 0.58 at $n = 3$), we calculate consistency ratio (CR)

$$CR = \frac{CI}{RI} = \frac{0.0043}{0.58} = 0.007413$$

As value of CR is also <0.1, so the evaluations are consistent.

Throughput = 0.5396 → first most important for m-QoS
Delay = 0.2969 → second most important for m-QoS
Jitter = 0.1634 → less important for m-QoS.

For further details see Fig. 4.

Now, for Telemedicine service selection at Level-3 as in Fig. 1.

Step-1: To build pair-wise comparison Matrix to obtain Throughput

$$M = \begin{matrix} \\ TeleSurgery \\ TeleConsultation \\ TeleEducation \\ TeleMonitoring \end{matrix} \begin{bmatrix} TeleSurgery & TeleConsultation & TeleEducation & TeleMonitoring \\ 1 & 2/1 & 3/1 & 4/1 \\ 1/2 & 1 & 2/1 & 3/1 \\ 1/3 & 1/2 & 1 & 2/1 \\ 1/4 & 1/3 & 1/2 & 1 \end{bmatrix}$$

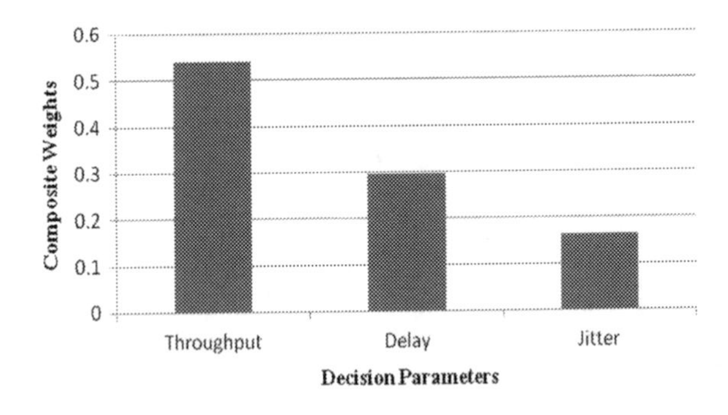

Fig. 4 Decision parameters and composite weights

Matrix M also can be written as shown below

$$M = \begin{bmatrix} 1.0 & 2.0 & 3.0 & 4.0 \\ 0.5 & 1.0 & 2.0 & 3.0 \\ 0.3333 & 0.5 & 1.0 & 2.0 \\ 0.25 & 0.3333 & 0.5 & 1.0 \end{bmatrix}$$

Step-2: Squaring the Matrix M (to four decimal places)

$$M = \begin{bmatrix} 1.0 & 2.0 & 3.0 & 4.0 \\ 0.5 & 1.0 & 2.0 & 3.0 \\ 0.3333 & 0.5 & 1.0 & 2.0 \\ 0.25 & 0.3333 & 0.5 & 1.0 \end{bmatrix} \begin{bmatrix} 1.0 & 2.0 & 3.0 & 4.0 \\ 0.5 & 1.0 & 2.0 & 3.0 \\ 0.3333 & 0.5 & 1.0 & 2.0 \\ 0.25 & 0.3333 & 0.5 & 1.0 \end{bmatrix}$$

$$= \begin{bmatrix} 4 & 6.8332 & 12 & 20 \\ 2.4166 & 4 & 7 & 12 \\ 1.4166 & 2.3332 & 4 & 6.8332 \\ 0.8332 & 1.4166 & 2.4166 & 4 \end{bmatrix}$$

$$\text{i.e. } (1.0 \times 1.0) + (2 \times 0.5) + (3 \times 0.3333) + (4 \times 0.25) = 4.0$$

Step-3: To find eigenvector by summing rows

$$\begin{bmatrix} 4+ & 6.8332+ & 12+ & 20 \\ 2.4166+ & 4+ & 7+ & 12 \\ 1.4166+ & 2.3332+ & 4+ & 6 \\ 0.8332+ & 1.4166+ & 2.4166+ & 4 \end{bmatrix}$$

$$\frac{SoR \begin{bmatrix} 42.8332 \\ 25.4166 \\ 14.5830 \\ 8.6664 \end{bmatrix}}{SoR\_total \; 91.4992}$$

$$\begin{bmatrix} 42.8332/91.4992 \\ 25.4166/91.4992 \\ 14.5830/91.4992 \\ 8.6664/91.4992 \end{bmatrix} = \begin{bmatrix} 0.4681 \\ 0.2777 \\ 0.1593 \\ 0.0947 \end{bmatrix} \rightarrow \text{Eigenvector} = \text{E1}$$

$$\frac{\begin{bmatrix} 0.4681 \\ 0.2777 \\ 0.1593 \\ 0.0947 \end{bmatrix}}{1.0}$$

Step-4: Construct and squaring pair-wise comparison Matrix for Delay

$$M = \begin{bmatrix} 1.0 & 2.0 & 2.0 & 3.0 \\ 2.0 & 1.0 & 2.0 & 2.0 \\ 0.5 & 0.5 & 1.0 & 2.0 \\ 0.3333 & 0.3333 & 0.5 & 1.0 \end{bmatrix}$$

$$M = \begin{bmatrix} 1.0 & 2.0 & 2.0 & 3.0 \\ 2.0 & 1.0 & 2.0 & 2.0 \\ 0.5 & 0.5 & 1.0 & 2.0 \\ 0.3333 & 0.3333 & 0.5 & 1.0 \end{bmatrix} \begin{bmatrix} 1.0 & 2.0 & 2.0 & 3.0 \\ 2.0 & 1.0 & 2.0 & 2.0 \\ 0.5 & 0.5 & 1.0 & 2.0 \\ 0.3333 & 0.3333 & 0.5 & 1.0 \end{bmatrix}$$

$$= \begin{bmatrix} 7 & 6 & 9.5 & 14 \\ 5.6666 & 6.6666 & 9.0 & 14 \\ 2.6666 & 2.6666 & 4 & 6.5 \\ 1.5832 & 1.5832 & 2.3332 & 3.6665 \end{bmatrix}$$

Step-5: Find the eigenvector of the services by summing rows

$$\begin{bmatrix} 7+ & 6+ & 9.5+ & 14 \\ 5.6666+ & 6.6666+ & 9.0+ & 14 \\ 2.6666+ & 2.6666+ & 4+ & 6.5 \\ 1.5832+ & 1.5832+ & 2.3332+ & 3.6665 \end{bmatrix}$$

$$\frac{SoR \begin{bmatrix} 36.5 \\ 35.3332 \\ 15.8332 \\ 9.1661 \end{bmatrix}}{SoR\_total\, 96.8325}$$

$$\begin{bmatrix} 36.5/96.8325 \\ 35.3332/96.8325 \\ 15.8332/96.8325 \\ 9.1661/96.8325 \end{bmatrix} = \begin{bmatrix} 0.3769 \\ 0.3648 \\ 0.1635 \\ 0.0946 \end{bmatrix} \rightarrow \text{Eigenvector} = \text{E2}$$

$$\frac{\begin{bmatrix} 0.3769 \\ 0.3648 \\ 0.1635 \\ 0.0946 \end{bmatrix}}{1.0}$$

Step-6: Construct and squaring pair-wise comparison Matrix for Jitter

$$M = \begin{bmatrix} 1.0 & 2.0 & 3.0 & 4.0 \\ 0.5 & 1.0 & 2.0 & 4.0 \\ 0.5 & 0.5 & 1.0 & 2.0 \\ 0.25 & 0.5 & 0.5 & 1.0 \end{bmatrix}$$

$$M = \begin{bmatrix} 1.0 & 2.0 & 3.0 & 4.0 \\ 0.5 & 1.0 & 2.0 & 4.0 \\ 0.5 & 0.5 & 1.0 & 2.0 \\ 0.25 & 0.5 & 0.5 & 1.0 \end{bmatrix} \begin{bmatrix} 1.0 & 2.0 & 3.0 & 4.0 \\ 0.5 & 1.0 & 2.0 & 4.0 \\ 0.5 & 0.5 & 1.0 & 2.0 \\ 0.25 & 0.5 & 0.5 & 1.0 \end{bmatrix} = \begin{bmatrix} 4.5 & 7.5 & 12 & 22 \\ 4 & 5 & 7.5 & 14 \\ 1.75 & 3.0 & 4.5 & 8.0 \\ 10 & 1.75 & 1.75 & 5.0 \end{bmatrix}$$

Step-7: Find the eigenvectors we will sum the rows

$$M = \begin{bmatrix} 4.5+ & 7.5+ & 12+ & 22 \\ 4+ & 5+ & 7.5+ & 14 \\ 1.75+ & 3.0+ & 4.5+ & 8.0 \\ 1.0+ & 1.75+ & 1.75+ & 5.0 \end{bmatrix}$$

$$\frac{SoR \begin{bmatrix} 46.0 \\ 30.5 \\ 17.25 \\ 9.5 \end{bmatrix}}{SoR\_Total\ 103.25}$$

$$\begin{bmatrix} 46.0/103.25 \\ 30.5/103.25 \\ 17.25/103.25 \\ 9.5/103.25 \end{bmatrix} = \begin{bmatrix} 0.4455 \\ 0.2953 \\ 0.1670 \\ 0.0920 \end{bmatrix} \rightarrow \text{Eigenvector} = \text{E3}$$

$$\frac{\begin{bmatrix} 0.4455 \\ 0.2953 \\ 0.1670 \\ 0.0920 \end{bmatrix}}{1.0}$$

Step-8: Find the composite eigenvector; we multiple the eigenvectors (E1, E2, E3) of the four services with the E1 of decisive factors and then sum them.

$$M = \begin{bmatrix} 0.4681 & 0.3769 & 0.4455 \\ 0.2777 & 0.3648 & 0.2953 \\ 0.1593 & 0.1635 & 0.1670 \\ 0.0947 & 0.0946 & 0.0920 \end{bmatrix}$$

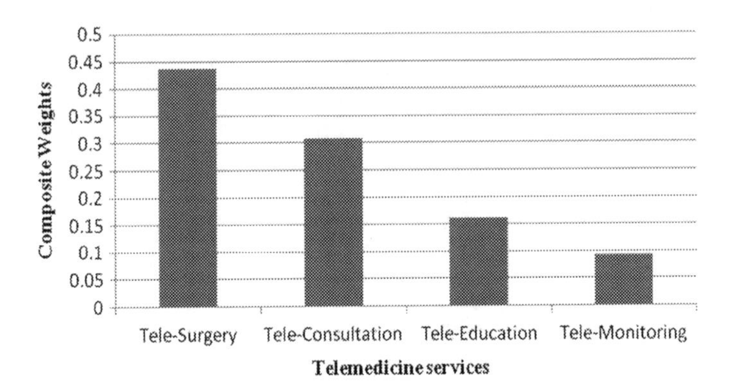

Fig. 5 Telemedicine services and composite weights

$$\begin{bmatrix} 0.2525+ & 0.1119+ & 0.07279 \\ 0.1498+ & 0.1083 & 0.0482 \\ 0.0859 & 0.0485 & 0.0272 \\ 0.0511 & 0.0280 & 0.0150 \end{bmatrix} = \begin{bmatrix} 0.4371 \\ 0.3063 \\ 0.1616 \\ 0.0941 \end{bmatrix}$$

Tele-Surgery = 0.4371 $\rightarrow$ first highest priority
Tele-Consultation = 0.3063 $\rightarrow$ second highest priority
Tele-Education = 0.1616 $\rightarrow$ third priority
Tele-Monitoring = 0.0941 $\rightarrow$ fourth priority
For further details see Fig. 5.

An AHP is analyzed for Level-2 with three decision making entities and Level-3 with four Telemedicine services. All of the above performance indicators for maintaining persistency proven to be consistent. Since, weights and average weights of the each decisive parameter and available services are determined.

In Level-2 and Level-3, the throughput and Tele-Surgery as decision making entities with maximum values of 0.5396 and 0.3063 respectively, are considered to be desired decisive factors for m-QoS management. Graphical representation of the composite weights of aforementioned levels and AHP strategy is shown in Figs. 4, 5 and 6, respectively.

6 Conclusions and Future Research

Large scale and distributed computing healthcare systems aim at extending the monitoring coverage from individuals who live at remote location. This chapter proposes a large scale and distributed systems for Telemedicine service selection

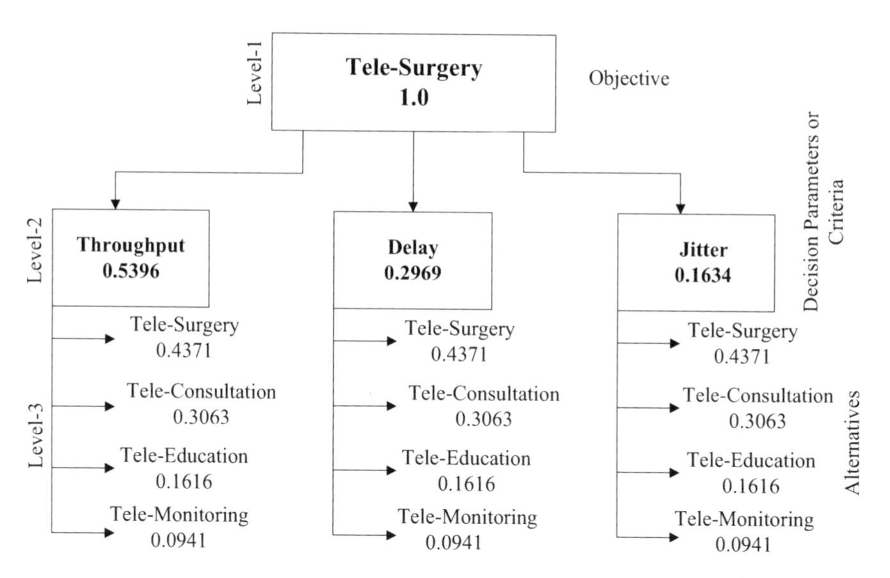

Fig. 6 AHP hierarchy with all weights

and m-QoS measurement at user end in a wide geographical area. The system is efficiently integrating many emerging technologies such as, mobile computing, wearable sensors, cloud computing, decision support systems, Telemedicine service selection, and m-QoS measurement. It can propose remote monitoring of patients at anytime and anywhere. Some unique functions that are of great importance for patients' health monitoring and diagnosing are deliberated. Furthermore, this chapter presents m-QoS management by selecting Telemedicine service from the pool of existing medical services on the priority and urgency basis. A structure of main challenge such as, service selection is formed by dividing that one into three levels. Level1 contains key goal, Level2 shows decision parameters and Level3 represents Telemedicine services as alternatives. An AHP pair-wise comparison matrix is formed then weights and composite weights of Level2 and Level3 elements are obtained. Since, the AHP algorithm measures and evaluates distinct entities such as, the objective, decision making parameters and criteria or alternatives from qualitative and quantitative aspect. The designed algorithm is simulated for three decision making parameters and four different Telemedicine services in which highest priority is assigned to decision parameter; Throughput and Telemedicine service; Tele-Surgery respectively. In near future, we intend to optimize the m-QoS over the joint network of WBSN and Telemedicine.

References

1. Qutaibah Althebyan, Qussai Yaseen, Yaser Jararweh, Mahmoud Al-Ayyoub, “Cloud support for large scale e-Healthcare Systems”, March 2016.
2. R. Trobec, M. Depolli, K. Skala, “Energy Efficiency in Large-Scale Distributed Computing Systems”, 36th International convention on ICT Electronics & Microelectronics (MIPRO), pp. 153–157, 2013.
3. Wu-Chun Chung, Chin-Jung Hsu, Kuan-Chou Lai, “Direction-aware resource discovery in large-scale distributed computing environments”, March 2013.
4. Denis Krivitski, Assaf Schuster, Ran Wolff, “A Local Facility Location Algorithm for Large-scale distributed systems”, April 2007.
5. Von Wangenheim A, Barcellos CL Jr, Andrade R, “Implementing DICOM structured reporting in a large-scale telemedicine network”, Telemed J E Health, Vol. 19, No. 7, pp. 535–541, July, 2013.
6. Kovendhan Ponnavaikko, D. Janakiram, Arogyashree: A distributed file system for large scale internet-based telemedicine, 2008.
7. Hafez Fouad, “Patient based web Telemedicine System for medical health Monitoring”, Journal of Communication and Computer, pp. 168–178, 2014.
8. Sriram Kailasam, Santosh Kumar, and Janakiram Dharanipragada, “Arogyasree: An Enhanced Grid-Based Approach to Mobile Telemedicine”, International Journal of Telemedicine and Applications Vol. 2010, pp. 1–11, 2010.
9. Jui-chien Hsieh, Meng-Wei Hsu, “A cloud computing based 12-lead ECG telemedicine service”, BMC Medical Informatics and Decision Making, 2012.
10. Topacan Umit, Basoglu A. Nuri, U. Daim Tugrul. “AHP application on evaluation of health information service attributes”, PICMET proceedings, 486–493, Portland, Oregon USA, 2009.
11. Anwar Sharna, Shusmita, M. Murshed Manzur, “Analysis of Performance of vertical handoff strategies with QoS indicators and separation”, 2010.
12. Tawil. R, Pujole. G, “A vertical handoff decision scheme in heterogeneous wireless systems”. In: IEEE vehicular Technology conference, 2626–2630, May 2008.
13. Yeh Li-Lun, “ Automated Devices in Taiwan’s Telemedicine Industry”, International Journal of Automation and Smart Technology, Vol. 3, No. 1, 2013.
14. Alharthi, Hana, “An AHP enabled method to Rank the Critical Success factors of Implementing a Pharmacy Barcode System”, Perspectives in Health Information management, 2015.
15. Ajami Sima, “Performance measurement of medical records departments by AHP strategy in the Selected Hospitals in Isfahan”. Journal of Medical Systems, Vol. 36, No. 3, pp. 1165–1171, New York, 2012.
16. Sri Kavya D. Manga, “Choice of wireless technologies for rural connectivity-in the context of Developing countries”, Journal of recent sciences, Vol. 3, No. 1, pp. 41–47, 2014.
17. Schiltz André, “Business model analysis of eHealth use cases in Europe and in Japan”. Journal of the International society for Telemedicine and eHealth, 2013.
18. Gao Cong, “A Collaborative QoS-Aware service evaluation method for service selection”, Journal of Networks, Vol. 8, No. 6, 2013.
19. Mirchandani Vinod. “Optimized Energy Management for Mixed Uplink Traffic in LTE UE”, Vol. 8, No. 3, 2013.
20. Al-Qurishi, Muhammad, “A Framework for Cloud-Based Healthcare Services to Monitor Non- communicable Diseases Patient”, International journal of distributed Sensor Networks, 2015.
21. Gülçin, “Strategic analysis of healthcare service quality using fuzzy AHP methodology”, Expert systems with application, Vol. 38, No. 8, pp. 940–942, 2011.
22. L Pecchia., “Analytic Hierarchy Process for examining healthcare professional’s assessments of risk Factors”, methods Inf medical, Vol. 50, No. 5, 2011.

23. Oltés Vincent, "The functionality comparison of the health care systems by the AHP methods", Ekonomica management, Vol. 17, No. 3, 2014.
24. Fengou Maria-Anna, "Group profile creation in ubiquitous healthcare environment applying the AHP", Chapter on wireless mobile communication and healthcare, Lecture notes of the Institute for computer science, social informatics and Telecommunications Engineering, Vol. 61, pp. 247–254, 2013.
25. Saaty T.L, "Decision making for leaders: The AHP for decision in a complex World", RWS publications, Int. J. Services Sciences, Vol. 1, No. 1, 2008.
26. Giancarlo Fortino, Stefano Galzarano, Raffaele Gravina, Wenfeng Li: A framework for collaborative computing and multi-sensor data fusion in BSN. Information Fusion, Vol. 22, pp. 50–70, 2015.
27. Hassan Ghasemzadeh, Pasquale Panuccio, Simone Trovato, Giancarlo Fortino, Roozbeh Jafari, Power-Aware Activity Monitoring Using Distributed Wearable Sensors. IEEE Trans. Human-Machine Systems. Vol. 44, No. 4, pp. 537–544, 2014.
28. G Fortino, V Giampa, PPG-based methods for non-invariance and continuous blood pressure measurement: an overview and development issues in BSNs, IEEE Conference on Medical Measurements and Applications Proceedings (MeMeA), 2010.
29. Raffaele Grayina, Parastoo Alinia, Hassan Ghasemzadeh, Giancarlo Fortino: Multi-sensor fusion in body sensor networks: State-of-the-art and research challenges. Information Fusion Vol. 35, pp. 68–80, 2017.
30. Raffaele Gravina, Giancaarlo Fortino: Automatic Methods for the Detection of Accelerative Cardiac Defense Response. IEEE Trans. Affective Computing Vol. 7, No. 3, pp. 286–298, 2016.
31. Stefano Galzarano, Roberta Giannantonio, Antonio Liotta, Giancarlo Fortino: A Task-Oriented Framework for Networked Wearable Computing. IEEE Trans. Automation Science and Engineering, Vol. 13, No. 2, pp. 621–638, 2016.
32. George Smart, Nikos Deligiannis, Rosario Surace, Valeria Loscrì, Giancarlo Fortino, Yiannis Andreopoulos: Decentralized Time-Synchronized Channel Swapping for Ad Hoc Wireless Networks. IEEE Trans. Vehicular Technology Vol. 65, No. 10, pp. 8538–8553, 2016.
33. Giancarlo Fortino, Paolo Trunfio: Internet of Things Based on Smart Objects, Technology, Middleware and Applications. Springer, ISBN 978-3-319-00490-7, 2014.
34. Giancarlo Fortino, Roberta Giannantonio, Raffaela Grayina, Philip Kuryloski, Roozbeh Jaffri: Enabling effective programming and flexible management of efficient BSN applications. IEEE Trans. Human-Machine Systems, Vol. 43, No. 1, pp. 115–133, 2013.

Development and Application of a Generic Methodology for the Construction of a Telemonitoring System

Amir Hajjam El Hassani, Amine Ahmed Benyahia, Emmanuel Andres, Samy Talha, Mohamed Hajjam El Hassani and Vincent Hilaire

Abstract Telemonitoring systems are nowadays being extensively developed and utilized, due to the fact that the worldwide elderly population is increasing. In fact, the use of a telemonitoring system alleviate the problem of health costs by providing a reliable way of alerting the healthcare personnel. The design of a telemonitoring system is a real challenge. In this context, the architecture of a telemonitoring system must be generic and flexible and its knowledge must be well defined so it can be shared between actors of the system. In this paper, we present a methodology for the design of a telemonitoring system. This methodology is based on the use of multi-agent system, ontologies and expert systems. The proposed approach relies on an existing multi-agent methodology known as ASPECS. The latter is adapted to construct a telemonitoring system by adding several activities that introduce ontologies and expert systems. This methodology is applied to E-care, a platform designed for a large scale computing. E-care is a telemonitoring

A. Hajjam El Hassani (✉)
Nanomedicine Lab, Univ. Bourgogne Franche-Comté, UTBM, 90010 Belfort, France
e-mail: amir.hajjam@utbm.fr

A. Ahmed Benyahia · M. Hajjam El Hassani
NEWEL, Le Trident 36 rue Paul Cézanne Mulhouse, Mulhouse, France
e-mail: amine.ahmed-benyahia@utbm.fr

M. Hajjam El Hassani
e-mail: mohamed.hajjam@newel.net

E. Andres
Service de médecine interne, médicale B, Université de Strasbourg (UdS), CHRU, Strasbourg, France
e-mail: emmanuel.andres@chru-strasbourg.f

S. Talha
Service de Physiologie et d'explorations fonctionnelles, Université de Strasbourg (UdS), CHRU, Strasbourg, France
e-mail: samy.talha@chru-strasbourg.fr

V. Hilaire
LE2I, Univ. Bourgogne Franche-Comté, UTBM, 90010 Belfort, France
e-mail: vincent.hilaire@utbm.fr

© Springer International Publishing AG 2017

S.U. Khan et al. (eds.), *Handbook of Large-Scale Distributed Computing in Smart Healthcare*, Scalable Computing and Communications,
DOI 10.1007/978-3-319-58280-1_22

platform for patients suffering from heart failure. As part of this platform, several experiments were conducted to validate this methodology at Strasbourg University Hospital (Strasbourg, France). Preliminary results show that this platform is able to assist health care professionals. E-care processes data sent from the sensors and generates automatically alerts in order to detect early risk situations of heart failure.

1 Introduction

The main objective of telemonitoring is to give people suffering from various pathologies, chronic diseases or disabilities, an independent quality of living in their homes. This objective can be realized by the use of telemonitoring systems. As a result, these systems offer a way to monitor patients and answer their needs within the comfort of their own homes [1].

Telemonitoring is based on the communication and the interpretation of medical indicators (e.g. clinical, biological or radiological data) [2]. The output of this interpretation may result in immediate intervention with the patient or may just end-up in providing medical advices and directives.

The current research proposes a methodological process to facilitate the design of a medical telemonitoring system. It also provides a scheme for early detection of signs of any complications. The proposed methodology is based on a multi-agent system using several types of ontologies associated with an expert system. In fact, ontologies are widely accepted as an appropriate mean for the conceptualization of knowledge through the use of adequate semantics to interpret information.

The multi-agent system used for medical monitoring, has a distributed architecture. The latter has the advantage to assure a certain level of autonomy to patients and provide habitats with an effective response in case of emergency.

The proposed method identifies the generic and the specific aspects of each multi-agent system. The designed architecture takes into account all the patient data such as: patient profile, medical history, drug treatment, physiological and behavioral data, as well as data relating to the patient's environment and lifestyle. This architecture should also be able to acquire new data sources (e.g. auscultation signal).

Our proposed approach is based on an adapted version of the ASPECS methodology [3]. It is based on multi-agent system which are applied to telemonitoring systems. ASPECS is a methodology [4] used to design complex systems using different activities in order to decompose the problem into sub-problems. Our modification consists in the definition of new activities that are proper to telemonitoring systems.

This methodology was then implemented using the E-care platform [5, 6] in order to define its information system. This information system is composed of two types of ontologies: The problem ontology and several domain ontologies. The information system integrates also an expert system for the detection of risk situations. The problem ontology was built to manage the system including users and their tasks. In fact, three domain ontologies have been built to represent, disease, drugs and cardiovascular risk factors. The expert system uses inference rules which are defined in collaboration with medical experts using their knowledge and using medical guidelines.

This methodology also defines the system architecture which consists of four autonomous agent types namely, the medical sensors to collect physiological measurements, etc. The gateway collects data from sensors and transmits them from the patients' homes, to the server. The server processes data and gives access to them. Finally, the patient data are stored and secured in the database.

The rest of the paper is structured as follows: Sect. 2 presents a general overview on ontologies and their advantages. This section also defines multi-agent systems and their components. Section 3 introduces the ASPECS methodology in designing complex systems with multi-agents. Section 4 describes our proposed readapted ASPECS scheme in designing telemonitoring systems. Section 5 describes the implementation of the telemonitoring scheme using E-care platform. Section 6 presents the experiments that were performed to validate the proposed telemonitoring scheme. Finally, Sect. 7 concludes the chapter.

2 Definition

2.1 *Ontology*

The first accepted definition for an ontology was proposed by Gruber in [7]. It is described as the "explicit specification of a conceptualization". This definition has also been clarified by Fensel et al. in [8] to be: "Ontology is an explicit formal specification and a shared conceptualization".

Ontologies make use of common semantics. All involved individuals and concepts can be explicitly defined in terms of their relationships and attributes. Ontologies are commonly interpreted by a machine. This improves the quality of the process of decision making and diagnosis. Moreover, ontologies share knowledge between several people or objects; As a result, they can work together without any ambiguity or loss of information.

Ontologies provide a model of high level of abstraction for the daily workflow inside an organization. This model can be readapted and each organisation can have an ontology adapted to its particular situation. Ontologies are generic and reusable. They are very easy to maintain with a minimal cost.

2.2 Multi-agent System

Multi-agent system (MAS) is associated to distributed intelligence. The goal of a multi-agent system is to solve a problem by associating each sub-problem to a sub-agent and coordinate the activities of these sub-agents. Following this principle, the challenge is to increase collective intelligence through the cooperation of agents.

Ferber et al. in [9], defined an agent as any physical or virtual entity with expertise that is capable of providing services. It is able to perceive its environment and limit its way of acting on it. It can communicate with other agents, perceive their actions, and respond accordingly. An agent is also an autonomous and a proactive entity. In other words, it is able to act without external intervention and ready to take new initiatives.

According to Ferber, a multi-agent system should consist of:

- An environment E, a space usually associated to a metric;
- A set of objects O. These objects have a location in the environment E. At some point, it is possible to associate an environment E to any object O;
- A set of agents A. These agents are specific objects (A can be included in O) and which represent the active entities of the system;
- A set of relations R. These define the relations between objects (and therefore between agents);
- A set of operators Op. These allow agents from set A to perceive, produce, consume, transform and manipulate objects O.

3 ASPECS

ASPECS is a step-by-step requirement to code software process for engineering Complex Systems using Multi-agent System and Holonic Multi-agent System [10].

To deal with all aspects of complex systems, multi-agent system must agree to multiple levels of abstractions and openness.

The authors of ASPECS tried to propose a set of organization-oriented abstractions. This set has been integrated into a complete methodological process. We can found in complex systems and especially hierarchical complex systems the target scope for the proposed approach. ASPECS offers the possibility to develop holonic (as well as non-holonic) multi-agent system societies.

ASPECS is based on three principal phases as shown in Fig. 1. These phases are described below:

1. The System Requirements Analysis phase: it identifies a hierarchy of organizations, whose behavior may fulfill the system requirements in the defined context.

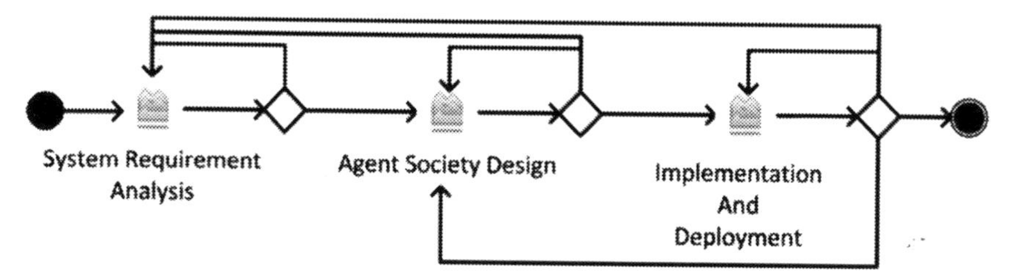

Fig. 1 The ASPECS process phases (and iterations) [10]

2. The Agent Society Design phase: it aims at designing a society of agents whose behavior can provide an effective solution to the problem described in the previous phase. This solution satisfies associated requirement.
3. The Implementation and Deployment phase: it aims at implementing the agent-oriented solution designed in the previous phase by deploying it to the chosen implementation platform.

4 Adaptation of Aspecs to Telemonitoring Systems

In our proposed methodology, the "System Requirement Analysis" phase was modified. As described in ASPECS, this phase is composed of several activities. Figure 2 illustrates these activities.

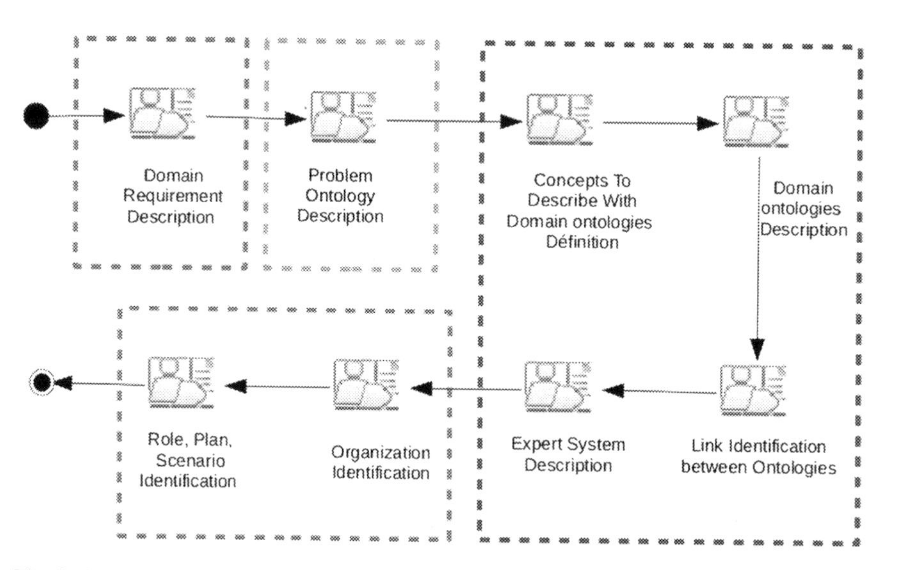

Fig. 2 System requirement phase adapted to telemonitoring

The green rectangle represents the activities that already existed in ASPECS. The orange rectangle represents the activities in ASPECS that have been changed. The red rectangle represents the new activities that were added to adapt ASPECS to telemonitoring systems. The following paragraphs will detail each set of activities.

4.1 Domain Requirements Description

The Domain Requirements Description activity consists of an initial requirements elicitation and provide a description of the application behavior.

Several approaches can be used, such as: use cases diagrams or documented version to introduce user annotations can specify functional and non-functional requirements.

4.2 Problem Ontology Description

The Problem Ontology Description activity defines conceptually the aforementioned domain requirements. This ontology tries to conceptualize the experts' knowledge that will provide the applications context. It helps to understand the problem and allows the refinement of the requirements.

We have adapted this activity to telemonitoring systems by defining a methodology to describe this ontology. This methodology is generic and can be used in other systems.

4.3 Definition of Concepts to Describe with Domain Ontologies

The purpose of this activity is to define the concepts of the problem ontology that can be represented by a domain ontology or part of a domain ontology.

The use of domain ontologies facilitates the understanding of concepts and knowledge and permits a more intuitive inference. Furthermore, the system's maintenance is easier.

4.4 Domain Ontologies Description

The Domain Ontologies Description activity aims to describe and build domain ontologies that provide a formal semantics in our medical telemonitoring system.

After studying various domain ontology construction methodologies, we proposed a generic method. This methodology can be used for the construction of any domain ontology and takes into account different types of resources like text corpus, thesaurus or classifications.

4.5 Link Identification Between Ontologies

The objective of this activity is to define relations between the problem ontology and the various domain ontologies. These links allow to have a connected ontological base, where the concepts of the problem ontology refer to domain ontology concepts. Moreover, every ontology can be individually updated without affecting other ontologies.

4.6 Expert System Description

The Expert system description activity aims to define an expert system for the detection of anomalies and changes in patient health conditions. An expert system infers new data using an inference engine, a fact base and a rule base.

The facts base consists of built ontologies (ontology of the problem and domain ontologies) and data about the patient (medical, analyzes, etc.). The inference engine must be compatible with the facts base, that is, it must be able to infer on ontologies.

A first level of reasoning is directly exploitable from the expressive power of OWL-DL. These reasoning are based, for example, on the characteristics of the relations in ontologies (reflexivity, transitivity, etc.).

For more complex reasoning of inference, rules must be defined in collaboration with medical experts or using expert guidelines.

4.7 Organization Identification

The Organization Identification activity assigns to each requirement a behavior represented by an organization. This behavior is the result of the interacting roles within a common context. A requirement should then be satisfied by an organization.

4.8 Role, Scenario and Plan Identification

The Role and interaction Identification should distribute the behaviour by finer actions represented by roles. The scenario should describe a set of possible interactions within an organization. The behaviour of each role is detailed by the Role Plan and represented by a general plan partial fulfilment of the objectives of the organization.

5 Implementation Using the E-care Platform

E-care is a medical monitoring platform for patients with Heart Failure (HF). The purpose of this platform is to contribute to a good level to the care of patients who are not necessarily under the supervisory framework of a medical personnel. For instance, the idea is that patients can stay at home while benefiting from ongoing monitoring.

The E-care platform's main objective is to optimize the monitoring of patients. This is achieved by detecting the early signs of cardiac decompensation in a telemonitoring system, combined with a motivational and an educational tool. In order to decentralize the data analysis tasks for a large scale computing, we opted for a service-oriented architecture.

To construct the E-care telemonitoring system, we applied the methodology described previously as well as its following activities.

In the first activity, we described the domain requirements namely heart failure and its specificities. In a second step, the activity of problem ontology description has allowed us to build a specific E-care ontology [11]. This ontology contains medical records of patients, physiological and biological screening, medical history, medications and other information related to heart failure like cardiovascular risk factor.

The third and the fourth activities, allowed us to construct three domain ontologies: (1) symptoms, (2) medications and (3) cardiovascular risk factor. To build these ontologies we used the ICD (International Classification of Diseases) and the ATC (Anatomical and Therapeutic Chemical Classification) classifications.

Using the expert system description activity, we built an expert system using the constructed ontologies and we added the different rules. Rules were defined using the knowledge of the domain experts by performing several working meetings and brainstorming sessions. Other rules were extracted from guidelines found in literature [12].

The remaining activities define the system architecture using four organizations. Each organization has its own roles and scenarios.

Finally, the E-care platform has been deployed and allowed the implementation of several experiments that were conducted in hospitals and in patients' homes [13].

These experiments validated the usability of the developed system and the reliability of the alert detection module.

6 Experiments and Results

The primary objective of the experiments was mainly the validation of the technological and medical choices. The first phase of the experiments was scheduled for 2 months' duration. The steps of the E-care experiments were: (1) to test the various functions of the system; (2) to improve the ergonomics; (3) to detect any vulnerability, (4) to identify its strengths; and last (5) to compare the output results with reference devices. We used, in the second phase, pre-determined indicators to test the E-care system. In order to assess improvements for a better patient management, we also verified the relevance of the triggered alerts. The goal was early cardiac impairment detection, before a degradation.

The system has been deployed during the period from October 2013 to November 2014 in Medical Clinic B of the Strasbourg University Hospital (in Strasbourg, France): Department of Internal Medicine, Diabetes and Metabolic Diseases of the. This unit is "open" to the emergency wards and takes care of 800 patients every year. More than 180 patients have been included in the study.

The patient profile included in this experiment was elderly patient, in 25% of cases, with a total loss of autonomy with:

- chronic HF > 60%;
- anemia > 40%;
- type 2 diabetes, chronic obstructive pulmonary disease and arrhythmia due to atrial fibrillation (AAF) > 30%;
- cancer > 20%;
- dementia and chronic renal failure > 15%.

We validated the selected sensors deployed as part of the E-care platform in the first experimental phase. We used a protocol of comparative measurements of the E-care system devices (Blood Pressure (BP), Weight, Heart Rate (HR) and Oxygen saturation (SPO_2)) and those of the conventional hospital (Fig. 3). We performed more than 150 measurements and these various measurements revealed a match between the different devices proposed by the E-care system and those used on a daily basis in the hospital. The E-care system operated as expected. The experimental phase has allowed us to validate the technological choices.

In the second phase, over 1,500 measurements were performed for about 180 patients. Nurses used the E-care measurement devices on a daily basis. This phase relies notably on the establishment of a new inference engine (Version 2 of E-care platform). Figure 4 shows the new human-machine interface. This second phase also includes a satisfaction survey of the system's ergonomics. The survey was filled out by caregivers and patients.

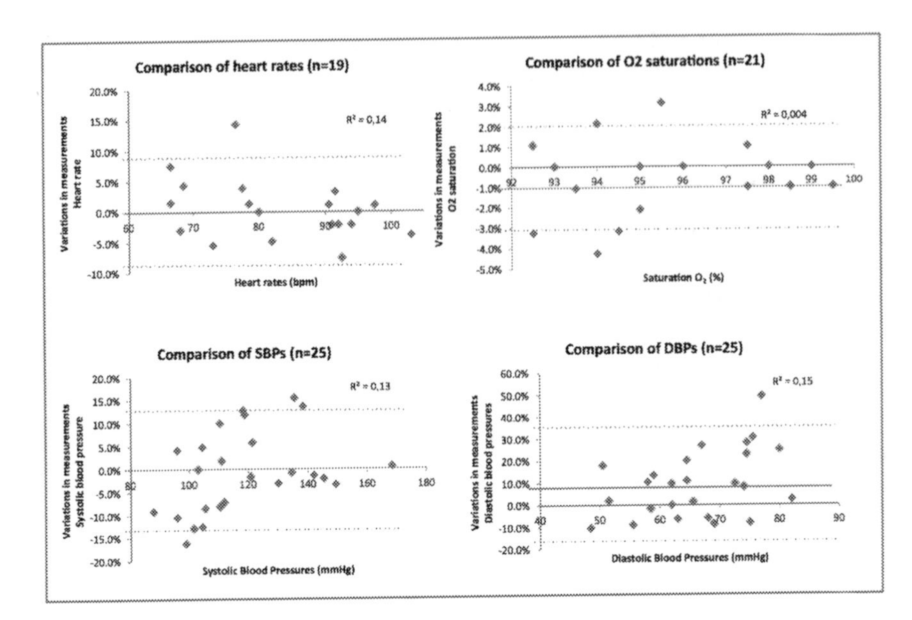

Fig. 3 Comparison of measurements performed by the sensors of the E-care system with those of the conventional hospital

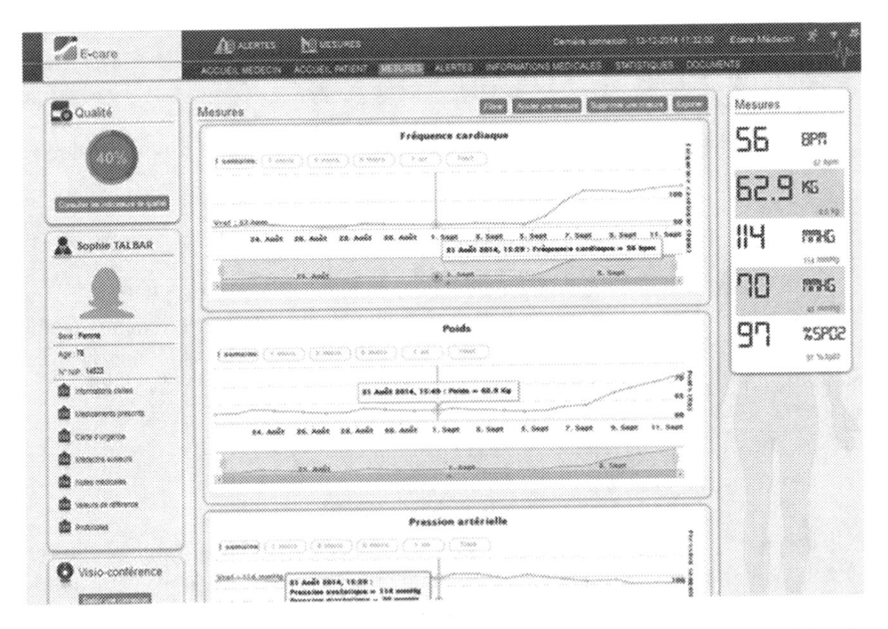

Fig. 4 New human-machine interface of the system (version 2) deployed in the University Hospital of Strasbourg (Strasbourg, France)

In parallel, E-care platform is deployed in patient's homes, in the Strasbourg area, as part of the project INCADO [14], Heart Failure at home (grant from the Alsace Regional Health Agency in Strasbourg, France: *Agence régionale de santé d'Alsace*). Several patients (n = 10) were included and with a daily use of the system. This project is expected to last at least 12 months before the solution can be marketed.

This experimentation is registered on the ClinicalTrials.gov site: *"Anticipation and Detection of Heart Failure Decompensation with Automatic Treatment of Information (e-INCA)" (No: NCT02411279).*

7 Conclusion

In this paper, we presented a generic methodology for the construction of telemonitoring systems. This methodology is based on the use of ontologies for knowledge representation and multi-agent system for system architecture.

We have adapted the ASPECS methodology to telemonitoring systems by adding new activities related to telemonitoring.

We applied this methodology to define and construct the E-care platform telemonitoring system. E-care enables the home monitoring of patients with chronic heart failure. It is an "intelligent" communicative platform using non-invasive sensors. It uses ontology process and advanced technology. E-care assists the health care professionals by providing a reliable way of alerting the healthcare personnel in order to early detect and report risk situations of HF impairment.

Several experiments were conducted on E-care platform that validated its architecture and its inference engine.

References

1. P. Barralon. 2005. Classification et fusion de données actimétriques pour la télésurveillance médicale. Projet de thèse, université Joseph Fourier.
2. La telesante: un nouvel atout au service de notre bien-être: Un plan quinquennal éco-responsable pour le déploiement de la télésanté en France. (2009), Rapport remis à Madame Roselyne Bachelot-Narquin, Ministre de la Santé et des Sports par Monsieur Pierre Lasbordes, Député de l'Essonne.
3. M. Cossentino, N. Gaud, V. Hilaire, S. Galland, A. Koukam, 2010. ASPECS: an agent-oriented software process for engineering complex systems. Autonomous Agents and Multi-Agent Systems 20, pages 260–304.
4. D. Isern, D. Sanchez, and A. Moreno. Organizational structures supported by agent-oriented methodologies. J. Syst. Softw., 84:169–184, February 2011.
5. Ahmed Benyahia, A. Hajjam, V. Hilaire, H. Hajjam "e-Care Ontological architecture for telemonitoring and alerts detection", 5 th IEEE International Symposium on Monitoring & Surveillance Research (ISMSR): Healthcare-Safety-Security, 2012.

6. Ahmed Benyahia, A. Hajjam, V. Hilaire, M. Hajjam, E Andres "E-Care Telemonitoring System: Extend the platform". The Fourth International Conference on Information, Intelligence, Systems and Applications (IISA), 2013, Piraeus, Greece.
7. T. Gruber, 2003. Towards principals for the design of ontologies used for knowledge sharing. Formal ontology in conceptual analysis and knowledge representation. Kluwer Academic pubishers.
8. Studer Benjamins Fensel. 1998. Knowledge Engineering: Principles and Methods. Data and Knowledge Engineering 25, 161–197.
9. J. Ferber, 1995. Les systèmes multi-agents. Vers une intelligence collective. InterEditions, Paris, 1995.
10. Massimo Cossentino, Vincent Hilaire, Nicolas Gaud, Stéphane Galland, and Abderrafiaa Koukam. 2014. Chapter in Handbook on Agent-Oriented Design Processes, chapter 4, pp. 65–114, Springer, 2014. ISBN: 978-3-642-39975-6.
11. A. Ahmed Benyahia, A. Hajjam, V. Hilaire, M. Hajjam "e-Care Ontological architecture for telemonitoring and alerts detection", 5 th IEEE International Symposium on Monitoring & Surveillance Research (ISMSR): Healthcare-Safety- Security, 2012.
12. A. Ahmed Benyahia, A. Hajjam, V. Hilaire, H. Hajjam "Ontological architecture for management of telemonitoring system and alerts detection", book chapter of: eHealth and Remote Monitoring, 2012, ISBN: 978-953-51-0734-7.
13. E. Andres, S. Talha, A. Ahmed Benyahia, O. Keller, M. Hajjam, A. Hajjam, A. Moukadem, J. Hajjam, S. Erve, A. Dieterlin. Projet E-care: déploiement d'un système de détection automatisé des situations à risque de décompensation cardiaque dans une unité de médecine interne. La Revue de Médecine Interne 35, A42–A43. 12/20.
14. Andrès E., Talha S., Ahmed Benyahia A. Monitoring patients with chronic heart failure using a telemedicine platform: contribution of the E-care and INCADO projects. *Int Arch Nurs Health Care*. 2015; 1:1–5.

Ontology-Based Contextual Information Gathering Tool for Collecting Patients Data Before, During and After a Digestive Surgery

Lamine Benmimoune, Amir Hajjam, Parisa Ghodous, Emmanuel Andres and Mohamed Hajjam

Abstract In the health domain, computer-based questionnaires are beneficial since they permit the collection of important elements regarding patients health status. These elements are generally used as input data for many medical systems such as health monitoring systems. The aim of this paper is to describe our contextual Information Gathering Tool (IGT). This tool permits to gather data by providing contextual questionnaires based on the question/answer mechanism and distributed architecture. Our proposed IGT is based on the use of an interrogation engine and ontologies. The engine provides contextual questionnaire as function of the user context and adapts questions depending on the users answer. The use of ontologies permits to model questionnaires and interrogations history. Moreover, ontologies are used to control the creation of questionnaires by offering meanings to the asked questions and then to the collected data. The proposed IGT is used in a clinical setting as a part of the E-care medical monitoring platform. It is applied to the rehabilitation process after a digestive surgery. The tool gathers contextual data relative to the patients hospitalization phase (i.e. before, during and after the surgery). The collected data are then represented graphically for statistical purposes and analyzed by the medical platform to make decisions regarding the patients health status

L. Benmimoune (✉) · A. Hajjam
IRTES-SET, Université de Technologie Belfort-Montbéliard, 90010 Belfort, France
e-mail: benmimoune.lamine@gmail.com

A. Hajjam
e-mail: amir.hajjam@utbm.fr

P. Ghodous
LIRIS, Université Claude Bernard Lyon 1, 69100 Villeurbanne, France
e-mail: parisa.ghodous@univ-lyon1.fr

L. Benmimoune · M. Hajjam
Newel, 68100 Mulhouse, France
e-mail: mha@newel.net

E. Andres
Hôpitaux Universitaires de Strasbourg, 67000 Strasbourg, France
e-mail: emmanuel.andres@chru-strasbourg.fr

© Springer International Publishing AG 2017

S.U. Khan et al. (eds.), *Handbook of Large-Scale Distributed Computing in Smart Healthcare*, Scalable Computing and Communications,
DOI 10.1007/978-3-319-58280-1_23

(i.e. warning medical staff if dangerous situations are detected, generating health status indicators, providing useful therapeutic recommendations, etc.).

Keywords Information gathering tool · Distributed architecture · Questionnaire · Clinical decision support system · Monitoring · Surgery · Ontology

1 Introduction

Nowadays, the growth of information technology has allowed the development of different data collection tools. These tools are designed to offer more advantages compared to classical oral interviews and paper-based questionnaires [1]. In fact, they offer a better structure with less time consuming and effort compared to classical methods [2].

In the medical field, the Information Gathering Tools (IGTs) have had significant benefits in reducing omissions and errors arising from traditional medical interviews [3]. IGTs advantages include: reducing paper trails, providing of centralized information leading to improved retrieval of patient medical data and save time [4].

Many research works are conducted to design and use the IGTs in a clinical setting within Clinical Decision Support Systems (CDSS). For instance, in [2, 5], authors proposed a generic model for context-sensitive self-adaptation of data gathering tool based on a questionnaire ontology. The proposed model is then implemented in [4] to collect patients medical data for preoperative risk assessment. In [6–8] authors proposed a questionnaire ontology based on the model of Bouamrane et al. [2]. This ontology is used to collect patients medical history, which is then integrated within CDSS for hypertension risk prediction. In [9] authors proposed an ontology-based CDSS for chest pain risk assessment based on [2]. The proposed CDSS integrates a IGT to gather patients clinical data. In [1] author proposed an approach to design an IGT based on the use of ontologies and inference engine. The approach consists to model a generic questionnaire by an ontology and use the Pellet inference engine in the questions selection process.

Despite the fact that the presented IGT in the literature allows the collection of patient data using ontologies, the created questionnaires are hard coded for specific domains. Moreover, the architectures of these tools are hard to maintain and update because of its rigidity. Unlike previous approaches, we propose an Information Gathering Tool based on an original approach that offers more flexibility by integrating a domain ontology to drive the creation of questionnaire models and separating ontologies. The domain ontology allows to give meaning to the created questions, and to be able to dynamically configure different models of questionnaires without hard coding and regardless of the content of the domain. Therefore, many CDSS can easily integrate the proposed IGT for their particular needs. Furthermore, the proposed approach allows to collect relevant data by providing contextual questionnaires depending on the patient context. The collected responses are also taken into consideration in the questions selection process. This improves the classical approach by adapting the interrogations related to the patient responses and context.

The proposed IGT is integrated within the E-care health monitoring platform [10, 11]. The application consists in gathering patients data before, during and after digestive surgery for follow-up purposes.

2 Information Gathering Tool Within E-care Surgery Platform

We have implemented our IGT as a data collector module within the E-care surgery platform for following-up with patients after digestive surgery by collecting their data in each hospitalization phase.

The E-care surgery platform is a component of the E-care health monitoring platform. The surgery module is applied to patients in each hospitalization phase of the digestive surgery. It works by collecting relevant data from the patient before, during and after the surgery and then by providing early detection of any anomaly. It is able to generate health status indicators and provide useful recommendations. The collected data are stored in the patients profile ontology. This profile models the health status of the patient and analyses by mean of medical engines the possible detection of anomalies while providing adequate recommendations.

3 Proposed Information Gathering Tool

The proposed IGT architecture (see Fig. 1) consists of four main components: Questionnaire Ontology, Interrogation History Ontology, Interrogation Engine and User Interfaces.

3.1 Questionnaire Ontology (QO)

This ontology aims to model two distinct aspects: (i) the structure of the questionnaire and (ii) the adaptive behavior of the questionnaire. This ontology is created based on research works presented in [2]. QO is designed as structured, generic and flexible to accept most of the questionnaire models (see Fig. 2).

The main concepts are: *Questionnaire*, *SubQuestionnaire*, *Question* and *PotentialAnswer*.

- *Questionnaire concept*: It is composed of Sub-questionnaires that represent a group of thematically related question concepts.

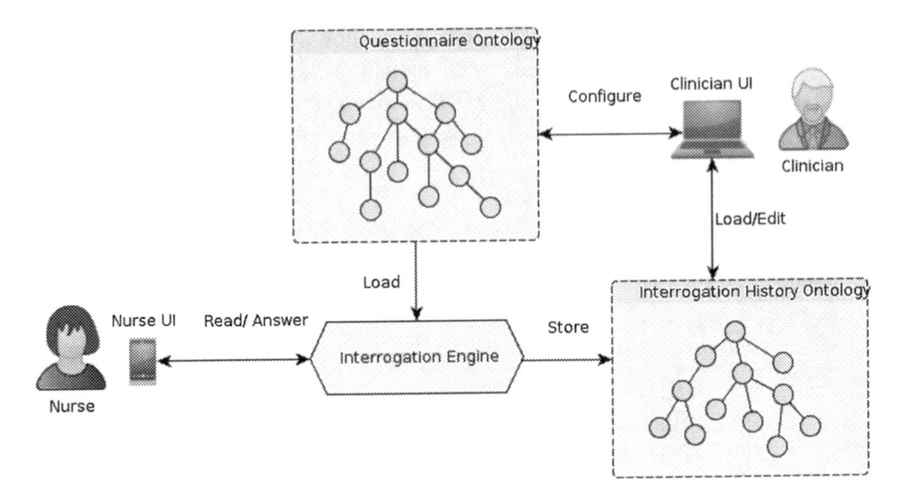

Fig. 1 Information Gathering Tool architecture

- *Subquestionnaire concept*: It aims to group semantic partitioning of the questionnaire under the same theme.
- *Question concept*: It encapsulates the necessary information for questionnaire implementation. The questions could be interrelated using adaptive properties such as *ifAnswerToThisQuestionEqualsTo*, *thenGoToQuestion* and structural properties such as *hasParent*, *hasChild* and *hasSibling*. Each question is characterized by a label to display the questions text, the questions order and the related questions data type concept from the data type ontology (DTOnto). The question has several types that are represented by the following concepts:

  – *MeasureQuestion concept*: This type of question is used to collect physiological data and laboratory tests. The response of this type of question is a numerical number (float).
  – *FreeTextQuestion concept*: This type of question is typically used to allow repliers to experiment information, or to provide them with the opportunity to explain a previous answer (i.e. complication details).
  – *MultiChoiceQuestion concept*: This type of question provides a list of potential answers. We distinguish 3 types of *multiChoiceQuestion*:
    TrueFalseQuestion: This type of question provides by default two potential answers yes and No with the possibility to select one answer.
    MultiChoiceQuestionWithSingleAnswer: This type of question pro- vides a list of potential answers with the possibility to select an answer.
    MultiChoiceQuestionWithMultiAnswers: This type of question pro- vides a list of potential answers with the possibility to select multiple answers.

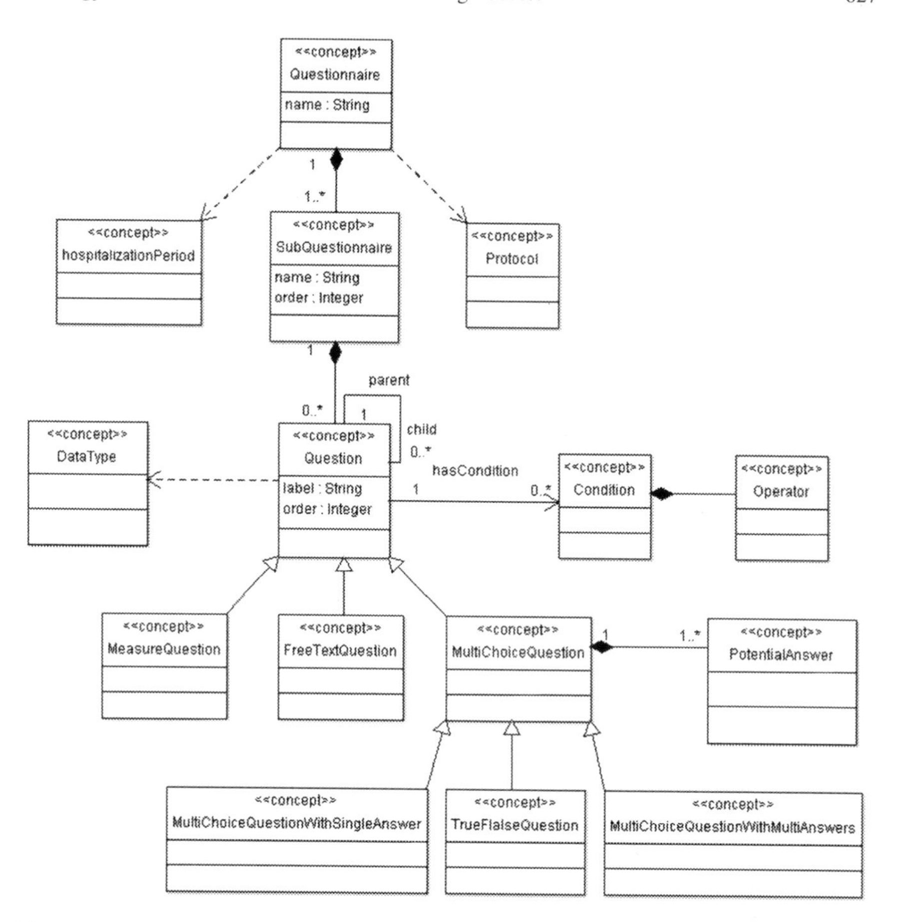

Fig. 2 Simplified representation of Questionnaire Ontology

3.2 Interrogations History Ontology (IHO)

It models medical interrogations and stores all asked questions, patient responses and the response date. It is composed of five main concepts, namely: *Interrogation*, *QuestionnaireHistory*, *SubQuestionnaireHistory*, *QuestionHistory* and *ResponseHistory* (see Fig. 3).

- *Interrogation concept*: This concept models the interrogations history. It handles the possibility to have multiple interrogations to a questionnaire. Recurring in postoperative follow-up where the same questionnaire could be asked for several times.
- *QuestionnaireHistory concept*: It models the questionnaire history related to the interrogation. At each new interrogation a new questionnaire history is created.

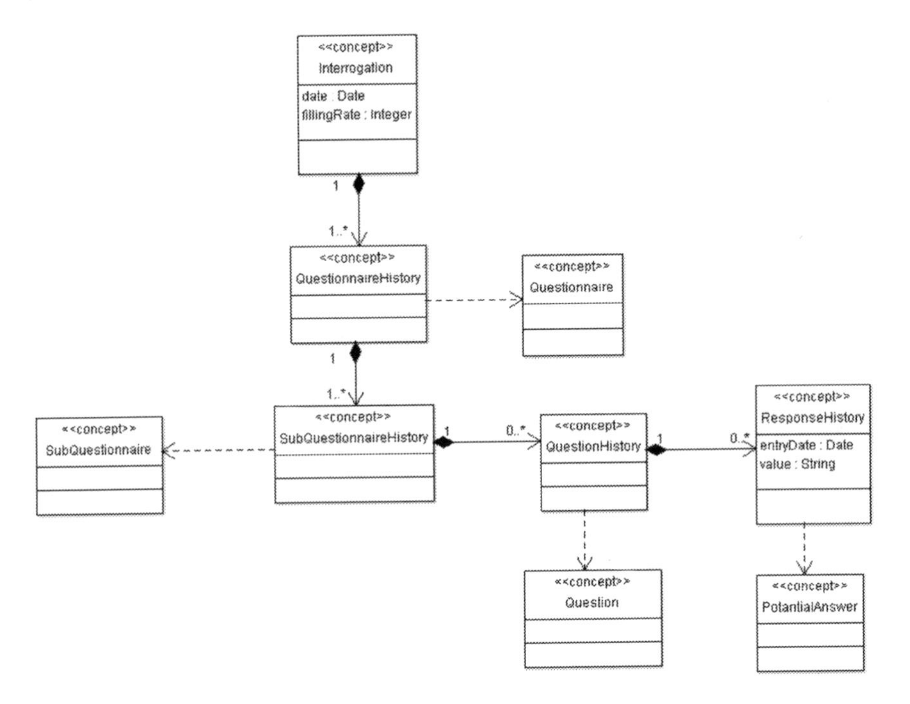

Fig. 3 Simplified representation of Interrogation Ontology

- *SubQuestionnaireHistory concept*: It models the sub-questionnaire history. It allows to save the same structure as the posed questionnaire structure Fig. 3. This concept is related to *SubQuestionnaire* from the Questionnaire Ontology.
- *QuestionnHistory concept*: It models the question history. This concept is related to the *Question* concept from the Questionnaire Ontology.
- *ResponseHistory concept*: It models the response history. This concept is related to *PotentialAnswer* concept from the Questionnaire Ontology in case the question has multi-potential answers.

3.3 Interrogation Engine (IE)

The IE interprets the properties asserted in the Questionnaire Ontology, provides the contextual questionnaires related to the current patient context, loads corresponding questions in connection with the collected responses and stores the user answers in the form of interrogations history.

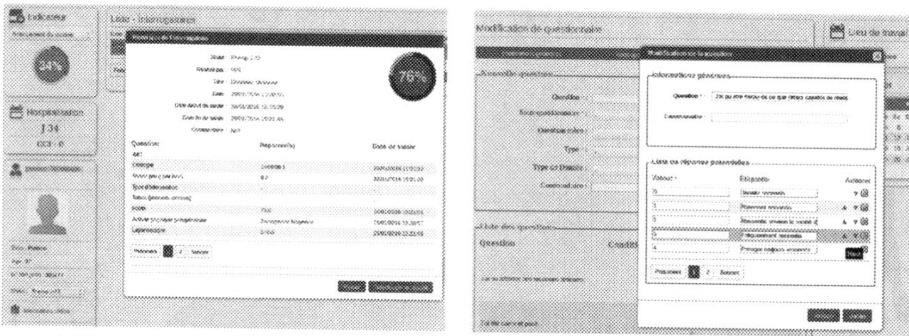

(a) Interrogations history consultation

(b) Questionnaire configuration

Fig. 4 Clinician UI Portal web access

The IE can act according to two questioning modes:

- *Sequential mode:* In this mode, questions are displayed one by one according to the order defined by the clinician. (See our previous work [12]). This mode is generally used by patients when they answer questions by themselves.
- *Instantaneous mode:* In this mode, the questions are all displayed in the form of a list. This mode is generally used by nurses.

3.4 User Interface (UI)

The User Interface consists of two parts, namely:

- **Clinician UI**: It allows clinicians to configure the IGT by defining questionnaire models and to consult the interrogations history (see Fig. 4).
- **Nurse UI**: It permits nurses to collect daily patient data using a mobile device (i.e. tablet). Nurse UI is a mobile application developed to give nurses more mobility when they collect patients daily information (see Fig. 5).

Depending on the hospitalization period of the patient, the IGT delivers more than one questionnaire. This allows to structure the collection of data and to avoid data losses. The storage of data is shown by the filling rate indicator (see Fig. 4a).

4 Collected Data Interpretation

In order to interpret the collected data. A Data type ontology (DTOnto) is created. It represents concepts that belong to a particular domain (i.e. digestive surgery domain in our case). We use this ontology to drive the creation of questionnaires. The main idea is to relate each created question to the corresponding concept in DTOnto (see

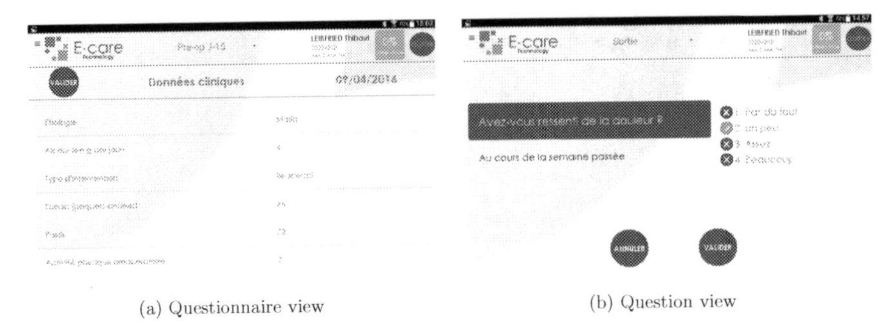

(a) Questionnaire view (b) Question view

Fig. 5 Nurse UI Mobile access

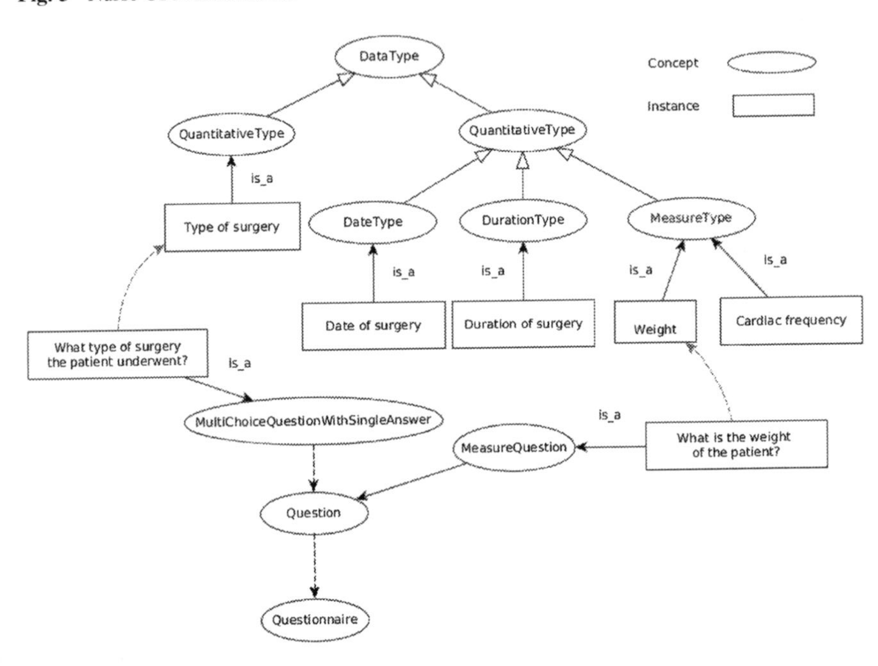

Fig. 6 Example of questionnaire guided by the domain ontology (DTOnto)

Fig. 6). This is useful to give meanings to the collected data for analysis purposes (i.e. similarity computing, rule executions, statistics, etc.). The collected data are stored into a database using the patient profiles ontology for interpretation and analysis. The latter step requires the representation of data using other modules, namely: statistical module, chart measures, rule engine, case engine, etc.

For example, the rule engine executes rules on the collected patient data to derive a number of scores. These scores range from simple formulas such as BMI (Body Mass Index) to more complex algorithms, such as CCI score (Comprehensive Complication Index) and ERAS score (Enhanced recovery after surgery).

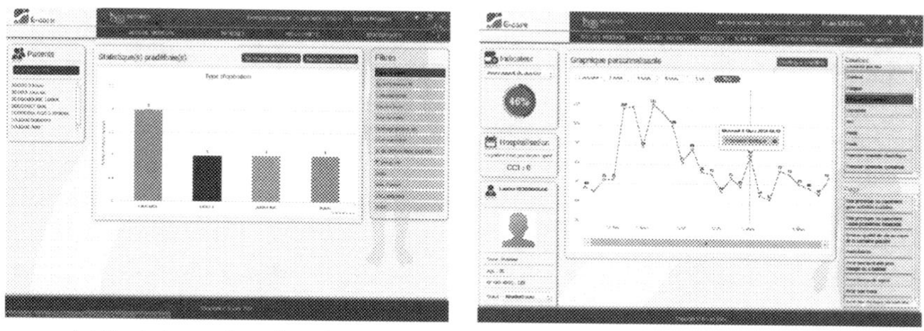

(a) Statistics on the collected data (b) Measures representation

Fig. 7 Collected data interpretation

The case engine uses the collected data of the current patient to search similar past patient profiles in the purpose of providing personalized medical acts. Future works will consider expanding this part. The collected data can have different natures and can be represented in different forms depending on their nature. Data measures such as physiological data (weight, blood pressure, etc.) can be represented by charts (see Fig. 7b).

5 Distributed Data Collection

In order to decentralize the data analysis tasks so as not to weigh down the system, we opted for a service-oriented architecture. The reasoning engine which comprises the case engine and the rule engine is implemented as a remote web service while the web application (clinician UI) and the mobile application (Nurse UI) of the system are considered as clients to the web service (see Fig. 8).

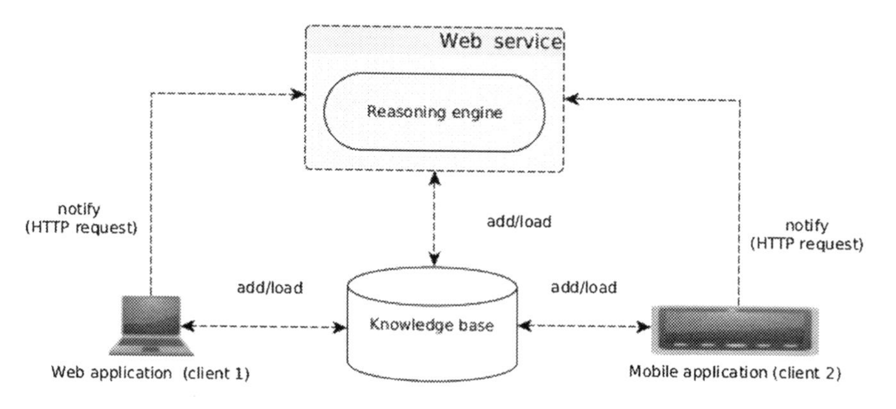

Fig. 8 Distributed data collection architecture

At each new data collected by the platform via the web application (client 1) or the mobile application (client 2), the engine is notified by an HTTP request containing the concerned patient identifier, the concerned data type and the data value. The requests are stored in a queue in their arrival order to avoid redundancy in the reasoning process.

The reasoning process is executed asynchronously, so as not to block clients (web portal and mobile application) during the data collection process. Once the process is complete, the inferred data is injected into the knowledge base which contains the patient profiles.

6 Experimentation

The proposed IGT is experimented as part of E-care platform within the REPOSE project at Strasbourg hospital, France. The goal of the REPOSE project is to follow-up patients before, during and after digestive surgery by automating the collection and analysis of patient data. The experimentation started in November 2015. It includes about 2500 patients over a period of 2 years with an average stay of 10 days.

6.1 E-care Platform Configuration

As a first step, we have defined with the medical experts 186 domain concepts for the knowledge representation of the digestive surgery. These concepts were created dynamically from the web portal of the platform and allowed to populate the domain ontology (DTOnto). The following table (see Table 1) shows the number of domain concepts created according to their types.

In a second step, we have created three hospitalized periods that allow to model the patient context before, during and after the surgery (see Fig. 9).

The created domain concepts have allowed the generation of 186 questions divided into 14 questionnaires and spread over the 3 hospitalized periods defined above. The generation of these questions was made available from the web portal of the platform. The following table (see Table 2) shows the number of questions with respect to their types.

Table 1 The created domain concepts

Domain concept	Number of concepts	%
Measure type	42	22.58
Duration type	7	3.76
Date type	5	2.68
Qualitative type	132	70.96

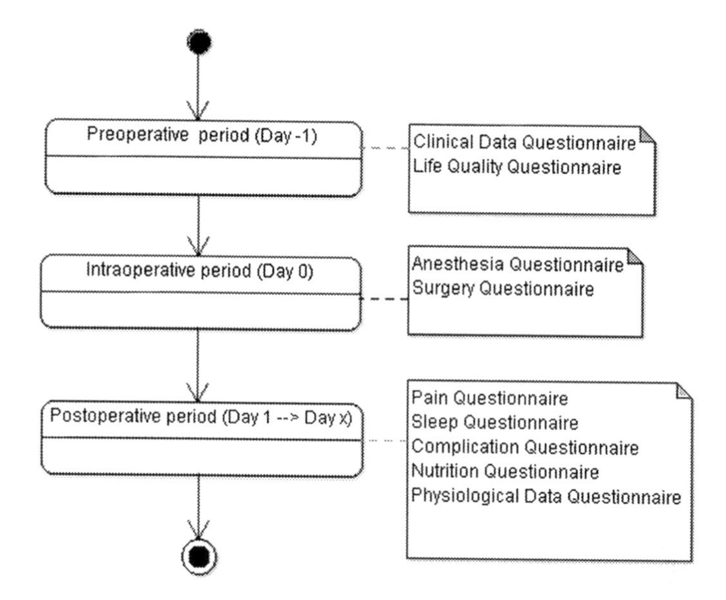

Fig. 9 Questionnaires related to hospitalization periods

Table 2 The created questions

Question type	Number of questions	%
Measure	42	22.58
Free text	24	12.9
Duration	7	3.76
Date	5	2.68
Multi-answers	4	2.15
Single answer	101	54.30
True false	3	1.61

The questionnaires created for the first two periods (Preoperative and Intraoperative) are configured to be asked one time. However, the postoperative questionnaires are configured to be asked several times during the third period (postoperative).

6.2 *Evaluation*

An evaluation survey was conducted by nurses to assess their satisfaction level over the use of the proposed IGT as part of their daily work. Several points were evaluated such as the ease of use, the ergonomy of the UI, the access speed to data and the improvement of the daily work. Results showed that the nurses were satisfied regarding all the evaluation points. Thus, the collection of medical data using our proposed IGT has proved advantageous compared to classical methods (i.e. paper-based questionnaire), since it allows a better organization of the data collection with respect to the patients context and saves time and effort.

7 Conclusion

In this paper, we presented our Ontology-Based Contextual Information Gathering Tool. The proposed tool provides contextual questionnaires according to the hospitalization period of the patients and adapts them according to their answers. On one hand, we have demonstrated the benefits of using the domain ontology DTOnto to give a meaning to the collected data. The creation of questionnaires using the configuration interface can be made easier and faster compared to the previous approaches. On the other hand, we have experimented the proposed IGT as a part of E-care platform in clinical setting to follow-up patients before, during and after digestive surgery as part of the REPOSE project. We have highlighted the interest of using such Tool to help nurses in the daily work with organizing the data collection.

References

1. M. Alipour, Aghdam. Ontology-driven generic questionnaire design. thesis for the degree of master of science in computer science. Master's thesis, University of Guelph, August 2014.
2. M. Bouamrane, A. Rector, and M. Hurrell. Ontology-driven adaptive medical information collection system. In *Foundations of Intelligent Systems*, volume 4994 of *Lecture Notes in Computer Science*, pages 574–584. Springer Berlin Heidelberg, 2008.
3. J.W. Bachman. The patient-computer interview: a neglected tool that can aid the clinician. In *Mayo Clin*, 2003.
4. M. Bouamrane, A. Rector, and M. Hurrell. Using ontologies for an intelligent patient modelling, adaptation and management system. In *On the Move to Meaningful Internet Systems: OTM 2008*, volume 5332 of *Lecture Notes in Computer Science*, pages 1458–1470. Springer Berlin Heidelberg, 2008.
5. M. Bouamrane, A. Rector, and M. Hurrell. Gathering precise patient medical history with an ontology-driven adaptive questionnaire. In *Computer-Based Medical Systems, 2008. CBMS '08. 21st IEEE International Symposium on*, pages 539–541, June 2008.
6. Vinu P.V. Krishnan R. Takroni Y Sherimon, P.C. Ontology based system architecture to predict the risk of hypertension in related diseases. *International Journal of Information Processing and Management*, 4(4):44–50, 2013.
7. P.C. Sherimon, P.V. Vinu, Reshmy Krishnan, Youssef Takroni, Yousuf AlKaabi, and Yousuf AlFars. Adaptive questionnaire ontology in gathering patient medical history in diabetes domain. In Tutut Herawan, Mustafa Mat Deris, and Jemal Abawajy, editors, *Proceedings of the First International Conference on Advanced Data and Information Engineering (DaEng-2013)*, volume 285 of *Lecture Notes in Electrical Engineering*, pages 453–460. Springer Singapore, 2014.

8. P.C Sherimon, Vinu P.V, R. Krishnan, and Y Saad. Ontology driven analysis and prediction of patient risk in diabetes. *Canadian Journal of Pure and Applied Sciences*, 8(3):3043–3050, October 2014.
9. K. Farooq, A. Hussain, S. Leslie, C. Eckl, and W. Slack. Ontology-driven cardiovascular decision support system. In *Pervasive Computing Technologies for Healthcare (PervasiveHealth), 2011 5th International Conference on*, pages 283–286, May 2011.
10. A. A. Benyahia, A. Hajjam, V. Hilaire, and M. Hajjam. e-care: Ontological architecture for telemonitoring and alerts detection. In *2012 IEEE 24th International Conference on Tools with Artificial Intelligence*, volume 2, pages 13–17, Nov 2012.
11. A. A. Benyahia, A. Hajjam, V. Hilaire, M. Hajjam, and E. Andres. E-care telemonitoring system: Extend the platform. In *Information, Intelligence, Systems and Applications (IISA), 2013 Fourth International Conference on*, pages 1–4, July 2013.
12. L. Benmimoune, A. Hajjam, P. Ghodous, E. Andres, S. Talha, and M. Hajjam. Ontology-based information gathering system for patients with chronic diseases: Lifestyle questionnaire design. In *Progress in Artificial Intelligence*, volume 9273 of *Lecture Notes in Computer Science*, pages 110–115. Springer International Publishing, 2015.

Printed in the United States
By Bookmasters